MUIR'S
TEXTBOOK OF
PATHOLOGY

MUIR'S
TEXTBOOK OF PATHOLOGY

FOURTEENTH EDITION

Edited by

David A Levison MD FRCPath
Professor of Pathology, University of Dundee, and Honorary Consultant Pathologist,
Ninewells Hospital and Medical School, Dundee, UK

Robin Reid BSc(Hons) MBChB FRCPath
Consultant Pathologist, Western Infirmary, Glasgow, and Honorary Senior Lecturer in
Pathology, University of Glasgow, Glasgow, UK

Alastair D Burt BSc(Hons) MBChB MD(Hons) FRCPath FI Biol
Professor of Pathology and Dean of Clinical Medicine, Newcastle University,
Royal Victoria Infirmary, Newcastle-upon-Tyne, UK

David J Harrison BSc(Hons) Ed MD MRCPath FRCPath FRCPEd FRCSEd
Professor of Pathology and Director of the Edinburgh Cancer Research Centre,
University of Edinburgh, Edinburgh, UK

Stewart Fleming MBChB BSc(Hons) MD(Hons) FRCPath
Professor of Cellular and Molecular Pathology, University of Dundee,
Ninewells Hospital, Dundee, UK

Hodder Arnold
www.hoddereducation.com

First published in Great Britain in 1924
Second edition 1929
Third edition 1933
Fourth edition 1936
Fifth edition 1941
Sixth edition 1951
Seventh edition 1958
Eighth edition 1964
Ninth edition 1971
Tenth edition 1976
Eleventh edition 1980
Twelfth edition 1985
Thirteenth edition 1992
This fourteenth edition published in Great Britain in 2008 by
Hodder Arnold, an imprint of Hodder Education, part of Hachette Livre UK
338 Euston Road, London NW1 3BH

http://www.hoddereducation.com

Whilst the advice and information in this book are believed to be true
and accurate at the date of going to press, neither the authors nor the
publisher can accept any legal responsibility or liability for any errors or
omissions that may be made. In particular (but without limiting the
generality of the preceding disclaimer) every effort has been made to
check drug dosages; however it is still possible that errors have been missed.
Furthermore, dosage schedules are constantly being revised and new
side-effects recognized. For these reasons the reader is strongly urged to
consult the drug companies' printed instructions before administering any
of the drugs recommended in this book.

British Library Cataloguing in Publication Data
A catalogue record for this book is available from the British Library

Library of Congress Cataloging-in-Publication Data
A catalog record for this book is available from the Library of Congress

ISBN [normal]   978 0 340 74062 0
ISBN [ISE]   978 0 340 81023 1 (International Students' Edition, restricted territorial availability)
ISBN [BookPower, formely ELST] 978 0 340 81024 8

1 2 3 4 5 6 7 8 9 10

Commissioning Editors: Georgina Bentliff and Sara Purdy
Development Editor: Heather Smith
Project Editors: Wendy Rooke and Jane Tod
Production Controllers: Jane Lawrence and Lindsay Smith
Cover Design: Amina Dudhia

Typeset in 10/12 Berling by Charon Tec Ltd (A Macmillan Company) www.charontec.com
Printed and bound in India

What do you think about this book? Or any other Hodder Arnold title? Please visit
our website at www.hoddereducation.com

CONTENTS

SECTION 1   MECHANISMS OF DISEASE: CELLULAR AND MOLECULAR

SECTION 2   SYSTEMIC PATHOLOGY

To download electronic files of the illustrations used in this book, go to the *Muir's Textbook of Pathology* homepage, www.muirspathology.com. Access to the files is password protected.

Your username is: student99
Your password is: pathology

CONTRIBUTORS

David Ansell MA MB BChir FRCPath
Consultant Histopathologist, Department of Histopathology, City Hospital, Nottingham, UK

Jonathan N Berg MB ChB MSc MD FRCP(Ed)
Senior Lecturer in Clinical Genetics, University of Dundee and Honorary Consultant in Clinical Genetics, Ninewells Hospital and Medical School, Dundee, UK

Alastair D Burt BSc(Hons) MD(Hons) FRCPath FIBiol
Professor of Pathology and Dean of Clinical Medicine, Newcastle University, Royal Victoria Infirmary, Newcastle-upon-Tyne, UK

Francis A Carey BSc(Hons) MB BCh BAO MD FRCPath
Consultant and Professor of Pathology, Department of Pathology, Ninewells Hospital and Medical School, Dundee, UK

Henry J Dargie MB ChB FRCP FESC FRSE
Consultant Cardiologist, Honorary Professor, University of Glasgow, Glasgow, UK

Ian O Ellis BMedSci BM BS MRCPath
Professor of Cancer Pathology and Honorary Consultant Pathologist, Faculty of Medicine and Health Sciences, Department of Histopathology, City Hospital Campus, Nottingham University Hospitals NHS Trust Nottingham, UK

Christopher W Elston MD FRCPath
Professor of Tumour Pathology and Consultant Histopathologist (Retired), City Hospital, Nottingham, UK

Alan T Evans BMedBiol(Hons) MD(Hons) FRCPath
Consultant Dermatopathologist, Department of Pathology, Ninewells Hospital and Medical School, Dundee, UK

Stewart Fleming MBChB BSc(Hons) MD(Hons) FRCPath
Professor of Cellular and Molecular Pathology, University of Dundee, Ninewells Hospital, Dundee, UK

Alan K Foulis BSc MD MRCPath FRCP(Ed)
Department of Pathology, Royal Infirmary, Glasgow, UK

David I Graham MBBch PhD FRCPath FRCP(G) FRS(Ed)
Emeritus Professor of Neuropathology, University Department of Neuropathology, Institute of Neurological Sciences, Southern General Hospital NHS Trust, Glasgow, UK

David J Harrison BSc(Hons) Ed MD FRCPath FRCP(Ed) FRCS(Ed)
Professor of Pathology and Director of the Edinburgh Cancer Research Centre, University of Edinburgh, Edinburgh, UK

Philip S Hasleton MD FRCPath
Professor of Pathology, Department of Histopathology, Manchester Royal Infirmary, Manchester, UK

C Simon Herrington MA MB BS DPhil MRCP FRCPath
Professor and Consultant in Pathology, Bute Medical School, University of St Andrews, St Andrews, UK

Robert Jackson
Department of Pathology, Royal Infirmary, Glasgow, UK

Frederick D Lee
Professor of Pathology, Department of Pathology, Royal Infirmary, Glasgow, UK

Andrew HS Lee MRCP FRCPath
Consultant Histopathologist, City Hospital, Nottingham, UK

David A Levison MD FRCPath FRCP(Ed)
Professor of Pathology, University of Dundee, and Honorary Consultant Pathologist, Ninewells Hospital and Medical School, Dundee, UK

George BM Lindop BSc(Hons) MBChB FRCP(Glas) FRCPath
Senior Consultant Pathologist, Sheikh Khalifa Hospital, Abu Dhabi, UAE

Sebastian B Lucas FRCP FRCPath
Professor, Department of Histopathology, King's College London School of Medicine, St Thomas' Hospital, London, UK

The late D Gordon MacDonald
Professor, Department of Oral Pathology, Glasgow Dental Hospital, Glasgow, UK

Anne Marie McNicol BSc MD MRCP(UK) FRCP Glas FRCPath
Reader, University Department of Pathology, Glasgow Royal Infirmary University NHS Trust, Glasgow, UK

Allan R McPhaden BSc(Hons) MBChB, MD, MRCPath
Department of Pathology, Glasgow Royal Infirmary, Glasgow, UK

Sarju Mehta BSc(Hons) MBBS MRCP(UK)
Consultant in Clinical Genetics, Department of Clinical Genetics, Addenbrooke's Hospital, Cambridge, UK

Wolter J Mooi MD PhD
Professor of Pathology, Department of Pathology, Vrye Universiteit Medical Centre, Amsterdam, the Netherlands

Ian AR More BSc PhD MD FRCP FRCPath
Department of Pathology, Western Infirmary, Glasgow, UK

James AR Nicoll BSc MD FRCPath
Professor of Neuropathology, Division of Clinical Neurosciences, University of Southampton and Honorary Consultant Neuropathologist, Southampton University Hospitals NHS Trust, Southampton, UK

Sarah E Pinder MBChB, FRCPath
Department of Histopathology, Addenbrooke's Hospital, Cambridge, UK

Robin Reid BSc(Hons) MBChB FRCPath
Consultant Pathologist, Western Infirmary, Glasgow, and Honorary Senior Lecturer in Pathology, University of Glasgow, Glasgow, UK

Fiona Roberts BSc MBChB MD FRCPath
Consultant Ophthalmic Pathologist, Department of Pathology, University of Glasgow, Western Infirmary, Glasgow, UK

R Stuart C Rodger MB FRCP
Consultant Nephrologist, Honorary Clinical Senior Lecturer in Medicine, Renal Unit, University of Glasgow, Western Infirmary, Glasgow, UK

Paul Van der Valk MD PhD
Professor of Pathology, Department of Pathology, Vrye Universiteit Medical Centre, Amsterdam, the Netherlands

PREFACE

This is the Fourteenth Edition of *Muir's Textbook of Pathology*, building upon the work of previous editions. It is different in a number of ways from previous editions, but we think it is similar enough to retain the traditional values of its predecessors. We trust we have produced a text that will be useful both to undergraduate medical students and to postgraduates who are interested in having a better understanding of disease upon which to base either their clinical practice or their research, or both.

This edition differs in the balance between general and systematic pathology from most earlier editions, with the general section being relatively shorter. This is deliberate; it is not meant to suggest that we think an understanding of the basic sciences is any less important to clinical practice than it used to be – quite the contrary. What we have tried to do is to focus on the most clinically relevant basic science and we have included some of that in the systematic chapters where its relevance is hopefully easier to appreciate.

We have also introduced into almost every chapter one or two special study topics where the information provided is rather more than most medical educators would include in the core curriculum of a medical undergraduate course. This is intended to interest and stimulate the best students to appreciate that undergraduate education is just the beginning – a window on the exciting and challenging world of disease. We have also included in most chapters, several case histories which illustrate and add to the information provided in the main text, in an attempt to emphasize the fundamental relevance of pathology to clinical medicine. By adopting this format of special study topics and case studies integrated into, but clearly distinguished from, the core text, we are adopting the approach taken to medical education in many medical schools. We strongly support the move in the UK to more integrated teaching of the disciplines in medicine. We, not unexpectedly, believe that the best doctors are knowledgeable about disease processes, and we hope that this belief is reflected in the level at which we have pitched the text.

It will be noted for this edition of the book that for the first time ever the majority of the editors are not based in Glasgow. However, three of us are Glasgow graduates, and we all acknowledge our debt to, and the inspiration we have drawn from, our predecessors in Glasgow Pathology. We are honoured to have had the opportunity to edit this latest edition of 'Muir' and hope that we have done justice to the task.

David A Levison
Robin Reid
Alastair D Burt
David J Harrison
Stewart Fleming

2008

ACKNOWLEDGEMENTS

We are extremely grateful to our fellow authors for their contributions and also for their patience through the extended gestation period of this work. We are fortunate that authors have been prepared to update texts submitted several years ago to ensure that the final text is as up-to-date as possible at the time of publication. We are grateful to the authors for their tolerance of our editing activities, and we trust we have not introduced errors of fact or judgement, and hope we have achieved a reasonable balance. The published text is the editors' final responsibility.

It is with sadness that we record the deaths of two of the originally selected authors. Professor DG MacDonald had completed his contribution to Chapter 9, the opening section on the mouth, salivary glands and oropharynx. The text he wrote is included with minimal editing and he remains a full author. Professor Wilhelmina Behan wrote the original draft text on muscle for Chapter 12. However, the required balance of that chapter changed as the book evolved and the muscle section was completely rewritten in shorter form by one of us (RR). We are grateful to Professor Behan for her early contribution and are greatly saddened by her passing.

In addition to named contributors we also wish to acknowledge the help of various colleagues for contributions as diverse as proof reading chapters e.g. Dr David Goudie who constructively criticised Chapter 3, and Dr Robert Doull who produced and sourced radiological images for Chapter 16. Numerous other contributors are acknowledged at specific points in the text.

We also wish to thank the staff of our publishers Hodder Arnold for their faith that this project would finally reach fruition, and we would particularly like to thank Jane Tod who, though she came late to the project, has been a pleasure to work with and has efficiently driven the production process through its final year.

Finally we wish to thank our families for their support and encouragement over yet another demand on time that could have been spent with them. We feel privileged to have been editors of the 14th edition of this iconic text and are grateful to our families for allowing us this indulgence.

David A Levison
Robin Reid
Alastair D Burt
David J Harrison
Stewart Fleming

2008

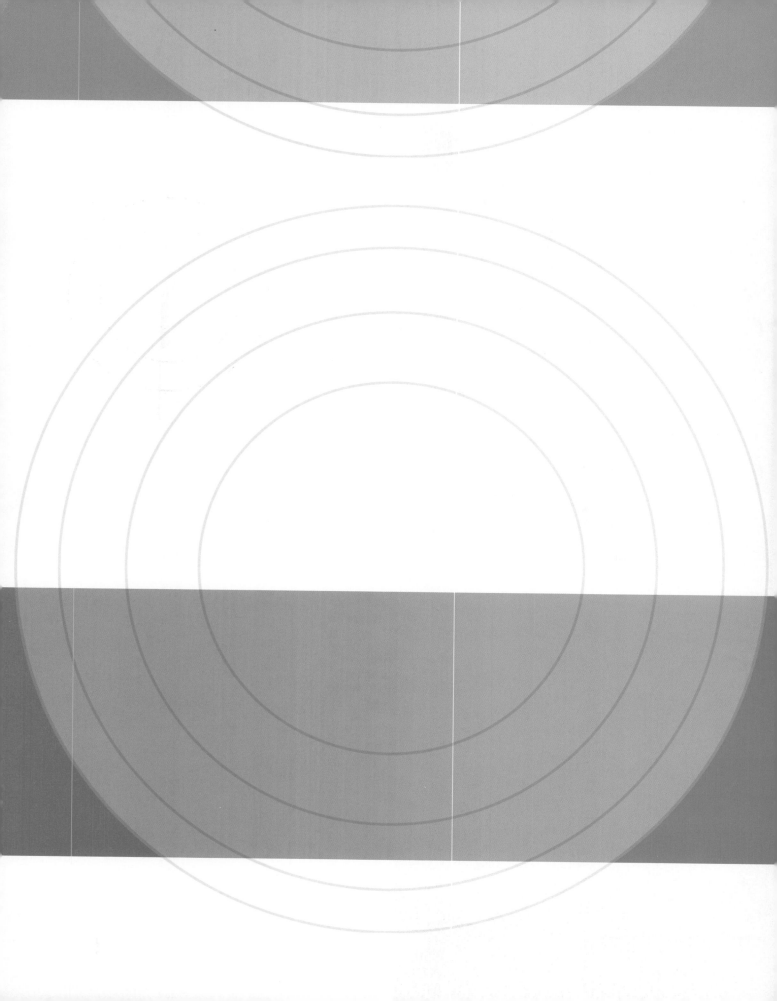

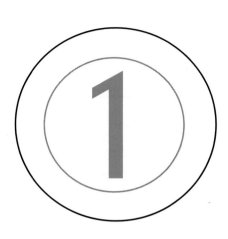

SECTION 1

Mechanisms of Disease: Cellular and Molecular

1 APPLICATIONS OF PATHOLOGY

Robin Reid and David J Harrison

WHAT IS PATHOLOGY?

Pathology is the study of disease. It is central to the whole practice of evidence-based medicine. Arguably, anyone who studies the mechanisms of a disease can be described as a pathologist, but traditionally the term is restricted to those who have a day-to-day involvement in providing a diagnostic service to a hospital or undertake research in a pathology department. Within the discipline there are numerous subspecialities:

- Cellular pathology, including histopathology (the study of tissues) and cytopathology (the branch in which diagnoses are made from the study of separated cells).
- Morbid anatomy is an old term which refers to postmortem dissection, and forensic pathology is the related branch concerned with medicolegal postmortem examinations. These are carried out under the aegis of a legal officer, for example the Coroner in England and Wales, the Procurator Fiscal in Scotland and the Medical Examiner in USA.
- Microbiology, the study of infectious diseases and their causes. This can be subdivided into bacteriology, virology, mycology (the study of fungi) and protozoology (the study of infections by protozoa).
- Haematology, the laboratory study of diseases of the blood. This is also a clinical discipline, its practitioners dealing with patients with these disorders. Most haematologists work in both clinical and laboratory arenas.
- Chemical pathology or clinical biochemistry is the study of body chemistry, usually by assaying the levels of substances – electrolytes, enzymes, lipids, trace elements – in the blood or urine. Increasing sophistication of analytical requirements often means that this discipline is at the cutting edge of new technology.
- Immunology is the study of host defences against external threats. Many of these are microbiological, but some are chemical, for example foodstuffs. In addition, this is also the study of autoimmunity, when the body's defence systems are turned on itself (see Chapter 2, p. 26).
- Genetics, the study of inheritance of characteristics and of diseases, or predisposition to diseases. Clinical geneticists, like haematologists, are directly involved with patients, while laboratory-based geneticists apply the traditional techniques of karyotyping, the microscopic examination of chromosomes in cells in mitosis, and the whole spectrum of modern molecular techniques, such as polymerase chain reaction (PCR), fluorescence in-situ hybridization (FISH), gene expression profiling and DNA sequencing.

Historically, these subjects emerged from the single discipline of 'pathology' which exploded in the mid-nineteenth century, especially in Germany where Rudolf Virchow introduced the term 'cellular pathology'. The divergence of specialities was largely on the basis of the different techniques used in each area. Today, the boundaries between these subspecialties are increasingly becoming blurred as modern techniques, especially those resulting from molecular biology, are applied to all. Cellular pathology remains a critical part of the clinical evaluation of a patient prior to definitive treatment being offered. Increasingly, some of the roles are also delivered by scientists who are not medically qualified, bringing new opportunities and challenges to building effective multidisciplinary teams.

The editors and almost all of the contributors to this book are primarily histopathologists and it is on this area that the book will focus.

DIAGNOSTIC HISTOPATHOLOGY AND CYTOPATHOLOGY: IMAGES OF DISEASES

Key Points

- Pathology is the study of disease.
- Naked eye examination and the light microscope are the traditional tools of the pathologist.
- Increasingly, molecular biological techniques are applied across the whole spectrum of study of diseases to explore underlying mechanisms.

Cellular pathology, i.e. both histopathology and cytology, are essentially imaging disciplines. Its practitioners interpret an image, usually obtained by microscopy, and from it deduce information about diagnosis and possible cause of disease, recommend treatment and predict likely outcome.

Preparing the Image

Tissues or cells are removed from a patient. The fairly simple technique of light microscopy is the bedrock of preparing images. A very thin slice of a tissue, usually about 3 μm thick, is prepared and stained so that the characteristics of the tissue, i.e. the types of cells and their relationships to one another, can be examined. To prevent the tissue digesting itself through release of proteolytic enzymes, the tissue is immersed in a fixative, usually formaldehyde, which cross-links the proteins and inactivates any enzymatic activity. It is impossible to cut very thin sections of even thickness without supporting the tissue in some medium. Usually the tissue is embedded in paraffin wax, but freezing the tissue (the principle of the frozen section) and embedding hard tissue in synthetic epoxy resins such as Araldite are also done. To stain the tissue section, the vegetable dyes haematoxylin and eosin are traditionally used to distinguish between nucleus and cytoplasm, and to identify some of the intracellular organelles (Figure 1.1). It is from examination of sections stained by these simple tinctorial techniques that normal histology (Figure 1.2) and the basic disease processes of inflammation, repair, degeneration and neoplasia were defined. In the past century numerous chemical stains have been developed to demonstrate, for example, carbohydrates, mucins, lipids and pigments such as melanin and the iron-containing pigment haemosiderin.

Refining the Image

Electron Microscopy

Pathological applications of this technique emerged in the 1960s as the technology of 'viewing' tissues by beams of electrons rather than visible light became available. This greatly increased the limits of resolution so that cellular

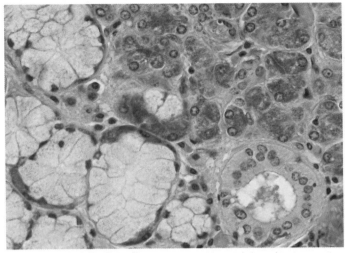

Figure 1.1 Haematoxylin and eosin stained section of the parotid allowing the serous cells (top right), mucinous cells (left) and salivary duct (lower right) to be readily distinguished.

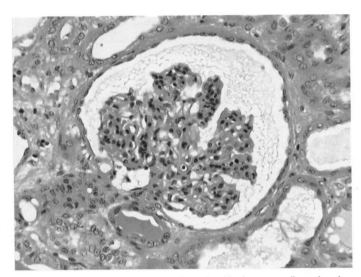

Figure 1.2 A section of renal glomerulus stained by haematoxylin and eosin. The nuclei have affinity for the basic dye haematoxylin and are blue. The cytoplasm has more affinity for the acidic dye eosin and is pink. This technique has not changed significantly in well over a century.

organelles could be identified and indeed their substructure defined. This allowed more precise diagnosis of tumour types and allowed the structure of proteins such as amyloid to be determined. Ultrastructural pathology now has only a limited place in tumour diagnosis, but still has a central role in the diagnosis of renal disease, especially glomerular diseases (Figure 1.3) (see Chapter 13, p. 373).

Immunohistochemistry

This technique evolved in the 1980s and gained a major boost from the development of monoclonal antibodies by the late Professor Cesar Milstein. It depends on the property of antibodies to bind specifically to cell-associated antigens. Of course one must beware of crossreactive

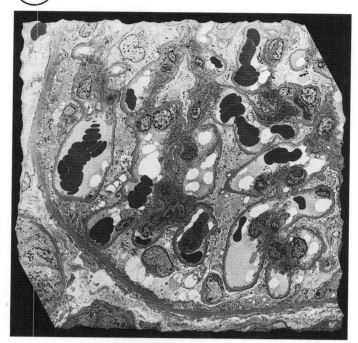

FIGURE 1.3 Electron micrograph showing the ultrastructure of a glomerulus. The increased detail is apparent even at this low power.

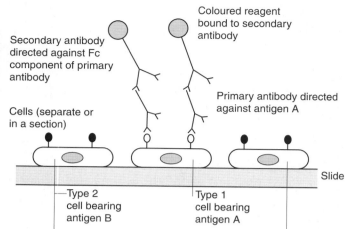

FIGURE 1.4 The principles of immunohistochemistry. The aim of the technique is to identify any cell bearing a specific antigen. The cell in the centre has antigens on its surface which are recognized by antibodies, often raised in mice, directed against that antigen. These are the primary antibodies. To demonstrate where these antibodies have bound, a secondary antibody is applied to the section. This antibody is raised in another species, e.g. rabbit, and directed against the Fc component of the primary antibody and therefore binds to it. An enzyme or fluorescent label is bound to the secondary antibody so that a coloured signal is produced. The cells on the left and right bear different surface antigens which are not recognized by the primary antibody and so no signal is produced in relation to them.

binding to other unrelated proteins. Tagging such an antibody with a fluorescent, radioactive or enzymatic label allows specific substances to be identified and localized in tissue sections or cytological preparations. This has proved particularly useful in the diagnosis of tumours, in which it is important to classify the tumour on the basis of the differentiation it shows to allow the most appropriate treatment to be given. The technique is outlined in Figure 1.4.

Molecular Pathology

Molecular techniques were the logical next step: rather than attempt to identify proteins within a cell, expression of the genes responsible could be identified if appropriate mRNA could be extracted from the cells or localized to them by *in-situ* hybridization techniques. In addition, expression of abnormal genes could be detected: for example in several forms of non-Hodgkin's lymphoma specific genetic rearrangements appear to be responsible for the proliferation of the tumour (see Chapter 8, p. 201); their identification allows precise subtyping (Figure 1.5).

Future Imaging in Pathology

Histopathology sets great store on making the correct diagnosis and gleaning information that is going to be useful in determining treatment options and likely clinical outcome. In parallel, oncologists now are increasingly aware how a patient's disease is unique to that patient and treatment must be 'individualized'. The image a pathologist sees down a microscope reflects the underlying differentiation of the cells and processes going on. The use of antibodies or RNA detection to identify different cell types and processes adds

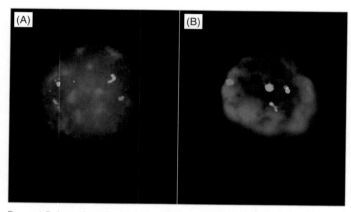

FIGURE 1.5 Interphase fluorescence *in-situ* hybridization (FISH) on a lymphoma using the IGH/CCND1 dual fusion probe (Vysis). (A) Normal pattern showing two green signals representing IGH on chromosome 14 and two red signals representing CCND1 on chromosome 11. (B) Abnormal pattern in a mantle cell lymphoma showing a single green IGH signal, a single red CCND1 signal and two fused signals representing the two derived chromosomes involved in the t(11;14) translocation. (For more information on the probe used see www.vysis.com/AnalyticSpecificReagents(ASR)_59424.asp (Part # 32-191017.)

to this basic knowledge. In recent years the techniques of genomics and proteomics have been developed. In these, the entire protein composition or gene expression profile of a diseased tissue can be established in comparison to the corresponding normal tissue (Figure 1.6). The next challenge is to be able not just to identify the genotype and phenotype but also the metabolic functions that are taking

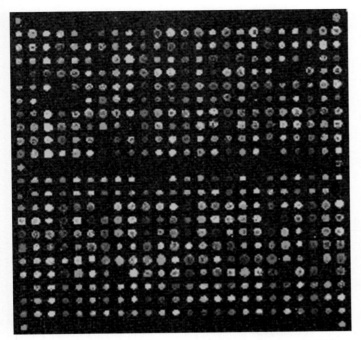

FIGURE 1.6 Gene expression microarrays were developed in the mid-1990s and have become a powerful tool to study global gene expression. Real time polymerase chain reaction (RT-PCR) is used to generate cDNA from mRNA extracted from test and control samples. The test and reference cDNAs are labelled with different fluorochromes, in this case represented by the red and green circles. These samples are then competitively hybridized to an array platform that comprises representations of known genes or expressed sequence tags (ESTs) which have been spotted onto a solid support, usually glass or nylon. The presence of specific cDNA sequences in each sample can then be determined by scanning the array at the excitation wavelength for each fluorochrome, with the ratio of the two signals providing an indication of the relative abundance of the mRNA species in the two original samples. Although spotted microarrays are still in use today, the market is now dominated by one-colour platforms such as the Affymetrix GeneChip in which a single sample is hybridized to each array. Gene expression microarrays have been used in numerous applications including identifying novel pathways of genes associated with certain cancers, classifying tumours and predicting patient outcome.

place and thereby provide even more relevant information to the clinician treating the patient and the researcher seeking new and effective therapies. Pathology thus has a key role in translational research and should remain at the forefront of medical advances.

HOW RELEVANT IS PATHOLOGY?

Is Histopathology Necessary?

It might be argued that with advances in radiological imaging and other laboratory techniques the role of the histopathologist has decreased. This misses the key point that pathology directly addresses the question of what disease process is occurring and is complemented by many other diagnostic modalities. This role is especially important in the management of patients suspected of having a tumour (see Case

History 1.1), but almost all tissues removed from a patient should be submitted for histopathological analysis.

What Can Cytology Achieve?

Unlike histology, where assessment of the tissue architecture is of prime importance, in cytology it is the characteristics of the individual cells which are of most value. Essentially, in diagnostic practice the cytologist looks for the cytological features of malignancy (see Figure 5.3D, p. 80). Admittedly, the relationships between adjacent cells can be appreciated to some extent: for example, in an aspirate from a breast lump loss of cohesion between cells is suggestive of malignancy, as is a high nucleus:cytoplasmic ratio of the cells (see Figure 1.10). In screening practice, for example in cervical cancer programmes, the cytologist seeks to identify the same changes but at an earlier stage and thus give a warning of incipient cancerous changes. The biological basis and efficacy of screening programmes continue to be hotly debated.

Is the Autopsy a Useful Investigation?

The popular image of a pathologist, perhaps fostered by television programmes, is of an individual who determines the cause of death, especially when foul play is suspected. From the early days of pathology, the post mortem has been of importance in understanding disease mechanisms, and in explaining the nature of the individual's final illness. However, advances in imaging and a cultural move not to accept autopsies in many countries have significantly reduced the number performed, other than those carried out for legal reasons. Enormous advances in imaging techniques, especially computed tomography (CT) and magnetic resonance imaging (MRI) when coupled with targeted needle biopsies have to some extent diminished the need for the autopsy, but publications continue to show that autopsies uncover hitherto unsuspected conditions.

Establishment of a robust, updated, scientific evidence base for post-mortem pathology remains a challenge. Recent events including the disclosure of widespread practices of retention of tissue and organs for research purposes have provoked a sea change in public attitudes to the autopsy. In some countries specific new legislation is attempting to find the balance of investigation versus prohibition and to provide a platform for education of the public and support of families. Nonetheless, the post-mortem examination remains the final arbiter of the cause of death in many cases, the key investigation in the forensic investigation of unexplained deaths and potentially an essential part of medical audit. This can only be so if it is carried out thoroughly and appropriately, realizing that no single investigation is the gold standard and that the autopsy is a much less effective way to examine death caused by metabolic 'failure' rather than due to a structural abnormality. The examples of new variant Creutzfeldt–Jacob disease (see Chapter 11, p. 307), acquired immune deficiency syndrome (AIDS) (see Chapter 19, p. 511) and severe acute respiratory syndrome

(SARS) (see Chapter 7, p. 178) emphasize that new diseases are still emerging. Meticulous post-mortem examinations can help clarify the disease mechanisms.

The Post Mortem Itself

The aim of a full post mortem is the examination first of the external aspects of the body, to look for injuries, haemorrhage, jaundice or other stigmata of disease. The body is then opened and the body cavities inspected, then the organs are removed so that each in turn can be weighed and examined both externally and on the cut surface. Ideally, if appropriate permission has been granted, small pieces of the major organs and any diseased tissues are taken for fixation and histological assessment, so that the impression gained on naked eye inspection may be confirmed (or refuted). For a detailed analysis of some organs, especially the brain, it is essential that the organ is retained intact, preserved in formaldehyde, and then cut into thin slices followed by histology, a process usually taking at least 3–4 weeks.

1.1 CASE HISTORY

The patient, a man of 55, presents with altered bowel habit. Both barium enema and colonoscopy show a stricture at the rectosigmoid junction. A biopsy is taken from this site.

WHAT DOES THE CLINICIAN (AND OF COURSE THE PATIENT) WANT TO KNOW?

Obviously, is this a benign stricture, perhaps due to diverticular disease or even Crohn's disease, or is this a tumour, and if so, is it benign or malignant? Figure 1.7 shows infiltration of the normal tissues by malignant cells arranged in glandular structures, this being an adenocarcinoma (see Chapter 5, pp. 82–83).

In the light of this diagnosis, the patient proceeds to have a resection of the rectum and sigmoid colon with anastomosis of the cut ends to restore bowel continuity. The specimen is submitted for pathology.

ONCE AGAIN, WHAT INFORMATION DO THE CLINICIAN AND PATIENT REQUIRE?

- First, confirmation of the diagnosis.
- Second, any information which would predict the likely prognosis of the patient and indicate whether any additional therapy should be given.

This information would include an indication of the type of tumour, an estimate of its biological potential – how malignant it is (its grade), how far it has spread (its stage), for example how far through the bowel wall the tumour has spread, and whether the tumour has been completely excised or is present in lymph nodes (Figure 1.8). To improve the collection of such information in a standard form, the concept of a 'minimum data set' has evolved. The data set recommended by the Royal College of Pathologists is shown in Figure 1.9.

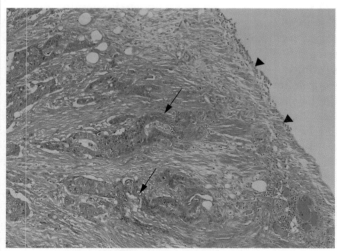

FIGURE 1.7 Adenocarcinoma of colon. Malignant glandular structures (arrows) have invaded the wall of the bowel and have almost reached the peritoneal surface (arrowheads).

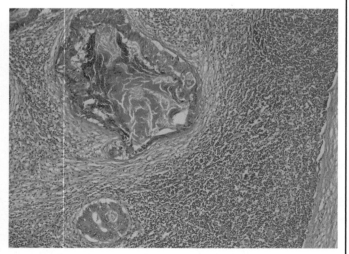

FIGURE 1.8 Secondary (metastatic) adenocarcinoma of colon in a lymph node. Two malignant glands can be seen, with surviving node to the right. A tumour that has reached nodes by the time of diagnosis has a worse prognosis.

NATIONAL MINIMUM DATA SET COLORECTAL CANCER HISTOPATHOLOGY REPORT

Surname....................... Forenames.......................... Date of birth..................... Sex.......................
Hospital...................... Hospital No.......................... NHS No....................
Date of receipt...................... Date of reporting...................... Report No......................
Pathologist...................... Surgeon......................

Gross Description

Site of tumour.......................

Maximum tumour
diameter.......................
Distance of tumour to nearer
margin (cut end).......
Presence of tumour perforation
(pT4) [ ] Yes [ ] No

For rectal tumours
Tumour is [ ] above [ ] at [ ]
below
the peritoneal reflection
Distance from the dentate
line.......................

Histology

Type

Adenocarcinoma [ ] Yes [ ] No
(to include mucinous and signet
ring adenocarcinomas)

If No,
other....................................
......

Differentiation by predominant
area
[ ] Well/moderate [ ] Poor

Local Invasion

[ ] Submucosa (pT1)
[ ] Muscularis propria (pT2)
[ ] Beyond muscularis propria
(pT3)
[ ] Tumour cells have breached
the peritoneal surface
or invaded adjacent organs
(pT4)

Margins

Tumour involvement N/A Yes No

Doughnut [ ] [ ] [ ]

Margins (cut end) [ ] [ ] [ ]

For rectal tumours [ ] [ ] [ ]

Circumferential margin [ ] [ ] [ ]
involvement
Histological measurement from
tumour to circumferential
margin ....mm

Metastatic Spread
No of lymph nodes
examined.......................
No of positive lymph
nodes.......................
(pN1 1–3 nodes, pN2 4+ nodes
involved) Yes No

Apical node positive (Dukes C2)[ ] [ ]

Extramural vascular invasion [ ] [ ]

Background Abnormalities

Yes No

Adenoma(s) [ ] [ ]
Synchronous carcinomas(s) [ ] [ ]
(Complete a separate form for each cancer)

Ulcerative colitis [ ] [ ]

Crohn's disease [ ] [ ]

Familial adenomatous polyposis [ ] [ ]

Other
comments.......................
....
....

Pathological Staging
Complete resection at all margins [ ]
Yes [ ] No

TNM

[ ] T [ ] N [ ] M

Dukes'

[ ] Dukes'A (Growth limited to wall, nodes negative)

[ ] Dukes'B (Growth beyond

muscularis propria, nodes negative)

[ ] Dukes'C1 (Nodes positive and apical node negative)

[ ] Dukes'C2 (Apical node positive)
Histologically confirmed liver
metastases [ ] Yes [ ] No

Signature...................................... Date...../...../.....
SNOMED Codes........./...............

FIGURE 1.9   National Minimum Data Set for Colorectal Cancer. (Reproduced with permission from the Royal College of Pathologists.)

Where is Pathology Going?

The past 20 years have seen major advances in our understanding of the underlying molecular mechanisms of disease. The completion of the human genome project, molecular genetics and cell biology, and more importantly the use of this information to allow construction of a functional framework of tissues in health and disease will inevitably lead to new approaches to basic research, and also to the day-to-day investigation of disease. Proteomic and functional genomic analysis of a few cells aspirated

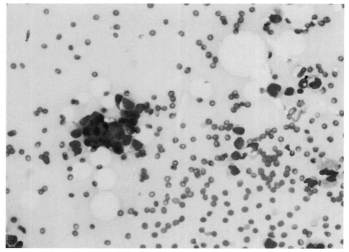

FIGURE 1.10 This breast aspirate shows cells with a high nucleus:cytoplasmic ratio and loss of cohesion indicating malignancy.

from a mass may give far more information on the nature of a tumour than conventional histopathological assessment of the entire specimen, which at present remains the gold standard. Virchow might be familiar with the workings of a twentieth century pathology department. It is doubtful if he would be as familiar with the evolving pathology department of the twenty-first century.

SUMMARY

- Pathology is the study of disease. Subspecialties include histopathology, cytopathology, post mortems, haematology, microbiology, chemical pathology, immunology and genetics.
- Techniques in pathology include light microscopy, electron microscopy, immunohistochemistry and molecular pathology.
- Genomics, proteomics and tests of metabolic function are entering practice.

FURTHER READING

Dobbs D. *Diagnostic Immunohistochemistry*, 2nd edn. Philadelphia: Churchill Livingstone, 2006.

Killeen AA. *Principles of Molecular Pathology*. Totowa, NJ: Humana Press, 2004.

Rosai J. *Rosai and Ackerman's Surgical Pathology*, 9th edn. Chapters 1–3, pp 1–91. London: Mosby, 2004.

NORMAL CELLULAR FUNCTIONS, DISEASE AND IMMUNOLOGY

David J Harrison and Stewart Fleming

INTRODUCTION

Disease may result from an abnormality in structure or function within a single cell, for example in cancer, but more often than not it manifests itself because of the way in which other cells and tissues are affected and take part in the response to the original cause.

Understanding the normal function of cells and tissues gives insight into both the cause and effect of disease, as well as beginning to allow rational design of therapy. Normal cellular function is encapsulated in the reproductive cycle. The body originates from a single fertilized ovum and generates different tissues, including germ cells in the gonads that ensure the survival of the species. This involves many processes: cell proliferation, cell deletion, intercellular communication, basic energy supply and use, oxygen delivery and combustion, protective mechanisms that may be active or passive and complex gene programming which can be overridden in certain circumstances by the environment in which a cell finds itself. For this complex organization to function there must be many checks and balances, and ways in which different cells and tissues can communicate with each other. At the heart of understanding the pathogenesis of disease is recognizing how different injuries and insults can subvert or overwhelm these normal physiological processes and lead to an imbalance in homeostasis. This principle is well illustrated by the normal and abnormal function of the immune system, which comprises the latter half of this chapter.

COMPONENTS OF THE CELL: STRUCTURE

With the exception of the red blood cells, all living cells in the human body contain a nucleus in which resides the majority of genetic information; the mitochondria harbour 37 genes, 13 of which code for proteins. The nucleus is not an inert structure cut off from the rest of the cell (Figure 2.1). The nuclear membrane is constantly crossed by factors which regulate the expression of genes and may repair DNA damage as soon as it occurs. The chromatin material that is the scaffold for the double-stranded DNA is packaged very tightly. It is critically important that this wrapped

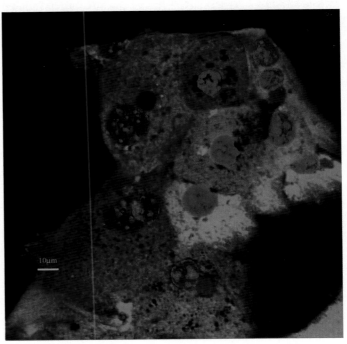

FIGURE 2.1 Nuclei in liver cells stained blue within cytoplasm. Nuclei communicate with cytoplasm, and cells connect intimately with one another through a variety of cell junctions. (Confocal fluorescence microscopy.)

DNA is protected from damage, and yet can be unravelled when needed for gene transcription, for replication and prior to cell division.

In the cytoplasm, a variety of organelles are responsible for the remainder of cellular function. In some cases these are permanent features, for example mitochondria (Figure 2.2), but in other cases a particular macromolecular complex may only be assembled when needed, for example the proteosome involved in protein degradation or 'apoptosome' which catalyses cell death by apoptosis. Ribosomes translate messenger RNA into peptide sequences and further processing, including splicing, glycosylation, and possible packaging for secretion in the endoplasmic reticulum. The mitochondria are the primary site of oxidative phosphorylation. As part of this function they generate free radicals, which in addition to potentially causing damage to membranes, enzymes and DNA, are also part of the ox–redox signalling system that indirectly regulates the expression of a number of genes involved in protection. The mitochondria are also key players in executing apoptosis in some situations.

appropriate levels in response to particular stimuli. In addition to control of gene expression, the cell uses a network of competing enzymes which regulate the activity, structure and function of other proteins. Thus phosphorylases and kinases compete at suitable amino acid residues to dephosphorylate or phosphorylate their targets. These cause pH-dependent conformational shifts that alter both structure and function. Thus enzymes can be used to flick switches after translation, providing a rapid response to the changing intracellular environment. Central to understanding many diseases is the realization that life in an oxygen-rich environment is a precarious business and that protection against oxidant-induced stress is key to cell survival.

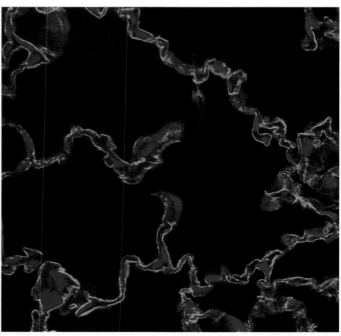

FIGURE 2.3 Lung alveolar epithelium. Nuclei are blue, flattened type 1 alveolar epithelial cells are green and type 2 cells are pink. The green and pink fluorescence depends on the expression of proteins specific to the different cell types identified by particular antibodies labelled with fluorescent dyes. (Courtesy of Dr Gareth Clegg.)

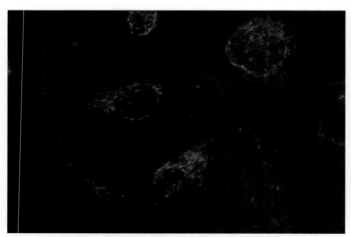

FIGURE 2.2 Mitochondria, visible as rod-like structures lying mostly around the nucleus, are demonstrated by a fluorescence technique. (Courtesy of Dr Rehab Al-Jemal.)

CELLULAR BIOCHEMISTRY: FUNCTION

Perhaps as many as 10 000 genes are actively expressed in a cell simply to maintain cell viability and function. These genes code for a variety of protein products involved directly and indirectly in energy production, protection against unwanted side effects of carbohydrate combustion in the presence of oxygen, and structural and waste disposal. It is clear that these many gene products interact with one another so that cell homeostasis is a complex interactive network (Figure 2.3). The regulation of gene expression is therefore complex, with many genes only being expressed when needed by the assembly of a complex of proteins including transcription factors. This gives the cell the ability to express selectively certain genes at

The balance between oxidation and reduction is central to many processes including the reduction of ribose acids to generate deoxyribose, which is a critical component of DNA. Antioxidant enzymes are positioned throughout the cell to maximize protection. Thus superoxide dismutase 2 (SOD2) is located in mitochondria where it quickly takes reactive superoxide anions and converts them to the less potent hydrogen peroxide. This diffuses from mitochondria and can be destroyed by catalase. Within the soluble component of the cytoplasm (the cytosol) many peroxidases and transferases protect against oxidative species or make use of them in other cell reactions. Lipid peroxidation can occur as a chain reaction, as is seen in alcoholic liver disease (p. 267), and there are many antioxidant enzymes associated with microsomes that can abort these reactions. In addition to enzymatic protection, which can also use hydrogen for reducing reactions, there are other molecules associated with nicotinamide adenine dinucleotide (NADH) and nicotinamide adenine dinucleotide phosphate (NADPH) which offer protection, notably the reduced tripeptide glutathione, uric acid, and vitamins E and C.

Protein Degradation and Removal

The half-life of cellular proteins varies from just a few moments to many months and perhaps even years. The haemoglobin protein in red blood cells lasts for more than 100 days before the effete cell is removed from the circulation. The regulation of cell proteins is a complex and important process for cell viability and function. If damaged protein accumulates it may inhibit normal protein and even injure the cell. Genetic abnormalities resulting in abnormal proteins are implicated in many diseases. In cystic fibrosis (see Chapter 7, p. 163) a transmembrane chloride channel is dysfunctional and this results in the phenotype seen clinically with abnormal secretion of mucus. In storage diseases, such α_1-antitrypsin disease, an abnormal protein is produced that cannot be efficiently secreted from the cell. The protein accumulates and can cause damage to the liver cells resulting in hepatitis, which may progress to cirrhosis (see Chapter 10, p. 265). In addition the absence of functional antiprotease in plasma leads to an increased risk of emphysema developing in the lungs (see Chapter 7, p. 168). Mutation of tumour suppressor genes results in formation of proteins with abnormal folding characteristics. Sometimes these inhibit the function of the corresponding normal protein (a dominant negative effect) and so contribute to the pathogenesis of cancer. Normally, damaged protein is marked for degradation by being bound to a carrier protein called ubiquitin, a process known as ubiquitination. This ubiquinated protein is then removed from the cellular pool and degraded in the proteosome.

INTERCELLULAR COMMUNICATION

For any multicellular organism it is essential that cells communicate with each other to allow proper functioning. This communication must occur at several different levels, starting with immediate direct cell-to-cell contact, extending through local communication networks to information passing around the whole body. Many distinct mechanisms exist to allow this to happen.

Cells are joined by cell junctions that are physical connections. These are of several types. Desmosomes and tight junctions join cell membranes, and gap junctions allow passage of chemical messages between cells. In addition, adhesion molecules are expressed on the cell surfaces, which not only join cells together but also transduce signals important for growth, migration and differentiation. The surface-bound major histocompatibility complex (MHC) molecules and immunoglobulin are specialized forms of recognition mechanism present in lymphocytes, without which an immune response would be impossible (see later in this chapter).

Another form of communication is the production and release of peptides and other mediators that act in a *paracrine* fashion; that is they pass messages to nearby cells. Examples of this include mediators of injury and inflammation and changes in extracellular matrix that occur during wound repair. Although cytokines are primarily locally acting paracrine factors they may also have systemic functions. Thus interleukin 1 (IL1) and IL6 are important mediators of the systemic response to injury. Hormones are of course *endocrine* mediators and act in a tissue-specific manner dependent on the presence of receptors on the target cells and tissues. Feedback loops that ensure coordination throughout the organism are a key feature of intercellular communication. Any dysregulation or interruption of these feedback loops can lead to disease, as discussed in Chapter 17.

Perhaps the most complex intercellular communication is found within the nervous system. It is a prerequisite of a nervous system that it will respond immediately to changes in the external environment for communication to be rapid, specific and geared to allow a direct pathway between sensory input on the one hand and effector output on the other hand. Neurones do not actually join to one another but instead have a close association through the synapse across which chemical neurotransmitters can pass causing depolarization of the adjacent cell and hence passage of a message. Many chemicals are neurotransmitters, including some more commonly thought of as hormones in the gastrointestinal tract (such as bombesin and gastrin).

STEM CELLS AND DIFFERENTIATION

Inevitably during life cells are damaged, die and must be replaced. For some tissues this is a continuous process and in these *labile* tissues cell loss occurs at a high rate. For example, mucosal cells in the colon and keratinocytes from the skin are constantly shed from the surface, neutrophils are constantly being phagocytosed and removed from the circulation and there is even a slow turnover of hepatocytes. To survive, an organism must therefore be able to produce cells to take the place of those that have been lost. Usually cell division is restricted to a small subpopulation of the total cell mass, a group of cells known as stem cells. A stem cell has a high capacity for self-renewal and for giving rise to daughter cells, which differentiate to replace those that have died.

In many tissues stem cells can only give rise to a single differentiated cell type, for example a keratinocyte, and are thus regarded as unipotential. Haemopoietic cells can give rise to cells of several lineages including monocytes and myeloid cells. These are called pluripotential. Stem cells necessary for passing on genetic information through the germline must be able to give rise to every cell type and are thus known as totipotential.

The importance of stem cells is their persistence as a pool of proliferating or potentially proliferating cells throughout life. They are exposed to many kinds of damage, some of which cause mutations leading eventually to cancer. Indeed most cancers are thought to arise from mutations accumulating in stem cell compartments rather than in morphologically recognizable differentiated cells. Stem cells are also important because they may be used to replenish cells that have been ablated. This may occur in the treatment of myeloid leukaemia, or in fulminant liver failure, in which the liver's prodigious ability to reconstitute itself may reduce the need for liver transplantation.

Stem Cells and Cloning

Until relatively recently it was assumed that pluripotent stem cells resided for the most part within specific organs. Thus bone marrow contains haemopoietic stem cells, the liver contains hepatocyte stem cells and so on. Recent data indicate the pool of stem cells is larger, more diverse and more potent than previously supposed. Thus stem cells have been found in bone marrow and umbilical blood which can generate, for example, hepatocytes, neurones or cardiomyocytes; these may be useful in treating specific diseases or used as part of gene replacement therapy.

An extension of this work, with important ethical implications, is the use of near-totipotent stem cells derived from human embryos fertilized *in vitro*. Basic genetics research is addressing how stem cells are controlled and in particular how many classes of genes can be switched on or off depending on differentiation status. This has led to the development of cloning, whereby a single nucleus from a differentiated cell can be conditioned to behave like a totipotent fertilized germ cell and give rise to a genetically identical offspring. This requires the pseudo-fertilization stimulation of a nucleus inserted into the empty cytoplasm of an ovum. To date cloned progeny have included sheep (e.g. Dolly the sheep), cats and mice. There is a high loss of embryos due to malformation, and the effects on ageing and disease susceptibility are being studied to determine whether the cloned animals retain memory of their originating cell's 'age' or whether their replicative clock is reset to zero.

MORPHOGENESIS AND DIFFERENTIATION

There is often a trade-off between a cell retaining the ability to proliferate and to exhibit differentiated functions necessary for the organism's wellbeing. In fetal development differentiation occurs during morphogenesis to allow formation of vital structures and organs. This involves cell migration, carefully regulated proliferation, cell differentiation to acquire new functional and structural characteristics and, as mentioned below, selective and highly regulated deletion of some cells by a form of cell death described morphologically as apoptosis (Figure 2.4). How this complex process is achieved in mammalian cells is only now beginning to be understood, having previously been extensively worked on in nematodes and fruit flies. It is clear that the whole process is under very tight genetic control. The master genes that are identified are very similar in higher order animals to those first identified in worms and flies; this indicates how conserved morphogenesis is in evolution. These genes are called homeobox genes and their primary purpose is to regulate the expression of groups of other genes and thus impose a discipline on the growing mass of cells. Mutations of these genes have been found, and these inevitably lead to developmental abnormalities. They have been implicated in some rare forms of childhood neoplasia. The main tumours of infancy are listed in Table 2.1.

More commonly morphogenesis and embryological development are adversely affected by damage caused by infection, metabolic, dietary or chemical action. In this situation, as would be predicted from the description of how whole groups of cells are herded to differentiate in unison, resulting malformations are often severe, for example

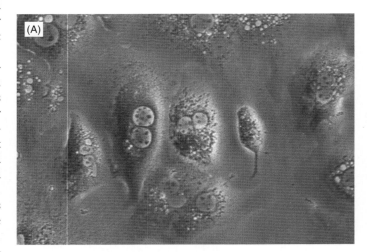

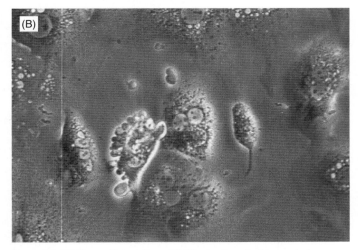

FIGURE 2.4 (A) Liver cells in culture. (B) After treatment with apoptosis-inducing injury, one cell has become shrunken and blebbed before completely disintegrating into apoptotic bodies. *In vivo* these apoptotic bodies are rapidly phagocytosed.

TABLE 2.1 Congenital and neonatal malignant neoplasms

Tumour type	Total (for four series)	% of total
Classic neuroblastoma	139	33
Sarcoma (not otherwise specified)	138	33
Renal tumours (mostly Wilms')	24	6
Retinoblastoma	20	5
Brain tumours	15	3
Germ cell tumours	8	2
Carcinoma	3	1
Liver tumours (mostly hepatoblastoma)	6	1
Leukaemia/lymphoma	24	5
Other	48	11
Total	**425**	**100**

Adapted from Stocker JT, Dehner LP (eds). *Pediatric Pathology*, Chapter 20, p. 325. Philadelphia: JP Lippincott, 1992.

resulting in the absence of a limb or failure of an eye to develop. This process is known as teratogenesis.

Dysmorphogenesis: Congenital Malformations

About 1 in 50 babies are born with malformations that may present with immediate problems or not declare themselves until later life (Table 2.2). Such congenital malformations are a heterogeneous group consisting of genetic disorders, effects of intrauterine infection or trauma and a variety of other conditions. The developing fetus is particularly susceptible to malformations because of the extremely rapid growth and the constraints of intrauterine existence. For example, an insufficiency of amniotic fluid caused by leakage from a damaged placenta compresses the developing fetus. The resulting appearance is characteristic: deformed, bent limbs; flattened face; and often poorly expanded chest with failure of normal lung development. Another mechanical cause of dysmorphogenesis is the presence of amniotic bands, strips of amniotic membrane that arise from tears in the amnion. These can constrict a limb or impede blood flow thus causing incomplete or absent development.

Infection and drugs taken during pregnancy are also important causes of fetal malformation. Rubella in the early stages of pregnancy can result in many abnormalities, including physical deformity, deafness and blindness. For this reason immunization against rubella is essential before pregnancy is likely to occur and teenage girls should be screened for evidence of immunity. Alcohol excess can lead to characteristic malformations and retarded growth, a constellation of features known as fetal alcohol syndrome.

Genetic disease, both chromosomal abnormalities and single gene defects, can cause physical and mental impairments. The commonest genetic malformation is associated with trisomy 21 and results in Down syndrome (see Chapter 3). This occurs in 1 in 1000 births and is commoner if the mother is over 35 years of age. Many cases of malformation are of unknown cause; these most likely represent a combination of genetic and envir-onmental factors, that is they are multifactorial. Even when detailed genetic analysis is performed many cases fail to show a recognizable genetic defect.

TABLE 2.2 Types of morphological abnormality

Defect	Descriptive term	Example
Failure of organ formation or development	Agenesis or hypoplasia	Drugs, e.g. thalidomide
Failure of differentiation	Dysplasia	Renal dysplasia in Potter syndrome
Failure of fusion of embryological structures	Dysraphism	Neural tube defects, e.g. meningocoele
Failure of programmed cell death, involution or luminization	Atresia	Syndactyly (webbed fingers), biliary atresia
Failure of migration, incomplete migration	Ectopia	Undescended testis
Chromosomal abnormalities	(multiple abnormalities)	Down syndrome
Single gene defects	(very varied effects)	Some forms of dwarfism; familial adenomatous polyposis (FAP)

CELL PROLIFERATION AND GROWTH

Mitosis results in daughter cells being produced, each containing the full complement of DNA (46 chromosomes, diploid) (Figure 2.5), whereas in meiosis the DNA content of a cell is halved and cells become haploid (Figure 2.6). Diploidy is achieved when two haploid cells combine, usually an egg and sperm. Although disturbance in cell cycle is widely known as important in the pathogenesis of cancer, an understanding of how cell proliferation is controlled is also needed to fully appreciate processes such as wound healing and atherosclerosis. Classically the cycle is divided into four states, G_1, S, G_2, M (mitosis), with an additional fifth state, G_0, which is in effect 'time out' for the cell (Figure 2.7). Despite the explosion of knowledge about the cell cycle control these five states remain the core of understanding how cells proliferate and, just as importantly, why they do not.

Mitosis

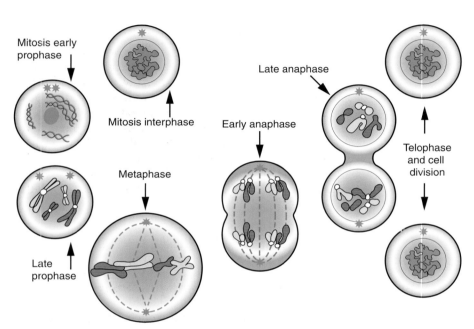

FIGURE 2.5 Summary of mitosis.

Meiosis

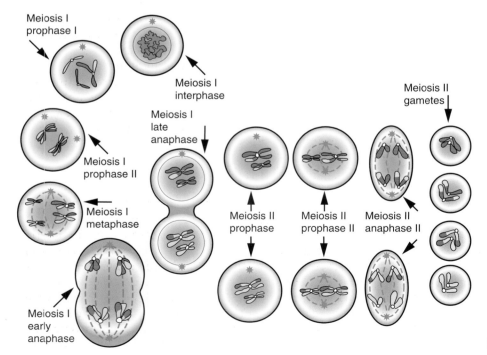

FIGURE 2.6 Summary of meiosis.

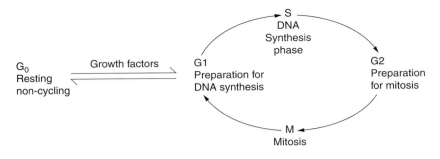

FIGURE 2.7 The cell cycle. Cells start at rest in G_0 and cycle through to mitosis or meiosis. At a number of steps there are checkpoints where the cycle can be stopped. Failing to activate cycle checkpoints may contribute to mutagenesis, ultimately leading to cancer.

Not all cells retain the ability to enter the cell cycle as they are terminally differentiated and permanently confined to G_0, for example neurones in the central nervous system (CNS) in adults. However, some cells in stable populations such as hepatocytes which normally have a very low rate of proliferation may be encouraged to proliferate under certain conditions in the presence of growth factors. Labile populations are constantly cycling even though a relatively small proportion of their cells is actively cycling at any given time. Because cell proliferation is such a key event in the life of an organism, and because inappropriate cycling activity could have such devastating effects, there are many tight controls over proliferation.

Cells normally reside in quiescent G_0 unless stimulated by an exogenous growth stimulus to enter the cycle and therefore be available for proliferation. The cell cycle is controlled by a complex network of competing gene products whose activities are frequently modulated by kinases and phosphorylases. Thus cyclins promote cell cycle activity but cyclin-dependent kinases and cyclin-dependent kinase inhibitors modulate their activity. There are several stages during the cell cycle in which a checkpoint has to be passed. This provides an opportunity for the cell cycle to be arrested, for example to allow repair of DNA damage. These checkpoints are in G_1, at the G_1/S boundary and in G_2, and they are critically important in the prevention of tumorigenesis. Some genes are particularly important in regulating these stages, notably *p53* and *Rb-1*, both well-known tumour suppressor genes (p. 98–99).

It is necessary that several genes are regulated and expressed simultaneously to allow the cycle to proceed. Without this temporal cooperation the correct players are not present and cycle activity is aborted. Disruption of the cell cycle may not simply arrest the growth of cells. Some genes involved in cell cycle activation, including *c*-myc and *H-ras*, if expressed aberrantly will cause the cell to engage apoptotic effector mechanisms and die. Thus genes involved in allowing cycle activity to proceed will directly lead to death if they are not expressed in the correct cellular context. We will return to this when we discuss cancer (see Chapter 5). It is apparent, however, that cells go to quite extreme lengths to prevent inappropriate cell proliferation. Cancer is very much the end stage of a series of extremely unlikely events and the evasion of a number of protective pathways.

Initiating Cell Cycle Activity

As discussed above cells communicate with each other directly, in the local neighbourhood by paracrine pathways and throughout the organism hormonally. It is unsurprising therefore that one of the major functions of these communication routes is to initiate cell proliferation. Selectivity is achieved by cell specific receptor expression coupled to an intracellular signalling pathway that will result in a permissive environment for proliferation to occur. Many growth factors are known and some when overexpressed aberrantly can act as oncogenes and promote excessive growth (Table 2.3).

TABLE 2.3 Growth factors and disease

Growth factor	Disease involvement
Platelet derived growth factor (PDGF)	Atherosclerosis
Insulin-like growth factors (IGF1, IGF2)	? Antiapoptotic effects in some tumours
Transforming growth factor α	Synergy with *c*-myc oncogene in transgenic models of liver cancer
Epidermal growth factor	Receptor overexpression in breast cancer
Interleukins	Autoimmune diseases
Fibroblast growth factors	Systemic response to injury ? Therapeutic use in vascular disease to promote new vessel formation

CELL DEATH BY ACCIDENT AND DESIGN

In general one assumes that a cell is a functional unit that should be kept alive as long as possible to maintain orderly functioning of the organism and to conserve energy and resources. Although this is often the case there are circumstances where this is neither possible nor even advisable. Under these circumstances cells die, either because they are overwhelmed by an injurious stimulus or because they are deliberately deleted as part of a master plan. At times the severity of an insult may be so great or the cell and tissue so vulnerable that normal homeostasis may be impossible to maintain. Under these circumstances a cell may lose metabolic control, rapidly decompensate and undergo catastrophic loss of viability leading to necrosis. *Necrosis* is thus defined as a collapse of membrane integrity and death of a cell or tissue. This results in the release of intracellular components. Many of these are reactive and can lead to the activation of the clotting cascade and the generation of mediators of inflammation. Necrosis is therefore always pathological and brings the risk of inflammation, scarring and may even be implicated in initiating autoreactive immune responses. Tissues rather than individual cells tend to be affected because the trigger for necrosis is usually a catastrophic exogenous event. A region of dead material is formed; this coagulum of protein is referred to as coagulative necrosis. In the brain where there are many lipid-containing cells and little supporting tissue architecture there is liquefaction, sometimes referred to as colliquative necrosis (see Chapter 11, p. 290). However, in each case the underlying pathology is the same.

In a multicellular organism cell death is an essential part of development and clearly it is advantageous to have a mechanism that is not likely to lead to inflammation and scarring, but which is conservative. Studies referred to earlier in worms and insects have revealed a process of selective and specific deletion of cells during embryogenesis known as programmed cell death. Through further studies of the effects of hormone withdrawal on the adrenal it became clear that this pattern of death also occurred in pathological situations not truly programmed in the sense of being morphogenetically determined. Thus, by analogy with leaves falling from a tree in autumn, the process was named apoptosis (*apo-* away from, *piptein* to fall). It is important to realize that although the morphology of apoptosis tends to be similar irrespective of the cause there are many different routes to apoptosis involving several different genetically regulated pathways. Thus the finding of apoptosis in a tissue is neither indicative of the cause nor of the particular biological significance in that situation.

One striking feature of apoptosis is the rapidity of removal of apoptotic cell fragments before their membrane integrity is lost. This is because of a number of changes in glycosylation and receptor expression on the surface of apoptotic cells that facilitate recognition and engulfment by macrophages. Intriguingly, phagocytosis of apoptotic debris does not elicit an inflammatory response; indeed macrophages may be prevented from producing pro-inflammatory cytokines by this process. Apoptosis is increasingly implicated in many diseases – from viral hepatitis, where it has long been suspected, to lymphocyte depletion in human immunodeficiency virus (HIV) infection and to type 2 diabetes and neurodegenerative disease. Inability to engage apoptosis following injury may result in the selection of cells in a developing tumour and in conferring resistance of cancer cells against chemotherapeutic drugs (Figure 2.8).

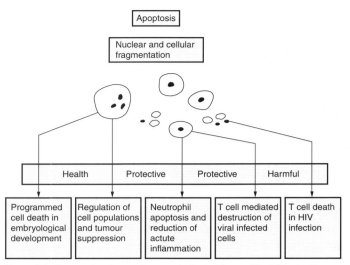

FIGURE 2.8 Apoptosis refers to the morphological form of individual cell death. It can occur as part of normal homeostasis in a variety of settings or as part of a disease. Programmed cell death, for example, when cells die during embryological development, usually occurs by apoptosis. HIV = human immunodeficiency virus.

DISORDERS OF GROWTH

Hypertrophy

Increased workload on a muscle may result in enlargement of individual cells by a process known as hypertrophy. In this situation increased cell number is not an option because the differentiated cells have lost the ability to proliferate and thus cannot increase in number. An important clinical example is the myocardium in hypertension (Figure 2.9), in which increased fibre size leads to increased oxygen requirements (see Chapter 6, p. 117–118). In the presence of atheromatous coronary artery disease it may be impossible to deliver sufficient oxygen and so ischaemic necrosis may occur. Hypertrophy is an active response, as the cell must synthesize extra proteins to allow increased cell size and activity. Hypertrophy itself cannot lead to neoplasia as no cell proliferation occurs.

Hyperplasia

In the presence of excessive growth factor or hormonal stimulation of growth a tissue which retains the ability to proliferate may be forced to undergo several rounds of cell cycle leading to an increase in cell number. This is called hyperplasia. This may be associated with an increase in size of the tissue that must be distinguished from hypertrophy. The cause may be apparent, such as overproduction of adrenocorticotropic hormone (ACTH) from a pituitary tumour causing adrenal hyperplasia (Figure 2.10).

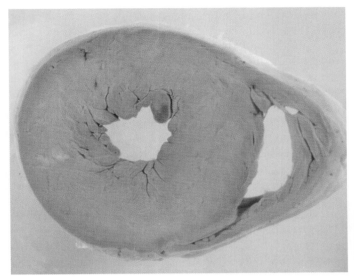

FIGURE 2.9 A slice of heart with the left ventricle to the left and right ventricle to the right. There is massive left ventricular hypertrophy. This occurs when an increased load is placed on the ventricle as in systemic hypertension or aortic valve stenosis.

Hyperplasia caused by abnormal growth factor stimulation should be distinguished from so-called reactive hyperplasia that may occur in response to tissue loss, for example in the liver following paracetamol-induced injury or in the gastric mucosa following acute gastritis. In the latter cases the proliferation is a healing response which is self-limiting and temporary.

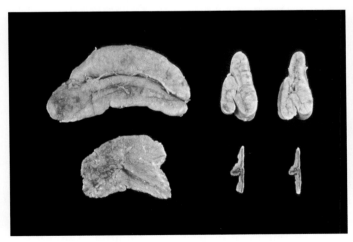

FIGURE 2.10 Normal (lower) and hyperplastic (upper) adrenal glands from different patients. The increased size of the upper glands is due to the presence of increased numbers of glucocorticoid-producing cells in response to sustained stimulation by adrenocorticotropic hormone from a pituitary adenoma.

Atrophy

This term refers to decrease in the size of a tissue or organ that may be caused by a combination of cell shrinkage (the opposite of hypertrophy) and fall in cell number (such as chronic hypoxia resulting in slow attrition of cell number). In some situations atrophy is physiological. Each month the breast and endometrium undergo hormonally induced proliferation followed by cell death (by apoptosis) and atrophy. Denervation of muscle (p. 371) or immobility results in disuse atrophy. Atrophy can be the result of destruction of cells as in the autoimmune damage resulting in primary myxoedema of the thyroid (Figure 2.11; see Chapter 17).

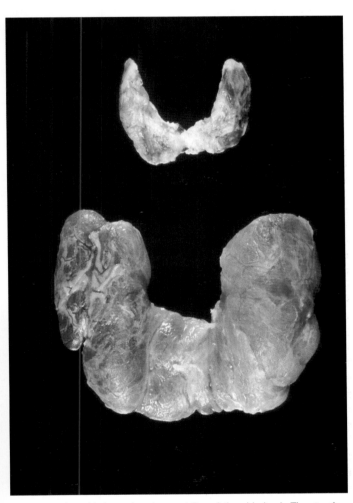

FIGURE 2.11 Atrophic (upper) and normal (lower) thyroid glands. The atrophy is the result of loss of normal thyroid tissue due to longstanding autoimmune disease.

Atrophy is thus a non-specific change which may occur when:

- blood flow is reduced
- nerve supply is interrupted
- there are changes in hormone concentrations
- the tissue experiences disuse or excessive pressure.

Metaplasia

Although it is usual for the precise differentiated state of a cell to be constant, under certain conditions one mature cell type may change into another. This process is known as metaplasia and is reversible. It is an adaptive response and may confer protection from a local injury. It often affects glandular epithelia, which may change to squamous epithelia when exposed to trauma or environmental insult. For example, in smokers the columnar epithelium of the bronchus may change to a more robust squamous epithelium (Figure 2.12). Exposure of the lower oesophagus to acid reflux is a factor resulting in the normal squamous epithelium of the oesophagus becoming glandular, like the stomach or intestine.

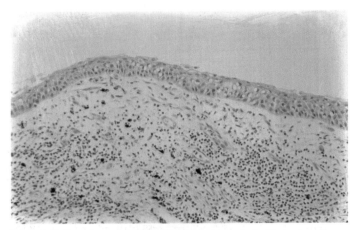

FIGURE 2.12 Squamous metaplasia. The normal pseudostratified columnar lining of the bronchus has been replaced by stratified squamous epithelium as a consequence of chronic exposure to cigarette smoke. The black flecks among the submucosal inflammatory cells are particles of carbon from the inhaled smoke.

Although the process of metaplasia is not in itself premalignant, metaplasia is sometimes associated with progression to malignancy. This can be explained by supposing that the new cell type, although not in any way cancerous, is more susceptible to injurious stimuli in the vicinity, which may lead to the development of cancer. Thus in the case of Barrett's oesophagus, in which glandular epithelium replaces squamous epithelium, continued follow-up is advised to ensure that malignant change does not superimpose itself on the banal metaplastic change. Metaplasia can also occur in mesenchymal tissues. In chronic scarring, fibrous tissue may exhibit focal metaplasia into bone, and this can be identified radiologically.

AGEING

Cellular Ageing

The lifespan of cells varies greatly according to cell type. Neutrophils may live for only a matter of hours, red blood cells for 100 days or more, and some mesenchymal cells for years. There has been much debate whether ageing of cells is a pathological process or a programmed physiological process. Judging from the factors that affect ageing it is clear that both programmable and non-programmable components are present. In rapidly proliferating cell populations cells eventually lose the capacity to divide any further and undergo a process known as cellular senescence.

For a long time it has been known that the number of replicative events a cell can undergo in tissue culture is fixed to around 50 divisions, the so-called Hayflick limit. This suggests a degree of inbuilt senescence although the equivalence of an *in vitro* phenomenon to the *in vivo* setting should not be assumed too readily. Every time a cell undergoes mitosis (with the exception of germ cells which express telomerase) DNA polymerization starts at the end of chromosomes at telomeres, which are tandem repeat sequences. This region is incompletely copied and so the telomere shortens each time. Eventually it becomes too short to allow replication and the cell ceases to undergo mitosis. This telomere-shortened cell is also more likely to permit translocations and be error prone, possibly increasing the risk of breakthrough proliferation leading to cancer. This seems plausible and indeed some cancers show re-expression of telomerase; this might explain why some cancer cells are immortalized and do not undergo senescence.

Further evidence that genetic control of ageing occurs comes from developmental genetic studies in the nematode *Caenorhabditis elegans* in which mutations of a gene called *clk-1* (the 'clock' gene) result in elongation of lifespan. Although homologues of these genes in primitive organisms may exist in humans, it is true that wear and tear is a major factor in ageing. Oxidative metabolism generates free radicals and over time these cause progressive damage to cell membranes, DNA, cytoskeleton and enzymes. Damaged lipids accumulate in cells in the form of lipofuscin, a giveaway sign of cellular ageing and damage. Although protective mechanisms exist to repair DNA, remove damaged protein and oxidized lipid there is a gradual attrition over time that eventually leads to the cell's demise.

Ageing of the Individual

Old age and the attendant increase in dependency and expenditure of resources is a major factor affecting the economies of every industrialized country and is now becoming important in developing countries. The features of ageing are of multisystem deterioration (Table 2.4), the effects of each compounding the others leading to gradual debility. In addition specific degenerative diseases may be superimposed on this 'normal' ageing further adding to the incapacity of the individual and the requirement for assistance. Just as is the case with cellular ageing there are both environmental and genetic factors in play. The earlier idea that environment and oxidant-induced injury were major players has been dashed following the failure of massive antioxidant consumption reliably to increase lifespan.

TABLE 2.4 Characteristics of ageing, showing a spectrum from genetically programmed to more overtly 'pathological' and environmentally linked

At the level of whole organism	Possible cause
Cardiovascular disease	Atherosclerosis, calcification
Loss of lung tissue resembling emphysema	Environmental pollution
Deafness	Repeated environmental trauma
Forgetfulness	Neurone loss due to ischaemia or other mechanisms
Elastotic, sagging skin	Solar damage
Frailty	Muscle wasting
Osteoporosis	Genetic, hormonal, ? previous diet

At the level of cells and tissues	Associations	
Cerebral atrophy	Loss of neurones	i.e. loss of permanent cells
Myocardial atrophy	Loss of cardiomyocytes	
Anaemia	Replication limit reached	
Atrophy of liver	Many, e.g. toxins, diet, hypoxia	

Features seen in ageing include atrophy, possibly as a result of disuse, reduced trophic supply and reduced ability to mount a new immune response or repair wounds quickly.

Growing old and ageing are often assumed to be synonymous, but different species, and different individuals within the same species, age at different rates. This indicates that although ageing is associated with the passage of time, it is not solely a function of time. Indeed, premature ageing syndromes such as progeria and Werner's syndrome indicate a strong genetic component, at least in disordered ageing. Recent genetic studies have identified regions of the genome where variation alters the propensity to age. Whereas yeasts and other single cell organisms that replicate by asexual means do not age, multicellular organisms and their constituent cells and tissues decline in function and eventually die. It is apparent that the clinical and cellular features of ageing are the result of a complex interaction between genes and the environment. For example, osteoporosis is strongly associated with ageing; however, it is very heavily influenced by genetic predisposition, menopausal status and previous dietary habits and calcium load. Perhaps half of ageing is genetically regulated (programmed or clonal senescence) with the other half influenced by environment, when cells simply lose the ability to respond to damage and the attrition of nature's ravages (replicative senescence).

There are many theories and putative remedies for ageing, many of which may have some validity, but none of which is sufficient to explain the phenomenon. There is still uncertainty how far ageing should be regarded as pathological and resisted or normal and accepted gracefully. Houseflies have a short lifespan, giant tortoises a long one. Humans, domestic animals and birds are intermediate in lifespan and in size. The generation of hydrogen peroxide as a function of body mass is inversely proportional to life expectancy, suggesting that oxygen free radical generation may be a major determinant in acquiring wear and tear injury. For some cells loss is irreplaceable, for example permanent cells such as neurones and cardiomyocytes, whereas other stable or labile cell populations may be regenerated, at least for a time. Oxygen free radicals damage proteins, membranes, RNA, DNA and perhaps mitochondrial DNA, in particular, which is repaired less efficiently than nuclear DNA and codes for proteins involved in oxidative phosphorylation. Thus ageing may be a curse imposed by living in an oxygen-rich environment and reliance on combustion of food for survival. Severe calorie restriction of laboratory rodents increases lifespan by up to 50%. A sedentary lifestyle, such as that enjoyed by the giant tortoise, may also be important but sloth has its own disadvantages as we shall see later in Chapter 6 (p. 114).

IMMUNOLOGY

Key Points

- The immune system is an adaptive defence mechanism.
- Immunoglobulins of five classes circulate in body fluids as a specific recognition and effector system.
- T lymphocytes provide the main cell-mediated defence.
- On occasion the immune system may cause disease such as hypersensitivity and autoimmunity.

The immune system is an adaptive defence mechanism protecting the body against the whole range of microbial pathogens which may be encountered. It is also involved in the recognition of self and non-self in transplantation. The immune system has another aspect, however, namely the capacity to cause disease and injury in certain circumstances; indeed some of our most common ailments such as asthma and hayfever are mediated by the immune system gone awry.

One of the most important properties of the immune system is its specificity, the capacity to recognize and respond appropriately to each pathogen separately and distinctly. The immune system has conventionally been divided in two parts, the humoral- and cell-mediated arms, the former consisting of a series of plasma proteins in the blood and tissue fluids and the latter the property of populations of cells which circulate throughout the body. In addition to this specific and sophisticated system there are many defence mechanisms that are general and non-specific and are often termed innate immunity.

Innate Immunity

Innate immunity is an immediate and important defence against many different microbial pathogens and toxins; it lacks specificity, i.e. the response is similar irrespective of the triggering agent.

Epithelial Surfaces

The interfaces between the body and external environment across which microbial pathogens may enter are lined by the epithelia of the skin, gastrointestinal tract, respiratory system and genitourinary tract. These epithelia consist of a continuous and tightly cohesive layer of cells; the cohesion of cells with each other and with the underlying connective tissue is achieved by the action of cell adhesion molecules. The epithelial cells form a physical barrier but through secretions complement this with antimicrobial chemicals. Fatty acids secreted by sebaceous glands in the skin maintain a low pH on this surface; in the gastrointestinal tract there is secretion of acid in the stomach, digestive enzymes from the pancreas and mucins produced by specialized cells throughout the tract. The respiratory epithelium secretes mucus to entrap bacteria which are then expelled due to the action of cilia on the cell surface. Urine produced in the kidney continually flows across the surface of the lower urinary tract impairing the adhesion of bacteria to the surface.

The importance of these features in defence against infection is illustrated by examining the consequences of their disruption in predisposing to disease. Thus stasis of urinary flow increases the risk of urinary tract infection. Likewise loss of gastric acid secretion allows pathogens to reside in the stomach.

Phagocytes

Once the epithelial layer is breached potential pathogens encounter a further defence, a population of cells capable of engulfing and destroying bacteria, the phagocytes named after the process which they use for such engulfment – phagocytosis. Phagocytes reside in tissues and can circulate in the bloodstream from where they are recruited to sites of tissue injury. During phagocytosis bacteria are engulfed, the cell membrane fuses around them to form a phagosome, this in turn fuses with a lysosome, an organelle containing bactericidal and digestive enzymes, to from a phagolysosome within which the bacteria are killed and degraded. The process of recognition of bacteria by phagocytes is a key step in this process. The phagocytes have on their surface recognition receptors which bind to microbial surface chemicals such as lipopolysaccharide and peptidoglycan. The phagocyte receptors include members of the toll-like receptor family. On binding of the toll-like receptor there is activation of a signalling cascade inside the phagocyte leading to the production of cytokines such as IL1, IL6 and tumour necrosis factor α. The toll-like pathway activation also results in the expression of so-called co-stimulatory signals on the surface of the phagocyte; these signals will become important in driving the adaptive and specific immune response.

Plasma Proteins

The cytokines produced by phagocytes have systemic as well as local effects. Prominent among the systemic effects is the release from the liver of proteins known collectively as acute phase reactants or proteins. C-reactive protein (CRP) is elevated in the plasma in a whole range of acute and subacute inflammatory disease. It enhances phagocytosis by binding to the phosphorylcholine component of lipopolysaccharide enabling recognition by the CRP receptor on the phagocyte surface.

Complement

Complement is a complex plasma protease cascade, the components of which are among the acute phase proteins released by the liver. It not only has an important role in mediating the protective effects of innate immunity, contributing in a major way to the effector arm of adaptive immunity but is also a significant factor in the tissue injury which occurs when the immune system goes awry. It can lead to direct cell (bacterial) killing, enhanced phagocytosis and amplification of the response by cell recruitment.

The components of complement circulate in the plasma in an inactive form; activation occurs on proteolytic cleavage by the relevant convertase. The important step in the complement cascade is the activation of C3 by cleavage to C3a and C3b. C3b then acts as the convertase for the activation of C5 which unleashes a cascade to complete the formation of a cell lytic complex C5–9. The key C3 activation may occur by the classical pathway, activated by immunoglobulin binding to antigen, or by an alternative pathway which can be activated by a number of triggers including bacterial cell surface and aggregated immunoglobulin. The complement cascade is also regulated by complement inhibitory or regulatory proteins. Genetic deficiencies in these lead to serious disorders of exaggerated complement activation and acute tissue injury. In addition to generating a cell lytic complex, various complement components have other properties. C3a and C5a are important chemotaxins, C3b bound on a bacterial cell surface enhances recognition and phagocytosis.

Adaptive Immunity

The adaptive immune response is divided into humoral- and cell-mediated components by the activity of B lymphocytes and T lymphocytes, respectively. Although in practice the immune response is a continuous process, for the sake of discussion and analysis it may conveniently be considered to have an afferent arm of initiation and stimulation of immuno-competent cells and an efferent or effector arm leading to the immune directed elimination of pathogens.

B Lymphocytes

B lymphocytes, originally so-called because in birds they develop in the bursa of Fabricius, develop in the bone marrow in mammals including humans and eventually comprise 10–20% of peripheral blood lymphocytes and provide for the humoral immune response. They are present in defined microanatomical compartments of lymph nodes, spleen and gut associated lymphoid tissue. In these sites, on stimulation they proliferate within roughly spherical germinal centres.

B lymphocytes are specifically activated by antigen, binding and crosslinking the B-cell receptor molecules on the surface. The B-cell receptor is composed of monomeric IgM existing in a transmembrane form with the antigen-binding fragment at the external surface and the Fc fragment at the cytoplasmic face. The crosslinking of the B-cell receptor provides one signal for B-cell activation but for complete activation and particularly isoform shift a second signal is needed. This may be provided by B-cell CD40 stimulated by CD40 ligand (CD154) on a helper T cell or by complement components associated with the antigen and acting via B-cell CD21.

On activation B cells proliferate to amplify the immune response and differentiate into plasma cells. Plasma cells are highly synthetic cells which synthesize and secret immuno-globulin, of the same specificity as its receptor, into the plasma. The different immunoglobulin isoforms are regulated in major part by signalling from T cells, resulting in the differing balance achieved in different immune responses.

Immunoglobulin

The main component of the humoral immune response is antibody or immunoglobulin. Broadly, these are tetrameric proteins composed of two identical heavy chains and two light chains. One heavy and one light chain combine to create the antigen-binding site that gives the antibody its specificity. The pairs of heavy and light chains mean that the typical immunoglobulin molecule is at least divalent (Figure 2.13). In addition to antibody binding, immunoglobulins have secondary properties including the activation of complement and enhancement of phagocytosis. Immunoglobulins are classified by their heavy chain type into one of five classes (Table 2.5).

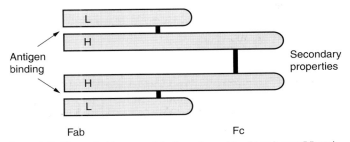

FIGURE 2.13 The typical immunoglobulin unit consists of two heavy (H) and two light (L) chains linked by disulphide bonds. The H and L chains both contribute to the antigen-binding site but the secondary properties reside in the H chain.

IgG is the most abundant immunoglobulin. It is present in plasma, tissue fluids and can cross the placenta. It exists as a monomer and in humans there are four subclasses of IgG, each with slightly different secondary properties. IgA is the second most abundant but exists in two slightly different forms in different body fluid compartments. In serum IgA exists as an immunoglobulin monomer but in secretions such as saliva and tears and gastrointestinal secretions it exists as a dimer, with an additional protective secretory piece which resists its digestion in these secretions. IgM is the largest of the immunoglobulins, found almost entirely in serum. It exists as a pentameric form which confers multivalency on each separate IgM molecule. It is also the first immunoglobulin to appear in immature B cells, and the first to appear in the initial immune response to any new antigen. IgE is a monomeric form which circulates in serum

TABLE 2.5 Immunoglobulin classes

	Heavy chain	Common form	Complement fixation	Location
IgG	γ	Monomer	Classical	Serum and tissue fluid
IgA	α	Monomer or dimer	Alternative	Secretions
IgM	μ	Pentamer	Classical	Plasma
IgE	ε	Monomer	No	Mast cells
IgD	δ	Monomer	No	B lymphocytes

but importantly is found bound to the surface of tissue mast cells and circulating basophils. It is involved in protection against parasites but is clinically most important as the mediator of allergic responses. IgD is a minor component of circulating immunoglobulin but is found on the cell surface of B lymphocytes where it acts as a cell surface receptor.

During the maturation of B cells and particularly during an immune response there is a phenomenon of heavy chain class switching. This involves the cessation of IgM production and a switch to IgG, IgA or IgE production but of antibodies with the same specificity. Heavy chain switching is dependent on a T-cell helper signal and some responses which are T independent such as the response to pneumococcal polysaccharide remain predominantly of an IgM type.

T Lymphocytes

T lymphocytes are responsible for cell-mediated immunity and are so called because they undergo a maturation process in the thymus. T lymphocytes start their development in the bone marrow but recirculate to the thymus. Here they become subdivided into CD4 helper T cells and CD8 cytotoxic T cells. These have different activities, a different pattern of cell-surface markers and respond to antigen in association with different MHC molecules. It is during thymic development that T cell receptor gene rearrangement (see below) occurs.

T cells recognize antigen presented to them on a cell surface and in association with molecules of the MHC class. There are two families of MHC molecules: MHC I and MHC II. MHC class I is expressed on the surface of most tissue cells as a heterodimer of an α chain and a common β_2 microglobulin. MHC class I is recognized by T lymphocytes of the CD8 class. In contrast MHC class II is only expressed on a limited range of immune accessory cells and endothelium. It exists as an $\alpha\beta$ heterodimer and is recognized by CD4 subclass T lymphocytes. Antigen is presented to T lymphocytes by these molecules in the form of small, partially degraded peptide held in molecular grooves on the MHC molecules (Figure 2.14).

MHC genes show extreme polymorphism within the population and are the major component of transplantation reaction. Hence in preparation for solid organ transplantation, patients are tissue typed for their MHC alleles and a match between donor and recipient is sought. Even with modern transplant immunosuppression the outcome remains best for optimally matched individuals.

On encounter with antigen, T cells proliferate to expand the reactive population. CD4 T lymphocytes after stimulation can be divided into Th1 and Th2 depending on the cytokine types they produce. Th1 lymphocytes produce interferon, a potent stimulator of macrophages in their capacity to aid antigen presentation and phagocytosis. Th2 lymphocytes produce a menu of cytokines including IL4 and IL5 which contribute to type 1 hypersensitivity. CD8 lymphocytes respond to cell-surface antigen by the production of a cell lytic molecule leading to cell killing. T-cell-mediated immune responses are particularly important in our defence against the first encounter with viruses and fungi.

Specificity and Diversity of the Immune Response

The immune response demonstrates specificity yet has the capacity to react to a whole range of pathogens, viruses, bacteria, fungi, parasites and transplantation antigens. How is this achieved? T cells and B cells must become committed to a specificity before activation, the specificity must be retained during expansion of the reactive population by cell division and the effector molecules such as immunoglobulin must share the same specificity. Immature B and T cells exhibit changes in the genetic material of the immunoglobulin and T cell receptor genes, respectively. There is gene rearrangement with excision of large parts of the genomic material of these receptors restricting the range of specificity but ensuring that rearrangement is inherited by daughter cells. During further maturation there is extreme hypermutation within the genomic components encoding the antigen-binding regions of the immunoglobulin molecules and T cell receptor. This ceases on maturation so diversity is expanded but remains inherited by daughter cells.

Hypersensitivity

Type 1 or Immediate Hypersensitivity

Type 1 hypersensitivity is a common clinical problem with up to 20% of the population having one or more allergies. It is the principal mechanism of disorders such as hay fever, asthma and anaphylactic shock. Typically there is a rapid onset of symptoms within less than 1 minute but if allergen exposure ceases the clinical effects wane.

The disease is mediated through binding of allergen to preformed IgE on the surface of mast cells usually within the submucosa of the respiratory tract or on the surface of basophils within the circulation. On first exposure to the specific allergen the atopic patient mounts a predominantly IgE response, whereas non-atopic individuals may mount an IgG or IgA response to the same allergen. The

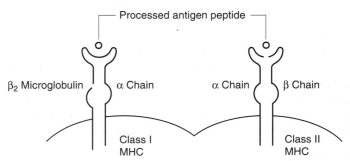

FIGURE 2.14 Major histocompatibility complex (MHC) class I and class II molecules present antigen on the cell surface as processed peptide. Class I MHC consists of an α chain and β_2 microglobulin, whereas class II consist of $\alpha\beta$ heterodimers.

factors regulating the balance of Ig subclass production in any immune response are incompletely understood. However, it appears that predisposed individuals mount a response driven by Th2 type helper T cells with the IL4 and IL13 produced by these cells influencing the isotype switch to IgE production. The Th2 response involving IL4, IL6 and IL9 also activates mast cells, priming them for their effector role in type 1 hypersensitivity. The circulating IgE thus formed binds to the surface of the submucosal mast cells via an IgE receptor, priming the mucosa for an allergic response.

On subsequent exposure the allergen, such as grass pollen or house dust mite, binds to the IgE crosslinking on the cell surface. The clustering of IgE receptors causes calcium influx and degranulation of the mast cell. The granules release several inflammatory mediators including histamine, chemokines and kallikrein generating factor. These substances act on microvascular smooth muscle and endothelium and on bronchial smooth muscle and mucous glands to trigger the characteristic symptoms. There is congestion, hyperaemia and leakage of a protein-rich exudate from the mucosal vessels. The mucosa becomes swollen and oedematous, and glandular production of watery mucus increases. Bronchial smooth muscle contraction causes the airway narrowing and bronchospasm of acute asthma. Once this acute phase is established the airway mucosa in particular becomes hyperresponsive to other inflammatory stimuli such as cigarette smoke or diesel fuel particulates that further accentuate and prolong the symptoms.

When a type 1 hypersensitivity reaction occurs in the general circulation the resulting anaphylactic shock is a serious life-threatening condition. This is the mechanism of acute collapse following peanut ingestion or bee stings in susceptible individuals. These two conditions alone may kill up to 100 people a year in the UK. There is generalized degranulation of mast cells and basophils with release of vasoactive mediators into the circulation. Generalized vasodilatation and plasma leakage occur with circulatory collapse. There is acute mucosal oedema of the larynx and respiratory tract with acute distressing dyspnoea. Unless reversed by immediate resuscitation measures, sudden death may supervene.

Type 2 or Cytolytic Hypersensitivity

Type 2 hypersensitivity reactions are triggered by antibody binding to an antigen on the cell surface and effector mechanisms lead to lysis of the cell. It is the type of reaction seen in some autoimmune disorders and in blood transfusion reactions. It is also the mechanism of certain forms of tissue damage in drug reactions. In these latter the drug binds to the cell surface, most commonly the red blood cell, and acts as a hapten with the cellular proteins in effect being carriers of the small drug molecule. Most commonly the antibody involved is either IgG or IgM.

Preformed antibody binds to the antigen at the cell surface locally activating complement. Completion of the complement cascade leads to insertion of the C_{56789} membrane attack complex in the cell wall and subsequent cell lysis. In haemolytic anaemia or in transfusion reactions the red blood cell lyses within the circulation releasing its contents into the plasma. In circumstances where complement is not activated cell injury may still occur. In Graves' disease antibody binding to the thyroid stimulating hormone (TSH) receptor mimics TSH binding leading to metabolic activation of the cell and hyperthyroidism (see Chapter 17).

Type 3 or Immune-complex-mediated Hypersensitivity

Type 3 reactions result from either the deposition or the formation *in situ* of immune complexes with subsequent activation of complement and recruitment of proinflammatory effector cells. They may exist as either local or generalized disease processes. The location of the disease is influenced by the route of exposure to the antigen, its size and charge and by genetic factors. The clinical features are also determined by whether the exposure is a single event or chronic repeated exposure, the former being typical of a reaction to an injectable drug or of diseases such as farmer's lung, the latter being typical of many autoimmune disorders including systemic lupus erythematosus (SLE) and rheumatoid arthritis. Briefly, immune complexes are deposited in tissue, usually within the walls of small blood vessels. At this site they activate complement by the classical pathway resulting in the liberation of chemotactic peptides. These in turn influence the accumulation of inflammatory cells, neutrophils and macrophages, which attempt to phagocytose and clear the immune complexes. As a bystander effect, tissue components are damaged by the proteolytic enzymes released by the inflammatory cells. The whole process takes 6–8 hours to develop in the acute setting but in many diseases there is persistence of the antigen and chronicity to the hypersensitivity reaction.

Type 4 or Delayed Hypersensitivity

Type 4 or delayed hypersensitivity tissue damage is mediated by T lymphocytes. Activated T lymphocytes directly kill cells or secrete cytokines leading to macrophage accumulation and activation. The aggregated macrophages may assemble into a granuloma. This form of hypersensitivity is independent of antibody and complement. It requires 24–48 hours to develop fully. If antigen persists there will be progressive tissue damage and eventually fibrosis.

Autoimmunity

A number of diseases are characterized by the immune system being targeted against self-antigens expressed in body tissues. The resulting tissue damage may be mediated by any of the various forms of hypersensitivity but most usually by type 2, 3 or 4. The self-autoreactivity occurs when the phenomenon of immunological tolerance breaks down.

Immunological Tolerance

Immunological tolerance is an active process that allows the immune system to maintain its protective role but avoid self-reactivating – during the generation of diversity of the immune repertoire T cell and B cell clones that detect self-antigens are actively eliminated. Tolerance occurs during the maturation of T cells in the thymus and B cells in the bone marrow. Self-reactive cells are eliminated by Fas-induced apoptosis, active T-cell-mediated suppression of self-directed immune responses, or T cell anergy, whereby antigen-stimulated T cells are inactive unless costimulation occurs simultaneously.

Tolerance may be bypassed by several mechanisms. Activation-induced cell death may be bypassed if Fas-induced apoptosis fails. This seems to increase with age as the efficiency of intrathymic elimination decreases. T-cell anergy is circumvented if tissue cells that normally do not express co-stimulatory molecules such as MHC class II are induced to do so. Thus, in the pancreas, induction of MHC class II molecules on the β cells of the islets triggers an immune response against self-antigens on these cells and the induction of both cell-mediated and antibody-mediated β-cell elimination and type 1 diabetes mellitus (Figure 2.15). Molecular mimicry occurs when a microbial antigen the patient encounters is sufficiently similar to a self-antigen so that crossreactivity with the self-antigen occurs. In rheumatic heart disease following throat infection with certain streptococcal strains the antibody formed to the bacterium crossreacts with an antigen present in the heart wall. The resulting antibody-mediated attack damages the myocardium and endocardium, leading to chronic valvular disease and potentially life-threatening long-term sequelae (see Chapter 6). In some circumstances, particularly exposure to Gram-negative endotoxin, there is a polyclonal and relatively non-specific activation of B cells. These B cells may be reactive against a number of different antigens including some self-antigens.

In the majority of clinically important autoimmune diseases it remains unclear how immune tolerance is bypassed.

Autoimmune Disease

Autoimmune diseases are common and may be either tissue specific or systemic (Table 2.6). They result from the breakdown of tolerance, generation of the autoimmune response and subsequent tissue damage. The autoimmune response may be humoral, cell mediated or more commonly due to both. Autoantibodies are mediators of injury but also useful in diagnostic assays. The tissue injury consequent to the autoimmune response may be mediated by any of the hypersensitivity reactions.

Tissue damage mediated by type 2 hypersensitivity in autoimmune disease is exemplified by autoimmune haemolytic anaemia. In this disease autoantibodies are formed against self-antigens on the surface of red blood cells. Autoantibody binds to these antigens leading to the local activation of complement. The red blood cells may then be either lysed by the lytic activity of complement or phagocytosed by mononuclear phagocytes in the spleen and liver, phagocytosis being enhanced by the presence of antibody and the C3b component of complement on the red cell surface. The red cells are destroyed and the patient presents with the signs and symptoms of anaemia and

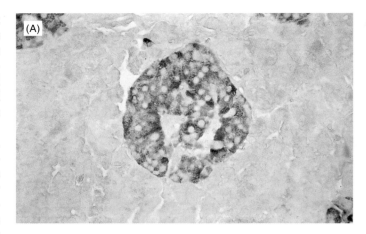

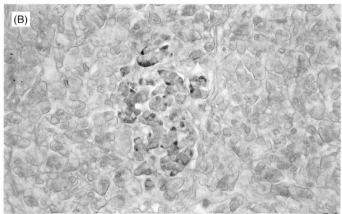

FIGURE 2.15 Double immunohistochemical staining of islets of Langerhans – insulin-producing cells brown, glucagon-producing cells blue. (A) is a normal islet and (B) from the pancreas of a patient with type 1 diabetes mellitus. There are virtually no surviving insulin-producing cells in (B).

TABLE 2.6 Autoimmune disease

Organ specific

Type 1 diabetes mellitus
Pernicious anaemia
Graves' disease
Hypothyroidism
Addison's disease
Autoimmune hepatitis

Multisystem disease

Rheumatoid disease
Systemic lupus erythematosus
Polyarteritis nodosa
Wegener's granulomatosis

usually with a spleen enlarged secondary to the increased phagocytic activity of its mononuclear cells.

In SLE the main mechanism of tissue injury is by a type 3 hypersensitivity mechanism. Soluble immune complexes, consisting of antibody directed against self nucleic acid and related antigen and double-stranded DNA, circulate in the

A 26-year-old woman presents with a short history of joint pain, a skin rash on her face and tiredness. On investigation she is also found to have urine abnormalities with both blood and protein excretion. Serological tests show that she has circulating antibodies to nuclear antigens including double-stranded DNA and a nucleic acid associated protein Rho. These features, especially the autoantibody profile, are diagnostic of systemic lupus erythematosus (SLE).

One of the most important prognostic features of SLE is the type, extent and activity of the renal involvement so a renal biopsy was done. Biopsy specimens from affected tissues may show a range of severity and acuteness, the assessment of which is an important part of the practice of histopathology of SLE. The biopsy specimens showed deposition of immune complexes in the wall of the glomerular capillaries (Figure 2.16A). The immune complexes contained IgG, IgM, IgA, and complement components. On light microscopy 80% of glomeruli were affected by an inflammatory process with infiltration by neutrophils and macrophages (Figure 2.16B). 30% of the glomeruli had crescents. This means that this woman's renal disease is of lupus nephritis type 4 with significant activity.

She started treatment with cyclophosphamide and steroids. Our understanding of the pathogenesis of SLE informs this therapy. Cyclophosphamide specifically targets the B lymphocytes that produce the autoantibody and the steroids suppress the activity of the effector neutrophils and macrophages. After 6 months of therapy the young woman is well with no blood and protein in her urine, her joint symptoms have improved and she does not have a skin rash.

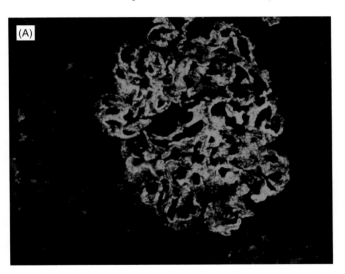

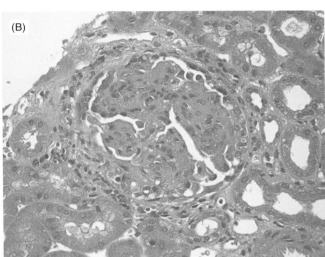

FIGURE 2.16 In the glomerulonephritis associated with systemic lupus erythematosus there is deposition of complement-activating immune complexes – IgG illustrated by immunofluoresence (A), with consequent infiltration by inflammatory cells (B).

blood and become deposited in the microcirculation of key tissues such as skin, joints and especially kidney. In these locations complement activation occurs, neutrophils and, in a chronic setting, macrophages infiltrate the tissues and elicit damage (see Case History 2.1 above).

Primary biliary cirrhosis is a chronic progressive disease of the liver with good evidence of an autoimmune aetiology. Although autoantibodies to mitochondria are present, the pattern of destruction of intrahepatic bile ducts is typical of a type 4 hypersensitivity. Autoreactive T lymphocytes directed against antigens on the epithelium of the bile duct trigger the activation of macrophages and formation of a granulomatous response. With the granulomas there is progressive destruction of bile ducts, obstruction to biliary secretion and fibrosis leading to cirrhosis and liver failure.

Attempts to suppress the autoimmune response and the inflammatory destruction of tissue form the basis of the medical management of these disorders. Understanding the type of autoimmune reaction and the type of hypersensitivity underlying the tissue injury is important in directing the rational treatment of autoimmune disease.

Immunodeficiency and Immunosuppression

Immunodeficiency may be primary or secondary, the primary immunodeficiencies being inherited abnormalities associated with a failure of development of components of the immune system, whereas secondary immunodeficiency occurs as a result of disease or its treatment.

Primary Immunodeficiency

These are rare often life-threatening diseases which nevertheless have contributed greatly to our understanding of the immune system. X-linked agammaglobulinaemia is the most common of these disorders and is caused by a failure of cell signalling and maturation of B cells with failure of the light chain gene rearrangement which normally allows the formation of immunoglobulin molecules. Circulating B cells are markedly reduced or absent, there is a failure to make antibody and once maternal antibody has declined the children become susceptible to recurrent episodes of bacterial infection.

Di George's syndrome occurs when there is failure of development of the thymus from the branchial arches, usually as a consequence of a deletion affecting chromosome 22q11, so there is no suitable microenvironment for the maturation of T cells. The patients are vulnerable to infection by viruses, fungi and parasites. There is also a marked propensity to infection by mycobacteria. Severe combined immune deficiency is the situation where both the T cell and B cell components of the immune system are defective. The affected individuals are susceptible to a whole range of microorganisms and frequently succumb to infection as infants. Several different genetic abnormalities have been demonstrated in these patients and different patterns of inheritance.

Secondary Immunodeficiency

Human immunodeficiency virus infection and acquired immune deficiency syndrome (AIDS) are a common worldwide cause of secondary immunodeficiency. The pathogenesis of this infection is dealt with in detail in Chapter 19. Briefly, HIV transmitted by blood or during sexual intercourse is capable of infecting the helper T cells of CD4 class. There is progressive and eventually profound loss of these helper T cells. This has detrimental effects on the capacity of the affected patients to mount an effective immune response. Helper T cells drive both cell-mediated and humoral responses. People with AIDS acquire a progressive susceptibility to a range of infections with various clinical consequences. They may develop intractable viral infections such as cytomegalovirus infections, but they are also often infected with tumour-promoting viruses – papilloma virus causing squamous carcinomas, Epstein–Barr virus (EBV) causing lymphomas and human herpes virus 8 causing Kaposi's sarcoma. They may develop overwhelming tuberculosis, which often lacks the formation of typical granulomas. They acquire protozoal infestation by organisms such as *Pneumocystis jirovecii* (*carinii*) or *Toxoplasma* species. Infective complications, including viral-induced malignancy, are the most common causes of death in the HIV/AIDS population.

Immunosuppression may result from specific therapy or may occur as a complication of therapy. To maintain the survival of transplanted organs, drugs and other therapies are administered to suppress the immune response. The main immunosuppressive drugs are designed to suppress specifically the afferent arm of the immune response, blocking the activation of immune cells reactive to the allogeneic

---

 2.1 SPECIAL STUDY TOPIC

PATHOGENESIS AND RATIONALE FOR THE MANAGEMENT OF POST-TRANSPLANT LYMPHOPROLIFERATIVE DISORDER

A 32-year-old man received a renal transplant for end-stage renal failure because of glomerulonephritis. He was immunosuppressed with tacrolimus and oral steroids. His clinical course was complicated by two acute rejection episodes. For these he was treated with high-dose steroids that on both occasions successfully suppressed the rejection. However, because of these episodes mycophenolate mofetil was added to his immunosuppression treatment in an attempt to prevent further rejection. Mycophenolate mofetil suppresses the proliferation of both B and T lymphocytes by the reversible inhibition of inosine monophosphate dehydrogenase, a key enzyme in the *de novo* synthetic pathway of guanine (Sievens *et al.* 1997).

Several months later the patient presented with enlarged lymph nodes in his groin. A biopsy was done on one of these. It showed a florid lymphoproliferative disorder, which was demonstrated to be of B-lymphocyte origin, to be monoclonal and the cells expressed Epstein–Barr virus (EBV) antigen. A diagnosis of post-transplant lymphoproliferative disorder (PTLD) in the monoclonal phase was made. This is an EBV-driven proliferation of B cells which progresses to a type of lymphoma (see Chapter 8). EBV survived in the infected B cells because the T cells that clear the body of the virus in a healthy individual were being suppressed by his transplant immunosuppression drugs.

Although PTLD is regarded as a neoplasm, chemotherapy is not usually the first choice of treatment as this would further immunosuppress the patient; instead the patient's transplant immunosuppression drug doses should be reduced. This was done with close monitoring of the lymph nodes, peripheral blood cells and transplant function. After 6 months he had no rejection episodes, his lymphadenopathy had regressed and his peripheral blood was free of EBV positive B cells. This is an instance of a viral-induced tumour in the context of immunosuppression being treated by allowing the host defence to clear the relevant virus.

Reference

Sievens TM, Rossie SJ, Ghobrial RM, *et al*. Mycophenolate mofetil. *Pharmacotherapy* 1997; **17**: 1178–1197.

MHC and other antigens present on the cells of the transplanted organ. Such drugs include tacrolimus, mycophenolate mofetil and azathioprine. However, if this suppression is overcome and the patient experiences an episode of transplant rejection the strategy shifts to one targeted at suppressing the effector arm of the response. In these clinical circumstances high-dose corticosteroids are used and if these are not wholly effective humanized monoclonal antibody may be used to deplete immunocompetent cells.

Comparable but undesirable immunosuppression may occur in patients receiving chemotherapy for malignancy or anti-inflammatory therapy for autoimmune or other chronic inflammatory disease. In these circumstances the immunosuppression is less specific, may affect the afferent or effector arms of the immune response and the outcomes are much less predictable.

Both groups of patients are susceptible to infection. The specific suppression of the afferent T cell response in transplantation renders these patients particularly susceptible to viral disease. Cytomegalovirus infection, by reactivation or *de novo* infection, is a well recognized and difficult problem in patients who have recevied transplants. Such patients are also at risk for two types of viral-induced malignancy. Those who have experienced several rounds of antirejection therapy have an especially high risk of developing EBV-induced B-cell proliferation and lymphoma called post-transplant lymphoproliferative disorder (PTLD). Patients with transplants also commonly develop multiple papilloma-virus-induced squamous cell carcinomas of the skin and genital tract. Chemotherapy patients have a tendency to more bacterial infection although may also experience viral infection. The risk of bacterial infection is particularly associated with bone marrow suppression and a fall in white blood cell count.

SUMMARY

- Understanding normal cellular structure and function is key to understanding disease.
- Stem cells form a small but fundamental subpopulation of the total cell mass.
- Morphogenesis occurs under tight genetic control which may be disrupted.
- The balance between cell proliferation (regulated through the cell cycle) and cell death (through apoptosis) is crucial for normal development and survival and is perturbed in many diseases.
- The main non-neoplastic disorders of growth are hypertrophy, hyperplasia, atrophy and metaplasia.
- Ageing is a complex process, aspects of which are still incompletely understood.
- The immune system has innate and adaptive components, the latter having humoral and cell mediated components.
- There are four classes of hypersensitivity reactions.
- Autoimmune disease occurs when immunological tolerance breaks down and is either tissue specific or systemic.
- Immunodeficiency may be primary (inherited) or secondary to disease (e.g. HIV infection) or its treatment (e.g. immunosuppression for organ transplantation).

FURTHER READING

Delves PJ, Martin SJ, Burton DR, Roitt IM. *Roitt's Essential Immunology*, 11th edn. Oxford: Blackwell Publishing, 2006.

Kumar V, Abbas AK, Fausto N. *Robbins and Cotran's Pathologic Basis of Disease*, 7th edn. Philadelphia: Elsevier Saunders, 2004.

Martin J, Sheaff M. The pathology of ageing. *J Pathol* 2007; **211**: 111–113.

Nairn R. *Immunology for Medical Students*. Edinburgh: Mosby, 2004.

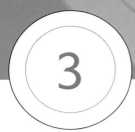

Jonathan N Berg and Sarju Mehta

INTRODUCTION

Clinical genetics is a branch of medicine concerned with the diagnosis, testing and management of diseases caused by changes in the human genome. Clinical geneticists must not only understand the molecular basis of genetic disease, but also identify clinical situations in which genetic testing is appropriate. A clinical geneticist must then communicate genetic information to family members so that they can understand the implications and make informed choices about gene testing and clinical management. Increasingly, clinical geneticists are also involved in identifying the best treatment for patients with rare genetic disorders, and in the testing for genetic predisposition to common disease.

Research in clinical genetics has led to the identification of the causative genes for many conditions, and has directed further research into the mechanisms of disease and understanding why certain genes and the proteins that they encode are important in a range of disease processes. Understanding the mechanisms of disease is an initial step in trying to identify new and specific treatments for disease. The practice of diagnostic pathology is intricately linked to the practice of clinical genetics. For example:

- A pathologist may be the first clinician to make a finding that suggests a genetic disorder running in a family, for example discovering at autopsy that a bowel cancer in a young man was caused by familial adenomatous polyposis (see Chapter 9). In such a case it would be important to arrange, referral of the affected individual to genetic services for gene testing and identification of other family members at risk. If this was a post-morten

finding it would be important to store a DNA sample, with appropriate consent.
- Pathology findings may be important in confirming a genetic diagnosis in an individual or a relative, such as Alport's syndrome on a renal biopsy (see Chapter 13).
- Pathology may be important in helping to establish a diagnosis, for example describing abnormal findings in a fetal post mortem that indicate a specific syndromic diagnosis.

BASIC STRUCTURE OF DNA

The DNA molecule consists of a sugar (deoxyribose) and phosphate backbone, with bases covalently bonded to each deoxyribose molecule. The base can be either adenine (A), cytosine (C), guanine (G) or thymine (T). The DNA double helix is formed by two strands running in opposite directions, held together by hydrogen bonds between the bases. Adenine always pairs with thymine, and guanine always pairs with cytosine. The basic structure of DNA is shown in Figure 3.1.

CHROMOSOMES

Chromosomes are the basic packages of DNA in the nucleus of a cell. In humans who have a diploid set (denoted 2n) of chromosomes, there are 22 pairs of chromosomes in every cell, called the autosomes, and two sex chromosomes. Females have two homologous sex chromosomes, the X chromosomes, denoted XX, and males have one X and one Y chromosome. Each chromosome has a long arm, designated the q arm, and a short arm, designated the p arm. At the ends of each chromosome are the telomeres. Chromosomes consist of a DNA strand that is wound

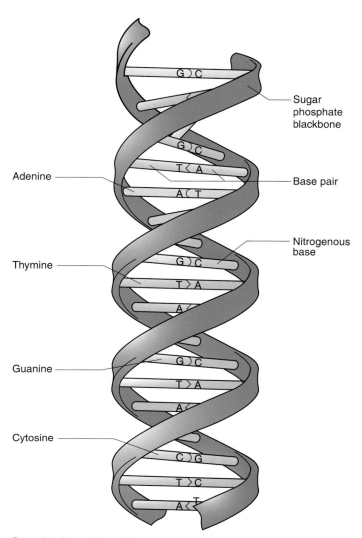

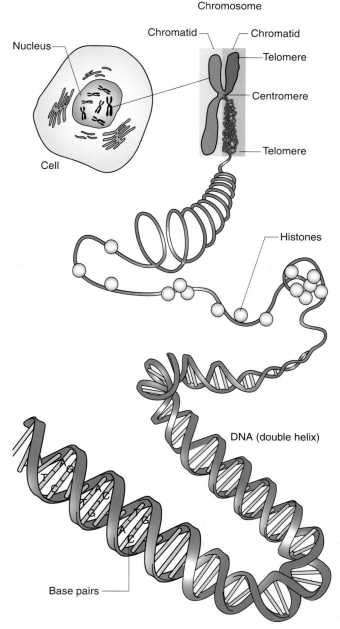

FIGURE 3.1 Deoxyribonucleic acid (DNA). (Redrawn with permission from the National Human Genome Research Institute, Division of Intramural Research.)

FIGURE 3.2 Structure of the chromosome. (Redrawn with permission from the National Human Genome Research Institute, Division of Intramural Research.)

around histones and packaged with other proteins into a compact structure (Figure 3.2). Figure 3.3 shows the chromosomes of a normal male, as seen during metaphase in mitosis.

CELL DIVISION

The cell cycle is discussed in Chapter 2. Although cell division takes place in the M phase (mitosis), DNA replication occurs during S phase. A number of checkpoints exist during the cell cycle to allow for repair of DNA damage and replication errors that have occurred in the S phase, and if repair of the DNA is not possible, for the cell to enter apoptosis.

Mitosis

In mitosis, the cell divides to produce two identical daughter cells. Both parent and daughter cells are diploid. The phases of mitosis are named interphase, prophase, prometaphase, metaphase, anaphase and telophase (Figure 3.4).

Meiosis

During meiosis, one diploid parent cell gives rise to four haploid daughter cells. In humans, it only occurs during gamete formation. It takes place in two stages, meiosis I and meiosis II (see Figure 3.5). One of the key features of meiosis is the formation of chiasmata between homologous chromosomes during meiosis I. This allows the exchange of

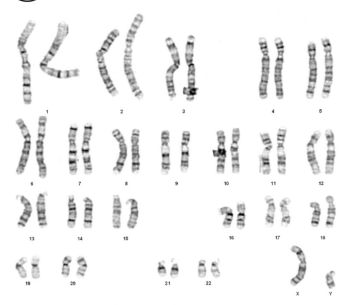

FIGURE 3.3 Normal male karyotype.

material or recombination between homologous chromosomes. Such recombination ensures that, although one of each chromosome is passed into the gamete, the chromosome is a mixture of parts of both parental chromosomes.

MOSAICISM

In theory, the usual state is that every somatic cell in an individual has the same genetic constitution. Mosaicism is the situation when there are two or more populations of cells with different genetic constitutions within the same individual. This arises during somatic cell division, at mitosis, after formation of the zygote. A mutation arises in one cell lineage. This mutation can be of any size from the change of a single base in a gene to a chromosomal aneuploidy in one cell lineage.

Sometimes this can be shown on analysis of DNA or chromosomes from blood, but detection of mosaicism may require analysis of another tissue. The other cell lineage most amenable to analysis are fibroblasts obtained from a

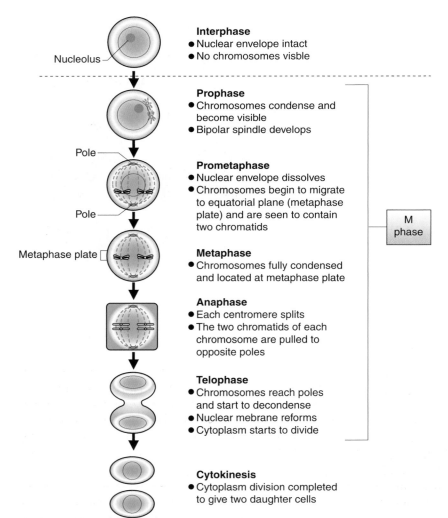

Interphase
- Nuclear envelope intact
- No chromosomes visble

Nucleolus

Prophase
- Chromosomes condense and become visible
- Bipolar spindle develops

Pole

Prometaphase
- Nuclear envelope dissolves
- Chromosomes begin to migrate to equatorial plane (metaphase plate) and are seen to contain two chromatids

Pole

Metaphase plate

Metaphase
- Chromosomes fully condensed and located at metaphase plate

Anaphase
- Each centromere splits
- The two chromatids of each chromosome are pulled to opposite poles

Telophase
- Chromosomes reach poles and start to decondense
- Nuclear mebrane reforms
- Cytoplasm starts to divide

M phase

Cytokinesis
- Cytoplasm division completed to give two daughter cells

FIGURE 3.4 Mitosis. (Redrawn with permission. This information was provided by Clinical Tools, Inc., and is copyrighted by Clinical Tools, Inc.).

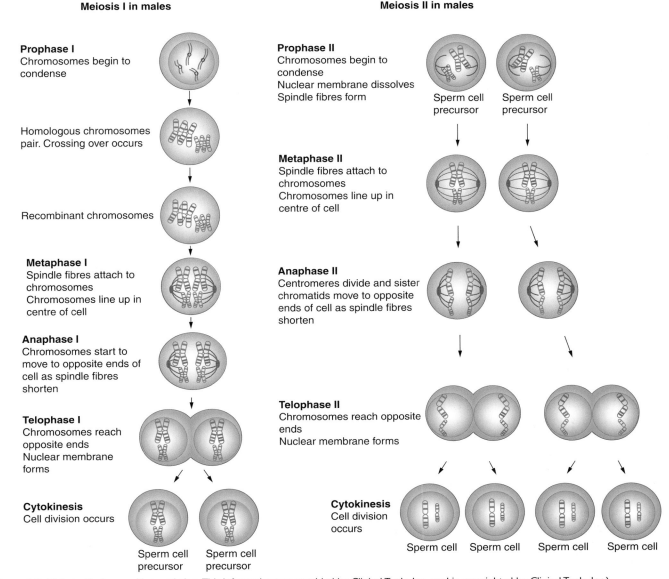

Meiosis I in males

Prophase I
Chromosomes begin to condense

Homologous chromosomes pair. Crossing over occurs

Recombinant chromosomes

Metaphase I
Spindle fibres attach to chromosomes
Chromosomes line up in centre of cell

Anaphase I
Chromosomes start to move to opposite ends of cell as spindle fibres shorten

Telophase I
Chromosomes reach opposite ends
Nuclear membrane forms

Cytokinesis
Cell division occurs

Sperm cell precursor   Sperm cell precursor

Meiosis II in males

Prophase II
Chromosomes begin to condense
Nuclear membrane dissolves
Spindle fibres form

Sperm cell precursor   Sperm cell precursor

Metaphase II
Spindle fibres attach to chromosomes
Chromosomes line up in centre of cell

Anaphase II
Centromeres divide and sister chromatids move to opposite ends of cell as spindle fibres shorten

Telophase II
Chromosomes reach opposite ends
Nuclear membrane forms

Cytokinesis
Cell division occurs

Sperm cell   Sperm cell   Sperm cell   Sperm cell

FIGURE 3.5 Meiosis. (Redrawn with permission. This information was provided by Clinical Tools, Inc., and is copyrighted by Clinical Tools, Inc.).

skin biopsy. It is also possible to analyse cells obtained from a buccal scrape, urinary sediment, or hair roots. The clinical effects of mosaicism are determined not only by genetic alteration but also by the tissue involved and the proportion of cells affected.

In germline mosaicism, a proportion of the gametes in an individual have the same mutation, even though other cells in the individual may not. A gamete which has the mutation will produce a child with an inherited disease. In this scenario, even if neither parent has the mutation in their blood or other tissues, there is a risk of having another child with the same mutation and therefore disease.

GENETIC CHANGES THAT CAUSE DISEASE

The genetic changes that cause human disease can vary in size from a whole additional or missing chromosome to a change of a single base in a gene sequence. The techniques required to detect such changes depend on the size of change being sought (Figure 3.6).

Chromosomal Aneuploidy

Chromosomal aneuploidy refers to the presence of an entire extra chromosome (trisomy) or absence of a whole

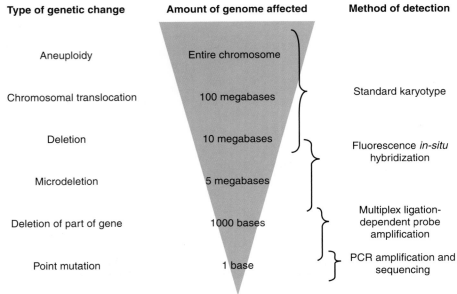

Type of genetic change	Amount of genome affected	Method of detection
Aneuploidy	Entire chromosome	
Chromosomal translocation	100 megabases	Standard karyotype
Deletion	10 megabases	Fluorescence in-situ hybridization
Microdeletion	5 megabases	
Deletion of part of gene	1000 bases	Multiplex ligation-dependent probe amplification
Point mutation	1 base	PCR amplification and sequencing

FIGURE 3.6 Types of gene change and methods for their detection. PCR = polymerase chain reaction.

chromosome (monosomy), usually arising as a consequence of non-disjunction during meiosis. The majority of conceptions with aneuploidy will miscarry, and only some chromosomal aneuploidies are viable. The commonest autosomal aneuploidy is trisomy 21 (Down syndrome). Infants with trisomy 18 (Edward syndrome) and trisomy 13 (Patau syndrome) can also survive to term. Aneuploidies involving the sex chromosomes are better tolerated by the fetus, and usually show a milder phenotype because of X chromosome inactivation. The most commonly detected sex chromosomal aneuploidies are Turner syndrome – in which a female has one X chromosome (45,X) and Klinefelter syndrome – in which a male has two X chromosomes and one Y chromosome (47,XXY). The 47,XXX and 47,XYY karyotypes are commonly detected as incidental findings on chromosome analysis. Affected individuals with 47,XXX and 47,XYY karyotypes usually show no obvious phenotypic features, although they may have subtle abnormalities of neurodevelopment.

Chromosome Translocations

Translocations are exchanges of chromosomal material between two or more chromosomes. If there is no significant loss or gain of chromosomal material it is described as a balanced translocation. If there is a significant gain or loss of chromosomal material, the translocation is described as unbalanced. A fetus with an unbalanced chromosome complement will often miscarry, sometimes before a pregnancy is recognized. If the pregnancy continues to term, the phenotypic effects of the imbalance involving the autosomes vary widely, but will usually include developmental delay, which may be severe, and may also include renal, gastrointestinal and cardiac malformations with facial dysmorphism.

The likelihood of chromosomal imbalance leading to miscarriage is determined by the size of the imbalance. A small imbalance is more likely to proceed to term, but the liveborn child would still be expected to have significant phenotypic abnormalities and developmental delay.

Robertsonian Translocations

In a Robertsonian translocation, the long arms of two acrocentric chromosomes become joined together, with loss of the short arms. The short arms of acrocentric chromosomes contain highly repetitive DNA sequences and ribosomal RNA genes, so the loss of this material does not cause any clinical phenotype. A (14;21) translocation and its inheritance is illustrated in Figure 3.7. An individual with a balanced Robertsonian translocation will usually be asymptomatic, but may have infertility (especially males), recurrent miscarriages (whether the translocation is carried by the mother or father) or a child affected with a chromosomal aneuploidy. If a parent carries a Robertsonian translocation involving chromosome 21, such as the (14;21) translocation shown in Figure 3.7, the risk of a child being affected with Down syndrome is increased (10–15% if the mother carries the balanced translocation, <1% if it is carried by the father).

Reciprocal Translocations

In a reciprocal translocation, there is exchange of material between two, usually non-homologous chromosomes. Again, in the balanced form, there is usually no phenotypic effect, although, rarely, the translocation may disrupt an important gene and cause a genetic disease. A person with a balanced reciprocal translocation may present with infertility, multiple miscarriages or have a child with multiple malformations and an unbalanced translocation. Figure 3.8 shows an example of an (8;9) reciprocal translocation.

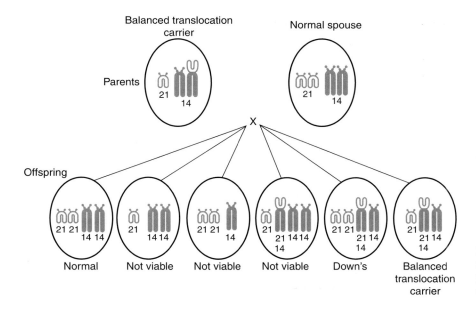

FIGURE 3.7 Possibilities for offspring in families with translocation Down syndrome. (Reproduced with permission from Harper PS. *Practical Genetic Counselling*, 6th edn. London: Hodder Arnold, 2005.)

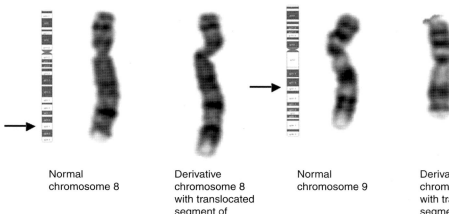

Normal chromosome 8

Derivative chromosome 8 with translocated segment of chromosome 9

Normal chromosome 9

Derivative chromosome 9 with translocated segment of chromosome 8

FIGURE 3.8 Chromosomes 8 and 9 from an individual with a reciprocal 8;9 translocation: 46,XX,t(8;9)(q24.1;q22.1).

Somatic Chromosomal Rearrangements

Chromosomal aneuploidies and chromosomal rearrangements may arise during mitosis. Normally, there are many checkpoints in the cell cycle at which chromosomal imbalance is identified, leading either to repair of the cell or apoptosis. However, loss of these checkpoints and subsequent accumulation of chromosomal abnormalities is one mechanism by which cells can start to transform into malignancy. Rarely, a somatic translocation may occur that activates an oncogene, a classical example of this is the Philadelphia chromosome.

 3.1 SPECIAL STUDY TOPIC

THE PHILADELPHIA CHROMOSOME

The Philadelphia chromosome results from a translocation between chromosomes 9 and 22. This was the first chromosome abnormality to be found in a tumour, after identification of an abnormally small chromosome, named the Philadelphia chromosome (Figure 3.9). The translocation occurs in a bone marrow cell, and then through clonal expansion leads to the uncontrolled production of mainly the granulocytic cell lineage, leading to leukaemia. This leads to the chronic phase of the disease, and additional genetic and epigenetic factors are required to transform chronic myeloid leukaemia (CML) from chronic to blast phase. The translocation leads to a fusion of the *ABL* gene, a proto-oncogene on chromosome 9 which encodes a tyrosine kinase enzyme, with the *BCR* gene on chromosome 22, denoted as t(9;22)(q34;q11). This fused gene encodes a protein with unregulated tyrosine kinase activity that ultimately leads to the leukaemia.

SPECIAL STUDY TOPIC CONTINUED . . .

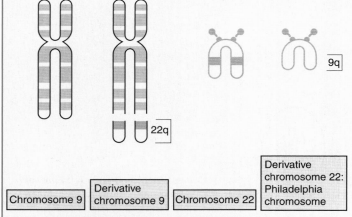

FIGURE 3.9 The Philadelphia chromosome results from a reciprocal translocation between chromosome 22 and chromosome 9, leading to fusion of the *ABL* oncogene with the *BCR* gene, activating *ABL* and contributing to malignant transformation. The other derivative chromosome is not important in the disease pathogenesis. (With permission from Haematological Malignancy Diagnostic Service, 'Molecular Diagnostics in Haematological Malignancies: Polymerase Chain Reaction (PCR)', www.hmds.org.uk.)

This discovery led to the development of imatinib mesylate (Gleevec), a specific tyrosine kinase inhibitor. In 80% of newly diagnosed cases of CML, imatinib induces the bone marrow to be totally free of the Philadelphia chromosome. Therefore the Philadelphia chromosome is a diagnostic marker and prognostic indicator for CML. The Philadelphia chromosome is also found in acute lymphoblastic leukaemia.

Further Reading

Ren R. Mechanisms of BCR-ABL in the pathogenesis of chronic myelogenous leukaemia. *Nat Rev Cancer* 2005; **5**: 172–183.

Chromosomal Deletions and Microdeletions

Deletion of a segment of a chromosome is likely to be visible microscopically if it is greater than approximately 5 megabases. A microdeletion can only be detected by more specialized techniques, such as fluorescence *in-situ* hybridization or microarray comparative genomic hybridization (CGH) described below.

Fluorescence In-situ Hybridization

The technique used to look rapidly for microdeletions and subtelomere deletions and also for gross alterations in chromosomal number is called FISH. In this technique a fluorescent dye is attached to a probe DNA that attaches to the chromosomal region of interest. The probe DNA can be designed to be specific to any particular genetic sequence. If that region is present, the dye fluoresces, which can be visualized microscopically, and if the region is absent, then no light is emitted. This technique is illustrated in Figure 3.10. An example of the use of this technique is shown in Figure 3.11.

As FISH just detects loss or gain of a specific small chromosomal region, it can only be used where clinical parameters have defined which chromosomal region should be analysed.

Microarray Comparative Genomic Hybridization

Microarray CGH is a technique that allows analysis of the entire genome for small losses or gains. It can be used to look at constitutional chromosome abnormalities or chromosomal abnormalities that have arisen in tumours. Although it is possible to look for deletions or gains of chromosomal material of smaller than 100 000 base pairs in size, there are many potential difficulties. It is becoming increasingly

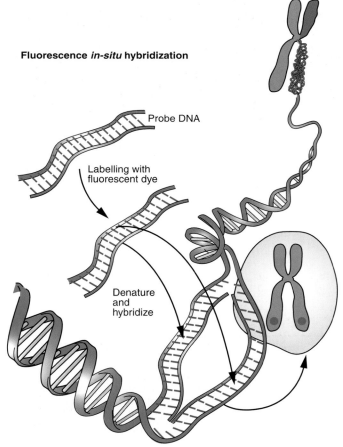

Fluorescence *in-situ* hybridization

Probe DNA

Labelling with fluorescent dye

Denature and hybridize

FIGURE 3.10 Fluorescence *in-situ* hybridization allows detection of the presence of specific genes. The principle of the technique is illustrated.

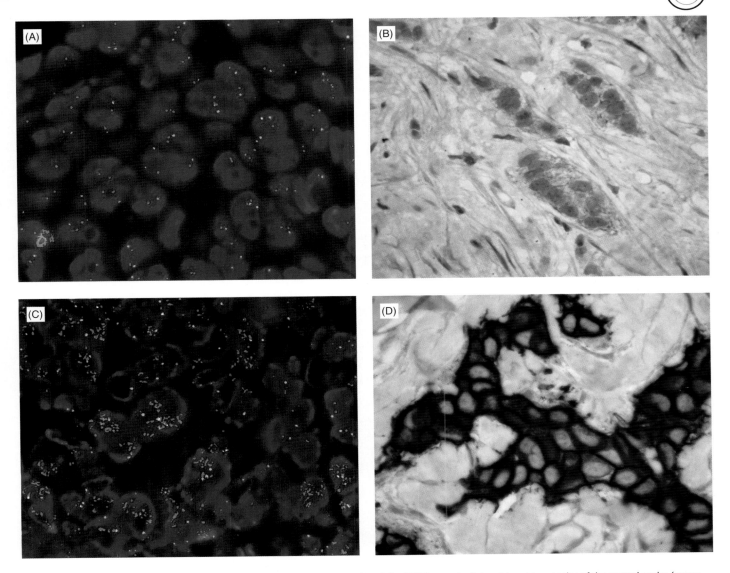

FIGURE 3.11 (A) FISH with a probe to the *HER2* gene shows the usual two copies of the *HER2* gene (red signals) and two copies of the control probe (green signal) in each cell. (B) Immunohistochemistry on this tumour with a normal *HER2* gene complement shows little expression of the epidermal growth factor receptor, which is encoded by the *HER2* gene. (C) FISH shows many copies of the *HER2* gene in each cell. (D) Immunohistochemistry on this tumour shows over-expression of the epidermal growth factor receptor, localized to the cell surface. Tumours showing overexpression of *HER2* show an improved prognosis following treatment with Trasumatab (Herceptin ™). (Images provided by Dr Lee Jordan, Department of Pathology, Ninewells Hospital and Medical School.)

recognized that there are copy number variations in the human genome that are not themselves disease causing.

SINGLE GENE (MENDELIAN) INHERITANCE

Single gene disorders are caused by mutations in a single gene. The inheritance of single gene disorders is determined by Mendel's laws of segregation and independent assortment. An autosomal gene is one that is carried on one of the autosomes (chromosomes 1 to 22, found in pairs in each cell), and an X-linked gene is one that is found on the X chromosome.

Alleles are the specific versions of a gene in an individual. For an autosomal gene, an individual will have two copies of that gene or two alleles. If one copy has a mutation, it is described as the mutant allele. The genotype is the genetic makeup of an individual. The phenotype is the effect of the genetic constitution. To visualize the inheritance of single-gene disorders in a family, it is often necessary to draw a family tree or pedigree (Figure 3.12).

Autosomal Dominant Inheritance

Autosomal dominant inheritance (Figure 3.13A) is a pattern of inheritance where an affected individual possesses one copy of a mutant allele and one copy of a normal allele. Individuals who have a disease which is autosomal dominant, have a 1 in 2 or 50% chance of passing the mutation to all their offspring. It should be remembered that many

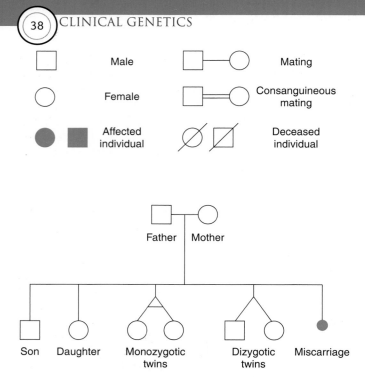

Male

Female

Affected individual

Mating

Consanguineous mating

Deceased individual

Father | Mother

Son | Daughter | Monozygotic twins | Dizygotic twins | Miscarriage

FIGURE 3.12 Drawing a family tree. A pedigree is drawn using standard symbols.

conditions that are autosomal dominant start with a new mutation in the person themselves and so their parents may be unaffected. In this case, the risk of recurrence for the parents is related to the germline mosaicism risk. Germline mosaicism accounts for the fact that if an individual has a child with a genetic disease yet they themselves do not carry the causative mutation, there is a risk that they bear a group of mutant germline cells (eggs or sperm) that could go on to produce another child with the same condition.

Autosomal Recessive Inheritance

In autosomal recessive inheritance (Figure 3.13B) both copies of the gene must harbour mutations for the disease to arise. This usually occurs when both parents are carriers, with one normal and one mutated copy of the gene, and they have each passed on their gene fault to a child. The risk of having a child with an autosomal recessive disease if both parents are carriers is 1 in 4 or 25%.

X-linked Disorders

X-linked disorders (Figure 3.13C) are caused by mutations in genes on the X chromosome. Females have two X chromosomes, and males have one X and one Y chromosome. In a female, to maintain chromosomal balance, one X chromosome becomes inactive in each cell. Usually, it is a random event which chromosome is inactivated (Figure 3.14A).

The Y chromosome contains few genes and has very little homology to the X chromosome. A male, therefore, has only a single copy of the majority of the genes on the X chromosome. In an X-linked recessive condition, a female with a mutation in a gene on the X chromosome shows few

(A)

Gene with mutation

Normal gene

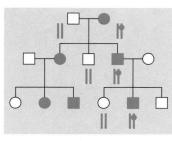

Autosomal dominant inheritance

- One faulty copy of gene is sufficient to cause disease
- Disease phenotype is seen in all generations
- Disease severity may be variable
- Males and females are equally likely to be affected
- If neither parent is affected, there may be a new mutation

(B)

Autosomal recessive inheritance

- Both copies of the gene are mutated to cause the disease
- Often only individuals in one generation are affected
- 1 in 4 risk of an affected child if both parents are carriers
- Higher incidence of recessive disorders in consanguineous families

(C)

X chromosome with mutation

Normal X chromosome

Y chromosome

Female carrier

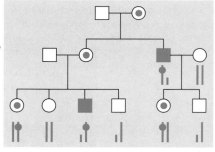

X-linked recessive inheritance

- The mutated gene lies on the X chromosome
- A female carrier:
    is unlikely to show significant features of disease
    half her male children will be affected
    half her female children will be carriers
- An affected male:
    all his male children will be unaffected
    all his daughters will be carriers of the condition

FIGURE 3.13 The three most common patterns of single gene inheritance for human disease. (A) Autosomal dominant inheritance; (B) autosomal recessive inheritance; and (C) X-linked recessive inheritance.

(A) Normal female

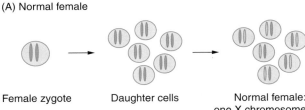

Female zygote   Daughter cells   Normal female:
one X chromosome has
inactivated in each cell

(B) Female carrier of mutation on X chromosome

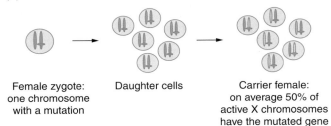

Female zygote: Daughter cells   Carrier female:
one chromosome   on average 50% of
with a mutation   active X chromosomes
have the mutated gene

FIGURE 3.14 X-inactivation. (A) Normal female. (B) Female carrier of mutation on X chromosome.

or no phenotypic effects, as she has a second functioning copy. A male with the same mutation will be affected as he has no functioning copy. Haemophilia A (see Chapter 8) is an example of such a condition. In an X-linked dominant condition, a female with a single faulty copy of the gene on the X-chromosome will show features of the disease. The effect of the same mutation on a male depends on the gene: in some cases, such as incontinentia pigmenti, the effect may be to make the male fetus non-viable, in other cases the phenotype in a male may be similar to that seen in a female, such as in X-linked rickets.

Females who carry an X-linked recessive disorder may display signs and symptoms of an X-linked disorder. This is most commonly because, due to X-inactivation, 50% of the nuclei in their cells contain the active X chromosome with the mutated gene (Figure 3.14B). For example, female carriers of haemophilia A, with mutations in the factor VIII gene may show mild coagulation disorders. Much less often, a female may show a phenotype of similar severity to an affected male. This arises because the mutated X chromosome is active in most or all of their cells. This may be either through non-random inactivation called skewed X-inactivation, or if they only have a single copy of the X chromosome that carries the mutation, as in a patient with Turner's syndrome (45,XO).

NON-MENDELIAN INHERITANCE

Mitochondrial Inheritance

The mitochondria are exclusively maternally inherited. Each mitochondrion has a genome of approximately 16.5 kb

in size. Therefore although a disease inherited through the mitochondrial genome can affect either sex, it can only be passed on by affected mothers. The mutation may be homoplasmic, affecting all mitochondria in a cell, or heteroplasmic, only affecting a proportion. Where there is heteroplasmy, the phenotypic effects can vary depending on what proportion of mitochondria have the mutation in each cell, and in which tissues.

Imprinting

Imprinted genes are ones that are differentially expressed depending on whether they are maternally or paternally inherited. Only certain genes in certain chromosomal regions are imprinted. For example, only the maternally inherited copy of the *UBE3A* gene on chromosome 15 is active. If a child does not inherit a functioning copy from their mother then they will be affected with Angelman's syndrome. The gene could be inactivated by a point mutation or deletion, or an unusual transmission of chromosomes may occur, so that the child inherits two chromosomes 15 from its father but no chromosome 15 from its mother (paternal uniparental disomy).

STRUCTURE OF A GENE AND HOW IT ENCODES A PROTEIN

Genes consist of a number of different components, shown in Figure 3.15. Upstream of the gene there are regulatory elements which may increase or decrease gene expression (enhancers and silencers). The promotor is the binding site for proteins that initiate transcription. Downstream from the promotor, a gene consists of many exons, which contain the DNA sequence that encodes the protein, and introns which do not. The production of protein from a gene requires the processes of transcription, splicing and translation (Figure 3.15).

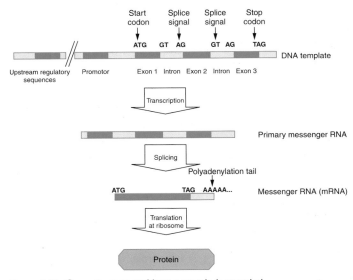

FIGURE 3.15 Gene structure and how a protein is encoded.

Transcription

A transcription factor binds to the promotor and a single RNA strand is synthesized using the DNA sequence as a template. RNA has a similar structure to DNA, with the minor differences that the sugar phosphate backbone contains ribose rather than deoxyribose and the base uracil (U) is substituted for the base thymine (T). In RNA, therefore, uracil pairs with adenine (A).

Splicing

The primary messenger RNA (mRNA) that is synthesized undergoes splicing to remove the intronic sequences, creating a mature mRNA. There are specific splicing recognition sequences, each intron starts with a GT sequence and ends with an AG sequence.

Translation

The mRNA is moved to the ribosome in the cytoplasm, where it is translated into a polypeptide. Every three bases (or codon) of the mRNA molecule encode an amino acid or a stop. Transfer RNAs transport the amino acids to the assembling peptide. The translation starts at a start codon, which is always AUG encoding methionine, and stops when a UAA, UAG or UGA is reached. The polypeptide then undergoes post-translational modification and is transported to its place of function as a mature protein.

The amount of a polypeptide produced is determined by many factors, including the rate of transcription and splicing of the mRNA, the stability of the mRNA, and the stability of the protein produced.

HOW MUTATIONS AFFECT GENE FUNCTION

Any change in DNA sequence that affects the processes of transcription, splicing or translation will affect the production of protein. A disease causing mutation may be a deletion of the entire gene, deletion of a part of the gene, or a change of a single base. When considering the effect of a mutation, it is important to work out how it will affect the processes of transcription, splicing, translation and post-translational modification of a protein (Table 3.1).

Loss of Function Mutations

The mutation abolishes production of protein. This can either be a deletion of the whole gene, or a smaller mutation in a gene that critically affects its ability to be transcribed or translated. Loss of function mutations would be expected to lead to complete loss of production of a protein in autosomal recessive and X-linked diseases.

TABLE 3.1 Types of mutations and their effects on protein function

Mutation	Possible effects on		
	mRNA	Protein production	Protein function
Deletion of whole gene	Loss of transcription	No protein produced	–
Deletion of promotor	Loss of transcription	No protein produced	–
Deletion of three base pairs from exon	Loss of one codon from mRNA	Loss of one amino acid from polypeptide sequence	May have no effect or severe effect depending on importance of amino acid deleted
Deletion of one or two base pairs	Loss of one or two base pairs from mRNA sequence. mRNA may be unstable	Frameshift at translation, leading to highly abnormal protein production after deletion	Likely to have severe effect or create unstable protein that is degraded
Single base change altering a splice signal	Abnormal splicing, creating highly abnormal mRNA. mRNA may be unstable	Production of an abnormal polypeptide	Likely to have severe effect or create unstable protein that is degraded
Single base change in an exon creating a premature stop codon	mRNA sequence includes a premature stop sequence. mRNA may be unstable	Production of polypeptide terminates early	Likely to have severe effect or create unstable protein that is degraded
Single base change in an exon altering amino acid sequence	mRNA produced incorporating mutant sequence	Production of a polypeptide containing an incorrect amino acid	May have no effect, may cause protein to be inactive or may activate protein

In autosomal dominant diseases, loss of function of one allele may reduce but it will not abolish protein production. In this case there are two possible mechanisms by which it may cause disease:

- Haploinsufficiency – the level of a protein is important, either in absolute terms or in relation to another protein. Loss of a single copy of the gene reduces the amount of protein produced sufficiently to cause a disease phenotype. This mechanism is more likely to be the case for signalling molecules where the exact level of a protein may be critical for normal cell function. Haploinsufficiency is also the mechanism whereby mutations in one of the collagen genes, COL1A1 or COL1A2, cause the milder form of osteogenesis imperfecta, osteogenesis imperfecta type 1. Loss of one copy of the collagen gene leads to reduced collagen levels in bone and a tendency to fractures in childhood.
- Loss of function of the second copy of the gene during somatic cell division, leading to a cell that has no functioning copy of the gene – this is a common mechanism in inherited cancer syndromes, such as in hereditary non-polyposis colorectal cancer (HNPCC) described in Case History 3.1.

Dominant Negative Mutations

A dominant negative mutation is one in which a mutation leads to creation of an abnormal protein that has an effect on the function of the normal version of the protein that is produced. An example of this is a point mutation in one of the collagen genes COL1A1 or COL1A2 that leads to production of an abnormal collagen protein. This abnormal protein is incorporated in the collagen fibril and disrupts formation of normal collagen in bone, leading to a severe deficiency of collagen. This severe collagen deficiency causes a severe form of osteogenesis imperfecta (osteogenesis imperfecta type II) that is usually lethal shortly after birth.

Gain-of-function Mutations

Rarely, a point mutation may alter the sequence of a gene, and subsequently the protein made, so as to activate the protein. This can occur in the germline, an example being mutations in the FGFR3 gene causing achondroplasia. Gain-of-function mutations may also arise somatically, and are commonly observed in the progression of cells to neoplasia.

CASE HISTORY 3.1

HEREDITARY NON-POLYPOSIS COLORECTAL CANCER

A 35-year-old man presented with a 4-week history of rectal bleeding. Clinical examination was entirely normal, but a colonoscopy identified a cancer of the transverse colon, which was removed surgically (Figure 3.16). Pathological examination of the resected colon showed a single 3-cm tumour with no polyps.

A family history was taken (Figure 3.17). The patient has a brother and a sister who are both in good health. His father died of bowel cancer at the age of 55, and his father's sister was affected with bowel cancer at the age of 48, but is still alive. The young age of onset of bowel cancer in the patient, and the number of affected relatives in the family is highly suggestive of a hereditary form of bowel cancer. The most common forms of hereditary bowel cancer are familial adenomatous polyposis (FAP) and hereditary non-polyposis colorectal cancer (HNPCC). The absence of polyps elsewhere in the bowel makes FAP unlikely. With three affected individuals, all of whom are first-degree relatives of each other, and at least one of whom is under 50, this family fulfils the modified Amsterdam criteria, and may, therefore have HNPCC.

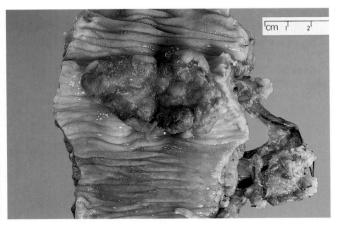

FIGURE 3.16 A plaque-like carcinoma in Transverse colon. (Image provided by Professor Jeremy Jass.)

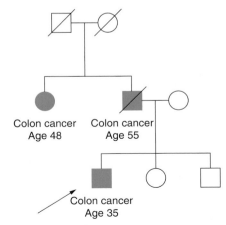

Colon cancer
Age 48

Colon cancer
Age 55

Colon cancer
Age 35

FIGURE 3.17 Family tree of the patient.

HNPCC is caused by mutations in genes that are responsible for repair of DNA mismatches. Mutations that cause HNPCC are usually found in the *MLH1*, *MSH2* and *MSH6* genes. These genes form a complex that scans DNA for mismatches (Figure 3.18). Patients with HNPCC have one normal and one mutated copy of one of these genes. The disease is, therefore, transmitted through families as an autosomal dominant condition.

As epithelial cells in the colon divide, they are subject to somatic mutations at random in the genome. A cell that loses its remaining functioning copy of the mismatch repair gene, will acquire mutations at other sites in the genome more easily (Figure 3.19). Loss of mismatch repair by cells in a tumour can be seen as microsatellite instability (Figure 3.20). Only 10–20% of sporadic colorectal tumours show microsatellite instability, whereas 80–90% of colorectal tumours in individuals with HNPCC show this. Tumours can also be immunostained for MLH1, MSH2 and MSH6. As loss of the remaining functioning copy of the gene is an early step in tumorigenesis, tumours from individuals with an HNPCC-causing mutation are expected to show absence of the protein in which the predisposing mutation lies.

Immunostaining for MLH1, MSH2 and PMS2 in the patient is shown with standard histological techniques in Figure 3.21. This shows complete loss of MLH1. The patient was referred to the local genetics service, where a DNA sample was taken and the *MLH1* gene sequenced to look for a mutation. Such a mutation was identified. As a result of this referral, the patient's sister was shown to have the same mutation in the *MLH1* gene and was referred for 2-yearly screening for bowel cancer by colonoscopy. The brother was shown not to carry the mutation, and did not, therefore, require any further investigation.

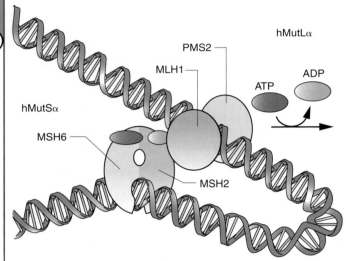

FIGURE 3.18 The proteins MSH6, MSH2, MLH1 and PMS2 form a complex that scans DNA for mismatched bases and repairs them. (Redrawn from www.uniklinikum-saarland.de.)

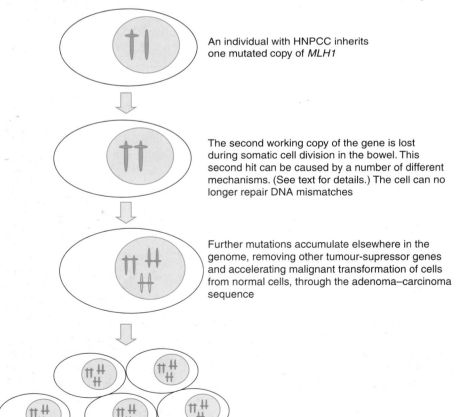

An individual with HNPCC inherits one mutated copy of *MLH1*

The second working copy of the gene is lost during somatic cell division in the bowel. This second hit can be caused by a number of different mechanisms. (See text for details.) The cell can no longer repair DNA mismatches

Further mutations accumulate elsewhere in the genome, removing other tumour-supressor genes and accelerating malignant transformation of cells from normal cells, through the adenoma–carcinoma sequence

FIGURE 3.19 Loss of the sole functioning copy of the *MLH1* gene during somatic cell division makes a colonic epithelial cell prone to developing further mutations.
HNPCC = hereditary non-polyposis colorectal cancer.

Key Points

- Pathological findings can indicate a genetic predisposition to disease in a family.
- DNA analysis techniques can be used to investigate tumours.
- Where pathological findings/clinical information suggest a genetic predisposition, this should be investigated with, at least, a family history.
- Immunohistochemistry can be used to identify loss of protein expression that may be due to a mutation in the gene.
- Such loss of a protein may guide diagnostic laboratories regarding which gene to test.
- Identifying a genetic predisposition in a family may have important implications for other family members.

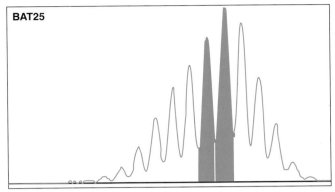

FIGURE 3.20　Analysis of microsatellite 'BAT25' in DNA from the patient. Microsatellites are short stretches of repetitive DNA that vary in length between individual copies of the genome. Analysis of DNA extracted from blood from the individual showed two different microsatellite lengths (shaded in the figure), reflecting the two copies of the genome in a diploid individual. Analysis of DNA extracted from the tumour showed multiple different lengths of microsatellite. This occurs because loss of the sole functional copy of *MLH1* causes failure of mismatch repair and the microsatellite length can change during cell division in multiple cell lineages in the tumour. The tumour is said to show 'microsatellite instability'.

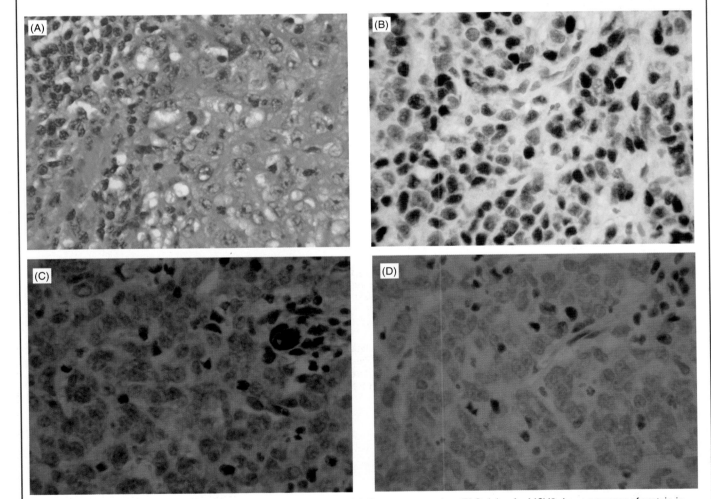

FIGURE 3.21　(A) Poorly differentiated adenocarcinoma of colon with chronic inflammatory reaction. (B) Staining for MSH2 shows presence of protein in tumour cells and inflammatory cells. (C) Staining for MLH1 shows loss of staining in tumour cells. Chronic inflammatory cells remain positive, providing an internal control. (D) Staining for PMS2 shows loss of protein. This occurs because PMS2 is stabilized by forming a complex with MLH1, which cannot take place when MLH1 expression is lost. Chronic inflammatory cells remain positive, acting as a positive internal control.

Triplet Repeat Disorders

These disorders are caused by a stretch of DNA that has a repeated three base pair sequence. In some individuals this 'trinucleotide' repeat has increased in length to cause disease. In conditions such as fragile X syndrome, there is a very large expansion of repeats outside the coding region of a gene, causing a loss of function by stopping transcription. In other conditions such as Huntington's disease, the expanded allele is translated into a polyglutamine tract in a protein. The expansion of this tract affects protein function and causes protein aggregation in cells.

THE GENETIC BASIS OF COMMON DISEASE

Although mutations in genes causing Mendelian inheritance of a disease are comparatively rare, most if not all human diseases are caused by a combination of environmental factors and genetic predisposition.

Normal Variation in the Genome

Every copy of the human genome contains multiple variations in sequence. These variations are described as polymorphisms, and they do not usually themselves cause disease. They may, however predispose an individual to disease.

Polymorphisms may be a single change of base sequence, in which case they are described as single nucleotide polymorphisms (SNPs) or they may involve deletion or duplication of larger regions of the genome, in which case they are described as copy number variations (CNVs).

An SNP in a gene may affect the amino acid sequence of a protein or its level of expression, but the majority of SNPs probably have no effect. To date, many SNPs have been identified in the human genome. The frequency of each polymorphism often varies depending on the population studied. The commonest method of identifying SNPs that may predispose to a human disease is an association study (see Special Study Topic 3.2). Even where a study shows that a SNP is associated with a disease, further study is required to confirm this. Where multiple different SNPs are tested and the effect of the SNP is weak, it is not uncommon to have a false positive result. Even if the result is correct, it may be a different unknown SNP that is in linkage disequilibrium with the one that is being studied. It is therefore essential that an association study is duplicated in a separate population, and that further experiments are carried out to identify the mechanism by which the SNP causes the predisposition to disease.

An association study can be carried out using a candidate gene approach, in which individual genes that are felt to be good candidates for causing a predisposition are studied. It is increasingly recognized that studies of many SNPs

MUTATIONS IN THE FILAGGRIN GENE CAUSE ICHTHYOSIS VULGARIS AND PREDISPOSE TO ATOPIC ECZEMA

Using a classic gene mapping approach it was shown that patients with severe dry and scaly skin (ichthyosis vulgaris) are homozygous for mutations in the filaggrin gene. The skin from a patient with ichthyosis vulgaris is shown in Figure 3.22. The two most common causative mutations both cause premature termination of the filaggrin polypeptide and lead to loss of production of the protein pro-filaggrin from that copy of the gene. There are a number of other mutations in the filaggrin gene which are less common. Up to 10% of the Caucasian population in the UK are carriers of one working and one mutated copy of the filaggrin gene.

The filaggrin gene encodes the pro-filaggrin protein that is expressed in skin epithelium during terminal differentiation. During formation of the cornified layer of the epithelium, it is cleaved into multiple peptides that cause the keratin filaments in the epithelium to aggregate. Loss of filaggrin, therefore, impairs this process (Figures 3.23 and 3.24).

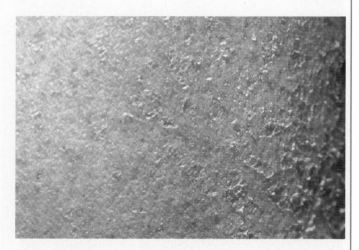

FIGURE 3.22 Skin of patient with ichthyosis vulgaris showing fine scaling and flaking. (Courtesy of Professor Colin Munro).

It has been noted that members of ichthyosis vulgaris families who are heterozygous for a filaggrin mutation can show mild ichthyosis. It was also suspected that they have a significantly increased risk of atopic dermatitis (eczema) and asthma. A formal study was carried out to look at

SPECIAL STUDY TOPIC CONTINUED . . .

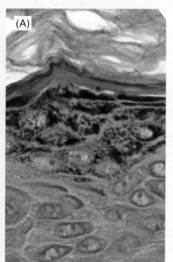

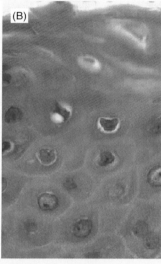

FIGURE 3.23 (A) Normal skin and (B) skin from a patient with ichthyosis vulgaris showing loss of normal keratinization in the upper epidermis.

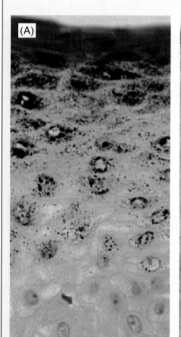

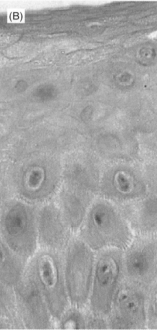

FIGURE 3.24 Immunohistochemical staining for filaggrin in (A) normal skin and (B) skin from a patient with ichthyosis vulgaris. There is no staining for the filaggrin protein in the upper epidermis from the patient, because the patient is homozygous for the R501X mutation in the *filaggrin* gene, abolishing protein production. (Courtesy of Professor McLean.)

frequency of the common filaggrin mutations in children with eczema or asthma when compared to the general population. An initial association study of 52 Irish children with atopic dermatitis compared to 186 population controls was carried out. The results of this are summarized in Table 3.2.

TABLE 3.2 Results

Filaggrin genotype	Atopic dermatitis patients	Population controls
normal/normal	23 (44%)	170 (91.5%)
normal/mutated	23 (44%)	16 (8.5%)
mutated/mutated	6 (12%)	0
Total	52	186

Using the chi-squared test with 2 degrees of freedom, these data show a highly significant association between mutations in the filaggrin gene and atopic dermatitis ($P < 3 \times 10^{-17}$). This is strongly suggestive, but does not in itself confirm that the mutations in filaggrin themselves cause a high risk of eczema in patients who carry them. Importantly this finding has been confirmed in other populations, both in this study and in others.

Proof of causation will require further studies demonstrating the mechanism by which filaggrin deficiency confers a predisposition to atopic disease. This mechanism is currently uncertain. Filaggrin deficiency may lead to a skin barrier that is more permeable to environmental antigens, leading to sensitization. This could explain why children who carry a filaggrin mutation also have a higher risk of asthma. The high prevalence of filaggrin mutations in the population suggests that it has conferred an evolutionary advantage in the past, possibly by improving immunity to severe infections.

Key Points

- All genes can contain polymorphisms, some of which affect protein function.
- This is the basis of genetic variation between humans, and genetic predisposition to common disease.
- A polymorphism in a gene can be tested for association with a common disease phenotype by comparing its frequency in affected and unaffected members of the same population.
- Where an association is found, this needs to be replicated and further studies carried out to demonstrate a biological effect of the polymorphism, before it can be said to be a predisposing factor for the disease process.

Further Reading

Palmer CN, Irvine AD, Terron-Kwiatkowski A, *et al.* Common loss-of-function variants of the epidermal barrier protein filaggrin are a major predisposing factor for atopic dermatitis. *Nat Genet* 2006; **38**: 441–446.

Smith FJ, Irvine AD, Terron-Kwiatkowski A, *et al.* Loss-of-function mutations in the gene encoding filaggrin cause ichthyosis vulgaris. *Nat Genet* 2006; **38**: 337–342.

(approximately 500 000) across the entire genome are feasible. There remain some problems with this approach including dealing with the large amount of data generated and correction for multiple testing. Using chip technology, it is now possible to analyse the majority of variations due to SNPs in the human genome in sufficient numbers of individuals for sensible whole genome association studies.

The extent of CNV in the human genome has only recently been realized. It is now thought that up to 12% of the human genome may have polymorphic duplications or deletions, often involving genes. The optimal methods for studying this as a cause of predisposition to human disease have yet to be established.

Use of Informatics

Given the diversity of human genetic diseases, electronic resources have become an essential tool for addressing clinical problems in genetics. Many websites provide information on genetic diseases, including PubMed, Online Mendelian Inheritance in Man or OMIM (www.ncbi.nlm.nih.gov/entrez/query.fcgi?db=OMIM) and GeneReviews (www.genereviews.org). Databases of laboratories performing mutation analysis of specific genes include the UK genetic testing network (www.ukgtn.org) and GeneTests (www.genetests.org). Information on DNA sequence, known polymorphisms and chromosomal location of genes can be accessed through Ensembl (www.ensembl.org) or the National Centre for Biotechnology Information (www. ncbi.nlm.nih.gov). Patient self-help group websites can also provide useful resources, particularly for patients, and many can be accessed through the contact-a-family website (www.cafamily.org.uk).

A clinical geneticist will usually have access to other more specialized informatics resources, including the London Dysmorphology and Neurogenetics Genetics databases, which allows identification of syndromes by specific clinical features, the REAMS Database for skeletal dysplasias and the European Skeletal Dysplasia Network.

SUMMARY

This chapter has described the basic structure of genes and the processes by which they are translated into proteins. This provides the essential information required to understand how gene changes (mutations and polymorphisms) cause, or predispose to, human disease. The case studies demonstrate the relationship between diagnostic pathology services and clinical genetics, how genetic testing techniques can be used in pathology, and how pathological findings can be important in management of patients in clinical genetics.

ACKNOWLEDGEMENTS

We thank the following people for assistance in preparation of this manuscript: Jacqueline Dunlop, Clinical Genetics, Ninewells Hospital and Medical School, for critical review of the manuscript. Chris Maliszewska and staff, Cytogenetics Laboratory, Ninewells Hospital and Medical School for review of the manuscript and cytogenetic images. Dr Alan Evans, Dr Shaun Walsh, Dr Lee Jordan and Professor D Levison, Department of Pathology for images of gross pathology, histology and immunohistochemistry. Professor Colin Munro, Department of Dermatology, Southern General Hospital, Glasgow, and Professor Irwin McLean, Dundee, for clinical images and tissue sections of ichthyosis vulgaris. Professor Jorens Jass, St Marks Hospital Park, London for Figure 3.16.

FURTHER READING

Eeles RA, Easton DF, Ponder BAJ, Eng C. *Genetic Predisposition to Cancer*, 2nd edn. London: Hodder, 2004.

Firth HV, Hurst JA, Hall JG. *Oxford Desk Reference – Clinical Genetics*. Oxford: Oxford University Press, 2005.

Strachan T, Read A. *Human Molecular Genetics*, 3rd edn. London: Garland Science, 2003.

Young ID. *Medical Genetics* (Oxford Core Texts). Oxford: Oxford University Press, 2005.

CELL INJURY, INFLAMMATION AND REPAIR

4

Alastair D Burt and Stewart Fleming

INTRODUCTION

Cells are generally able to cope with a range of normal physiological demands, a state referred to as homeostasis. When fluctuations in the environment around the cell are more severe, leading to cellular stress, a number of adaptive responses may occur. These allow the cell to remain viable but may modify its structure and function. Some of these adaptive responses are characterized by changes in cell size or number. An increase in cell size in response to a stimulus is termed hypertrophy, whereas an increase in the number of cells is called hyperplasia. Atrophy is the process by which there is a decrease in the size of cells in response to a stimulus. Cells may also adapt by changing their differentiation, so-called metaplasia. These phenomena have been considered in Chapter 2 and will also be dealt with in Chapter 5 along with other growth disorders.

In some circumstances, particularly in the face of a pathological stimulus, the capacity for adaptation is exceeded, leading to cell injury. Initially the events that follow may be reversible and the cell may return to its previously normal state, particularly if the injurious agent is removed. If the pathological stimulus, however, is severe enough or if it is persistent, a point of no return is reached beyond which the cell loses its viability and cell death occurs. This has been discussed in Chapter 2 in the context of normal cellular functions but here we consider the causes and mechanisms of cell injury and death and then look at the tissue responses to these.

CELL INJURY AND DEATH

Causes of Cell Injury

There are many diverse causes of cell injury, from subtle changes occurring because of a genetic mutation leading to

a single amino acid change in a polypeptide chain to massive burns:

- hypoxia (deficiency of oxygen)
- chemical agents and poisons
- infectious agents
- immune-mediated processes
- genetic abnormalities
- nutritional imbalances
- physical agents.

The commonest cause in clinical practice is hypoxia where the cell is damaged because aerobic respiration is diminished. Hypoxia can occur when there is a reduction in the blood supply to a tissue, as occurs in myocardial infarction for example (Figure 4.1). Such an impairment in blood supply, ischaemia, clearly leads to a reduction in the availability of key substances other than oxygen (e.g. glucose).

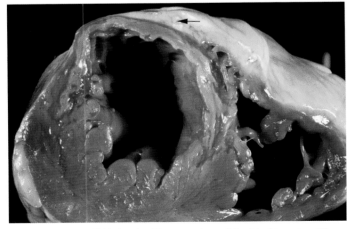

FIGURE 4.1 Myocardial infarction. The posterior wall (top) is thinned and there is an area of yellow discoloration representing dead myocardium. A coronary artery (arrow) is seen; this is occluded by complicated atheroma.

Hypoxia can also occur when there is a reduction in the overall oxygenation of the blood as occurs in cardiorespiratory failure and in carbon monoxide poisoning.

Many chemical agents can cause cell injury; even some apparently innocuous substances (e.g. salt) in certain situations and concentrations may bring about cell death. Other agents that can be considered in this category include adverse effects of prescribed medications, poisons such as arsenic, environmental pollutants and recreational drugs such as alcohol. The range of infectious agents that cause cell and tissue injury, and some of the mechanisms by which this occurs, are discussed in Chapter 19. With some pathogenic organisms cell injury is a direct result of products of the infectious agent whereas in others much of the injury is a 'bystander' phenomenon where the cell gets in the way of the host's immune response to the pathogen. Immunological reactions are also a cause of cell injury when there is an exaggerated response to a foreign protein (anaphylaxis) or when there is breakdown of the normal tolerance mechanisms to self-antigens (auto-immune disease).

Genetic diseases can lead to cell injury by a variety of mechanisms. At one extreme there are gross chromosomal abnormalities which lead to major congenital malformations (e.g. trisomy 21) and at the other extreme, single base mutations in a gene leading to a protein product which is abnormally folded and which cannot be exported from the cell (e.g. α_1-antitrypsin deficiency). Many inherited metabolic abnormalities are caused by there being a genetically determined enzyme defect or deficiency; these may have consequences for only one tissue or organ system but most commonly have systemic effects.

Nutritional imbalances can also be gross, such as that seen in protein-calorie malnutrition (kwashiorkor) which sadly remains a common condition in certain parts of the world, or more subtle, for example a vitamin deficiency. It is important to recognize, however, that nutritional imbalances are not always due to a lack of nutrients but increasingly common is the cell injury associated with excess of nutrients. Obesity and the associated metabolic syndrome are a major cause of serious disease, particularly in Western countries. Physical agents which cause cell injury include extremes of temperature and atmospheric pressure, radiation, direct and indirect mechanical trauma and electrical currents.

Mechanisms of Cell Injury

Key Points

- Subcellular targets of injury include mitochondria, membranes, DNA and the cytoskeleton.
- Some changes of cell injury are potentially reversible.
- Examples of sublethal injury include vacuolar degeneration, fatty change and accumulation of cytoskeletal proteins.

Cell injury results from disruption to the structure and function of one or more subcellular components; the precise mechanisms vary depending on the nature, duration and severity of the injurious stimulus. The key targets for injury are: interference with aerobic respiration in mitochondria; cell membranes (both at the surface and those of intracellular organelles); DNA; protein synthetic pathways; and the cytoskeleton (Figure 4.2).

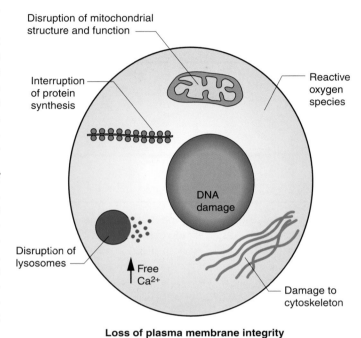

FIGURE 4.2 Key targets of cellular injury. Individual agents may disrupt more than one subcellular compartment.

Interference with the process of oxidative phosphorylation in mitochondria leads to a reduction in adenosine triphosphate (ATP) and therefore impairs many key biochemical processes in the cell. This is a central mechanism in hypoxic injury and is also a feature of some chemical injury. Reduction in ATP reduces the activity of the sodium pump at the cell membrane leading to gross changes in intracellular sodium and potassium concentrations, the net result of which is an influx of water across the membranes, causing the cell to swell. Continued ATP depletion interferes with protein production. There is also failure of intracellular calcium homeostasis. Normally calcium concentrations in the cytosol are low. This is important because calcium can activate cytosolic enzymes that could destroy cellular components. The calcium levels are kept in check by ATP-dependent enzymes. With a reduction in ATP as occurs in hypoxia there is a dramatic increase in cellular calcium leading to activation of (i) phospholipases which break down membranes; (ii) endonucleases which degrade DNA; and (iii) proteases which also destroy membranes and other cytosolic components such as the cytoskeleton. Increased cytosolic calcium can also further damage mitochondria leading to a vicious cycle; this can be a key event in progression to a point of no return for the cell – irreversible injury or cell death (Figure 4.3).

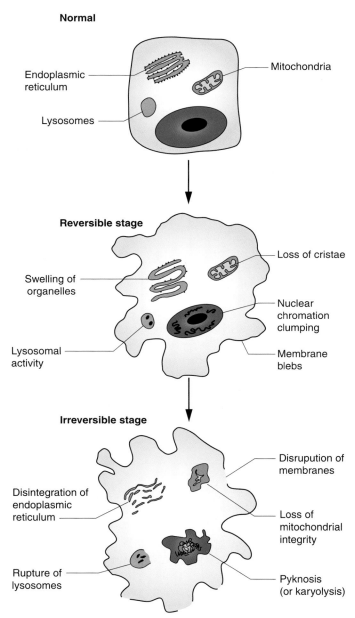

Normal

Endoplasmic reticulum

Mitochondria

Lysosomes

Reversible stage

Swelling of organelles

Loss of cristae

Nuclear chromation clumping

Lysosomal activity

Membrane blebs

Irreversible stage

Disintegration of endoplasmic reticulum

Disrupution of membranes

Loss of mitochondrial integrity

Rupture of lysosomes

Pyknosis (or karyolysis)

FIGURE 4.3 Overview of changes during the reversible and irreversible phases of cellular injury. Note that the precise point of no return is not fully established but loss of membrane integrity appears to be an important factor.

Another biochemical pathway which is now recognized to be important in cell injury involves so-called reactive oxygen species (Figure 4.4). These are byproducts of normal cellular respiration and are partially reduced oxygen molecules including OH^-, O_2^- and H_2O_2. These are free radicals, that is they are chemical compounds with a single unpaired

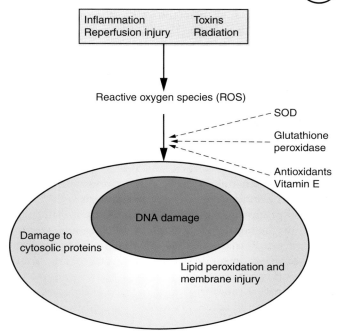

Inflammation
Reperfusion injury

Toxins
Radiation

Reactive oxygen species (ROS)

SOD

Glutathione peroxidase

Antioxidants Vitamin E

DNA damage

Damage to cytosolic proteins

Lipid peroxidation and membrane injury

FIGURE 4.4 Role of reactive oxygen species in cellular injury. Several molecular structures are generated during cellular injury that can damage membranes, proteins and nucleic acids. A number of inherent antioxidant compounds are present within the cell to limit the damage. Cellular injury due to reactive oxygen species occurs when these normal defence mechanisms are overwhelmed. SOD = superoxide dismutase.

electron; they are highly reactive and interact with adjacent molecules releasing energy but also potentially altering the molecules. Normally, there are efficient intracellular homeostatic mechanisms that prevent injury by such free radicals but in some situations the normal defence mechanisms (which include antioxidants such as vitamin E and enzymes such as glutathione peroxidase and superoxide dismutase) are overwhelmed and free radicals interact with lipids in cell membranes (peroxidation), cellular proteins, and DNA leading to breaks in its continuity. The imbalance between free radical generation and scavenging which occurs in injury is referred to as oxidative stress. Free radicals can be generated by a variety of processes and are thought to be important in so-called reperfusion injury (this occurs following restoration of blood flow in ischaemic tissues), chemical injury and radiation damage.

It is important to recognize that although the relative importance of these various mechanisms varies depending on the injurious agent, a common theme is the disruption of membranes. We have already seen that ATP depletion affects the plasma membrane whereas the calcium-modulated activation of phospholipases interferes with all membranes. Free-radical-induced lipid peroxidation further damages their structures. Activation of proteases can also disrupt the cytoskeleton and as this is anchored to the plasma membrane there is further damage to the overall structure of the cell. Disruption of lysosomal membranes leads to escalation of the cell injury. These organelles are packets of highly reactive enzymes including DNAses and proteases; release of these enzymes into the cytosol almost inevitably leads to the demise of the cell.

Reversible and Sublethal Injury

As noted above some of the changes that occur in cell injury are thought to be potentially reversible. Several manifestations of this sublethal injury can be recognized histologically; some of these may in fact be adaptive responses of the cell. One of the earliest changes detected is swelling of the cytoplasm. The cells may become vacuolated (hence the term vacuolar degeneration). This is a reflection of the inability of the cell to regulate the ionic and fluid balance across the plasma membrane reflecting ATP depletion. There is electron microscopic evidence of disruption of the membranes; blebs are seen and points of contact with adjacent cells become loosened. Mitochondria may also be swollen and there may be subtle changes in the nuclear structure. Another common manifestation of sublethal injury is the accumulation of triglycerides in the cell – fatty change or steatosis. This is most commonly seen in liver injury (Figure 4.5) but can occur at other sites such as heart and skeletal muscle. The mechanisms for the accumulation are complex but include impairment of fatty acid oxidation, increased generation of free fatty acids and reduction in apolipoprotein production.

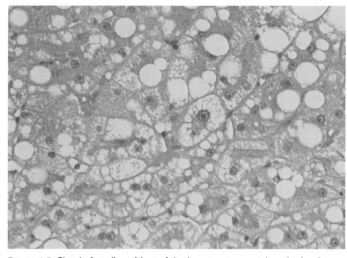

FIGURE 4.5 Simple fatty liver. Most of the hepatocytes contain pale droplets; in some cells this is a large single droplet, in others there are smaller droplets. In this case lipid accumulation in hepatocytes has occurred as a consequence of excess alcohol.

Cytoskeletal abnormalities can also be seen microscopically. The commonest forms are an accumulation of intermediate filaments. This is the basis for the so-called Mallory bodies seen in liver disease (p. 267) and the neurofibrillary tangles seen in neurodegenerative disorders such as Alzheimer's disease (Figure 4.6). This is in part thought to be a consequence of misfolding of the intermediate filament proteins as a consequence of the injury and in part a failure of the normal mechanisms for getting rid of abnormal

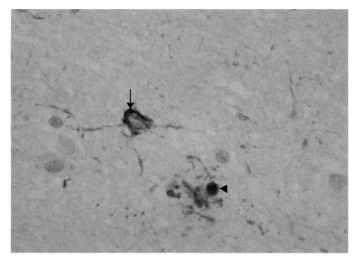

FIGURE 4.6 Neurofibrillary tangles in Alzheimer's disease. Tau protein is seen in an astrocyte (arrow) and in a plaque (arrowhead). (Courtesy of Professor David Ellison.)

intracellular proteins – the so-called sequestrome. Other compounds can accumulate within cells: these include cholesterol and cholesterol esters (an important process in the development of atherosclerosis); glycogen (seen in some inborn errors of metabolism); and pigments. The latter includes lipofuscin, a yellow-brown pigment present in lysosomes which occurs where there has been previous lipid peroxidation. Iron may also accumulate in cells as a response to injury; it may be a localized phenomenon, for example surrounding an area of haemorrhage or form part of a systemic disorder where iron is deposited in different tissues as occurs in genetic haemochromatosis (p. 271). In the latter the accumulation in cells is referred to as haemosiderosis or iron overload.

Cell Death

Key Points

- Two distinct pathways of irreversible cell death exist – necrosis and apoptosis.
- Necrosis is always a consequence of injury and is associated with loss of membrane integrity.
- Apoptosis is a more regulated process – programmed cell death – which may be physiological or pathological.

The precise point beyond which reversible injury becomes irreversible is not yet fully defined. As noted above a pathway common to most forms of injury is disruption to membranes and there may be a level beyond which cell viability is no longer possible. Another may be irreversible mitochondrial dysfunction. Loss of cell viability – cell death – is thought to occur through two major and distinct pathways: necrosis and apoptosis. These are different biological processes, occur in different disease states and are morphologically distinguishable. Necrosis is the form of cell death which generally follows the sequence of events described above with ultimately loss of membrane integrity, whereas apoptosis is a more tightly regulated pathway often described as programmed cell death if it occurs as part of a predetermined, genetically regulated process (see Chapter 2). Necrosis often involves a group of cells within a tissue whereas apoptosis involves single cells and necrosis is generally accompanied by a host inflammatory response whereas this does not happen with apoptosis. Apoptosis may be a physiological phenomenon. It is thought to play a key role in the programmed remodelling of tissues during embryogenesis and in the shaping of the immune system with the programmed deletion of auto-reactive T cells; it also occurs in the endometrium during the menstrual cycle.

Necrosis

Necrosis is the death of cells with loss of membrane integrity and with enzymatic destruction of the cellular constituents. This leads to leakage of cell constituents into the surrounding tissue and the circulation. There is an inflammatory response to these cellular constituents and the initiation of a repair process.

The microscopic changes that occur in necrosis reflect these key processes. Necrotic cells stain pink with routine (haematoxylin and eosin) stains: this is demonstrating denatured proteins produced by action of lysosomal enzymes. The cells lose definition under the microscope; this reflects loss of organelles again because of the effects of phospholipases and proteases. Nuclear changes are an important feature: there may be loss of staining of the nucleus (karyolysis); shrinkage of the nucleus (pyknosis: more characteristically seen in apoptosis) and fragmentation of the nucleus (karyorrhexis). Eventually the nucleus disappears completely. Calcium may be deposited in the dead cells, a process referred to as dystrophic calcification. It is important to recognize that the histological changes are only identifiable microscopically after several hours. There are several different types of necrosis defined by morphological features (Figures 4.7 and 4.8).

The most frequently encountered is coagulative necrosis in which cell outlines are initially maintained but the protein constituents coagulate. The area of necrosis appears pale yellow/white but initially of normal consistency. Histological examination shows loss of nuclear staining with increased eosinophilia of the cytoplasm but retention of the cellular outlines. These are gradually lost and eventually the extracellular tissue architecture breaks down. At this stage the tissue is soft and autolysed. Inflammatory cells infiltrate the necrotic tissue to phagocytose and digest the dead cellular debris.

Colliquative or liquefactive necrosis is seen in the lipid rich tissues of the central nervous system. The lack of extracellular architecture and the high lipid content lead to liquefaction of the necrotic nervous tissue. Caseous necrosis is seen in tuberculosis. There is an amorphous white centre to

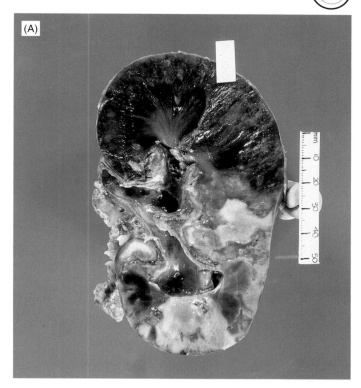

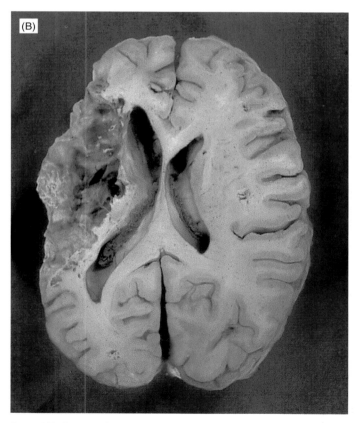

Figure 4.7 Common forms of necrosis. (A) Renal infarction. A well-defined area of renal parenchyma has undergone necrosis due to an embolus in a renal artery. (Courtesy of Dr Katrina Wood.) (B) Cerebral infarction. (Courtesy of Professor David Ellison.)

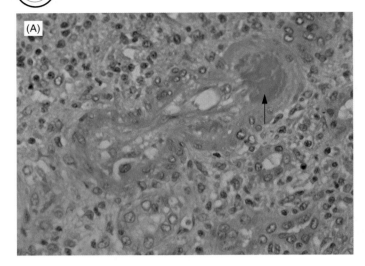

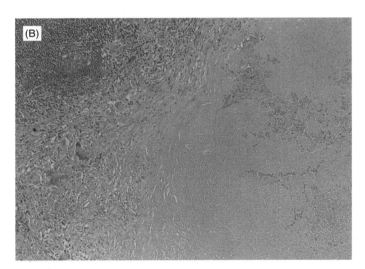

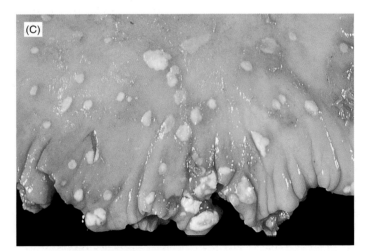

FIGURE 4.8 Other forms of necrosis. (A) Fibrinoid necrosis. In this artery there is accumulation of a fibrin-like substance (arrow) in the media. In this case it is part of a generalized systemic vasculitis. (Courtesy of Dr Katrina Wood.) (B) Caseous necrosis. This is granulomatous inflammation with degeneration at the centre of the lesion, a characteristic feature of tuberculosis. (Courtesy of Dr Fiona Black.) (C) Fat necrosis. In this case destruction of the peritoneal fatty tissue has resulted from the release of lipases following pancreatitis.

the granulomas in tuberculosis as a consequence of the tissue digestion by activated macrophages. Fibrinoid necrosis is seen in the special circumstances of vascular damage. It is characterized by platelet activation, fibrin deposition and usually cell death of the vascular smooth muscle. The terms gangrenous and fat necrosis are commonly used in clinical practice.

Apoptosis

Apoptosis is programmed cell death in which the cell initiates a genetic cell death programme in response to external stimuli. It leads to the deletion of individual cells, the membrane remaining intact, with engulfment and destruction of the cellular remains by adjacent cells or macrophages (Figure 4.9). An inflammatory response is not generally seen in apoptosis. The cells are seen to undergo shrinkage with condensation and fragmentation of the nuclear chromatin. Individual cells are affected rather than numerous adjacent cells as seen in necrosis. As noted above, apoptosis may occur under physiological circumstances. In some situations it could be thought of as a defence mechanism, providing a means of eliminating cells that are no longer required or which have acquired potentially dangerous properties, for example significant DNA damage. It is, however, also the mechanism for cell loss in a number of pathological conditions:

- some forms of radiation injury
- elimination of tumour cells (including action of anti-cancer agents)
- elimination of cells infected with virus (for example hepatitis)
- neurodegenerative conditions.

(A)

Dense apoptotic cell

Liberated cellular debris

Mitochondrion

Macrophage

Nucleus

Apoptotic body (secondary lysosomes containing phagocytosed material)

FIGURE 4.9 (A) Scheme of events in apoptosis. The accompanying electron micrographs in (B), (C) and (D) demonstrate the changes at an ultrastructural level. (B) Cellular shrinkage and blebbing. (C) Nuclear condensation. (D) Phagocytosis within a neighbouring cell whose own nucleus (N) is normal. The boundaries of the phagosome are arrowed. (Courtesy of Professor Andrew Wiley.)

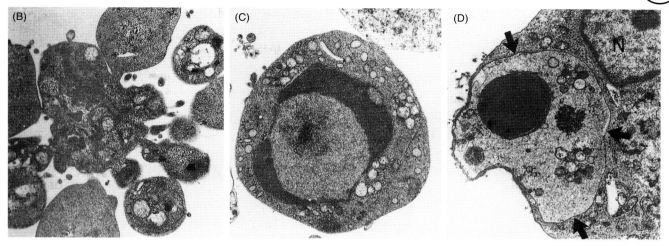

FIGURE 4.9 (Continued)

Apoptotic cells may be difficult to detect by conventional light microscopy. A number of cellular markers such as the binding of dyes (annexin V) and the demonstration of fragmented DNA using the TUNEL method can help (Figure 4.10) and DNA fragmentation can also be shown in cellular extracts by the technique of DNA laddering but it is probably best identified by electron microscopy. The cells are smaller than their normal counterparts and have a dense cytoplasm with tightly packed organelles. The most dramatic features are seen in the nucleus where there is condensation of the chromatin; the nucleus may become fragmented. Small fragments of the cell bud off: these are called apoptotic bodies. The apoptotic cells and the apoptotic bodies are then engulfed by macrophages or other adjacent cells. By contrast with necrosis there is not thought to be appreciable loss of membrane integrity until the very last stages of the process.

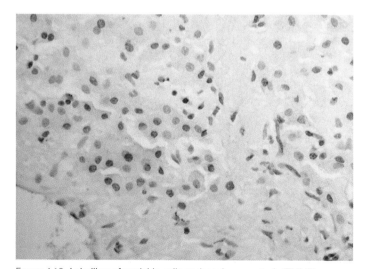

FIGURE 4.10 Labelling of nuclei in cells undergoing apoptosis (TUNEL method). In this case the injury has been induced in the liver during radiofrequency ablation of a tumour. (Courtesy of Dr Helen Robertson.)

In common with necrosis, apoptosis involves the activation of cellular enzymes. With apoptosis however it is not the 'blunderbus' approach seen in necrosis but it involves a group of proteases which are particularly active in destroying the proteins of the nuclear membranes and skeleton and can in turn activate DNases which degrade nuclear DNA. These so-called caspases are found in normal cells but apoptosis is only initiated when these become catalytically active. There are three major phases of apoptosis: (i) initiation or induction; (ii) execution; and (iii) phagocytosis.

The first phase principally involves two distinct but overlapping pathways which both lead to activated caspases that go on to stimulate the execution phase (Figure 4.11). One pathway involves cell surface 'death receptors' that span the membranes of many cells. These are members of the tumour necrosis factor (TNF) receptor family of proteins of which the best characterized are type I TNFR and a related protein, Fas. When these are linked to their ligands, several molecules come together to form a binding site for another protein which also has a cytoplasmic 'death domain' (so-called Fas-associated death domain or FADD). This in turn activates one of the caspases (caspase 8) and there is then a cascade reaction whereby other pro-caspases are sequentially and rapidly activated.

The other pathway involves mitochondria. In normal cells, there are antiapoptotic molecules present in the membranes of mitochondria. These belong to the Bcl-2 family of proteins most notably Bcl-2 itself and Bcl-x. Their presence is stimulated by growth factors and other normal survival signals. In circumstances of cellular stress or where the cell is deprived of its normal survival signals, there is loss of the antiapoptotic proteins and these are replaced by pro-apoptotic members of the same family such as Bax. With the reduction in Bcl-2 and Bcl-x, the mitochondrial membranes become leaky (so-called mitochondrial permeability transition). One of the proteins that then escapes from the mitochondria is cytochrome C, an enzyme involved in respiration. In the cytosol, this protein binds to

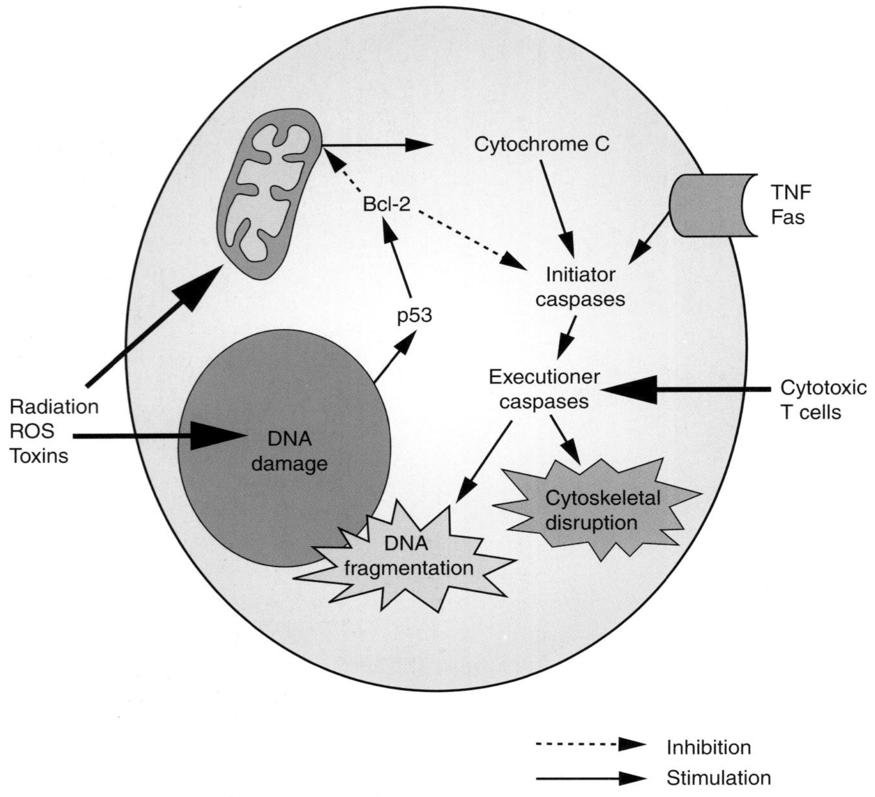

FIGURE 4.11 Role of caspases in apoptosis. Note: the caspase system can be activated via a variety of routes. The common result is DNA fragmentation and disruption of the cytoskeleton. TNF = tumour necrosis factor; ROS = reactive oxygen species.

another protein Apaf-1 (apoptosis activating factor 1) which is capable of activating caspases. At the same time other proteins leak out from the mitochondria which further encourage apoptosis.

It is now recognized that there are other ways to stimulate the initiation pathway. We know for example that cytotoxic T lymphocytes release compounds such as granzyme B which lead to the executioner phase without the involvement of a transmembrane death receptor complex or mitochondrial changes. Radiation and free radicals can also set the pathways in motion by inducing DNA damage involving the tumour suppressor gene *p53*. As we shall see in Chapter 5, p53 is the guardian of the genome, arresting the cell cycle under these circumstances allowing time for DNA repair. If there is no repair, p53 induces apoptosis by upregulating the proapoptotic signals, Bax and Apaf-1.

The final common pathway which comprises the execution phase involves more members of the caspase family. These are all proteases which have a cysteine amino acid at their active site. The members of the family involved in the executioner phase are caspases 3 and 6; on catalytic activation these enzymes degrade nuclear proteins including those involved in regulating gene transcription and DNA repair and activate DNases leading to cleavage of nuclear DNA. Other effects include alteration of cytoskeletal proteins, contributing to cell shrinkage.

Cells undergoing apoptosis secrete factors and express molecules on their surface which facilitate uptake either by macrophages or by adjacent cells; it is this efficient uptake of apoptotic cells that explains the lack of a significant inflammatory response compared with necrosis.

INFLAMMATION

Inflammation and repair are the local responses initiated to limit the damage caused by tissue injury, infection, toxins and ischaemia and to aid recovery from tissue damage. Despite the primary role as defence mechanisms the inflammatory response and repair processes may contribute to the tissue damage seen in many diseases.

The term 'inflammatory response' encompasses a whole range of processes designed to limit tissue injury. For convenience and to aid understanding the inflammatory response is divided into acute inflammation and chronic inflammation based largely on temporal features but also on the different cells involved in the process.

Acute Inflammation

Initial Response to Tissue Injury

● Vascular phase of increased flow.
● Exudate formation.
● Neutrophil polymorph infiltration of tissue.
● Bacterial phagocytosis and killing.
● Resolution, suppuration, organization or chronicity.

Acute inflammation is the initial response to tissue injury in most circumstances and the main causes are:

- bacterial infection
- hypersensitivity reactions
- physical agents such as radiation
- chemical reagents including toxins
- tissue necrosis following infarction.

It is of short duration initiated within minutes and lasting for several hours or a few days. Its main function is the delivery of cells and mediators to the site of injury by the blood stream, therefore vasculature has a central role in coordinating the inflammatory response. Acute inflammation can be considered to comprise two phases, the vascular phase and the cellular phase. These usually coexist in any one inflammatory response with the vascular phase occurring earlier and merging with the later cellular phase of acute inflammation. Inflamed tissue has characteristic morphological features as a consequence of the vascular and cellular changes described classically as the cardinal signs of inflammation (Figure 4.12):

- redness
- heat
- swelling
- pain
- loss of function.

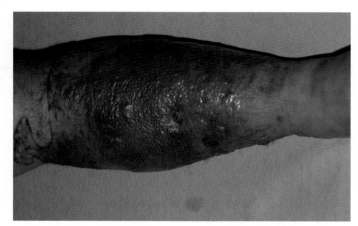

FIGURE 4.12 Cellulitis. Note: swelling and reddening of the skin. (Courtesy of Dr Clifford Lawrence.)

Vascular Phase of Acute Inflammation

Key Points

- At sites of injury there are marked changes in blood flow.
- An initial phase of vasoconstriction is followed by prolonged vasodilatation.
- Increased vascular permeability accompanies the vasodilatation and this leads to the formation of a protein-rich exudate and tissue oedema.

Changes in Blood Flow

One of the earliest features of the acute inflammatory response is an alteration in the flow of blood to the injured site. It consists of an early transient vasoconstriction, mediated by contraction of smooth muscles within the arterioles, which leads to a short-lived reduction in blood flow to the injured site. This is followed by vasodilatation, achieved by relaxation of arteriolar smooth muscle and by distension of capillaries within the injured site. This vasodilatation is more sustained and can last for many hours. There is also increased blood flow to inflamed tissue giving the characteristic red and warm appearance. This series of events allows the increased delivery of molecules and cells involved in acute inflammation (Figure 4.13).

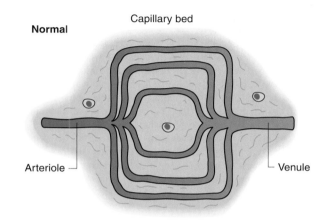
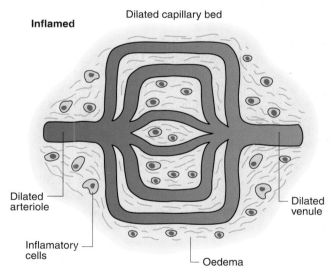

FIGURE 4.13 Overview of vascular changes in acute inflammation.

Following on increased blood flow there is a gradual slowing of the circulation through inflamed tissue. This is achieved partly by the dilatation of capillaries and partly by altered vascular permeability as capillary endothelium becomes more permeable to plasma proteins. The leakage of protein into the interstitium contributes to oedema formation. Increased flow through arterioles causes an increase in hydrostatic pressure at the arterial end of the tissue microcirculation (Figure 4.14).

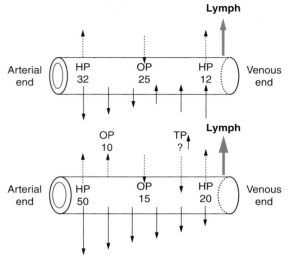

FIGURE 4.14 Exchange of fluid by extra-filtration across the wall of small blood vessels. HP and OP represent the difference between the hydrostatic and colloid osmotic pressures (mmHg) of plasma and extravascular space. The solid arrows indicate the net movement of fluid in and out of vessels along their length. The interrupted arrows indicate the direction of forces exerted by HP, OP and tissue pressure (TP). Upper figure, normal tissue: fluid movement across vessel wall approximates to equilibrium. Lower figure, acute inflammation: much more fluid leaves vessels than is returned to them. The values of HP and OP are approximations. In inflammation, HP may be less than indicated because of rise of TP and OP will also be reduced due to escape of plasma protein (via endothelial gaps) into the extravascular space which increases OP in the extravascular fluid (shown as 10 mmHg). The level of TP varies depending upon the nature of the tissue involved. In loose tissue TP will show no increase, whereas in tissues which are tightly tethered or have fibrous capsules TP can rise considerably (hence the question mark in this figure).

Combined with increased capillary permeability this causes an increase in fluid moving from within the blood vessels to the tissue spaces. The fluid is rich in protein so there is a loss of the normal osmotic gradient which opposes the accumulation of tissue fluid.

Increased Vascular Permeability

There are several different mechanisms of increased vascular permeability, depending on the nature of the injurious agent. Endothelial cell contraction is probably the most common mechanism. It occurs predominantly in venules and is a response to inflammatory mediators including histamine, bradykinin and leukotrienes. It is a rapidly occurring event and is short lived of duration up to 30 minutes. Typically this alteration affects venules between 20 μm and 60 μm in diameter but does not appear to affect capillaries or arterioles.

Direct endothelial injury may occur in diseases in which vascular damage is part of the tissue injury. This type of alteration in vascular permeability is seen following burns and in some bacterial infections. There may be some delay between the time of injury and the leakage of protein rich exudate to allow the development of the full process of cell death and detachment from the vessel wall. These changes

can affect all of the microvessels, arterioles, capillaries and venules. The leakage of a protein-rich exudate is sustained until the vessels either become occluded with thrombus or are repaired.

Leucocyte-mediated injury to vessels occurs when the white blood cell release of cytotoxic agents causes endothelial damage. This is characteristically seen in vasculitis. The leakage of an exudate occurs from the time of endothelial loss and is sustained throughout the duration of the disease activity as new endothelial cells become targets for leucocyte mediate damage. In the neoangiogenesis associated with the repair process (see below) there is loss of a protein-rich exudate from these healthy but immature capillaries. There are many mediators of these different mechanisms of vascular phase of the inflammatory response. The biochemical nature of these agents is discussed in detail below.

These properties of the vascular phase of the acute inflammatory response lead to the formation of a protein-rich exudate, consequent tissue oedema and increased blood viscosity coupled with reduced flow leading to stasis. The proteins within the exudates include immunoglobulins, complement components, coagulation factors and kinins, all of which contribute to the inflammatory response. These events allow the next stage, the cellular phase of acute inflammation, to occur. This cellular phase involves the migration of white blood cells, particularly neutrophils, from the circulation into the site of tissue injury.

Cellular Phase of the Acute Inflammatory Response

The cellular phase of acute inflammation involves the movement of white blood cells, particularly neutrophils, from the circulation into the site of tissue damage where they act to limit the extent of injury. This involves several different stages and again the endothelial cells play a key role (Figure 4.15).

Margination and Adhesion

During the slowing of blood flow which occurs as part of the vascular phase of the acute inflammatory response the larger white blood cells move from a central axial position in flowing blood to a peripheral position. In the microcirculation these white blood cells can be seen adjacent to the endothelium. As the blood flows slowly along the microcirculation the white blood cells roll on the endothelial surface. This process is known as margination. During rolling the white blood cells become increasingly adherent to the endothelial cell surface. This leucocyte endothelial adhesion is achieved by the expression on the surface of activated endothelial cells of a family of molecules known as selectins. Selectins recognize specific carbohydrate groups found on the surface of neutrophils and macrophages, the most important of which ise the sialyl-Lewis X molecule. The interactions between s-Lewis X and selectins increase the stickiness between leucocytes and endothelial cells. The adhesion between leucocytes and endothelial cells become firmer by interactions between other adhesion molecules, especially members of the immunoglobulin supergene family on the endothelial surface and integrins on the leucocytes.

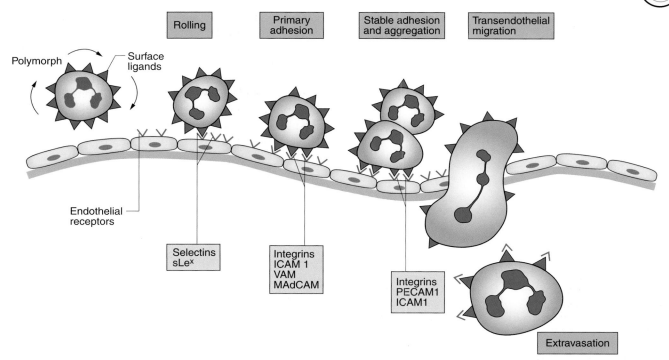

FIGURE 4.15 Margination of leucocytes, endothelial adhesion and leucocyte emigration. PECAM = platelet/endothelial cell adhesion molecule; ICAM = intercellular adhesion molecule.

The immunoglobulin gene superfamily adhesion molecules include intercellular adhesion molecule-1 (ICAM-1) and vascular cell adhesion molecule-1 (VCAM-1), whereas the main integrins are members of the β1 family expressed on the surface of leucocytes. These molecules allow a much tighter adhesion and stabilize the interactions between leucocytes and endothelial cells.

Obviously the response of endothelial cells on activation adjacent to tissue injury is critical in signalling to leucocytes in the circulation. Expression of cell adhesion molecules is controlled in several different ways in these cell types. Molecules such as P selectin are stored preformed in endothelial cells in Weibel–Palade bodies. On stimulation of the endothelial cells by histamine or by platelet activating factor the P selectin within these cytoplasmic storage granules is rapidly redistributed to the cell surface within minutes. Thus the expression of P selectin on the endothelium is an important early mechanism for attracting leucocytes to a site of inflammation. Other adhesion molecules, including E selectin, ICAM-1 and VCAM-1, are expressed by *de novo* protein synthesis. On stimulation of the endothelial cells by proinflammatory cytokines such as tumour necrosis factor (TNF) or interleukin 1 (IL1) there is transcriptional activation of the genes encoding these proteins. This level of control of adhesion molecules requires between 4 and 6 hours of stimulation but can be sustained for hours or days.

Finally in the regulation of leucocyte endothelial interactions there may be alteration in the relative avidity of the two groups of molecules for each other. This is particularly seen during the activation of leucocytes when integrins of the β1 family undergo conformational changes which increase their avidity for adhesion molecules on the endothelial surface such as ICAM-1.

The importance of leucocyte endothelial interactions is emphasized in a group of diseases collectively known as leucocyte adhesion deficiencies. Of these the best described is deficiency of the leucocyte expression of β1 integrin. Patients with this inherited disorder are susceptible to recurrent bacterial infections, which they clear rather poorly, suffering more extensive tissue damage than would be seen in unaffected individuals.

Leucocyte Migration (Figure 4.15)

After attachment leucocytes pass between adjacent endothelial cells and exit from the circulation. The endothelial cells retract and the leucocytes migrate on the endothelial surface using the above adhesion molecules and possibly others, including platelet/endothelial cell adhesion molecule-1 (PECAM-1 or CD31). Leucocytes pass through the endothelial basement membrane probably by enzymatic degradation of the extracellular matrix and then migrate towards the site of injury by a process known as chemotaxis. This is directional migration in which the leucocytes sense and respond to a concentration gradient of chemotaxins. A variety of important molecules in the inflammatory process behave as chemotaxins, in particular the C3a and C5a components of complement, leukotriene B4 and IL8. Leucocyte migration further into the inflamed site occurs on the extracellular matrix. The cells move by the extension of an anterior pseudopod with attachment to extracellular matrix molecules such as fibronectin mediated via adhesion molecules at the anterior end of the pseudopod. The cell body is then pulled forward by the action of actin and myosin filaments that insert into the adhesion complex.

Phagocytosis

Once neutrophils accumulate within the inflammatory focus they are involved in clearing the injurious agent, for example bacteria, by the process known as phagocytosis (Figures 4.16 and 4.17). This involves the cellular events of attachment, engulfment and killing of bacteria by inflammatory cells.

The first event is recognition and attachment. Most microorganisms and particles to be phagocytosed by neutrophils and by macrophages require to be coated by opsonins of which there are three main families: immunoglobulin,

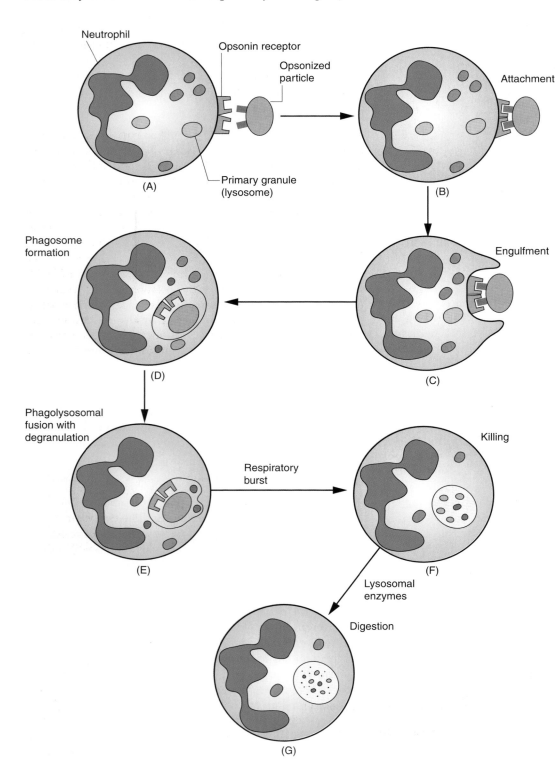

FIGURE 4.16 (A) Phagocytosis and killing of microorganisms. The microorganism is opsonized with antibody or complement. (B) The opsonized particle becomes attached to neutrophil membrane receptors for the opsonin. (C) Engulfment. (D) The opsonized microorganism is internalized into a phagocytic vacuole (phagosome). (E) Fusion of the lysosomes (primary granules) with the phagosome allows the discharge of lysosomal enzymes into the phagolysosome and triggers the respiratory burst which results in bacterial killing. (F) Lysosomal enzymes degrade the dead microorganism (G).

complement and carbohydrate molecules. Immuno-globulins may bind specifically to antigens on the bacterial surface leaving exposed their Fc fragments which are recognized by Fc receptors on the neutrophil surface. Activation of complement (directly by bacterial surfaces by the alternative pathway or by the classical pathway following antibody binding to bacterial surfaces) generates the C3b fragment of complement. This, the opsonic fragment, can be recognized by C3b receptors on the neutrophil surface. Finally carbohydrate binding proteins or lectins circulating in plasma may bind to sugar residues on bacterial cell walls particularly via mannose sugars. These receptors in turn can be recognized by neutrophils. For all three of these recognition phenomena binding and crosslinking of receptors allows progression to engulfment.

During engulfment, cytoplasmic extensions or pseudopods flow around the bacterium and fusion of the membranes of the pseudopods leads to complete enclosure of the bacterium within a membrane bound phagosome. This is internalized and fusion of the membrane of the phagosome with the limiting membrane of lysosomal granules results in secretion of the granule contents into what is now known as the phagolysosome. This leads to the final stage of phagocytosis, namely bacterial killing.

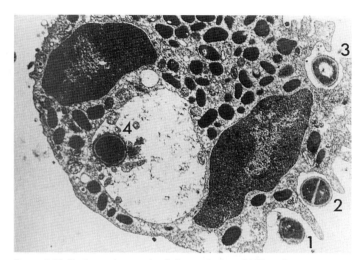

FIGURE 4.17 Electron micrograph of phagocytosis and killing of *Staphylococcus aureus* by a neutrophil: 1, 2 and 3 are the different stages of engulfment of the microorganisms, leading to their presence in a phagolysosome (4).

Bacterial Killing

The microorganismal killing mechanisms of neutrophils and macrophages may be either oxygen dependent or oxygen independent (Figure 4.18). Although both probably co-exist during the phagocytosis of most organisms, the oxygen dependent mechanism is the more important. In oxygen dependent killing, reactive oxygen metabolites are generated during phagocytosis because of the rapid activation of nicotinamide adenosine dinucleotide phosphate (reduced form) (NADPH) oxidase on NADPH. This enzyme activity reduces oxygen molecules to the superoxide anion (O^{2-}). These superoxide anions are then converted into hydrogen peroxide mostly by spontaneous dismutation. Hydrogen peroxide is produced within the lysosome during the phagocytic metabolic burst. Although the concentration of hydrogen peroxide rises considerably within the

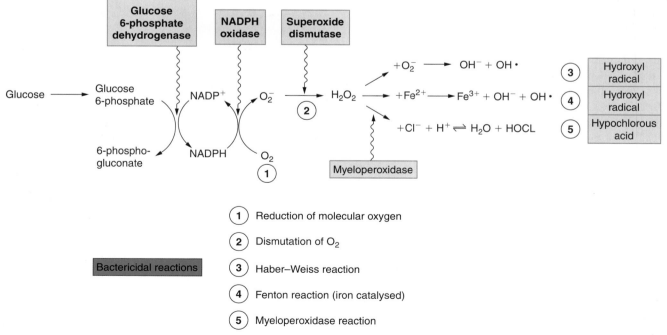

FIGURE 4.18 Pathways of intracellular killing of microorganisms.

phagolysosome this may be insufficient to kill many bacteria. However, the granules of neutrophils also contain the enzyme myeloperoxidase which in the presence of chloride ions converts hydrogen peroxide to HOCl$^-$, a potent antimicrobial agent. This hydrogen peroxide myeloperoxidase halide system is the major bactericidal system in neutrophils but is also effective against fungi, viruses and parasites. Hydrogen peroxide is eventually detoxified into water and oxygen by the action of catalase and the dead micro-organisms are degraded by lysosomal enzymes. Oxygen-independent killing also occurs through the action of substances within the phagolysosome. Lysozyme, an enzyme which degrades the glycopeptide coat of bacteria, lactoferrin an iron-binding protein, and the major basic protein particularly found in eosinophils all have bacteriocidal and bacteriostatic activity.

Diseases in which these defence mechanisms are deficient again illustrate their importance in infection. There is deficient phagocytosis in the Chediak–Higashi syndrome, an autosomal recessive condition in which there is increased risk of bacterial infection. In chronic granulomatous disease, an X-linked recessive disorder, there are defects in the capacity of the neutrophils to generate the superoxide anion leading to deficient bacterial killing and chronic bacterial infections. During these processes a number of reactive, potentially toxic, substances are released into the environment of the inflammatory focus. Although their primary role is as a defence mechanism they may contribute to tissue injury by lipid peroxidation, extracellular matrix degradation and cytocidal properties. In some disease situations, for example immune complex mediated disorders such as Goodpasture's syndrome (see Chapter 13), neutrophil infiltration of the affected organs is the major pathological event. Their action leads to cell death and degradation of the extracellular matrix of critical structures such as the glomerulus.

Outcomes of the Inflammatory Response

Acute inflammation has both beneficial and harmful consequences. As a protective mechanism inflammation allows ingress of phagocytes to the inflammatory focus; the oedema formation dilutes toxic substances; antibodies are delivered to sites of infection and fibrin forms a substratum for cell migration. The harmful effects of inflammation include the digestion of adjacent viable tissue, and local tissue swelling of hollow viscera can be detrimental, for example acute epiglottitis may be life-threatening. There may be loss of function of affected organs and, when generalized, the increased vascular permeability can cause shock as seen in some hypersensitivity reactions (anaphylaxis).

Sequelae of Acute Inflammation

There are four main possible sequelae of acute inflammation:

- resolution
- abscess formation
- healing by fibrosis and scar formation
- chronic inflammation.

Complete resolution occurs following short-lived tissue injury in which there has been little tissue damage. The offending bacterium may be neutralized, killed and cleared by the acute inflammatory response and the affected tissues return entirely to normal. This occurs in some acute bacterial infections and is the ideal outcome. Abscess formation occurs when a localized collection of pus forms, often surrounded by granulation tissue and fibrosis. This is characteristically seen with certain pyogenic organisms such as staphylococci. An abscess may discharge spontaneously or require drainage by surgical intervention (Figure 4.19).

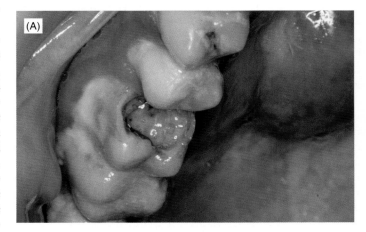

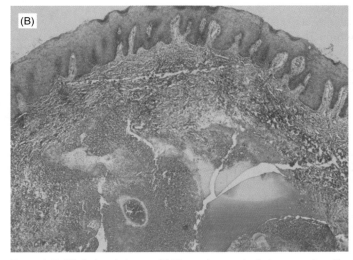

FIGURE 4.19 (A) A dental abscess. (B) Photomicrograph of abscess cavity with accumulation of neutrophils and fibrin. (Courtesy of Dr Max Robinson.)

Healing by fibrosis and scar formation occurs when substantial tissue destruction is seen during the acute phase. The damaged tissues are unable to regenerate and are replaced by fibrous tissue. This process is dealt with in more detail below. Progression to a chronic inflammatory response occurs in several circumstances which are also discussed below.

Chronic Inflammation

Key Points

- Chronic inflammation is characterized by an infiltration of lymphocytes and macrophages.
- Granulomatous inflammation is a specific form of chronic inflammation seen in diseases such as tuberculosis and sarcoidosis.
- Chronic inflammation may follow acute inflammation or may arise *de novo*.

Chronic inflammation occurs over a more prolonged and sustained course than the acute inflammatory response and although it shares many features in its vascular and leucocyte biology the major leucocytes involved are the peripheral blood monocytes or macrophages. Chronic inflammation may supervene on an acute inflammatory response in two main instances or may arise *de novo*.

Persistence of the microorganism or toxic agent is particularly seen with microorganisms that are not cleared by neutrophils, for example *Mycobacterium tuberculosis*, the causative agent of tuberculosis. Recurrent episodes of acute inflammation may lead to tissue destruction and the inflammatory response then enters a chronic phase. This is seen in repeated episodes of acute cholecystitis associated with gallstones (p. 274). Eventually this leads to chronic cholecystitis, thickening of the gall bladder wall, infiltration by macrophages and persistence of symptoms. Finally, chronic inflammation may be seen in certain diseases in which the immune system reacts against the individual's own tissues. Autoimmune diseases are relatively common and in these the chronic inflammatory response is the major cause of tissue damage.

Features of Chronic Inflammation

The chronic inflammatory response is characterized by less oedema formation and changes in blood flow than acute inflammation. But the major difference is infiltration of the tissues by peripheral blood monocytes and lymphocytes (Figure 4.20). Chronic inflammation is almost uniformly accompanied by tissue destruction followed by attempts at healing by fibrosis.

Macrophages in Chronic Inflammation

The macrophage is a key cell in the chronic inflammatory response. It undergoes extravasation from the circulation, chemotaxis and phagocytosis in the same way as neutrophils although some of the mediators differ. Compared with neutrophils, the time course of exit of monocytes into the inflammatory focus is delayed and is more prolonged. This sustained monocyte and macrophage infiltration may be achieved by continued recruitment, prolonged survival and immobilization of macrophages or by local proliferation of macrophages within the inflammatory focus.

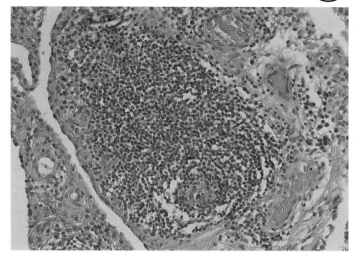

FIGURE 4.20 Chronic inflammation in a joint from a patient with rheumatoid arthritis. The inflammatory infiltrate includes lymphocytes and plasma cells with few neutrophils. (Courtesy of Dr Petra Dildey.)

Macrophages are large cells that can react to chemotactic stimuli by migration. They are capable of phagocytosis and intracellular killing of bacteria by mechanisms similar to those seen in neutrophils. However, they may be activated by interactions with T lymphocytes during inflammatory responses, enhancing their intracellular killing and degradation capacity. In the response to particularly resistant organisms, such as *M. tuberculosis*, macrophages have the capacity to fuse together to form multinucleated giant cells during granulomatous inflammation. Macrophages are capable of releasing a variety of potent proteolytic enzymes important both in defence against bacterial infection and in causing tissue injury during chronic inflammation. These products include proteases, elastase, collagenase, plasminogen activators and lipases. The secretion of these substances by macrophages leads to extensive degradation of the extracellular matrix resulting in the tissue damage which is such a prominent feature of chronic inflammation.

Macrophages can influence the repair process by the production of a variety of growth factors including platelet-derived growth factor (PDGF), epidermal growth factor (EGF), fibroblast growth factor (FGF) and transforming growth factor β (TGFβ). They can also secrete a number of proinflammatory cytokines and plasma proteins which contribute to the development of the inflammatory response. Macrophages are also important in directing the early induction of the specific immune response. Following intracellular killing and degradation of bacteria certain macrophages can then express antigenic peptides on their cell surface in association with major histocompatibility complex (MHC) molecules. This combination of antigenic peptide and MHC is required for the activation of T lymphocytes. Macrophages thus have an important role in both the recognition and effector arms of inflammatory and immunological responses.

Ulricka was a 56-year-old married woman who spent the first 30 years of her life in Sweden. She then came to the UK as a student and is now a chemical engineer. She had always been fit and well and had no previous ailments of any significance. She had had all relevant immunizations as a child including BCG.

Ulricka presented to her general practitioner with increasing breathlessness which had developed over a period of approximately 3 months. She complained of some tightness in her chest and had occasional bouts of a dry cough but there was no haemoptysis. She had also developed some stiffness of her knee and ankle joints and also noticed that she had dry eyes and on occasions sensitivity to light (photophobia). On examination there were no abnormal chest signs, and no finger clubbing or cyanosis. She did, however, have palpable lymph nodes in her neck and evidence of hepatosplenomegaly.

A chest X-ray was taken which showed some shadowing in both lungs, particularly around the mid-zones and there was marked bilateral hilar lymphadenopathy. She underwent a series of lung function tests which demonstrated a restrictive lung disease with decreased compliance and mild impairment of diffusion capacity. All routine blood tests, including full blood count, urea and electrolytes were in the normal range but there was mild derangement of liver function tests including elevation of alkaline phosphatase (p. 262). There was elevation of inflammatory markers, in particular C-reactive protein and a markedly elevated serum angiotensin-converting enzyme. Mantoux's test for active tuberculosis was negative.

She underwent biopsy of one of the lymph nodes identified in her neck. It showed replacement of the node by granulomas characterized by the presence of large multinucleated giant cells, epithelioid macrophages and lymphocytes (Figure 4.21). Some of the granulomas showed accompanying scarring but there was no necrosis. Staining for mycobacteria was negative.

The appearances on biopsy and the constellation of clinical signs and symptoms together with the finding of high serum angiotensin-converting enzyme levels led to a diagnosis of sarcoidosis. Ulricka was treated with corticosteroids and within 2 months the lung symptoms had disappeared and the lymph node swelling in the neck had also reduced. Over time the joint stiffness improved and she was able to lead a normal life again.

Sarcoidosis is a multisystem disorder characterized by granulomatous infiltration in various tissues. The precise

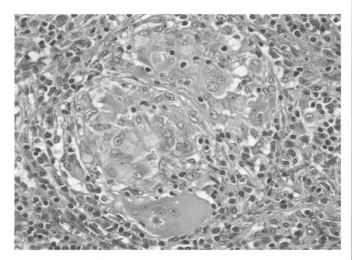

FIGURE 4.21 A well-formed sarcoid granuloma. It is composed of epithelioid and giant cells with surrounding lymphocytes. The giant cell at the lower border contains an asteroid body (most often seen in sarcoidosis).

aetiology remains uncertain but it has long been considered to be likely due to an abnormal response to some external agent such as bacteria or chemicals. It is a disease which occurs worldwide but there are some areas with a much higher prevalence, in particular Scandinavia. Lymph nodes and liver are the most commonly affected sites but, as with Ulricka, there can be ocular involvement and joint involvement. In addition some patients develop cardiac sarcoidosis, and involvement of the nervous system and brain may lead to cranial nerve palsies including facial palsy.

A number of conditions need to be distinguished from sarcoidosis in patients such as Ulricka. In particular it was important to consider whether she may have had another condition characterized by granulomatous inflammation – tuberculosis – and the other concern was that she may have developed a lymphoma. It was clearly therefore extremely important to obtain a histological diagnosis by sampling the enlarged node in her neck. Although Ulricka showed an impressive response to the corticosteroid therapy, in the longer term there is a high chance of relapse, particularly when steroids are stopped, and interestingly little difference is demonstrable in the long-term outcome, comparing patients who have been treated with steroids with those who have not.

Granulomatous Inflammation

Granulomatous inflammation is a specific pattern of chronic inflammatory response defined by the localized aggregation of activated macrophages around an inflammatory focus. It is encountered in a small number of highly characteristic diseases including tuberculosis, leprosy, brucellosis and Crohn's disease. In clinical practice the recognition of granuloma formation is therefore a major diagnostic criterion for these diseases.

A granuloma is a localized aggregate of macrophages which are activated and transformed into so-called epithelioid cells, usually surrounded by a cuff of lymphocytes and occasionally plasma cells (see Figure 4.21). In haematoxylin and eosin stained histological sections epithelioid cells have abundant pale pink granular cytoplasm with indistinct cell boundaries. In some instances multiple macrophages may fuse together to form a multinucleated giant cell. As granulomatous inflammation progresses it may eventually be surrounded by fibroblasts and scar tissue. Granulomas form in response to two quite different mechanisms: immune-mediated granulomas, of which the main clinical diseases discussed above are examples, and foreign body granulomas, elicited by inert foreign particles that have proved difficult for macrophages to clear.

Granulomas form after macrophages have initially digested the pathogenic organism. During the killing and partial degradation of the organism antigenic peptides are expressed on the macrophage surface. They pass through the draining lymphatics to the adjacent lymph nodes where the antigenic peptides stimulate specific antigen-recognizing T lymphocytes. These are activated and migrate to the inflammatory focus, where they secrete proinflammatory cytokines. These cytokines in turn activate macrophages which accumulate, immobilized within the inflammatory focus. Macrophage activation causes increased production of a variety of proteases and lysosomal enzymes increasing the cytoplasmic volume and resulting in the pale granular eosinophilic staining seen in histological preparations. In some granulomas, tissue associated with the release of digestive enzymes leaves the centre of the granuloma necrotic. In tuberculosis this is the characteristic caseous (cheese-like) necrosis.

Granulomas form relatively slowly over a period of days and are dependent on the integrity of the immune system as well as the chronic inflammatory response. They are an important defence mechanism against several major infections and patients with defective cell-mediated immunity (e.g. in acquired immune deficiency syndrome [AIDS], may have overwhelming tuberculosis or leprosy (Chapter 19). Nevertheless the process of granuloma formation, with central necrosis and tissue destruction, consequent on macrophage degranulation, leads to significant tissue damage and scar formation and therefore contributes to the pathogenesis of the disease.

Systemic Effects of Inflammation

There are many systemic effects of inflammation, some of which may be symptomatic and some of which are a response to injury only demonstrated by laboratory testing. Fever is one of the most commonly encountered consequences of an acute inflammatory illness (Figure 4.22). It is a consequence of the effect of the cytokines IL1 and TNF directly acting on the hypothalamus to reset the thermoregulatory mechanisms in the body leading to a rise in

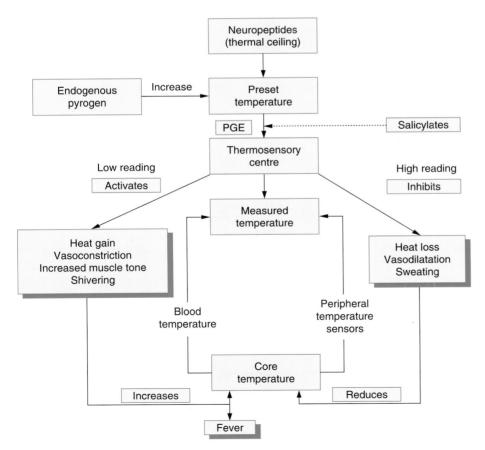

Figure 4.22 Mechanisms of pyrexia.
PGE = prostaglandin E.

body temperature through increased sympathetic nerve stimuli of cutaneous arterioles, vasoconstriction and reduced heat loss. The liver produces a number of acute phase proteins including C-reactive protein, serum amyloid A, serum amyloid P protein and the important complement and coagulation proteins. There is increased production of the stress-related glucocorticoids and there may be a diuresis as a consequence of reduced vasopressin production. One of the consequences of these effects is a catabolic state with increased breakdown of fat and protein stores in the body. Leucocytosis, an increase in the number of white blood cells within the circulation, is an important part of the defence mechanism in inflammatory illness. The release of increased numbers of white cells, initially from bone marrow stores, and in a more prolonged inflammatory illness because of increased bone marrow turnover and differentiation towards leucocytes, can lead to white cell counts two to three times the normal level. This leucocytosis may be regulated by IL1 and TNF acting on the bone marrow stores but a more prolonged leucocytosis requiring increased bone marrow turnover is dependent on the production of colony-stimulating factors.

Mediators of the Inflammatory Response

Key Points

- The processes of acute and chronic inflammation are mediated by a variety of small molecules.
- Some of these are found circulating in plasma while others are produced by inflammatory cells.
- Activation of many of these mediators involves a cascade of kinase reactions.
- The activation pathways are tightly regulated.

A variety of chemical mediators of acute and chronic inflammation have been described. These may circulate in plasma or be synthesized and secreted by inflammatory cells. In general plasma-derived mediators require to be activated, usually by proteolytic cleavage, to an active form. Cell-derived mediators tend to be stored in the active form within intracellular granules or are synthesized *de novo* in the active form in response to an external stimulus. Most of these mediators exert their biological property by binding to specific receptors on target cells leading to a characteristic biological response. Some mediators can act on several target cells within the inflammatory focus. Most mediators are rather short lived and are degraded to inactive forms within minutes. The importance of many of these mediators is that they provide an important point for therapeutic intervention, for example the use of antihistamines in the treatment of hay fever.

Histamine

This is widely distributed in tissues mostly stored within the granules of mast cells present in connective tissue. It is also found in circulating basophils and platelets. The preformed histamine is released by mast cell degranulation in response to a variety of signals including trauma, cold, IgE binding by antigen, anaphylotoxic elements of complement, C3a and C5a, and cytokines such as IL1 and IL8. In the acute inflammatory response histamine causes dilatation of arterioles by relaxation of vascular smooth muscle and increases the endothelial permeability in venules. It is thought to be one of the major mediators of the early stages of the acute inflammatory response particularly the increased vascular permeability.

Serotonin

This is another preformed vasoactive mediator similar to histamine but present in platelets. Serotonin is released from platelets during platelet activation and aggregation following platelet contact with collagen, thrombus or antigen-antibody complexes. Serotonin has target organ properties similar to histamine, causing dilatation of arterioles and increased vascular permeability of venules.

Platelet Activating Factor

Platelet activating factor is a bioactive phospholipid synthesized *de novo* in leucocytes and endothelial cells in response to inflammatory stimuli. It is an extremely powerful activator of platelets and of venular endothelial permeability with a potency at least 1000 times greater than that of histamine. Platelet-activating factor can also increase leucocyte adhesion to endothelium, is probably chemotactic and can influence the degranulation of neutrophils. It is one of the important elements of inflammation and in certain experimental models the inflammatory response may be considerably subdued by the use of platelet activating factor antagonists.

Metabolites of Arachidonic Acid (prostaglandins, leukotrienes and lipoxins)

During the activation of cells as part of the inflammatory response membrane lipids are metabolized to produce inflammatory mediators. The major category of these is derivatives of arachidonic acid (Figure 4.23) derived from phospholipids by the action of phospholipases. Arachidonic acid is an unsaturated fatty acid which is a constituent of many cell membrane phospholipids. There are two main pathways of metabolism of arachidonic acid, namely the cyclooxygenase (COX) pathway and lipoxygenase pathway. The two main enzymes in the cyclooxygenase pathway are COX1 and COX2, the enzyme activity of which leads to the generation of prostaglandins. Prostaglandins may be further metabolized into three main groups of molecules, prostacyclin, thromboxane and other members of the prostaglandin family. The metabolism of prostaglandins towards these substances is dependent on the action of other enzymes, many of which have a tissue-specific distribution. Platelets contain thromboxane synthetase and metabolize prostaglandins to thromboxane A_2, which causes vasoconstriction and promotes platelet aggregation. It is short acting and rapidly converted to an inactive form.

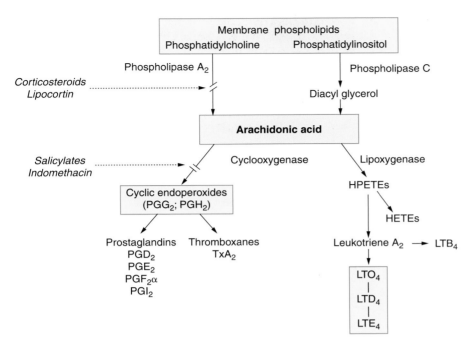

FIGURE 4.23 Formation of arachidonic metabolites. HPETE = cyclic hydroperodixes.

Vascular endothelial cells lack thromboxane synthetase but rather express prostacyclin synthetase which metabolizes prostaglandins to prostacyclin. Prostacyclin is a potent vasodilator and an inhibitor of platelet aggregation and therefore has the opposite properties to thromboxane. Some molecules remain as part of the prostaglandin family, notably prostaglandin D_2, E_2 and $F_{2\alpha}$ which promote vasodilatation and enhance the formation of inflammatory oedema through alterations in vascular endothelial permeability.

Metabolites of the lipoxygenase pathway are members of the leukotriene family. These again fall into main groups depending on their subsequent metabolism. Leukotriene B_4 is a potent chemotactic agent produced by inflammatory cells. The other leukotrienes C_4, D_4 and E_4 all promote smooth muscle contraction and endothelial cell contraction therefore enhancing vasoconstriction and causing increased vascular permeability.

Many anti-inflammatory drugs used in clinical practice act on this group of molecules. Steroids inhibit the phospholipases required for the generation of arachidonic acid. Aspirin, indomethacin and other non-steroidal anti-inflammatory drugs inhibit COX thereby reducing the generation of prostacyclin, thromboxane and prostaglandins. The anti-inflammatory properties of dietary fish oils are dependent on the metabolism of the phospholipids derived from these oils to leukotrienes, which are less potent as proinflammatory agents.

Plasma Protease Pathways

Complement

The complement system consists of more than 20 components circulating within the plasma (Figure 4.24). It is a major defence mechanism contributing to the inflammatory response and to damage of bacteria following immunologically mediated attack. There are two main pathways for the activation of complement: the classical pathway involving activation of C1 the first complement component by antigen antibody complexes, or the alternative pathway in which C3 activation occurs on microbial surfaces, polysaccharides or other microbial products. The most important step in the complement cascade is the cleavage of C3 to C3a and C3b and is the essential element to both the alternative and classical pathways. Complement activation influences three different biological functions within the inflammatory response.

C3a and C5a, the cleavage products of C3 and C5 respectively, may increase vascular permeability and cause vasodilatation by acting via release of histamine from mast cells. C5a can also activate the metabolism of arachidonic acid causing the release of further inflammatory mediators. C3a and C5a are both powerful chemotactic agents for neutrophils and monocytes and enhance the adhesion of leucocytes to endothelium thereby influencing the cellular phase of the acute inflammatory response. C3b is an important opsonin enhancing the phagocytosis of bacteria by fixation to the bacterial cell wall; C3b is recognized by receptors on the macrophage surface. Finally the membrane attack complex C5–9 may insert into bacterial cell walls leading to cell lysis. The cascade of complement activation allows amplification at each stage further enhancing its proinflammatory properties. This, however, requires regulatory mechanisms to prevent overactivity. Protein inhibitors, including the inhibitors of C3 and C5 convertases, closely regulate the activity of the complement system. There are also circulating proteins in the plasma which combine with complement components thus inactivating them. Among the most important of these is the C1 complement inhibitor.

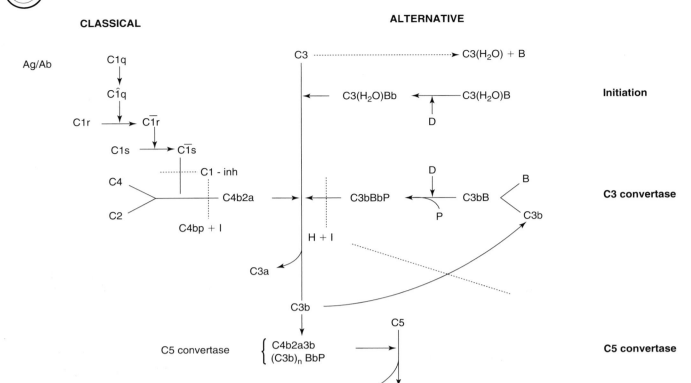

FIGURE 4.24 Outline of complement activation pathways.

Clotting and Fibrinolytic Systems

Although the major function of the clotting system is haemostatic control there are intimate links with the inflammatory response and many clotting factors are involved either with the complement or kinin cascades (Figure 4.25). Particularly important in inflammation is the activation of Hageman factor, a protein synthesized in its inactive form by the liver as part of the acute phase response. When Hageman factor is exposed to collagen in basement membranes or activated by platelets it undergoes a conformational change to become factor XIIa exposing an enzymatically active site that can act on downstream components of both the clotting and kinin cascades. Two further components of the coagulation system provide links between blood clotting and inflammation. Thrombin, which is the cleavage product of the inactive precursor prothrombin, cleaves the plasma protein fibrinogen to form fibrin, an important component of blood clot formation. However, during this process small fibrin peptides are formed which can increase vascular permeability and are chemotactic for leucocytes. Thrombin itself may activate leucocytes directly causing increased leucocyte adhesion to endothelial cells and may cause fibroblast proliferation during the healing response. Factor X when activated to factor Xa may also increase vascular permeability and enhance leucocyte exudation. During the activation of the coagulation cascade the fibrinolytic regulatory mechanism is activated. This second cascade generates the proteolytic enzyme plasmin to degrade fibrin, but it is also capable of activating the complement cascade.

The Kinin System

The kinin system generates vasoactive peptides from a group of plasma protein kininogens. These kininogens are cleaved by enzymes called kallikreins, which are formed from the cleavage of prekallikrein by factor XIIa of the coagulation system. The resulting activation of the kinin cascade releases bradykinin, a potent vascular permeability agent. Bradykinin also causes vasodilatation and excites nerve endings causing pain. The properties of bradykinin are therefore similar to those of histamine but the rate of production of bradykinin is slower because of the multiple steps involved in activating the kinin proteolytic cascade. Other elements of the kinin cascade, in particular kallikrein, have not only chemotactic activity, but also activate the complement component C5 to C5a.

There are therefore four plasma protease cascades which are intimately interlinked regulating both the inflammatory response and haemostatic properties of blood.

Cytokines

Cytokines are a variety of soluble mediators produced by inflammatory cells and by endothelium, epithelium and connective tissue during the inflammatory response. They are locally acting with rapid degradation although a few also have systemic effects. They usually act by binding to cell

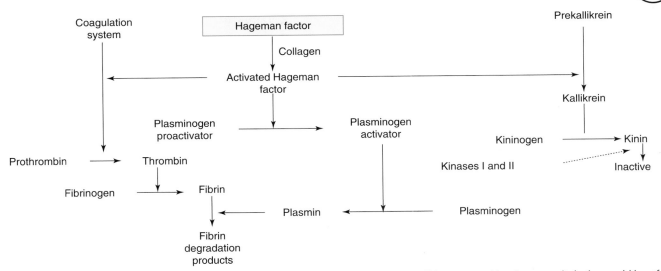

FIGURE 4.25 Hageman-factor-dependent pathways. Activation of Hageman factor (coagulation factor XII) by contact with collagen results in the acquisition of protease activity which is able enzymatically to activate the coagulation system, the fibrinolytic system and the kallikrein–kinin system. Kallikrein, an enzyme which converts kininogen to kinin, also amplifies the system by activating for Hageman factor. Kininases I and II inactivate kinins rapidly.

membrane receptors on the target cells promoting proliferation, activation and differentiation. A large number of cytokines have been described and more continue to be identified but their general properties and functional classes are of more importance than the recognition of individual molecules. Some cytokines regulate the function of lymphocytes: lymphocyte activation, proliferation and terminal differentiation. Among the most important of this category are IL2 and IL4 both of which stimulate lymphocyte proliferation whereas IL10 and TGFβ suppress lymphocyte proliferation. There are cytokines that activate effector cells within the inflammatory response particularly macrophages. Many of these cytokines are released by T lymphocytes or by target cells damaged during inflammation. Macrophage-activating cytokines include interferon γ and TNFα. Some cytokines stimulate inflammatory responses and immune responses in a non-specific manner including TNFα and IL1β, both of which are responsible for many of the systemic effects of the inflammatory response. Other cytokines stimulate the generation of white blood cells required for the leucocytosis seen in inflammation.

Chemokines are a family of small proteins acting as activators and chemotactic agents for specific leucocytes. They are divided into several groups depending on their amino-acid sequence, in particular the grouping of cystine residues. These different groups have different biological properties. CXC chemokines such as IL8 act primarily on neutrophils having been secreted by macrophages or endothelial cells attracting neutrophils to the inflammatory focus. These chemokines may be induced by other cytokines, in particular, general proinflammatory cytokines such as IL1 and TGF. C-C chemokines act mostly on macrophages and comprise the main monocyte chemoattractant proteins MCP1 (macrophage chemotactic protein) and RANTES (Regulated on Activation, Normal T-cell Expressed and Secreted). Both of

these are responsible for attracting and immobilizing monocytes within the inflammatory focus, and they also act on eosinophils and lymphocytes. They do not possess chemotactic properties for neutrophils. C chemokines possess only one of the conserved cystine residues of the chemokine family and are specific for lymphocytes. CX3C is a more recently described family and appears to exist mostly as cell surface bound chemokines promoting the adhesion between monocytes and T cells which is an important part of the inflammatory and immune responses.

Most chemokine activity is highly localized and these are therefore paracrine regulators of the inflammatory response.

Nitric Oxide

Nitric oxide is an important mediator of inflammation. It was first identified as a substance released from endothelial cells which caused smooth muscle cell relaxation and was known as endothelium-derived relaxing factor. It is produced not only by endothelial cells but also by macrophages and by certain neurones in the brain. Nitric oxide is synthesized from L-arginine, oxygen and other cofactors by the enzyme nitric oxide synthase. There are three different types of nitrous oxide synthase: endothelial, neuronal and inducible. Both endothelial and neuronal nitric oxide synthase are constitutively expressed but their level may be enhanced following stimulation of the appropriate cells. Inducible nitric oxide synthase by contrast is only up-regulated when macrophages are activated by cytokines or other agents. In the inflammatory response endothelial and macrophage generation of nitric oxide appears to be important. Nitric oxide may influence the vascular phase of the inflammatory response by causing vascular smooth muscle relaxation and hence vasodilatation. Nitric oxide is also an important part of the pathway of the generation of free oxygen radicals, which are important in macrophage killing of bacteria.

Repair

When cellular injury has resulted in necrosis of cells a repair process occurs, the aim of which is to attempt to replace the dead cells by healthy tissue. This response is referred to as healing. It involves two distinct processes:

- regeneration – in which there is replacement of injured cells by proliferation of surviving cells of the same type
- a connective tissue response characterized initially by the formation of granulation tissue (see below) and its subsequent maturation which may include scar formation (fibrosis).

The mechanisms which control the regenerative and connective tissue responses are similar and involve cell proliferation, differentiation, interactions between cells and the surrounding matrix and cell migration. The relative roles of regeneration and the connective tissue response vary in different tissues. In some tissues, for example skin, there may be complete restoration of the epithelial architecture after healing, particularly if the injury is very superficial. Elsewhere (e.g. in the central nervous system) the specialized cells cannot regenerate and the healing process is dominated by a connective tissue response. This is clearly a less satisfactory outcome for, although healing may have restored structural defects, there will be residual functional abnormalities because the specialized cells will have been replaced by scar tissue.

The outcome of a healing process is also affected by the nature, severity and duration of the injury (Figure 4.26). For example, the liver shows a remarkable capacity for regeneration. Two-thirds of the liver can be removed surgically and the remaining parenchyma will in time regenerate to the original mass and will show a normal structure. A similar remarkable degree of regeneration can occur when there is acute necrosis such as occurs following paracetamol (acetaminophen) overdose. This is a serious condition and many patients either die or require a liver transplant. However, those patients who survive without the need for liver transplantation have an essentially normal liver within a few weeks with no fibrosis. In contrast, in chronic liver injury such as occurs with hepatitis C virus, although there is ongoing regeneration, it is the connective tissue response which predominates and leads to severe scarring. A combination of liver cell regeneration and fibrosis results in the formation of liver nodules, a condition called cirrhosis (Chapter 10). In this section we shall consider the mechanisms of regeneration and the connective tissue response and see how these relate to important and common forms of healing – skin wounds and bone fractures. Before considering basic mechanisms however, we review the composition of the extracellular matrix.

Extracellular Matrix

Composition of the Matrix

The extracellular matrix is a complex structure of interacting molecules which provides structural support for tissues. It also modulates the function of surrounding cells and has an effect on proliferation, differentiation, movement and structure. The proteins which comprise the matrix are well hydrated providing turgor for soft tissues and act as a sink for growth factors which control the proliferation of surrounding cells. It also provides a base on which cells adhere and can migrate.

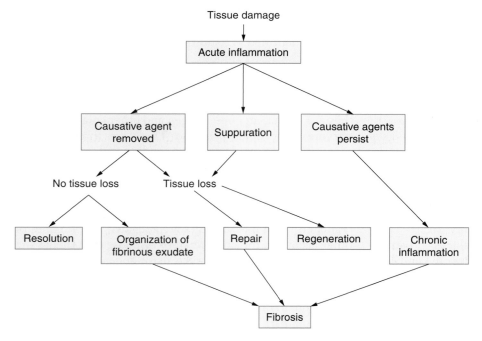

FIGURE 4.26 Sequelae of acute inflammation.

(A)

Fibroblast

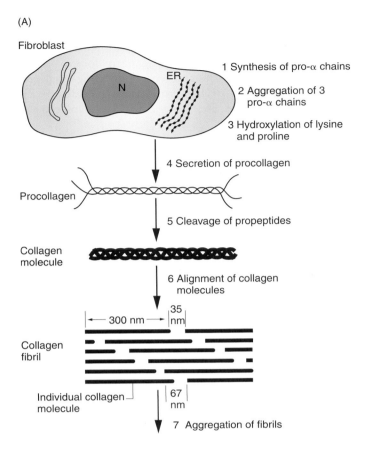

1 Synthesis of pro-α chains

2 Aggregation of 3 pro-α chains

3 Hydroxylation of lysine and proline

4 Secretion of procollagen

Procollagen

5 Cleavage of propeptides

Collagen molecule

6 Alignment of collagen molecules

←— 300 nm —→ |35 nm|

Collagen fibril

Individual collagen molecule ⌐ |67 nm|

7 Aggregation of fibrils

Collagen fibre

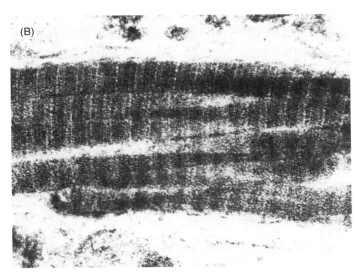

(B)

FIGURE 4.27 Principal steps in biosynthesis of interstitial collagens: (A) 1, Synthesis of pro-α chains in rough endoplasmic reticulum; 2, aggregation of three pro-α chains; 3, hydroxylation of lysine and proline residues; 4, secretion of procollagen molecule; 5, cleavage of propeptides; 6, alignment of collagen molecules to form fibrils; 7, aggregation of fibrils to form collagen fibre, seen here in longitudinal section and showing regular crossbanding (B). N = nucleus; ER = endoplasmic reticulum.

Four main groups of compounds form the extracellular matrix: (i) collagens; (ii) elastin and related proteins; (iii) structural glycoproteins; and (iv) proteoglycans/hyaluronic acid. There are two major forms of connective tissue – the interstitial extracellular matrix and basement membranes. The most common matrix protein is collagen. Collagens are a family of closely related proteins with common structural properties unique to this group of molecules. To date some 18 collagens have been described. The common property is that they all contain (at least in part), a triple helical structure formed from three protein chains (α chains). Along a substantial length of the amino acid sequence of these chains there is the repeating sequence gly-x-y. They are rich in hydroxyproline and hydroxylysine; these amino acids are formed by hydroxylation of proline and lysine, a process which requires vitamin C. In this context it is of interest that scurvy (vitamin C deficiency) results in abnormal healing.

In the case of some collagens the individual chains are identical. In others such as type I collagen, which is the most abundant form, the molecule is composed of two identical chains and one non-identical chain. Collagens are produced on the endoplasmic reticulum of mesenchymal cells such as fibroblasts and osteoblasts. The sequence of events in collagen biosynthesis is outlined in Figure 4.27. Individual collagen molecules formed line up to form fibrils and these have a banded appearance ultrastructurally. There is crosslinking of the different molecules and this stabilizes the fibrils. The sites of the major forms of collagen are summarized in Table 4.1.

Some tissues require elasticity for their function and this is facilitated by another matrix protein, elastin. This forms the core of elastic fibres found in blood vessels, skin and the lung. The elastin molecules are surrounded by a microfibrillar network containing the protein fibrillin. Elastic fibres can recoil after transient stretching and this is important in tissues such as large blood vessels and the skin.

TABLE 4.1 Types of collagen

Collagen type	Localization
I	Skin, bone, tendons (accounts for 90% of all collagen)
II	Cartilage
III	Internal organs, skin, blood vessels
IV	Basement membranes
V	Blood vessels, internal organs
VI	Widespread distribution
VII	Dermal, epidermal junction in skin
VIII	Descemet's membrane in eye
IX	Cartilage

The extracellular matrix contains several large glycoproteins which act as adhesion molecules that link matrix components to one another and to surrounding cells. The most abundant of these is fibronectin. This protein binds to other matrix components such as collagens via specific peptide domains on its molecule and to cells via a three amino acid sequence (arginine–glycine–aspartic acid) (RGD). Laminin is the principal structural glycoprotein of basement membranes. This also has cell-binding and matrix-binding domains. It has the capacity to alter the morphology and differentiation of a wide range of cell types. A new group of related proteins – so-called matricellular proteins – have been described which do not function as structural proteins, but rather appear to disrupt cell matrix interactions. These may be important during tissue remodelling and include osteonectin and tenascin.

Another important component of the extracellular matrix is a heterogeneous group of negatively charged polysaccharide chains, known as glycosaminoglycans. The most abundant of these are hyaluronic acid, chondroitin sulphate, dermatan sulphate and heparin sulphate. With the exception of hyaluronic acid, all of the compounds are linked to a core protein to form proteoglycans. These are long unbranched structures which form a water replete gel. Proteoglycans may also be found within cell membranes (e.g. syndecan).

Turnover of the Extracellular Matrix

The extracellular matrix is not a static structure. During development, for example, there needs to be substantial remodelling and even in adult tissues there is a constant (albeit low level) turnover of all matrix proteins. So-called degradation of matrix proteins is achieved by a family of metalloproteinases. Various forms exist which degrade either interstitial collagen, basement membrane collagen (type IV) or other matrix components such as the structural glycoproteins. All of the matrix metalloproteinases are produced as inactive precursors. Once activated, metalloproteinases are controlled by a family of tissue inhibitors of metalloproteinase (TIMPs).

Cell Receptors for Matrix Proteins

Integrins are the principal form of cell surface receptor by which cells can attach to the matrix. This family of proteins is also important in cell–cell interactions such as those occurring in leucocyte adhesion (p. 56). Integrins are transmembrane proteins comprisng an α and a β chain. There are over 20 different forms of integrin molecule and these have different matrix binding properties. The extracellular part of the integrin molecule binds to several of the matrix components by recognizing the RGD sequence referred to above. The integrins not only act by anchoring cells to the matrix but they transmit the effect of surrounding matrix on the structure and shape of the cells by their interaction with cytoskeletal proteins. There is also recent evidence to suggest that the binding of matrix to the integrins leads to the activation of intracellular pathways similar to those activated by cytokines and growth factors (see below), thereby influencing cell behaviour such as gene expression.

Regeneration

Proliferation of parenchymal cells forms an important part of the healing of any injured organ. The capacity for such regeneration varies between tissues, in general reflecting the degree of proliferative activity of the normal tissue (see Chapter 2).

The control of cell division and regulation of the cell cycle is discussed elsewhere. In broad terms, cell proliferation is controlled by binding of extracellular growth factors to specific receptors on the cell surface of the cells. Ligand–receptor binding in turn sets in motion a series of cascade processes or signal transduction pathways by which signals are transferred to the nucleus leading to activation of transcription factors, ultimately influencing gene expression. Of particular importance are the changes in the expression of genes which control entry into the cell cycle. This includes a number of proto-oncogenes such as c-*myc* and tumour suppressor genes such as *p53*. The cell surface receptors are of three types: (i) those which act through intrinsic tyrosine kinase activity; (ii) transmembrane receptors without intrinsic enzyme activity; and (iii) receptors linked to G proteins. There are several different forms of signal transduction pathway which link these receptors to nuclear events. The principal pathways are the MAP kinase pathway, inositol phosphate pathway, cyclic-AMP pathway, the Janus kinases (JAK)/signal transducers and activators of transcription (STATs) pathway and integrin-mediated pathways. This is almost certainly an oversimplification and there is evidence of crosstalk between the different pathways.

At least three types of extracellular signal can initiate these events. First, there are substances which are secreted by the cells themselves, i.e. a cell produces a growth factor together with the relevant receptor and can therefore control its own proliferation. This is referred to as autocrine signalling and occurs in epithelial proliferation in skin wounds and in liver regeneration and is also a feature of some tumours. The second form is where the molecules stimulating proliferation are produced by cells in the vicinity of the target cell. As we shall see, this occurs in the connective tissue response of repair where for example growth factors produced by inflammatory cells can stimulate the proliferation of endothelial and mesenchymal cells. This is referred to as paracrine signalling. Finally, substances produced at a distant site, such as a completely separate organ can also control cell proliferation. This is referred to as endocrine signalling (Figure 4.28).

There is now a wealth of information on a large number of growth factors that may be involved in regeneration. Some of these act on a wide range of cell types, but others are more specific. Many influence not only proliferation but also cell motility and differentiation. The most important factors in regeneration (particularly that of epithelial tissues) are epidermal growth factor (EGF) and the related TGFα, insulin-like growth factors (IGFs), so-called hepatocyte growth factor (HGF) and some of the fibroblast growth factor (FGF) family. In some tissues, for example in the gastrointestinal tract, there are other peptides that may

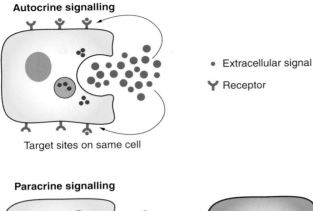

Autocrine signalling

- Extracellular signal
- Y Receptor

Target sites on same cell

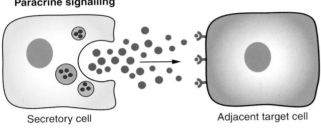

Paracrine signalling

Secretory cell

Adjacent target cell

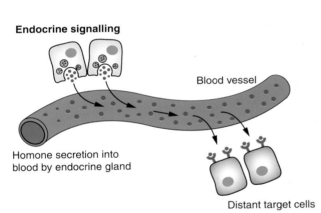

Endocrine signalling

Blood vessel

Homone secretion into
blood by endocrine gland

Distant target cells

FIGURE 4.28 Comparison of autocrine, paracrine and endocrine signalling.

of regulation when healing has occurred, for example in compensatory liver hyperplasia following hepatectomy, it is important that proliferation does not get out of control and is kept in check by inhibitory signals. There is less known about growth inhibition than proliferation, although it appears to be regulated through autocrine and paracrine means by growth factors such as TGFβ.

Connective Tissue Response

When tissues are injured there is damage not only to the epithelial cells but also to the surrounding matrix. Therefore there needs to be restoration not only of the epithelial mass, but also of the normal structural framework. It follows that in all forms of repair there is at least some connective tissue response, although as noted above the balance between regeneration and connective tissue is influenced by a number of factors including the severity and duration of the injury. The connective tissue response consists of four main processes. The first is a formation of new blood vessels, a process referred to as angiogenesis. The second is the activation and proliferation of fibroblasts and related mesenchymal cells (myofibroblasts). The third (and a consequence of the second) is the deposition of extracellular matrix proteins, in particular collagens. Finally, there is remodelling of the matrix and this includes gradual changes in the relative abundance of different matrix proteins. The processes of angiogenesis and fibroblast proliferation lead to the development of so-called granulation tissue (Figure 4.29). This name derives from the red granular appearance seen on the surface of skin wounds, but it is a process which occurs in the healing of most tissues.

play an important role. These have a unique structure – the so-called trefoil peptides.

Epidermal growth factor and TGF-α share a common receptor – the EGF receptor. This has inherent tyrosine kinase activity, and ligand–receptor binding leads to the series of signal transduction events referred to above. Epidermal growth factor is found in abundance in tissue secretions such as sweat, saliva and urine, whereas TGF-α is probably more important in the regeneration of solid organs such as liver and kidney. Another growth factor which signals through a similar pathway is HGF. This is a misnomer in that it has a wide ranging proliferative effect on a variety of cells in different tissues. Its receptor *c*-met is expressed by many epithelial cells including those of the breast and kidney. This growth factor not only controls cell proliferation, but also acts as a morphogen (controlling cell differentiation during development), controlling cell motility, particularly during regeneration. Because of the latter property HGF has also been referred to as 'scatter factor'.

It is important to recognize that there are also signals which inhibit cell proliferation. This is an important form

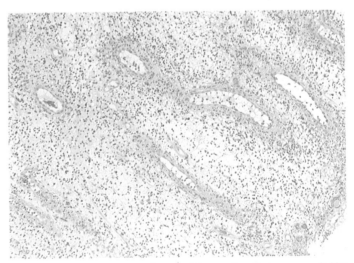

FIGURE 4.29 Granulation tissue. Note parallel rows of capillaries surrounded by oedema and inflammatory cells, many of which are neutrophils.

Angiogenesis

The process of angiogenesis involves the formation of new capillary buds (sprouts) from pre-existing vessels. It follows a sequence of events which includes (i) breakdown of the basement membrane of the pre-existing vessel; (ii) migration of endothelial cells; (iii) proliferation of endothelial cells behind the migrating cells; (iv) maturation of endothelial cells with the formation of capillary tubes; and (v) recruitment of supporting cells (pericytes) to surround the endothelial cells. The new vessel formation is thought to be critical in healing as it supplies oxygen and nutrients to the injured tissue and it ensures the delivery of both humoral and cell-mediated arms of the immune system to help prevent infection in the injured tissue. Several growth factors have been found to stimulate angiogenesis but the principal factor involved in the formation of new vessels in granulation tissue is a peptide known as vascular endothelial growth factor (VEGF). Matricellular proteins such as tenascin are also thought to have an important role in the formation and maintenance of new vessels; and there are also factors in the extracellular compartment (e.g. endostatin) that regulate angiogenesis and which act by inhibiting endothelial proliferation.

Fibrosis

One of the key elements in the development of granulation tissue is the migration, activation and proliferation of fibroblasts. This is controlled by a number of growth factors including PDGF, TGFβ, IL1, FGFs and TNFα. These are released by platelets, inflammatory cells, injured epithelial cells and endothelial cells. Other cells may also contribute, such as mast cells and eosinophils. It is thought that TGFβ is the most important profibrogenic peptide. As noted above, it acts principally as an inhibitor of cell proliferation, but in granulation tissue its main action is in switching on the fibroblasts to produce extracellular matrix proteins. Some of the fibroblasts which are involved in granulation tissue formation contain myofibrils and express the cytoskeletal protein α-smooth muscle actin. These are so-called myofibroblasts which may have contractile properties and are thought to play a role in contraction of wounds (see below).

4.1   SPECIAL STUDY TOPIC

CELL AND MOLECULAR BIOLOGY OF LIVER FIBROSIS

Fibrosis of the liver is an end result of most forms of chronic liver disease including that associated with alcohol misuse, chronic viral hepatitis and inherited metabolic diseases such as haemochromatosis. In the fibrotic liver, there is a substantial increase in most matrix proteins but in particular the interstitial collagens type I and III. These are not only present in greater amounts but are deposited in abnormal sites within the liver microanatomy. This leads to replacement of functional parenchymal tissue by scarring and to disruption of the intrahepatic blood flow as a space occupying effect.

It is now clear that the principal cell involved in liver fibrosis is a special form of mesenchymal cell which acts as a facultative (myo) fibroblast and which is now referred to as the hepatic stellate cell (Figure 4.30). This was previously called the Ito cell or fat-storing cell and is found within the perisinusoidal space of Disse (the area between the hepatocytes and the endothelium of the liver sinusoids). These cells resemble pericytes in other tissues, but have some unique properties including the expression (at least in some species) of intermediate filament proteins normally seen in either muscle cells or cells of the central

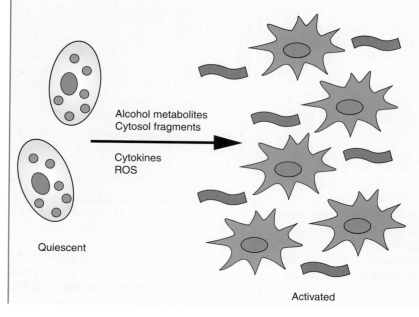

Quiescent

Alcohol metabolites
Cytosol fragments

Cytokines
ROS

Activated

FIGURE 4.30 Role of hepatic stellate cells in liver injury. Quiescent stellate cells contain abundant cytoplasmic lipid (vitamin A). In response to a number of cytokines, reactive oxygen species (ROS), proteins from dead hepatocytes and acetaldehyde, the cells proliferate, lose cytoplasmic fat and begin to resemble myofibroblasts. There is increased production of matrix proteins together with a reduction in activity of metalloproteinases which degrade the matrix. The net result is accumulation of collagen and other matrix proteins.

nervous system. In the normal liver, their principal functions are storage of vitamin A (they are the main site of storage for retinoids in the body) and regulation of the intersinusoidal blood flow through contraction and relaxation in response to vasoactive mediators.

Hepatic stellate cells are thought to be responsible for producing extracellular matrix proteins in the normal liver and contribute to the low level turnover required for maintaining the structural integrity of the liver microcirculation. However, in response to most forms of liver injury these cells become activated and undergo phenotypic transformation to become myofibroblast-like cells. They are then much more active in producing matrix proteins, in particular the interstitial collagens, become more contractile and are more responsive to vasoactive mediators. They are thus the principal driving force behind the progressive scarring that occurs in chronic liver disease, but as the result of their increased contractility they also lead to reduction of blood flow through the liver sinusoids and this contributes to the development of portal hypertension (see Chapter 10). Not only do they produce increased amounts of collagens, but on activation they produce tissue inhibitors of metalloproteinases (TIMPs), which inhibit the breakdown of collagens and other matrix proteins.

There has been recent interest in unravelling the molecular events which are associated with activation of these cells. They can be readily isolated from liver tissues and grown in primary culture. Studies using such an approach have shown that they proliferate in response to PDGF and TGFα and undergo phenotypic changes including increased collagen production in response to TGFβ and TNFα. Numerous other growth factors may also have a role, but on an equimolar basis, these four are considered to be the most important. Hepatic stellate cells however can also be activated by reactive oxygen species and other low-molecular-weight compounds including metabolites of alcohol metabolism.

The intracellular signalling cascades involved in bringing about the biological changes in activated hepatic stellate cells include the mitogen activated protein kinase (MAPK) pathway, inositol lipid pathway, the JAK/STAT pathway and integrin mediated pathway. Some of the growth factors stimulate more than one cascade pathway and this may explain why they are more active than others. For example, PDGF is more mitogenic than TGFα and recent evidence suggests that this is because whereas TGFα signals through the extracellular signal-regulated protein kinase (ERK) and stress activated protein kinase forms of the MAPK pathway, PDGF signals through these and inositol lipid pathways.

The interest in identifying the cell and molecular biological events in fibrosis is driven largely as a consequence of the current lack of specific therapies for treating liver fibrosis. Strategies are now being designed which target inhibitors of the signalling pathways to hepatic stellate cells in an attempt to prevent activation of the cells. There is also the development of strategies to not only reduce collagen production, but enhance its resorption by stimulating matrix metalloproteinases. Core aspects of liver damage and cirrhosis are discussed in Chapter 10.

HEALING OF SKIN WOUNDS

The simplest form of wound healing occurs when uninfected skin incisions are closed promptly by suturing. This is referred to as healing by first intention (or primary union). It is characterized by the formation of only minimal amounts of granulation tissue. It is a rapid process and contrasts with healing by second intention, which occurs in an open wound, the edges of which are not brought together and where there is loss of epithelium.

When an incision is made in the skin and subcutaneous tissue, blood escaping from cut vessels clots on the wound surface and fills the gap between the wound edges (Figure 4.31). In sutured wounds, this gap is narrow. Fibrin in the clot acts as a glue which holds the cut surfaces together. The dehydrated blood clot on the surface forms a scab which seals the wound. After 24 hours there is a mild inflammatory reaction at the wound edges with exudation of fluid and migration of polymorphs. Blood clot is digested by lysosomal enzymes released from polymorphs and this is contributed to from day 3 by macrophages. These cells phagocytose cellular debris, fibrin and red cells. Within 24–48 hours there is enlargement of the basal cells of the epidermis with some loss of their normally close adherence to the underlying tissue and with flattening of rete ridges. Close to the cut edge, cells from the deeper part of the epithelium begin to proliferate and slide over each other; they migrate out along the exposed surface of the dermis and become flattened to form a continuous advancing sheet. Whereas the advancing edge of the sheet of new epidermis consists of a single layer of flat cells the older part at the periphery of the wound becomes stratified so there is a gradient of thickness. The cells will only migrate over viable tissue. There may be some growth of cells down the cut edges of the dermis. This is later resorbed, although occasionally a small implantation cyst, which contains epithelium, may form.

The dermis and subcutaneous tissues are repaired by the formation of small amounts of granulation tissue. From about day 3 angiogenesis occurs at the wound margins. The newly formed capillaries are delicate and lack a basement

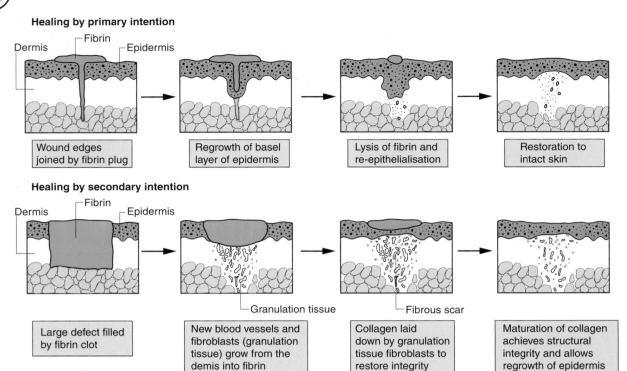

Healing by primary intention

| Wound edges joined by fibrin plug | Regrowth of basel layer of epidermis | Lysis of fibrin and re-epithelialisation | Restoration to intact skin |

Healing by secondary intention

| Large defect filled by fibrin clot | New blood vessels and fibroblasts (granulation tissue) grow from the demis into fibrin | Collagen laid down by granulation tissue fibroblasts to restore integrity | Maturation of collagen achieves structural integrity and allows regrowth of epidermis |

FIGURE 4.31 Outline of stages involved in healing of skin wounds, and comparison of primary and secondary intention.

membrane. They leak protein-rich fluid and neutrophils emigrate from them. Within a few days however, these structures differentiate into arterioles and venules. Fibroblasts stream from the perivascular connective tissue and begin to proliferate and move into the wound. Collagen and other matrix proteins are produced and these help to unite the cut edges from about day 7. By 3 weeks the total amount of collagen in the wound has reached a maximum. At this stage the tensile strength is still low, but this increases over a period of months by further modification to the matrix proteins including crosslinking between collagen fibrils. From the second week onwards there is devascularization, a process by which the newly formed blood vessels and proliferated fibroblasts gradually disappear. Some sensory nerves may gradually grow into the scar from about 4 weeks, but specialized nerve endings such as Pacinian corpuscles do not re-form. The end result of healing by first intention is usually a fine pale linear scar which is level with the adjacent surface. Occasionally, the connective tissue component of the healing process is excessive leading to a hypertrophic scar or keloid (Figure 4.32).

Healing of an open gaping wound where there has been loss of tissue occurs by the formation of more substantial amounts of granulation tissue which grows from the base of the wound to fill the defect. Angiogenesis and fibroblast proliferation are more abundant and healing takes longer than that following first intention healing. Initially, there is haemorrhage and exudation of fibrin from the cut surfaces. This is followed by a massive emigration of neutrophils and subsequently macrophages. These cells soften and remove the fibrin and other debris. As in the incised wound, epithelial cells at the margins enlarge and begin to migrate down

the walls of the wound after 24–48 hours. Migration and proliferation together produce a sheet of cells which advances in a series of tongue-like projections beneath any

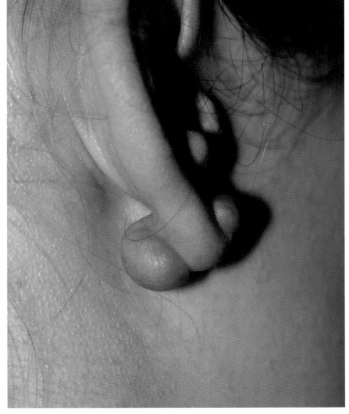

FIGURE 4.32 Keloid scar after ear piercing. (Courtesy of Dr Clifford Lawrence.)

residual blood clot on the wound surface. As the single layer of cells moves inwards towards the wound centre there is stratification of the cells near to the wound margin. As the denuded area is large, the advancing epithelial sheet does not completely cover the wound until the granulation tissue from the base has started to fill the wound space. Within a few days pre-existing vessels in the wound bed produce vascular sprouts which grow upwards forming loops and coils near the wound surface. From these new, more permeable vessels, small haemorrhages occur and neutrophils migrate reinforcing those already present in the exudate on the wound surface and help to keep down bacterial growth. This fibrovascular granulation tissue continues to proliferate and to fill the wound space until the epithelium grows over its surface, at which time the exudative inflammatory changes subside. As soon as the wound surface is covered, epithelial cell migration ceases and proliferation, stratification and keratinization are then rapidly completed although rete ridges are not re-formed.

The fibroblasts become oriented parallel to the wound surface and by the end of week 1, collagen is being actively produced which rapidly increases in amount. There is subsequently devascularization and remodelling of the collagen as described above and the dermis over a period of months becomes progressively less cellular. Healing of an open, excised wound is aided by contraction of the surface area at sites where the skin is mobile and loosely attached to underlying tissue. This movement of the edges towards the centre of the wound is brought about by so-called myofibroblasts which develop from mesenchymal cells within the connective tissue of the wound. The term 'contracture' is used when the repair process ultimately leads to distortion or limitation of movement of the tissues. This may result either from contraction of the wound itself or from scarring of the deeper muscle and soft tissues.

Several factors can alter the rate and efficiency of wound healing – local and systemic factors which can interfere with healing are outlined in Table 4.2.

HEALING OF FRACTURES

TABLE 4.2 Factors that slow down healing

Local	Systemic
Poor local blood supply and infection	Diabetes mellitus; renal failure
Excessive movement	Malnutrition
Ionizing radiation	Vitamin C deficiency

The basic processes involved in the healing of bone fractures bear resemblance to many of those seen in skin wounds (Figure 4.33). Primary union is rarely found, however, and there is usually a marked connective tissue response involving osteogenic cells. Continuity between bone fragments is first established by a mass of new bony

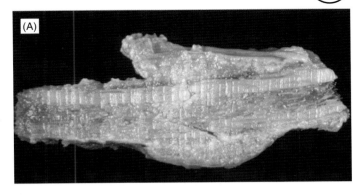

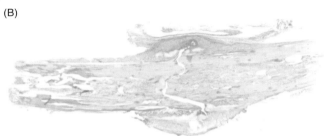

FIGURE 4.33 Fracture healing. This segment of rib was excised from a woman aged 22 years, who complained of a painful swelling in the chest wall, of a few weeks' duration. The preoperative diagnosis was of a tumour of bone. (A) The gross specimen shows an irregular fracture line involving both cortices and the medullary canal. The fracture is bridged by periosteal callus, which is particularly marked on the superior surface. (B) Histological examination shows that the periosteal callus consists of arcades of reactive bone and a mass of cartilage overlaying the fracture line. There is also callus within the medullary canal. At this relatively early stage of fracture healing, the fracture gap remains unrepaired.

trabeculae and cartilaginous tissue (provisional callus). This undergoes slow remodelling with resorption, so that under favourable conditions firm bony union is achieved. Sometimes this is so efficient that the original fracture site can hardly be identified.

A good deal of force is required to break a bone. The fragments are usually displaced and there may be haemorrhage between the bone ends. There may also be substantial haemorrhage into the adjacent tissues. Inflammatory changes take place with exudation of protein-rich fluid from which fibrin is deposited. Neutrophils are scanty unless there is infection and this is common only in compound fractures when a bone fragment has torn the overlying skin. Macrophages invade and phagocytose the clot and tissue debris. Bone necrosis occurs chiefly as a result of tearing of blood vessels in the medullary cavity, cortex and periosteum. Damage to the bone marrow may have serious results when globules of fat enter torn local vessels, producing fat emboli (see p. 108). When there is splintering of bone (comminuted fracture) some of the fragments may lose their blood supply. These become necrotic and if small enough are eventually resorbed by osteoclasts. Bone death is recognizable histologically by the loss of osteocytes from bone lacunae.

There are three components to the formation of provisional callus:

- Periosteal reaction. The cells of the inner layer of the periosteum proliferate in a wide zone overlying the cortex of each fractured bone end. A cuff of bone trabeculae is formed around each bone at right angles to the cortex and anchored to it. Mixed with this there may be nodules of cartilage formed. The two enlarging cuffs of callus advance towards each other and finally unite to bridge the fracture line. This bandage of external callus helps to immobilize the fragments in an unstable or poorly fixed fracture. The amount of bridging periosteal callus varies greatly between different sites. In fractures occurring within a joint capsule (e.g. some fractures of the neck of femur) there is no periosteum and union occurs almost entirely due to internal callus formed by osteoblasts lying in the medullary cavity (see below). In contrast fractures of the long bones such as humerus form large amounts of external callus with relatively little internal callus.

- Medullary reaction. The first evidence of healing in the medullary cavity is the advance of capillaries from viable marrow into necrotic marrow. This is followed by emigration of macrophages and proliferation of fibroblasts and osteoblasts. The osteoblasts produce new woven bone in the marrow spaces. The new bone is deposited partly on the surface of dead trabeculae which when surrounded by new bone may remain unabsorbed for months or even years.

- Cortical reaction. In viable cortex adjacent to the fracture there is an increase in osteoclastic resorption with widening of the Haversian canals. This may be followed later by some osteoblastic activity. Similar changes are seen in the dead cortex of the bone ends once there has been revascularization of the Haversian canals from adjacent vessels in viable bone, or from periosteal and medullary vessels.

The periosteal callus unites the fragments externally, but there remains a gap within the fracture itself. This is initially filled with blood clot. This becomes replaced by granulation tissue in which there are varying amounts of osteoblasts and fibroblasts. Bony union of the fracture gap may occur through two processes. Direct ossification is brought about by osteogenic cells from the medullary and periosteal callus and is rapid and effective. By contrast a process of fibrous union may occur initially in which there is initially collagen laid down and this is only later ossified to become bony tissue. This slower form of union occurs when there is instability or separation of the bone ends. It also occurs more often when there is poor blood supply or infection. Occasionally ossification fails to occur leading to an unstable healed fracture (non-union).

Once bony union has occurred and function has been regained, the bone begins to be remodelled in response to mechanical stresses. Excess callus is resorbed, slowly formed lamellar bone begins to replace the hastily laid down woven bone and any remaining necrotic bone is removed and replaced. The cortex is re-formed across the fracture gap and gradually medullary callus is removed and the marrow cavity restored. The whole process may take about a year and is more rapid and complete in children.

SUMMARY

- Cellular and tissue stress may lead to adaptation responses which include hypertrophy, hyperplasia, atrophy and metaplasia.
- When the capacity for adaptation is exceeded, there is cellular injury which may be reversible or irreversible.
- Cell death (irreversible injury) occurs through two distinct mechanisms – necrosis and apoptosis.
- Inflammatory and repair processes are designed to limit the adverse effects of cellular injury and death but may themselves contribute to tissue damage.
- Acute inflammation is the initial response to most forms of tissue injury and comprises a vascular phase and a cellular phase in which neutrophil polymorphs have an important role.
- Acute inflammatory processes may be followed by resolution, abscess formation, development of chronic inflammation and/or healing with fibrosis.
- Chronic inflammation lacks the vascular component of acute inflammation and is characterized by an infiltrate of lymphocytes and macrophages.
- Repair processes are designed to restore tissue integrity and consist of both regenerative and connective tissue responses.
- The balance between regeneration and fibrosis varies depending on the tissue and nature of injury as does the outcome.
- Some repair processes lead to complete restitution of tissue integrity whereas in others there is replacement of functional tissue by dense scar tissue.

FURTHER READING

Kumar V, Abbas AK, Fausto N. *Robbins and Cotran Pathologic Basis of Disease*, 7th edn. Philadelphia: Saunders, 2004.

Majno G, Joris I. *Cells, Tissues and Disease. Principles of General Pathology*, 2nd edn. Oxford: Oxford University Press, 2004.

Solomon L, Warwick DJ, Nayagan S. *Apley's Concise System of Orthopaedics and Fractures*, 3rd edn. Hodder Arnold, 2005.

CANCER AND BENIGN TUMOURS

5

Robin Reid and David J Harrison

CASE HISTORY 5.1

NEOPLASIA (CANCER AND BENIGN TUMOURS)

History

A 63-year-old man presented to his general practitioner with a history of 3 months' increasing breathlessness and a non-productive cough. He was an electrician, and had worked in a shipbuilding yard for over 40 years. He admitted to having smoked 25 cigarettes per day since the age of 16 years.

On clinical examination he was noted to have finger clubbing; his fingers were heavily stained with nicotine. On examining the chest, there was evidence of diminished air entry at the left base.

Investigations

A left-sided hilar mass was seen in the chest X-ray. Bronchial biopsy showed a moderately differentiated squamous cell carcinoma (Figure 5.1).

The recommended treatment was surgical, and a left pneumonectomy was done (Figure 5.2). Histological examination confirmed the biopsy diagnosis and showed that the surgical resection margins were free of tumour. Tumour had, however, involved the parietal pleura and the lymph node metastases suspected on gross examination were confirmed histologically. The tumour was staged as T3 N1 M0.

The patient made a good recovery from surgery, but at a routine outpatient clinic appointment 18 months later,

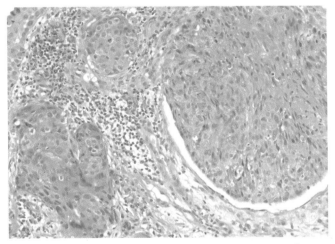

FIGURE 5.1 This bronchial biopsy shows islands of large tumour cells which are cohesive and have long cell-to-cell borders. Keratin production is not, however, prominent.

he complained of fatigue and recent onset of backache. On examination, his liver was found to be enlarged, and a radiograph of his spine showed multiple areas of bone destruction with collapse of the body of T8. Palliative radiotherapy was given to the spine with good pain relief, but the patient died 3 months later. At post mortem, multiple bony metastases (secondaries) were found in his liver and spine.

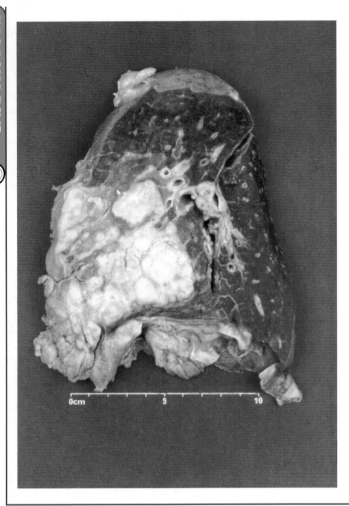

COMMENTARY

This patient died of lung cancer, the commonest malignant tumour in the Western world. The case raises a number of points including:

- What is a cancer?
- How do tumours develop?
- Why did this patient develop this tumour? Were his cigarette smoking and his occupation in any way responsible? If so, why did he develop the tumour when many equally heavy smokers do not?
- How do metastases develop, and why do they occur in the sites they do?

FIGURE 5.2 This section of left lung shows a large white tumour which extends to the pleural surface to which parietal pleura is attached. Two peribronchial lymph nodes contain what appears to be white tumour.

CANCER EPIDEMIOLOGY

Key Points

- Cancer is predominantly a disease of the middle aged and elderly.
- The varying incidence of cancer in different populations may indicate the underlying causes of these tumours.
- Environment and genetics are important in determining cancer risk but the former is more significant.
- Smoking and diet are major predisposing causes.

Epidemiology is the branch of medicine which describes the prevalence of a disease. It was formerly known as 'geographical pathology'. Through studying the geographical distribution of a type of cancer, its racial prevalence and the occupations of those who have developed it, much can be understood both about the risk factors and underlying pathogenic mechanisms. To draw meaningful epidemiological conclusions about cancer, precise diagnoses must be made, then accurately registered with cancer registration organizations and, ideally, there should be good follow-up information to determine mortality.

The Global Cancer Burden

The World Health Organization publishes annual cancer mortality statistics for most countries, and its subsidiary, the International Agency for Research on Cancer, issues a regular statistical analysis known as Cancer Incidence in Five Continents. It is estimated that about 10 million new cases of cancer are diagnosed each year and cancer accounts for around 12% of all deaths worldwide. The annual total is predicted to rise to 15 million per year in 2020 as the population increases and ages; cancer is predominantly a disease of the middle-aged and elderly.

Taking all forms together, cancer is the second commonest cause of death in developed countries and has recently overtaken heart disease to become the major killer in some Western societies, killing around 25% of the population. The major human cancers are carcinomas (malignant epithelial tumours); lymphoma (malignant lymphoid tumours) ranks about tenth, and sarcomas (malignant connective tissue tumours) are rarer still. The commonest cancer in men is bronchial (lung) carcinoma, followed by stomach, colorectal and prostate carcinomas. Worldwide, carcinoma of the breast is the commonest cancer in women, but in some areas, for example west Scotland, the incidence of lung cancer in women exceeds breast as smoking habits of women have changed. Cervical, colorectal and endometrial carcinomas are also relatively common.

The risk of developing a cancer depends on many different factors, among them age, sex, geographical location, race, occupational history, social habits and socio-economic class. Some of the factors that influence the risk of cancer are discussed below.

Age

Overall, cancer particularly affects the middle aged and elderly, but different tumour types have different age profiles. Some particularly affect infants (e.g. neuroblastoma, nephroblastoma), childhood (e.g. acute lymphoblastic leukaemia) and adolescence (e.g. osteosarcoma). Hodgkin's disease, a form of lymphoma, has a bimodal peak affecting young adults and then the middle aged to elderly. Carcinomas, the commonest cancers, tend to affect the middle aged and elderly, the incidence generally increasing with age.

Geographical Variations

There are striking regional variations in cancer incidence throughout the world. Many of these variations appear to be due to environmental factors such as carcinogens rather than genetic factors. In southeast Asia and Africa, hepatocellular carcinoma is common due to the high prevalence of hepatitis B infection and environmental exposure to carcinogens, for example aflatoxins present in mouldy groundnuts. Chewing betel-quid and areca-nut, a practice common in Asia, is recognized to be carcinogenic. Malignant melanoma is mainly a disease of white-skinned people and is especially common in sunny climates such as Queensland, Australia, where many of the population are fair-skinned individuals of northern European extraction. Exposure to high levels of ultraviolet light can cause cancer. Gastric carcinoma is common in the former Soviet Union, in Japan and in China, whereas its incidence in Western countries has progressively fallen, perhaps due to altered dietary habits and to the decline of infection with *Helicobacter pylori*. Breast and colorectal carcinoma are far commoner in Western countries than in Asia.

Changing Patterns of Disease and Effects of Migration

Careful epidemiological studies of large populations who have migrated around the world have demonstrated that the incidence of cancers in migrant populations rapidly moves towards that of the recipient country. For example, the incidence of gastric carcinoma in Japanese migrants to the west coast of America falls from the high level seen in Japan to the lower incidence in the USA by the second generation of immigrant families. These data strongly suggest that environment is more important than heredity in determining geographical variation in cancer risk. It is thought that environmental factors account for over 80% of human tumours.

Diet

In general, diets rich in fruit and vegetables are associated with lower risks of many major forms of cancer including tumours of the lung, stomach, breast and colon. In contrast, a diet rich in animal fat is statistically linked to increased incidence of cancers of breast, colon, prostate, pancreas and endometrium. The risk of colon cancer in a population is directly proportional to the extent of meat consumption. A diet rich in salted fish is associated with high incidence of gastric and nasopharyngeal carcinoma. Alcohol consumption is linked to tumours of the breast, colon and liver and acts in a synergistic manner with smoking in tumours of the aerodigestive tract.

Cigarette Smoking

It is now generally acknowledged that cigarette smoking is responsible for at least a quarter of cancer deaths, especially from cancers of the lung, larynx, oral cavity and to a lesser extent the urinary tract. Most of the effects are due to direct contact with carcinogens in smoke, but these are also absorbed and excreted through the kidneys. Many carcinogens are present in smoke including benzopyrene and dimethylnitrosamine. There is a direct relationship between the number of cigarettes smoked and the risk of lung cancer, and, although stopping smoking reduces this risk, its effects are not totally reversible.

GENERAL FEATURES OF TUMOURS

A neoplasm, literally a new growth, is classically defined as an abnormal mass of tissue, whose growth is uncoordinated with and exceeds that of the normal tissues. It results from aberration of the normal mechanisms which control cell number: these are cell production by cell division and cell loss by the process of apoptosis. Most tumours are monoclonal, i.e. all the cells in a tumour appear to have risen from one parent cell which has undergone a genetic change, which is then passed on to all its progeny. Because the tumour cells lack the normal control mechanisms, the clone expands due to uncontrolled proliferation. Although the tumour is derived from one clone, further genetic changes develop in some of the progeny, so that the tumour may become heterogeneous, a property described as clonal evolution.

Classification of Tumours

Tumours are divided into two major groups according to their behaviour: benign and malignant. Benign tumours remain localized at their site of origin. They grow by expansion, pushing the normal tissues away, often with the formation of a capsule of compressed fibrous tissue. Benign tumours usually grow slowly, but despite their name, are not always benign in clinical terms. Their effects are described on p. 91.

Malignant tumours, also known as cancers, grow by infiltrating into the surrounding normal tissues and have the ability to spread to distant sites, to metastasize, where secondary deposits, metastases, form. The histological appearance of metastases resembles that of the primary tumour. While malignant tumours usually grow rapidly, it should be recognized that not all malignant tumours are equally malignant. Some are highly aggressive and metastasize early, for example small cell carcinoma of bronchus. Others are slow growing and although they are locally infiltrative, they rarely metastasize. Basal cell carcinoma (p. 498) and chondrosarcoma are good examples of this. The degree of malignancy, described as tumour grade, usually correlates well with survival. The features of benign and malignant tumours are shown in Figure 5.3 and summarized in Table 5.1.

Histogenesis of Tumours

Tumours are further classified according to the differentiation they show. This property is usually determined by the tumour's appearance on light microscopy, i.e. its phenotype. The term 'histogenesis' – meaning tissue of origin – is used because most tumours resemble to some extent the tissue from which they arise, although tumours of course arise from primitive stem cells so the concept of histogenesis is not very helpful scientifically. It is now clear that the phenotype and

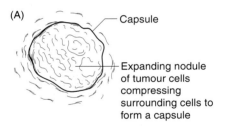

(A)
— Capsule

— Expanding nodule of tumour cells compressing surrounding cells to form a capsule

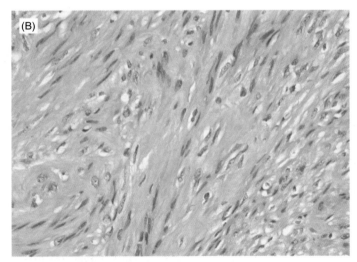

(B)

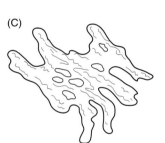

(C)

Infiltrating crab-like processes invading surrounding normal tissue

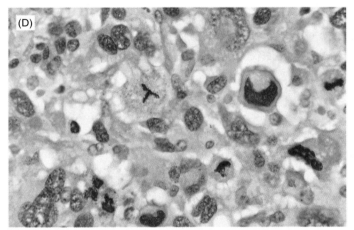

(D)

FIGURE 5.3 (A) Benign tumours are well circumscribed and the surrounding tissue often forms a capsule of fibrous tissue. (B) The cells of benign tumours closely resemble those of the normal tissue in which they arise. The nuclei are normal. As growth is slow, mitoses are uncommon, and as division is normal mitotic figures are of normal appearance. (C) Malignant tumours have infiltrative margins both on naked eye and on microscopic examination. (D) The nuclei are usually enlarged and the nucleoli active, indicating that the cell is active. The nuclei are often darkly staining – hyperchromatic – and variable in size and shape – pleomorphic – as the DNA content of the nucleus is frequently increased. Mitoses are often numerous and they are frequently abnormal in form indicating that the process of cell division may be abnormal. A tripolar mitosis is one in which the chromosomes are attempting to segregate towards three daughter cells.

TABLE 5.1 Differences between benign and malignant tumours

	Benign	**Malignant**
Growth pattern	Expansion, remain localized	Infiltrate locally, spread to distant sites (metastasize)
Growth rate	Slower	Faster
Clinical effects	Local pressure effects; hormone secretion	Local pressure and destruction; inappropriate hormone secretion; distant metastases
Histology	Resembles tissue of origin	Many differ from tissue of origin (less well differentiated)
Nuclei	Small, regular, uniform	Larger, pleomorphic
Mitoses	Few, normal	Numerous, including atypical forms
Treatment	Local excision	Local excision and systemic therapy if metastases present

histogenesis of a tumour are not necessarily synonymous: thus rhabdomyosarcoma, a malignant tumour showing skeletal muscle differentiation, may arise at sites in which no skeletal muscle is normally found. Increasingly, traditional histological ways of defining the phenotype of a tumour are being complemented by molecular biology techniques such as the polymerase chain reaction and gene chip array technology to determine the genes expressed by tumour cells.

It is important to understand that some highly malignant tumours do not show any definite form of differentiation. These tumours are described as poorly differentiated or as anaplastic.

Epithelial Tumours

Benign Epithelial Tumours

Benign tumours may arise from both covering epithelium, for example of squamous type, forming papillomas, and from glandular epithelium, for example of colon or thyroid, forming adenomas.

Papillomas

Papillomas are warty growths in which the proliferating epithelium is thrown upwards into folds, and does not invade into the underlying connective tissue. Between these folds of epithelium are cores of fibrous tissue and blood vessels which bring nutrition to the epithelium. In general, the epithelium is well differentiated and closely resembles the normal epithelium from which it arises. Typical examples are squamous papillomas of skin or larynx (Figure 5.4) which are usually viral in origin. Papillomas may arise within duct structures, for example intraduct papillomas of the breast which often cause a blood-stained nipple discharge.

Adenomas

Adenomas are benign tumours of glandular epithelium. The tumour cells in such a tumour form glandular structures mimicking the arrangement of the normal tissue (Figure 5.5).

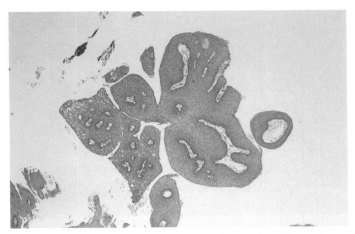

FIGURE 5.4 Squamous papilloma, larynx. This lesion consists of finger-like projections of squamous epithelium with central connective tissue cores.

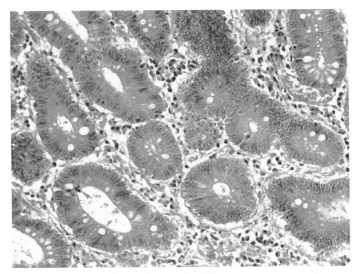

FIGURE 5.5 Adenoma of colon. Several gland-like structures are present, mimicking the structure of normal colonic mucosa.

The cells are well differentiated and often continue to secrete the normal product of the gland; thus the cells of a colonic adenoma may produce mucin or a thyroid adenoma thyroglobulin. If the glands become distended by secretion they may form cysts – resulting in a multiloculated lesion described as a cystadenoma, which may be found in the ovary or pancreas. Sometimes, especially in the ovary, there is proliferation of epithelium within the cyst, often in the form of papillary structures – papilloma-like growths with central fibrovascular cores – and the term papillary cystadenoma is used.

Adenomas of viscera such as the colon tend to grow into the lumen, and often adopt a papillary architecture. Some are sessile and are thrown into greatly thickened papillary folds – so called villous adenoma – whereas others become pedunculated with a stalk of normal mucosa – these are known as tubular adenomas (Figure 5.6).

Squamous Carcinomas

These are tumours showing squamous differentiation (Figure 5.7) in the form of keratin production or the presence of intercellular bridges, which on electron microscopy can be seen to be desmosomes. Squamous carcinomas can arise from pre-existing squamous epithelium, for example of skin or larynx, but some, for example of bronchus and cervical transformation zone, arise at sites where there is normally glandular epithelium, but where squamous metaplasia has been followed by malignant change. Squamous carcinomas resemble normal squamous epithelium to varying extent. Well-differentiated tumours show maturation from proliferating basal cells through acanthotic cells resembling the stratum spinosum to heavily keratinized cells. Poorly differentiated tumours show much less maturation, often with no keratin production, but consist of sheets of cells joined by intercellular bridges.

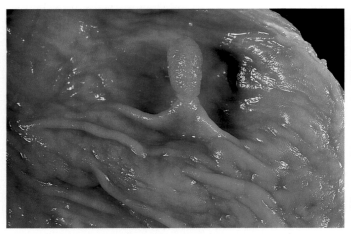

FIGURE 5.6 Tubular adenoma of colon. This is a small pedunculated polyp on a slender stalk.

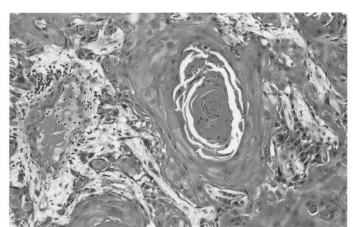

FIGURE 5.7 Squamous carcinoma. This is an example of a well-differentiated tumour with irregular islands of squamous epithelium, and one showing central keratinization.

In most benign tumours, the cytological features closely resemble those of the normal tissue from which they arise. Colonic adenomas are an exception – they usually show a varying degree of cytological atypia with a high nuclear: cytoplasmic ratio and increased mitotic activity – features known as dysplasia. The importance of this lies in the risk of malignant change to carcinoma. This is described as the adenoma–carcinoma sequence; the underlying molecular biology of this process is now well understood (p. 256). It is important to realize that the paradigm does not mean that every single tumour follows the same route or necessarily harbours identical genetic abnormalities.

Malignant Epithelial Tumours (Carcinomas)

Carcinomas are the commonest type of malignant tumour in humans. They fall into several different subtypes, depending on the form of differentiation they show.

Adenocarcinomas

These are tumours showing glandular differentiation. They usually arise from glandular epithelium, for example within the stomach, endometrium or colon, and may arise from metaplastic glandular tissue, for example at the lower end of the oesophagus in Barrett's oesophagus when chronic acid reflux has resulted in metaplasia. Adenocarcinomas may be well differentiated – forming well-defined glandular structures known as acini (Figure 5.8) – but in poorly differentiated forms there may be only occasional glandular structures or evidence of mucin production. In some tumours, typically of stomach, individual cells contain intracytoplasmic globules of mucin; these push the nucleus to one side – the tumour cells are known as signet-ring cells (Figure 5.9). In other mucin-producing tumours there is extensive extracellular accumulation of mucin that forms large lakes in which scattered epithelial cells are seen. These are known as mucoid carcinomas, and are seen in stomach, colon and breast.

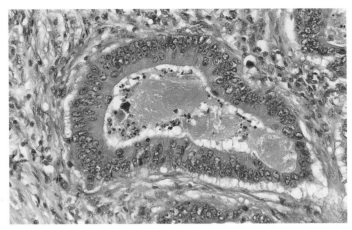

FIGURE 5.8 **Adenocarcinoma.** The tumour cells form an acinar structure. The nuclei contain prominent nucleoli.

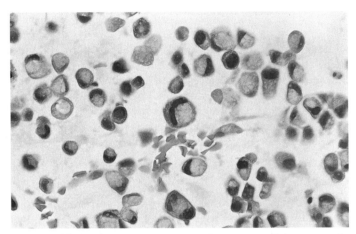

FIGURE 5.9 **Signet-ring cell cancer of stomach.** The tumour cells have eccentric nuclei, pushed to the side by a central globule of mucus.

Some adenocarcinomas, like cystadenomas, form large cystic spaces (cystadenocarcinoma) and may have papillary ingrowths (papillary cystadenocarcinomas); these are typically found in the ovaries.

Transitional Cell Carcinoma

Transitional cell carcinoma arises from the transitional epithelium of the urogenital tract. It too may show considerable variation in appearance: well-differentiated papillary transitional cell carcinomas resemble papillomas, and may not show any invasion of the underlying stroma, but they are regarded as malignant for practical purposes because they have a high risk of recurrence, often in a more aggressive form. Poorly differentiated transitional cell carcinomas have a more solid architecture and frequently invade deeply within the wall of the bladder or ureter.

Small Cell Carcinoma

Small cell carcinoma is a tumour which shows neuro-endocrine differentiation in the form of neurosecretory granules which may be found on electron microscopy or immunostaining for vesicle membrane proteins such as synaptophysin. Typically, it arises in the bronchus, where it is the most aggressive form of lung cancer, but occasionally in other sites such as the cervix and oesophagus.

Other forms of carcinoma include hepatocellular carcinoma, the malignant tumour of the hepatocytes, and basal cell carcinoma, a variety of skin cancer which is often locally destructive, but which seldom metastasizes.

Connective Tissue Tumours

The connective tissues are fibrous tissue, fat, nerve, muscle, blood vessels, bone and cartilage. Both benign and malignant tumours can be found, which show differentiation towards one of these forms. It is likely that all arise from primitive mesenchymal stem cells which retain the ability to differentiate in many directions.

Benign Connective Tissue Tumours

The nomenclature of these tumours is straightforward – the name consists of a prefix indicating the type of differentiation, for example lipo- (fat), chondro- (cartilage), haemangio- (blood vessel), with the suffix -oma denoting a benign tumour. Most are slowly growing encapsulated tumours composed of the appropriate differentiated tissue. The commonest form is a leiomyoma, a benign tumour showing smooth muscle differentiation, often occurring in the uterine muscle (p. 409). Lipomas are also common tumours, usually occurring in the subcutaneous tissues of adults, typically on the back and shoulders. They consist of an encapsulated mass of mature fat. These, and other benign tumours, are discussed in appropriate chapters in this volume.

Malignant Connective Tissue Tumours

These are known as sarcomas (Greek *sark* = flesh). They are far less common than carcinomas. Most occur within the deep soft tissue of the limbs and trunk, although some arise within viscera. There are numerous different types. Like benign tumours, the nomenclature indicates the form of differentiation shown: for example a leiomyosarcoma is a malignant tumour showing smooth muscle differentiation (Figure 5.10).

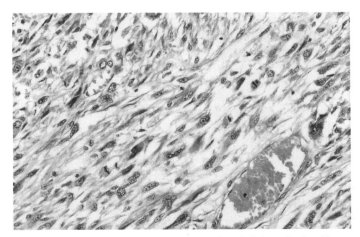

FIGURE 5.10 **Leiomyosarcoma.** This tumour consists of elongated cells with a cigar-shaped nucleus and eosinophilic cytoplasm. There are several mitoses in this field.

Rhabdomyosarcomas show skeletal muscle differentiation and are among the commonest tumours of childhood. Well-differentiated examples contain myosin and actin myofilaments so well orientated that cross-striations similar to those found in normal skeletal muscle can be seen. In poorly differentiated tumours, the diagnosis is made on the basis that proteins found in skeletal muscle (e.g. desmin, myoglobin) or involved in skeletal muscle differentiation (e.g. $MyoD_1$) can be demonstrated by immunochemistry.

Some sarcomas tend to occur in soft tissue, for example liposarcoma, leiomyosarcoma and malignant peripheral nerve sheath tumours; soft tissue sarcomas are discussed on p. 363. Some, such as osteosarcoma and chondrosarcoma, occur preferentially within bone (p. 345).

Tumours of Haemopoietic and Lymphoid Tissues

Leukaemias

These are malignant tumours of haemopoietic cells, derived from stem cells within the bone marrow. From the marrow the malignant cells, like their normal white cell counterparts, tend to migrate into the peripheral blood so that there is usually an elevated white cell count (leukaemia – *leukos* [white], *hamia* – blood). There is often widespread infiltration of other organs such as liver and spleen. Leukaemia is therefore a diffuse form of tumour, and the usual concepts of tumour spread do not apply. Leukaemias fall into two broad categories – tumours of lymphoid and myeloid cells, and within each group the cells may be primitive or fairly mature and associated with a rapidly progressing or indolent natural history, respectively. The four main types – acute lymphoblastic leukaemia, chronic lymphocytic leukaemia, acute myeloblastic leukaemia and chronic myelocytic leukaemia, together with less common variants are discussed on p. 215.

Lymphomas

These are malignant solid tumours of lymphocytic origin, most of which arise in lymph nodes, spleen, thymus or bone marrow. A smaller proportion, around 30%, arise in other organs such as the gastrointestinal tract, thyroid and brain, usually within lymphoid tissue resulting from chronic inflammatory conditions, such as *Helicobacter* gastritis and Hashimoto's thyroiditis. Lymphomas may remain localized to the site of origin for some time or they may be widely disseminated. They are broadly divided into two groups – Hodgkin lymphoma and non-Hodgkin lymphoma, on the basis of the distinctive large cells known as Reed–Sternberg cells (Figure 5.11) present in Hodgkin lymphoma. Non-Hodgkin lymphoma falls into two main groups – those derived from B cells or T cells. In recent years immunocytochemical and molecular biological techniques have been applied to these tumours to determine the form of differentiation of the cells in different types, in comparison with normal lymphoid cells; for example it is now apparent that Reed–Sternberg cells of Hodgkin lymphoma, are of B cell lineage. Lymphomas are discussed in detail on p. 191.

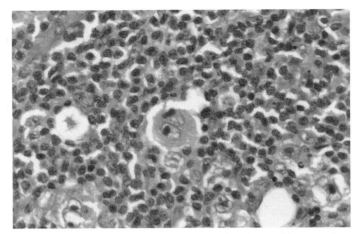

FIGURE 5.11 Hodgkin lymphoma. A typical Reed–Sternberg cell is present in the middle of the field. It is binucleate with an 'owl's eye' appearance due to the large eosinophilic nucleoli.

Leukaemias and lymphomas are related tumours, and there is some overlap: for example chronic lymphocytic leukaemia and well-differentiated lymphocytic lymphoma are essentially the same disease, but one label is applied when the disease predominantly affects marrow and peripheral blood, and the other when enlarged lymph nodes are the presenting complaint. No true benign tumours have been described in either group.

Germ Cell Tumours

Tumours may arise from the germ cells, and are therefore usually found within the testis or ovary. Occasionally, however, they may arise from nests of germ cells which have been left behind during embryonic migration of germ cells from the posterior dorsal ridges. Germ cell tumours can therefore be found, usually in the midline, from the pineal, base of skull, mediastinum and retroperitoneum to the sacro-coccygeal region.

Normal germ cells are totipotent – they give rise to all tissues found within the body and to the placenta and yolk sac, tissues described as extraembryonic. Unsurprisingly, therefore germ cell tumours may contain differentiated tissue from any of the three layers of the embryo – ectoderm, mesoderm and endoderm – and from the extra-embryonic tissues. Tumours of this type are teratomas. These are commonest in the ovary (Figure 5.12), where they are almost always benign, and, less commonly but with a rapidly rising incidence, within the testis where they are almost always malignant. In benign tumours, such as those of the ovary, the tissues may be very well differentiated resembling normal skin, thyroid, brain or cartilage. Malignant tumours, as might be predicted, contain much less well-differentiated tissues, but curiously often form differentiated tissues under the influence of chemotherapeutic drugs.

Some germ cell tumours consist of undifferentiated cells which resemble primitive germ cells. These are known as seminomas when they arise in the testis and dysgerminomas when they arise in the ovary.

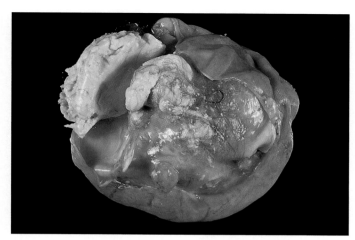

FIGURE 5.12 Benign cystic teratoma of ovary. This cyst is lined by squamous epithelium and is filled with sebaceous material and hair.

Tumours of Neuroectoderm

Many tissues of the body are derived from neuroectoderm – the brain, neurones and supporting glia, peripheral nerves, including axons and their supporting Schwann cells, and melanocytes. Tumours derived from these cells are discussed in detail in the appropriate chapters.

The nomenclature of tumours is summarized in Table 5.2.

SPREAD OF MALIGNANT TUMOURS

> **Key Point**
>
> Forms of tumour spread include:
> - local spread
> - lymphatic spread
> - blood (haematogenous spread)
> - transcoelomic spread
> - intraepithelial spread.

Malignant tumours spread in several ways which will first be described in general terms and then the complex underlying mechanisms will be outlined.

Local Spread

Malignant cells have the ability to insinuate themselves between adjacent normal cells and invade the surrounding tissues. For epithelial tumours the first step is for the tumour cells to breach the basement membrane, i.e. to proceed from the stage of intraepithelial neoplasia to that of an invasive tumour (Figure 5.13). It is at this point that the cells of the tumour can be said to have become malignant. Tumour cells follow the paths of least resistance and spread easily through loose fibrous and adipose tissue (Figure 5.14). Dense fibrous tissue such as fascia and periosteum tend to form more of a barrier, but are eventually also penetrated.

TABLE 5.2 Tumour nomenclature

Tissue of origin	Benign	Malignant
Epithelial		
Covering epithelia	Papilloma	Carcinoma, typically squamous
Glandular epithelia	Adenoma (cystadenoma)	Adenocarcinoma (cystadeno-carcinoma)
Connective tissue	Benign (*-oma*)	Malignant (*-sarcoma*)
Muscle		
Smooth	Leiomyoma	Leiomyosarcoma
Skeletal	Rhabdomyoma	Rhabdomyosarcoma
Bone forming	Osteoma	Osteosarcoma
Cartilage	Chondroma	Chondrosarcoma
Fibrous	Fibroma	Fibrosarcoma
Blood vessels	(Haem)angioma	Angiosarcoma
Adipose	Lipoma	Liposarcoma
Other tissues		
Lymphoid	No benign lymphoid tumours recognized	Lymphoma (Hodgkin lymphoma or non-Hodgkin lymphoma)
Haemopoietic	No benign ones recognized	Leukaemia
Primitive nerve cells	Ganglioneuroma	Neuroblastoma, retinoblastoma and others
Glial cells	None benign	Glioma (e.g. astrocytoma)
Melanocytes	Pigmented naevi (moles)	Malignant melanoma
Mesothelium	None	Malignant mesothelioma
Germ cells	Teratoma	Teratoma, seminoma

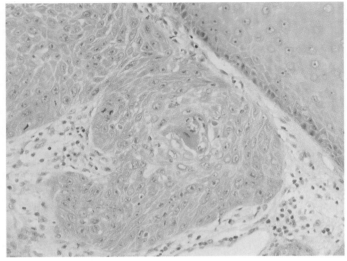

FIGURE 5.13 Early invasive squamous carcinoma. Small groups of tumour cells have broken free from the overlying epithelium and have invaded the underlying connective tissue.

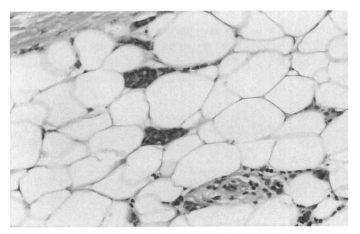

FIGURE 5.14 Local invasion by breast carcinoma. The tumour cells have spread along paths of least resistance, here through adipose tissue.

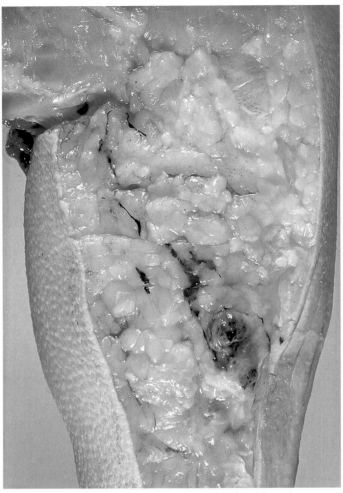

FIGURE 5.15 Lymphatic spread. This malignant melanoma has spread extensively through the lymphatics (outlined in black by melanin) in the leg.

Lymphatic Spread

This is the principal mode by which carcinomas spread. The very thin walls of lymphatics are readily penetrated by tumour cell tissue (Figure 5.15), which is carried along in the lymph to the first lymph node in the lymph node chain, the sentinel node. Whether this node is involved by tumour is now recognized to be important in planning the extent of surgery, for example melanoma or carcinoma of the breast. At first, the tumour cells are seen in small groups in the subcapsular sinus tissue (Figure 5.16), but they extend through the sinuses and gradually replace the node; they then spread proximally along the chain of lymph nodes (Figure 5.17). Ultimately they may reach the thoracic duct and enter the superior vena cava from which further dissemination through the blood stream may occur.

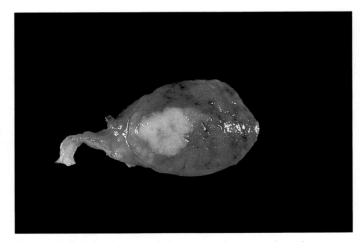

FIGURE 5.16 Early involvement of a lymph node by metastatic carcinoma. A nodule of white tumour is present under the subcapsular sinus.

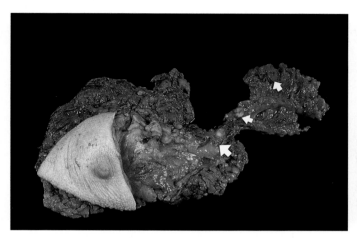

FIGURE 5.17 Breast carcinoma showing lymph node involvement. The tumour lies just lateral to the nipple. The largest arrow indicates the first node in the chain. This and the node marked by the next arrow are both involved by metastatic carcinoma. The third node is free from tumour.

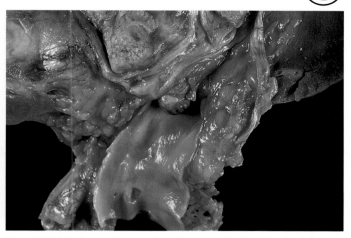

FIGURE 5.18 This large yellow renal carcinoma is seen invading along the opened renal vein. Tumour can propagate via the inferior vena cava and reach the heart.

Blood (Haematogenous) Spread

Tumour cells are also able to invade thin walled veins and grow along the venous system or embolize into the blood stream. The site of initial metastasis (first-pass organ) depends on the venous drainage of the location of the tumour. Most tumour emboli pass through the right heart and impact in the pulmonary capillary bed, whereas many tumours of splanchnic origin, for example of bowel, metastasize by blood to the liver along the portal vein. Visceral tumours also invade blood vessels which communicate with the paravertebral venous plexus of Batson, a complex system of valveless veins. Retrograde flow occurring, for example when intra-abdominal pressure is raised, is responsible for the common metastases to the spine seen for example in prostate carcinoma. Tumour emboli from the lungs enter the systemic circulation and may be widely disseminated to the brain or elsewhere. In contrast to the thin-walled veins, the thick walls of arteries are resistant to invasion by tumours.

It is not only the anatomical features of blood flow which explain the sites of metastases. The term 'seed and soil' was coined in the nineteenth century to describe the tendency of some cancers to spread to specific sites. This is now explicable in terms of tissues bearing the appropriate extracellular matrix and cell adhesion molecules.

Sarcomas usually spread through the blood stream and carcinomas, which usually initially spread through lymphatics, often spread by blood in the later stages. Renal carcinoma shows a particular tendency to invade the renal vein (Figure 5.18).

Transcoelomic Spread

Transcoelomic spread means spread across body cavities, the peritoneal, pleural and pericardial spaces. These provide no planes of resistance so that once tumour cells gain access to the open spaces they readily spread widely. This is best seen in intra-abdominal tumours, especially ovarian carcinoma,

which disseminates throughout the abdomen often resulting in a mass of tumour matting loops of gut together. Gastric carcinoma can spread in a similar fashion, to involve the peritoneal cavity, often seeding in the ovaries. When these ovarian metastases are bilateral in premenopausal women they are known as Krukenberg's tumours.

Intraepithelial Spread

This is the process by which tumour cells can infiltrate between the cells of a normal epithelium, without invading the underlying stroma. It is best seen in Paget's disease of the nipple (p. 430) in which the cells of ductal carcinoma *in situ*

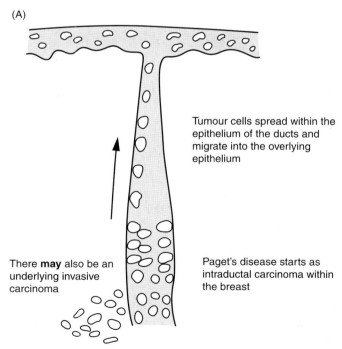

(A)

Tumour cells spread within the epithelium of the ducts and migrate into the overlying epithelium

There **may** also be an underlying invasive carcinoma

Paget's disease starts as intraductal carcinoma within the breast

FIGURE 5.19 Paget's disease of the nipple. The mechanism of development is shown in (A) and the resulting eczema-like appearance of the overlying skin in (B).

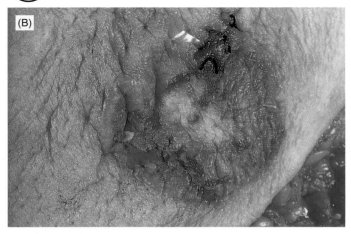

FIGURE 5.19 (Continued)

TABLE 5.3 Spread of tumours

Tumour	Blood	Lymphatic	Transcoelomic
Carcinoma	Common, late	Common, early	Stomach, ovary
Melanoma	Common, late	Common, early	Rare
Sarcoma	Common, early	Rare	Rare

grow into the nipple skin (Figure 5.19) giving an appearance resembling eczema. Extramammary Paget's disease is seen in the vulva and anorectal region and may complicate malignant skin adnexal tumours.

The mechanisms of tumour spread (Table 5.3) and the process of metastasis (Figure 5.20) are complex and not simply due to the anatomy of blood flow.

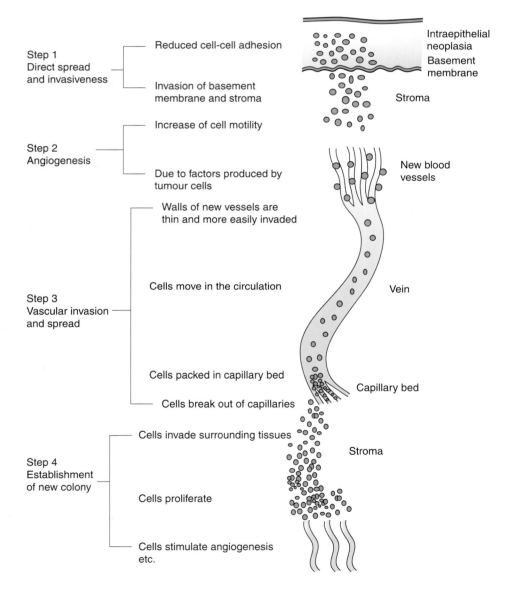

Step 1
Direct spread
and invasiveness
— Reduced cell-cell adhesion
— Invasion of basement membrane and stroma

Step 2
Angiogenesis
— Increase of cell motility
— Due to factors produced by tumour cells

Step 3
Vascular invasion
and spread
— Walls of new vessels are thin and more easily invaded
— Cells move in the circulation
— Cells packed in capillary bed
— Cells break out of capillaries

Step 4
Establishment
of new colony
— Cells invade surrounding tissues
— Cells proliferate
— Cells stimulate angiogenesis etc.

Intraepithelial neoplasia
Basement membrane
Stroma
New blood vessels
Vein
Capillary bed
Stroma

FIGURE 5.20 The process of tumour spread (metastasis). This diagram outlines the basic process of blood-borne metastasis. More detail is provided in the accompanying Special Study Topic 5.1.

SPECIAL STUDY TOPIC

MECHANISMS OF TUMOUR SPREAD

Invasion and metastasis are part of a complex multistep process involving cell:cell and cell:matrix interactions in which cell adhesion molecules of various types are involved. Here the spread of carcinomas is described, but similar concepts apply to other tumours.

Step 1 Direct Spread and Invasiveness

Reduction in Cell:Cell Adhesion

Normal epithelial cells bind tightly to one another by molecules such as E-cadherin (epithelial cadherin), a member of a family of calcium dependent cell–cell adhesion molecules. Malignant epithelial cells are less firmly attached to one another, due at least in part to reduced expression of E-cadherin, and this correlates with the invasiveness of the tumour, for example in breast carcinoma. In colonic carcinoma and gliomas loss of N-CAM (neural cell adhesion molecule) plays a similar part.

Invasion of Basement Membrane and Stroma

Initially, the tumour cell must attach to the basement membrane by interaction between cell surface integrins and matrix proteins such as laminin and fibronectin. A wide variety of alterations in integrin expression are seen in cancer cells. Next, the tumour cells produce proteolytic enzymes such as collagenase and stromelysin (members of the group of zinc-containing matrix metalloproteinases [MMPs]), which break up the matrix proteins laminin, fibronectin and collagen. These proteolytic enzymes are under complex control mechanisms; they are produced in an inactive form (proenzyme) and require activation. MMP inhibitors are being developed for clinical use. In addition, there is a group of naturally occurring antagonists known as tissue inhibitors of metalloproteinases (TIMPs). Other proteins including plasminogen activators and cathepsins are involved in matrix breakdown.

Tumour Cell Motility

Invasion of the basement membrane and underlying stroma requires that the tumour cells are motile. The cells extrude pseudopodia at the front and attach to stromal proteins. Movement is generated by the cytoskeleton of crosslinked actin molecules, and is stimulated by a wide variety of growth factors, stromal components and cytokines, for example autotaxin.

Step 2 Angiogenesis

Angiogenesis is the process by which new blood vessels are formed. It is seen in embryogenesis, in wound healing and in chronic inflammation. In recent years its importance in tumour development has been recognized. The development of a rich blood supply around the tumour is a critical step (described as the 'angiogenic switch') in the progression from a small localized tumour to a large one with the potential for metastasis. The mechanisms involved are complex and are summarized here.

Initially, the tumour consists of a morula of cells, deriving nutrition from pre-existing blood vessels. The distance over which nutrients can diffuse limits the tumour size. New blood vessels are formed by outgrowth of endothelial cells from post-capillary venules into the tumour mass. The stimulus for this is the increased production of angiogenic factors by the tumour cells, especially vascular endothelial growth factor (VEGF), fibroblast growth factors and angiogenin. Normally, angiogenesis is controlled by a balance between these angiogenesis promoting factors and inhibitors of angiogenesis such as angiostatin and endostatin. The steps involved in angiogenesis include:

- proteolytic digestion of basement membrane by plasminogen activators and matrix metalloproteinases
- migration of endothelial cells, initially as a solid cord
- proliferation of endothelial cells
- organization of the cords of endothelial cells into new blood vessels with lumens.

Although these mechanisms are not yet fully understood, inhibition of angiogenesis is being investigated as a potential new form of anticancer therapy.

Step 3 Vascular Invasion

Tumour cells must breach the basement membrane and penetrate between endothelial cells; the thin walls and poorly formed basement membranes of newly formed blood vessels are easy to penetrate. Once tumour cells are free within the lumen of the blood vessel they are carried into the circulation and lodge in a capillary bed.

At this site, further complex interactions are required. The tumour cells bind to endothelial cells, mediated by selectins and certain isoforms of CD44, a hyaluronic binding protein. The cells then penetrate the capillary basement membrane by mechanisms similar to those described above. Angiogenesis is again necessary for the establishment of any metastasis greater than 1 mm or so.

Step 4 Establishment of a New Colony

This involves cell proliferation and the development of a tumour blood supply by stimulation of angiogenesis as previously described.

It will be apparent that the process of metastasis is not simply determined by simple mechanical factors. It has long been recognized that some sites are much more prone to metastasis than would be determined simply by their blood flow – the role of the tumour and the recipient tissue being described as 'seed and soil'. In addition, not all cells in a tumour are equally likely to metastasize: the acquisition of the ability to metastasize is determined by the expression of a series of genes whose normal function appears to be the control of cell migration during embryogenesis, normal tissue homeostasis and inflammation and repair. Finally, it should be noted that some metastases can lie dormant for many years before becoming apparent. This phenomenon of 'latency' involves balance between cell proliferation and cell loss by apoptosis, but also the extent of angiogenesis.

PREMALIGNANCY

Key Points

Three main groups of lesions can be regarded as premalignant:
- malignant change in benign tumours
- intraepithelial malignancy/dysplasia
- malignancy developing in chronic inflammation.

Familial syndromes in which there is an increased risk of malignancy are described on p. 97.

Benign Tumours which Undergo Malignant Change

Examples include colonic adenomas which may become adenocarcinomas, a relationship described as the adenoma:carcinoma sequence, the molecular basis of which is dealt with in Chapter 9. Polyps may be solitary (or few) in sporadic cases or more numerous in inherited susceptibility syndromes. Other benign tumours which may undergo malignant change are neurofibromas (p. 319).

Intra-epithelial Malignancy: Carcinoma *In Situ* and Dysplasia

This is a key concept in understanding carcinomas. At numerous sites (Table 5.4) it is possible to identify a stage of pre-invasive neoplasia, where the epithelial cells show the cytological features of malignancy but have not yet developed the ability to invade adjacent normal tissues. This process has been known as dysplasia, carcinoma *in situ* and more recently as 'intraepithelial neoplasia'. It can affect epithelia of all types – squamous, transitional (e.g. bladder) and glandular (e.g. stomach). In squamous epithelia the key feature is a loss of the normal maturation which occurs from the basal layer, where proliferation normally takes place, to the surface where fully mature cells are found. Detection at this early stage allows treatment to be given before local invasion occurs and metastasis is possible. This is the basis of the cervical screening programme (p. 404) in which the abnormal cells from cervical intraepithelial neoplasia (CIN) can be seen in cervical smears.

TABLE 5.4 Major sites of intraepithelial neoplasia

Site	Terminology
Cervix	CIN (cervical intraepithelial neoplasia)
Vulva	VIN (vulval intraepithelial neoplasia)
Vagina	VAIN (vaginal intraepithelial neoplasia)
Prostate	PIN (prostatic intraepithelial neoplasia)
Skin	Carcinoma *in situ*
Breast	Ductal and lobular carcinoma *in situ*

Similar changes can be seen in the vulva, the vagina, the bladder, the skin, but none of these is currently part of a screening programme. In other tissues, for example endometrium and breast, a range of proliferative lesions can be seen, from simple hyperplasia through hyperplasia with cytological atypia to *in-situ* malignancy (carcinoma *in situ*). Like CIN, if these are diagnosed and treated at a preinvasive stage, the prognosis is much improved.

Breast screening aims to detect carcinoma *in situ* and also small invasive carcinomas, with the hope of diagnosis before metastases have occurred. Dysplastic changes can also be seen in the metaplastic intestinal epithelium found in the oesophagus in Barrett's oesophagus, an important precursor of adenocarcinoma of the oesophagus (p. 232).

Chronic Inflammatory Conditions

The increased proliferation found in inflammatory and reparative conditions appears to predispose to the development of malignancy. Examples include longstanding ulcerative colitis in which there is an increased risk of colonic cancer and Hashimoto's thyroiditis in which lymphoma may develop. Hepatocellular carcinomas typically arise in livers affected by cirrhosis (Figure 5.21).

CLINICAL EFFECTS OF TUMOURS

Not all tumours are symptomatic. Many are found incidentally on X-ray or at post mortem and all tumours pass through a stage when they are too small to cause any effects.

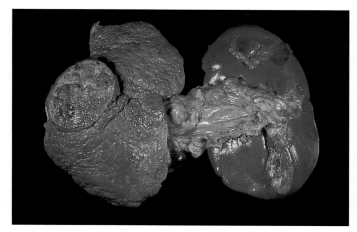

FIGURE 5.21 Cirrhotic liver on left with large spleen (due to portal hypertension) on right. A large hepatocellular carcinoma has arisen in the cirrhotic liver.

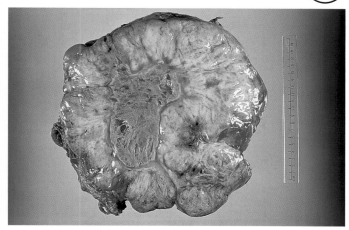

FIGURE 5.22 Central necrosis is a feature of many highly malignant tumours such as this large soft tissue sarcoma.

Benign Tumours

Despite their name these are not always harmless. As they remain localized at their site of origin, the effects fall into three broad categories:

- The presence of a palpable lump, often painless, but occasionally causing discomfort.
- The effects of substances produced by a tumour. The cells of a benign tumour are well differentiated and often retain the function of the tissue of origin such as production of hormones. This is usually outwith the normal feedback mechanisms and overactivity may result, e.g. a thyroid adenoma may lead to hyperthyroidism.
- The effects on adjacent tissues due to pressure from expansion of the tumour. This is seen particularly when the tumour arises in a confined area, e.g. within the cranial cavity. Thus, a pituitary adenoma may cause hypopituitarism by compressing the surrounding normal glandular tissue. The distortion of the uterine cavity by a fibroid (leiomyoma) often results in heavy menstrual blood loss, while a benign tumour may block a hollow viscus, e.g. by causing intussusception (p. 253).

Malignant Tumours

Direct Effects

Malignant tumours may cause a palpable mass which often grows rapidly and compresses adjacent structures such as nerves with resulting pain. Despite the angiogenesis they induce, cancers often outgrow their blood supply so that there is central necrosis (Figure 5.22). Blood loss due to haemorrhage from an ulcerated carcinoma may be acute or chronic, thus leading to iron deficiency anaemia. Carcinomas often cause narrowing (stenosis) or complete obstruction of a hollow viscus (Figure 5.23).

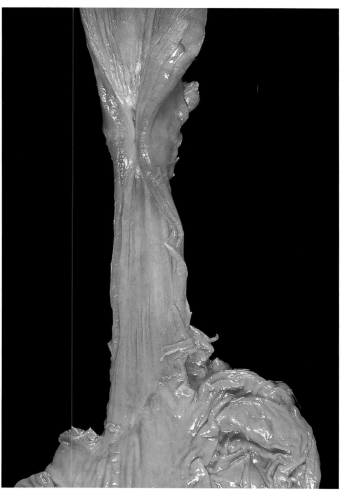

FIGURE 5.23 This carcinoma of the oesophagus had caused a tight stricture, resulting in dysphagia.

Metastatic Effects

Metastases can cause similar mass effects to primary tumours, but because they are usually multiple (Figure 5.24) the

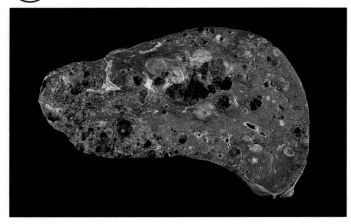

FIGURE 5.24 Metastatic melanoma in the liver. Note the numerous deposits of tumour, some deeply pigmented and others more pale. The liver was greatly enlarged. The patient had had an eye removed for a malignant melanoma many years before.

TABLE 5.5 Common sites of metastases and their effects

Site	Effects
Lung	Haemoptysis, pneumonia, pleural effusion
Bone	Pain, fracture, spinal cord compression
Liver	Hepatomegaly, jaundice, hepatic failure
Brain	Seizures, stroke, raised intracranial pressure
Bone marrow	Anaemia, leucopenia, thrombocytopenia

consequences tend to be more severe. The common sites of metastases and their effects are summarized in Table 5.5.

Non-metastatic Effects

This is a heterogeneous group of disorders, many due to release of cytokines such as interleukin 1 (IL1) and tumour necrosis factor α (TNFα) from tumour cells. Patients with advanced cancer are often wasted (cachectic) with weight loss, anorexia and fever. Immunosuppression, abnormalities of coagulation, for example thrombophlebitis migrans, and neurological disorders, for example neuropathy, cerebellar degeneration and the Eaton-Lambert syndrome, a syndrome resembling myasthenia gravis, may all be seen.

Inappropriate Hormone Production

Many tumours produce hormones not normally produced by their tissue of origin. These include antidiuretic hormone (ADH) and adrenocorticotrophin (ACTH) typically secreted by small cell carcinoma of the bronchus. Many tumours including squamous carcinomas produce parathyroid hormone related peptide which has a parathormone-like action and results in humoral hypercalcaemia of malignancy.

The typical effects of common cancers are summarized in Table 5.6.

TABLE 5.6 Common cancers and their effects

Cancer	Effects
Lung	Cough, haemoptysis, chest pain, pneumonia, pleural effusion, obstruction of the superior vena cava, metastases to bone, liver, brain
Breast	Lump, early spread to nodes, bone, lung, liver
Colon	Altered bowel habit, obstruction, anaemia; metastases to liver
Prostate	Urinary symptoms, metastases to bone
Pancreas	Obstructive jaundice, back pain
Kidney	Mass, haematuria, metastases to lung, bone
Oesophagus	Dysphagia, anaemia, early local spread and metastases
Lymphoma	Lymph node enlargement, infection, marrow replacement
Leukaemia	Anaemia, infection, bleeding (marrow replacement)

PATHOLOGICAL DIAGNOSIS OF TUMOURS

Although clinical, radiological and biochemical findings all contribute towards the diagnosis of a tumour, the final diagnosis is made in almost all cases by microscopic examination: a so-called tissue diagnosis. Depending on the procedure used to obtain a sample for examination, the entire lesion, a large or small sample, or a few cells may be studied.

Biopsies for Histopathological Assessment

These allow assessment both of the appearance of the tumour cells and of their relationship to normal tissues, i.e. the tissue architecture.

Excisional Biopsy

In this process, usually performed for relatively small tumours, the entire lesion is removed and submitted for examination.

Incisional Biopsy

In this process, the surgeon exposes the tumour and removes a wedge of tissue giving a fairly large and hopefully representative specimen. On the basis of the biopsy result, either immediately by frozen section or after a day or so, the appropriate therapy can be instituted.

Needle Biopsy

Many tumours, including deep-seated ones under radiological control, can be sampled by needle biopsy in which a thin core of tissue is removed (Figures 5.25 and 5.26). This technique provides small amounts of tissue. This may not be representative of the entire lesion, i.e. there is a potential for sampling error.

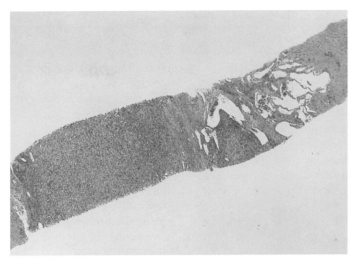

FIGURE 5.25 Needle biopsy of mass in thigh shows a highly cellular tumour. There was enough tissue for immunohistochemistry to confirm the diagnosis of Ewing's sarcoma (see Chapter 12).

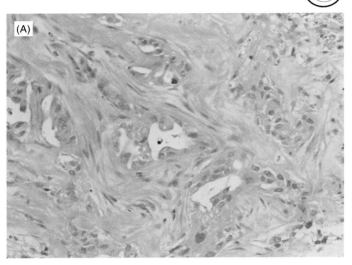

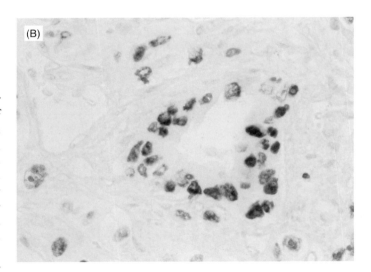

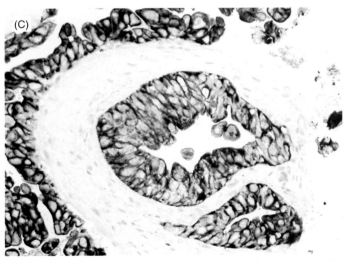

Cytology

In recent years there has been an explosion in the use of cytology to obtain cells for study. This technique relies largely on interpretation of the appearance of the individual cells, although the degree of cohesion of the tumour cells (a feature of epithelial tumours) can also be assessed. Cells can be found easily in body fluids, for example extracted by syringe and needle from the pleural or peritoneal cavities, or in urine or sputum. Fine needle aspiration of solid tumours is now routine; it has the benefit of being relatively atraumatic to the patient who usually does not require an anaesthetic. It is a simple procedure for superficial lesions, for example breast lumps, and deeply located lesions can be sampled under imaging control.

Conventional Diagnosis and Additional Techniques

In most cases, for example carcinomas of breast, colon or lung the diagnosis is made on H&E-stained sections applying the conventional criteria of malignancy. Simple histochemical techniques, for example for the detection of glycogen, mucopolysaccharides and pigments such as melanin help in some cases. Immunohistochemistry, using antibodies to cell constituents, contributes much to the diagnosis of poorly differentiated tumours (Figure 5.27) and often allows a precise diagnosis to be made on small needle biopsies. Some of the commoner markers are listed in Table 5.7. Immunostaining has largely superseded electron microscopy in this regard. Recently, molecular biology techniques such as *in-situ* hybridization have been used to detect gene expression as a way of determining tumour type, but this is of limited clinical usefulness so far. A number of tumour types, especially lymphomas, leukaemias and sarcomas have been

FIGURE 5.26 This needle biopsy is from the paraspinal tissue of a 40-year-old woman. The H&E-stained section (A) shows an adenocarcinoma. Strongly positive immunostaining for thyroid transcription factor 1 in the nuclei (B), and cytokeratin 7 in the cytoplasm (C), indicate that the likely primary is in the lung.

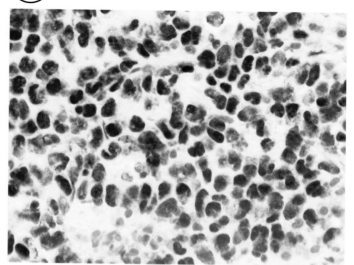

FIGURE 5.27 Immunocytochemistry is a powerful tool in determining the histogenesis of poorly differentiated tumours. Here, the nuclei stain strongly for myoD$_1$, a marker of skeletal muscle differentiation, allowing the diagnosis of rhabdomyosarcoma to be made with confidence.

TABLE 5.8 Commonly used tumour markers

Marker	Tumour
α-Fetoprotein	Teratoma; hepatocellular carcinoma
Human chorionic gonadotrophin (hCG)	Choriocarcinoma; teratoma
Prostate-specific antigen	Prostatic carcinoma
CA125	Ovarian carcinoma
Carcinoembryonic antigen	Carcinoma, e.g. gut, lung
Calcitonin	Medullary carcinoma of thyroid
Thyroglobulin	Follicular and papillary carcinomas of thyroid

TABLE 5.7 Common immunocytochemical markers of value in cancer diagnosis

Marker	Nature	Tumour
Cytokeratins	Intermediate filaments	Carcinomas*, rare sarcomas
Desmin	Intermediate filament	Muscle tumours
Glial fibrillary acid protein	Intermediate filament	Gliomas
CD45	Glycoprotein	Lymphomas
α- Fetoprotein	Oncofetal antigen	Teratoma; hepatocellular carcinoma
Human chorionic gonadotrophin (hCG)	Hormone	Choriocarcinoma; teratoma
Prostate-specific antigen	Protein	Prostatic carcinoma
CA125	Glycoprotein	Ovarian carcinoma
Calcitonin	Hormone	Medullary carcinoma of thyroid
Thyroglobulin	Hormone	Follicular and papillary carcinomas of thyroid

*In recent years it has become common practice to determine the cytokeratin profile of a metastatic carcinoma in an attempt to determine the site of origin; for example colonic carcinoma typically expresses CK20 and not CK7, whereas ovarian carcinoma is CK7 positive and CK20 negative.

shown to have characteristic chromosomal rearrangements which can be detected by karyotyping, i.e. examination of chromosomes, or by nucleic acid techniques (Chapter 3).

Tumour Markers

These substances are produced by tumour cells, are detectable in the blood, and are of value in diagnosis and in monitoring progress following treatment. Many are oncofetal antigens, proteins that are usually produced by fetal cells but not by normal mature adult cells. Examples are given in Table 5.8, and are discussed in more detail in appropriate chapters.

TUMOUR STAGING AND GRADING

Once the diagnosis of cancer is made, it is important to predict the likely behaviour of a tumour, both to decide the appropriate therapy and to estimate the patient's survival. The two main factors are the biological nature of the tumour, the grade, and its extent, the stage.

Different grading systems have been developed for various tumour types. The main parameters are:

- mitotic activity
- nuclear pleomorphism
- degree of differentiation
- extent of necrosis.

TABLE 5.9 TNM staging of gastric carcinoma

Stage	Explanation
T1	Tumour in mucosa or submucosa
T2	Tumour penetrates muscularis propria
T3	Tumour erodes through serosa
T4	Tumour involves adjacent organs
N0	No nodal metastases
N1	Metastases in 1–6 regional lymph nodes
N2	Metastases in 7–15 regional lymph nodes
N3	Metastases in more than 15 regional lymph nodes
M0	No distant metastases
M1	Distant metastases

Tumour stage can also be assessed in a number of ways. The TNM system, developed by the Union Internationale Contre le Cancer (UICC) is applied to many tumour types especially carcinomas. In this scoring system an increasing number is ascribed to more extensive disease, at the primary site *T*, in the draining lymph nodes *N* and distant sites of metastasis *M* (Table 5.9). Other systems include the Dukes' staging system for colonic carcinoma (p. 255). Tumour stage correlates well with outcome in most tumour types.

CARCINOGENESIS

Aetiology of Cancer

Cancer is not a single disease, and different cancers have different causes. In some tumours a single major factor is implicated, but in most tumours multiple factors are involved. The clues to our understanding of the causes of cancer come from several sources, but it is clear that environment, genetic predisposition and interindividual variability in coping with toxic injuries are all important.

Environmental Factors

Chemical Carcinogenesis

Many chemicals have been implicated in causing cancer in humans. Sometimes this is based on strong epidemiological evidence, for example lung cancer and cigarette smoking or bladder cancer in aniline dye workers, but it may also be assumed from animal experiments. A list of some chemicals associated with human cancer is given in Table 5.10.

From animal studies it became apparent that chemicals acted in different ways to cause cancer. Some acted directly, while others required metabolic conversion to an active form. Many chemicals are weakly carcinogenic but that potency is much increased when chemicals are given in combination or sequentially. From these observations the multistep theory of carcinogenesis evolved. Initiation leads to

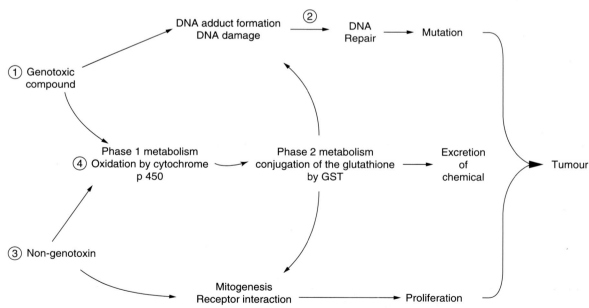

FIGURE 5.28 (1) A genotoxin may directly interact with DNA or do so following metabolic activation, e.g. by one of the cytochrome P450 enzymes. DNA adducts are formed or direct DNA strand breakage occurs. (2) Defective DNA repair may result in mutations which affect key genes such as those involved in regulating the cell cycle, apoptosis or differentiation leading to tumour formation. (3) Non-genotoxins do not have direct effects on DNA but cause cell proliferation by deregulating normal cell cycle activity. (4) Many of the enzymes involved are polymorphic, that is there is a sequence variation in the gene that may reflect a change in expression, inducibility of the gene or function. At each stage of metabolism there is variability between individuals in terms of exposure levels and also the metabolic activity determined both by the genotype of the individual and level of expression and function of the enzymes. GST = glutathione S-transferase.

TABLE 5.10 Some chemicals associated with human cancer

Chemical	Occurrence	Tumour
Alkylating agents	Chemotherapy	Leukaemia
Asbestos	Insulation	Mesothelioma
Benzene	Solvents	Leukaemia
Nickel	Mining	Lung cancer
Nitrosamines	Dietary	Gastric carcinoma
Polycyclic hydrocarbons	Incomplete burning of organic material	Lung, bladder carcinoma
Radon	Mining	Lung cancer
Vinyl chloride	PVC monomer	Angiosarcoma of liver

DNA damage and mutation of cells followed by promotion where there is clonal expansion of the abnormal cell eventually giving rise to cancer. Although useful conceptually it has become apparent that this model is too simple. Some chemicals appear to be initiators and promoters, so-called complete carcinogens, but not all of these cause DNA damage. A further complication is extrapolation from animal experiments to the human state for several reasons. First, humans and rodents have markedly different metabolic pathways in some respects and may therefore cope with a potential carcinogen in quite different ways. Second, the capacity of human cells to repair damage may differ. Third, animal experiments tend to rely on a constant, relatively high exposure to one or a few agents whereas in the human context exposure to potential carcinogens occurs intermittently, frequently at low dose, and as complex mixtures rather than single agents.

It is perhaps more useful therefore to think of carcinogens as being either genotoxic, that is causing DNA damage, or non-genotoxic. This concept is illustrated and explained in Figure 5.28. Of critical importance is being able to recognize and identify carcinogens and use the information to plan accordingly. They may be present in the environment as pollutants, derived during preparation of food, produced as a byproduct of industry or a therapeutic drug.

Radiation

There is much evidence that ionizing radiation can induce cancers. Radiation-induced cancers were seen in early radiologists, who used their own hands to calibrate their equipment. Many of the survivors of the atomic bombs which fell on Hiroshima and Nagasaki in 1945 later succumbed to tumours, especially carcinomas and leukaemias. An increased incidence of cancer, especially of the thyroid, was seen in the aftermath of the nuclear explosion at Chernobyl in 1986. Therapeutic irradiation, principally in the treatment of cancer may be followed several years later by the development of second tumours, both carcinomas and sarcomas.

Ionizing irradiation acts by damaging DNA. Both single- and double-strand cleavage is seen. Breaks in a single strand of DNA are repaired but, especially in rapidly growing cells this may be inaccurate leading to single base mutations. In contrast, double strand damage leads to chromosomal breakage, and repair of multiple such breaks may lead to major chromosomal rearrangements such as translocations and deletions.

Ultraviolet irradiation is strongly implicated in the aetiology of skin tumours especially malignant melanoma of which 90% of cases can be attributed to exposure. Because ultraviolet light is of low energy it does not penetrate deeply and the effects are confined to the skin. Ultraviolet rays induce the formation of pyrimidine dimers, which lead to base–pair substitutions during replication. Abnormalities of DNA repair systems, for example xeroderma pigmentosum, lead to greatly increased risk of skin cancer.

Viruses and Cancers

It has been recognized that viruses are responsible for some cancers for 90 years, since the pioneering work of Peyton Rous who demonstrated that 'cell-free filtrates' could transmit leukaemia and sarcomas in experimental animals. Viruses contribute to the development of cancers in different ways. Some RNA tumour viruses (retroviruses) contain genes – viral oncogenes – which are directly responsible for transforming cells to malignancy. The viral RNA genome is copied into DNA by the enzyme reverse transcriptase and this is then inserted into the host genome. Viral genes can thus influence the expression of adjacent cellular genes. Other viruses, for example hepatitis C virus, act indirectly by causing tissue damage, leading to increased proliferation and an increased risk of mutations. The major viruses thought to be involved in human cancers are given in Table 5.11.

TABLE 5.11 Viruses implicated in human cancers

Virus	Human tumour
Papilloma viruses, especially types 16 and 18	Cervical carcinoma Anal and penile carcinomas
Epstein–Barr virus	Nasopharyngeal carcinoma Burkitt's lymphoma Hodgkin lymphoma
Hepatitis B and C viruses	Hepatocellular carcinoma
Human T-lymphotropic virus 1	T-cell leukaemia
Herpes virus 8	Kaposi's sarcoma

The final common pathway of many of these precipitating factors is mutation of DNA. Other factors such as chronic infection or hormonal stimulation cause increased cell turnover and may therefore make mutations more likely. Immunosuppression is associated with an increase particularly of lymphomas, a common complication of AIDS.

Genetic Factors

Undoubtedly there are individuals with significant genetic predispositions to various tumours, including the common cancers of breast, lung, and colon. There are three broad categories of familial cancer.

Familial Cancer Syndromes

In this group of disorders the increased risk of cancer is due to transmission of a single gene which appears to act in an autosomal dominant manner, although in fact both copies of the gene must be inactivated before a tumour develops.

Familial adenomatous polyposis coli is characterized by the growth of numerous adenomas in the colon (Figure 5.29) and the almost inevitable development of colonic carcinoma by middle age. The responsible gene (*APC*) has been identified and its function as an inhibitor of growth promoting signal transduction molecules established. The normal APC protein binds β-catenin and promotes its proteolytic destruction; mutations of *APC* tend therefore to increase the concentration of β-catenin, which is important in carcinogenesis.

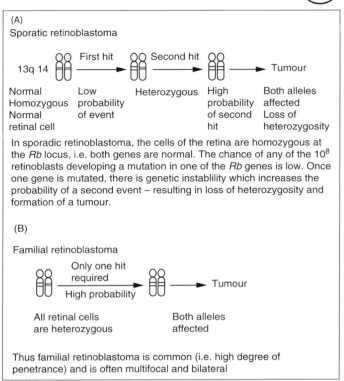

(A)
Sporatic retinoblastoma

In sporadic retinoblastoma, the cells of the retina are homozygous at the *Rb* locus, i.e. both genes are normal. The chance of any of the 10^8 retinoblasts developing a mutation in one of the *Rb* genes is low. Once one gene is mutated, there is genetic instablility which increases the probability of a second event – resulting in loss of heterozygosity and formation of a tumour.

(B)
Familial retinoblastoma

Thus familial retinoblastoma is common (i.e. high degree of penetrance) and is often multifocal and bilateral

FIGURE 5.30 Inheritance of retinoblastoma. The retinoblastoma gene lies on the long arm of chromosome 13. (A) The sporadic form of retinoblastoma occurs in individuals who have two normal *Rb* genes. Loss of both alleles is required before a tumour will develop, therefore the risk of this is very small and the tumour, which is unilateral, often occurs in older children. (B) In contrast, in patients with familial retinoblastoma one *Rb* allele is mutated in the germ line, and therefore in every cell in the body. Only one mutation in the remaining normal *Rb* gene is required for a tumour to develop. Accordingly, this almost invariably occurs, and most patients develop bilateral tumours at an early age. Unfortunately, they also develop a variety of other tumours in later life.

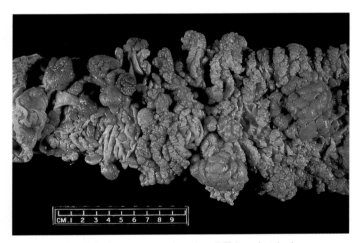

FIGURE 5.29 Familial adenomatous polyposis coli. This patient had a pancolectomy at the age of 25. Innumerable polyps are present throughout the colon. Fortunately no invasive carcinomas were identified. The patient's mother was less fortunate and died at the age of 43 from metastatic carcinoma of the colon.

In the Li–Fraumeni syndrome family members have an increased propensity to premature development of a variety of different tumour types; for example the early development of breast carcinoma and childhood sarcoma, typically in mother and child. It is due to mutation of the *p53* gene. Familial retinoblastoma is characterized by the almost inevitable development, usually bilaterally, of the rare retinal tumour retinoblastoma. This is due to inheritance of one abnormal copy of the retinoblastoma (*Rb*) gene (Figure 5.30 and see also p. 99).

Familial Cancers

In some families there is a striking increase in the incidence of a common cancer, for example of breast, colon or ovary. In some cases the responsible gene can be discovered, for exmaple the *BRCA1* and *BRCA2* genes associated with familial breast carcinoma.

Autosomal Recessive Disorders due to Defects in DNA Repair

In ataxia-telangiectasia, an autosomal recessive condition, there is an increased risk of developing lymphoma or leukaemia. This is related to excessive fragility of the chromosomes, either spontaneously or following radiation. The responsible gene (*AT*) is thought to act as a sensor of DNA damage which activates the *p53* gene causing the cell to enter G_0 until DNA repair is complete. In its absence, the mutated cell continues to proliferate increasing the chance of malignancy.

Hereditary non-polyposis colon cancer is another disorder due to impaired DNA repair. The relevant genes are known as 'mismatch repair genes'; they detect point mutations where the nucleotides on complementary DNA strands do not match correctly (i.e. normally A:T, C:G) and excise the abnormal base. Failure of these mismatch repair genes can be detected by the accumulation of variable microsatellites, short sequences which are normally identical in any individual; microsatellite instability is an indication of mismatch repair. Xeroderma pigmentosum is due to loss of the genes involved in excision of so-called pyrimidine dimers caused by ultraviolet damage. It leads to a greatly increased risk of skin cancer.

Oncogenes

The sections above indicate that mutations of DNA are fundamental to the causation of tumours. The topic of oncogenes and tumour suppressor genes can be difficult and confusing. In simple terms: cancer is due to excessive and uncontrolled cellular proliferation or insufficient cell loss, i.e. it results from defects in the normal control mechanisms for cell populations (see Chapter 2). Normal genes which are switched on when cell division is needed and which when expressed promote cell division are known as cellular proto-oncogenes. If these genes are inappropriately switched on, the cell will divide at the wrong time: the abnormal variant is called an oncogene, and produces an oncoprotein. Only one of the two cellular copies has to be affected as the oncogene acts in a dominant manner. The numerous proto-oncogenes fall into at least four main categories:

- Genes which produce growth factors, for example the *sis* gene encoding PDGF.
- Genes which produce growth factor receptors, for example the *erbB1* gene which encodes a receptor with tyrosine kinase activity for epidermal growth factor. There may be overexpression of the gene or it may be mutated and the conformation of the receptor is altered so that it does not require binding of its growth factor to be activated. The cell is therefore 'switched on' permanently.
- Genes which encode 'signal transducers', i.e. proteins which transmit the growth signal to the nucleus. Mutations may cause the signal to be *on* permanently. The *ras* group of genes encode for GTP-binding proteins.
- Genes which activate other genes to promote growth (transcription activators), for example the *fos* and *myc* genes.

Oncogene Activation

Oncogenes can be activated in a variety of ways. Point mutations may change the structure of the oncoprotein so that it becomes permanently active. The *ras* gene encodes a cell membrane associated signal transduction protein which exists in two forms: an inactive form bound to GDP and an active form bound to GTP. Normally, GTPase activity cleaves GTP to GDP so that activation of *ras* is short lasting. Mutations of *ras* result in a reduction of GTPase activity, so that the *ras* protein remains bound to GTP and is therefore locked into its active form.

Gene amplification is a process whereby multiple copies of an oncogene are formed by reduplication. Transcription of these extra copies of the gene results in increased production of the oncoprotein. For example, the N-*myc* gene on chromosome 2 is greatly amplified in many cases of neuroblastoma, a rare childhood tumour of primitive neurones. The extra copies may be located on the correct chromosome, where they can be recognized as a 'homogeneously staining region', or as numerous extra chromosomal structures known as 'double minutes'. The consequence in either case is of increased synthesis of the *myc* protein, a transcription factor for genes involved in cell proliferation.

Translocations between chromosomes may also cause overexpression of oncoproteins. There are two main mechanisms. In some lymphomas, for example Burkitt's lymphoma and mantle cell lymphoma, an oncoprotein (c-*myc* and cyclin D_1, respectively) is moved so that it lies under the control sequences of the immunoglobulin heavy chain, which is constitutively expressed in active B lymphocytes. Thus the oncoprotein is permanently switched on. The second mechanism, commonly seen in sarcomas (p. 366) results in the fusion of two genes, thus producing a new hybrid molecule which has increased transcription activity. Several well-recognized translocations and the resulting tumours are listed in Table 5.12.

TABLE 5.12 **Some tumours associated with specific chromosomal translocation**

Tumour	Translocation	Genes involved
Burkitt's lymphoma	t(8;14)(q24;q32)	c-*myc*; Ig heavy chain
Chronic myeloid leukaemia	t(9;22)(q34;q11)	*Abl*; *bcr*
Ewing's sarcoma	t(11;22)(q24;q12)	*Fli*-1; *EWS*
Follicular lymphoma	t(8;14)(q24;q32)	Ig heavy chain; *bcl*-2
Mantle cell lymphoma	t(11;14)(q13;q32)	cyclin D_1; Ig heavy chain
Alveolar rhabdomyosarcoma	t(2;13)(q35;q14)	*PAX*-3; *FKHR*
Synovial sarcoma	t(X;18)(p11;q11)	*SSX*; *SYT*

Tumour Suppressor Genes

Tumour suppressor genes are genes whose products normally stop a cell growing, or promote differentiation of a cell to a terminal end state, or trigger checkpoints that cause cell cycle arrest if DNA damage occurs. Thus, tumour suppressor genes are cell cycle arrest genes or DNA repair genes. It also follows that tumour suppressor genes cause problems when they are absent, i.e. when their normal protective function has been lost. This can occur by inactivating mutations, deletion or even when they form a complex with viral proteins resulting in their deactivation. It follows that to lose their tumour suppressor function it may be necessary to lose both functional copies of a gene.

Inherited cancers, although not common, have given valuable insight into the role of tumour suppressor genes and how they are implicated in disease. Alfred Knudson studied retinoblastoma, a rare cancer of the retina of the eye. Retinoblastoma may be familial (approximately 40% of cases) or sporadic (approximately 60% of cases). In familial cases the child affected is usually under 3 years of age and both eyes may be affected. In sporadic cases the child tends to be older and the disease is unilateral. Knudson reasoned that if there was an inherited element then it was perhaps a similar genetic mechanism in both familial and sporadic cases. He further argued that as the familial cases occur at younger ages and the occurrence of disease was more frequent in members of families affected by the familial disease, it was possible that the inherited trait meant that these cases were already 'halfway' to cancer. Since then the gene *RB1* (retinoblastoma 1) has been identified. This is a tumour suppressor gene, the normal function of which is to regulate entry of cells into the cell cycle. Disruption of the function of the *RB1* product results in inappropriate cell proliferation, eventually leading to cancer. In cases of familial retinoblastoma the sufferer inherits one normal copy of *RB1* and one copy that is non-functional. In retinoblasts (why in these cells in particular you may wish to enquire) a further mutation may occur in which case there is loss of function of the normal gene resulting in dysregulated entry into cell cycle. The same happens in sporadic cases: there must be loss of function. However, in sporadic cases cells must suffer two mutations or deletions in the same cell to knock out each copy of *RB1*. This may happen but is much less likely than a single hit. Therefore, in sporadic cases the disease occurs at a later age, indicating that many more chances of mutation must have occurred. This theory also explains why multiple tumours are generally not found in the sporadic form because the chance of more than one retinoblast receiving mutations in both *RB1* genes is very unlikely, whereas in the hereditary form all the retinoblasts have one hit from the outset. This is Knudson's two-hit hypothesis.

It then becomes apparent that other cancers do have familial and sporadic forms though the precise organ type, age at onset, penetrance of disease and pattern of hereditary are more ill defined. However, in these diseases there is indication that an inherited trait, a dysfunctional tumour suppressor gene, has been acquired. A number of important tumour suppressor genes are listed in Table 5.13.

TABLE 5.13 **Tumour suppressor genes**

Gene	Tumour
APC	Familial adenomatosis coli, colon cancer
BRCA-1	Breast, ovarian cancer
BRCA-2	Breast cancer
NF-1	Neurofibromatosis type 1
p53	Li–Fraumeni syndrome, sporadic cancers
Rb	Retinoblastoma, osteosarcoma, sporadic cancers
WT-1	Wilms' tumour

Apoptosis and Cancer

Oncogenes and tumour suppressor genes are important because they regulate cell number by controlling cell proliferation. Cell number also depends on the rate of cell loss. Apoptosis, or programmed cell death, is also governed by a number of genes, and aberrant function of these is important in the cause of some cancers. In follicular B cell lymphomas, a translocation t(14;18)(q32;q31) causes the *bcl-2* gene to come under the control of the immunoglobulin heavy chain regulatory sequences and to become overexpressed. This inhibits apoptosis so that the cells are immortalized. Even though the tumour cells are growing very slowly, the tumour increases in size due to the lower rate of cell loss. A number of other similar genes are thought to be important in other tumours.

Telomerases and Cancer

Much experimental work is currently directed at clarifying the role of telomerases in cancers. Telomeres are repeating DNA sequences found at the ends of chromosomes which are important in regulating the number of cell divisions of which a cell is capable, the so-called Hayflick limit (see Chapter 2). Each time a cell divides, the telomere is shortened until eventually the cell is incapable of further replication, a phenomenon thought to be important in cellular senescence. This does not apply to stem cells, because they contain a mechanism for lengthening telomeres, an enzyme called telomerase. Theoretically, overexpression of telomerase might immortalize tumour cells. Indeed, many tumours do appear to express increased enzyme activity. This may open novel therapeutic approaches to cancer, with the development of telomerase-inhibiting drugs. At present, the role of telomerase is exciting, but not yet proved.

SUMMARY

Cancer epidemiology, the study of the prevalence of different tumour types, has demonstrated that cancer is a major health problem in all countries although the ageing populations of Western countries are particularly affected. This importance is reflected in the large share of healthcare budgets spent on care of patients with cancer, in attempts at cancer prevention and by the widespread development of cancer screening programmes which may detect both preinvasive and invasive tumours. Appropriate clinical management depends on an understanding of the classification of tumours, both benign and malignant, and of their biological behaviours, including effects both local and distant, and knowledge of modes of spread dictates a rational approach to staging of tumours. It is important that all clinicians involved in cancer care have some understanding of the processes involved in laboratory diagnosis of tumours, the strengths and limitations of existing techniques and newer immunological and molecular techniques, and the necessity of close clinicopathological

DNA REPAIR MECHANISMS

DNA damage is an obligatory risk of being alive and so it is important that repair mechanisms exist. In general they are extremely effective and it is only when they fail that we become aware of how stressful an environment we inhabit. DNA repair has similarities irrespective of whether we are looking at yeast or people. Repair machinery is always linked to replication and so it is no surprise that induction of repair is associated with cessation of replication (lest erroneous sequence replication takes place). At several points in the cell cycle (see Chapter 2), known as checkpoints, damage sensing and repair induction have a particularly effective influence over cell cycle progression. Driving through cell cycle checkpoints is a bad idea!

Basic Repair Principles

Cells Die by Apoptosis

Basically it is better to have no cell than a cell with potentially harmful damage and mutation. This is not simply a matter of dose of injury; it is also dependent on the importance or stage of differentiation of the cell type.

Tolerance of Damage

We will consider three examples to illustrate, not so much that these mechanisms occur, but rather to demonstrate that a lot of eukaryotic DNA repair is still speculative and based on the much more robust science of yeast:

- Neurones in the brain are susceptible to damage. They cannot be repaired easily and cannot replicate. They adapt to live with damage.
- An alternative mechanism may occur in hepatocytes. These cells are constantly under attack by free radicals generated by respiration and metabolism of xenobiotics. As the liver cells age and sustain damage they undergo polyploidy. This process, which is not fully understood, results in cells that instead of having a diploid content of DNA become polyploid: doubling, quadrupling and more their cellular DNA content. Instead of having two copies of genes they have four, eight, sixteen or more copies. The reasoning is that the polyploid cell has more copies of each gene and so can still produce protein even if numerous gene-inactivating mutations are sustained. This is a persuasive argument if the liver cell is regarded as a protein factory where the production line output is the major driving force in existence, but largely without an evidence base to support it.
- DNA repair may be delayed because replication is not imminent. For example, a pyrimidine dimer caused by UV light may persist and act as a brake on replication.

If there is no involvement of a transcriptionally active gene that may not matter in a cell for some time. But there is a danger that because DNA replication can have multiple start sites a gap may be formed around the damaged area resulting in a frameshift type mutation. In these circumstances recombination using undamaged DNA as a template may be useful. Many genes are involved in this fairly complex scenario including *BRCA1*, implicated when defective in causing breast and ovarian cancer. In essence the repair refers back to the original sequence manual, and uses it to cut and paste – well actually to fuse – back the correct sequence, thereby bypassing the replicative block posed by the intercalation or pyrimidine dimer.

Removal of Damage

A single base or a stretch of damaged DNA is excised and repaired.

Base Excision Repair

If a damaged base is present the easiest repair method is simply to excise it and replace it with a correct base. This is the principle of base excision repair. It is conservative, i.e. minimal effort is required, and is not error prone.

Nucleotide Excision Repair

If the damage is more severe, for example a pyrimidine dimer, then the DNA configuration is altered, not just a single base. The same basic idea of base excision is relevant but the processes of recognition, excision and replacement are more complex. Instead of a single base being excised a strip of nucleotides on one strand are excised and DNA polymerase enzymes replicate the gap using the other strand as a template. Defects of nucleotide excision repair have serious effects. In the condition xeroderma pigmentosum skin cannot repair UV-induced damage and there is a high incidence of mutation and skin cancer.

Mismatch Repair

Think of the spellchecker on your computer. It is generally useful but if you are dealing with specialist material the spellchecker is sometimes less helpful as it tends to insert a suggestion that is perhaps erroneous. This is because the dictionary available to the software is limited. Similarly when DNA is replicated it is checked for spelling errors. The trouble is that the only comparator available is the original strand from which replication started. The repair mechanism checks for mismatches and corrects those it finds, or deletes the cell altogether. Some areas of DNA are more error prone than others, for example regions having multiple repeat short sequences, and defects of mismatch repair are more likely to be found in these regions. Defects of mismatch repair are implicated in susceptibility to a number of cancers, in particular colon cancer.

Reversal of Damage

This can be envisaged as a cosmetic exercise smoothing over the bumps or gaps in damaged DNA. If DNA suffers a single strand break the most simple option is to recognize damage and then simply to ligate it with a DNA ligase enzyme. It sounds simple of course but within that straightforward mechanism there must be recognition, specificity, distinguishing normal strand breakage (e.g. uncoiling DNA during replication) and catalytic activity to actually anneal the ends.

Conclusion

It is worth emphasizing that prevention is better than correction – but most DNA damage is an obligatory part of being alive. Inherited or acquired defects in DNA repair are important in causing cancer, allowing progression and potentially in inducing resistance of cancer cells to therapy.

cooperation, not least in multidisciplinary team review of cancer management.

Our understanding of the underlying molecular mechanisms underlying the development of tumours (carcinogenesis) and the spread of malignant cells has greatly increased in recent years. As well as being of scientific interest, this offers alternative strategies for cancer prevention including genetic testing in families of cancer patients and has led to the development of novel therapies, some already in clinical use and many others in development and assessment.

FURTHER READING

Fletcher CDM. *Diagnostic Histopathology of Tumours*, 3rd edn. Edinburgh: Churchill Livingstone, 2007.

Hall PA, Lowe SW. Molecular and cellular themes in cancer research 2. *J Pathol Annu Rev* 2005; **205**: 121–292.

Kufe DW, Bast RC, Hait WN, *et al. Holland and Frei Cancer 7 Medicine*. Hamilton: BC Decker, 2006.

Skarin AT, Canellas GP. *Atlas of Diagnostic Oncology*, 3rd edn. Edinburgh: Mosby, 2003.

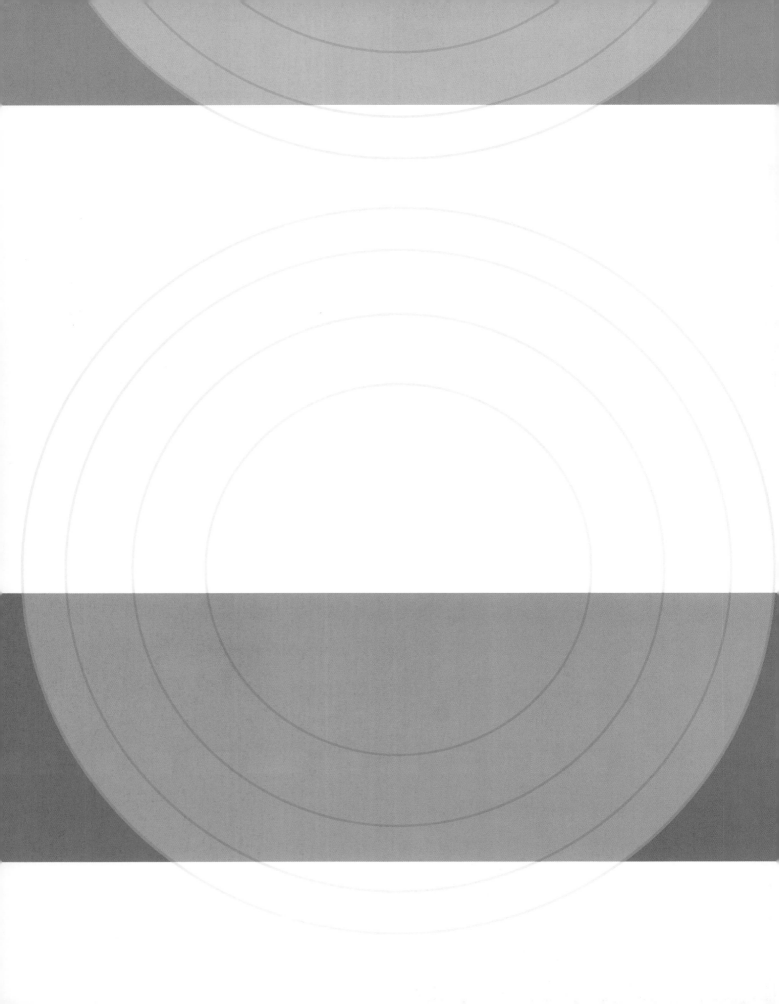

SECTION

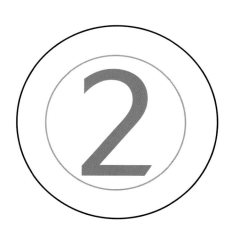

Systemic Pathology

THE CARDIOVASCULAR SYSTEM

6

George BM Lindop, Allan R McPhaden and Henry J Dargie

INTRODUCTION

The cardiovascular system maintains the circulation of the blood. The arterial tree distributes blood to the microcirculation, where exchange of fluid and solutes takes place with the interstitial fluid that bathes and nourishes the cells. Oxygen and nutrients are delivered to tissue cells and waste products are removed by the flow of interstitial fluid. Excess interstitial fluid is drained by the lymphatic system and returned to the venous blood. After the microcirculation, blood returns through the venous system to the heart, which maintains the pressure and hence the flow of blood. Each part of the circulation is structurally adapted to the pressure and flow of blood within it. This chapter begins by examining some effects of altered blood flow, and goes on to consider diseases of arteries, abnormalities in the microcirculation, interstitial fluid and veins, and finishes by discussing diseases of the heart.

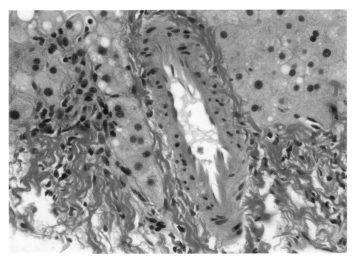

FIGURE 6.1 A normal medium-sized artery in transverse section. The wall is composed mainly of smooth muscle (van Geison).

STRUCTURE AND FUNCTION OF THE COMPONENTS

As systemic arteries distribute the blood at high flow rates and high pressure (about 100 mmHg) they require thick muscular walls. Conductance arteries absorb the impulse of cardiac systole and their elastic recoil maintains blood flow in diastole whereas the more muscular medium-sized arteries (Figures 6.1 and 6.2) regulate the distribution of blood to the various tissues by vasoconstriction and vasodilation. Excessive vasoconstriction in arteries and arterioles can damage cells by diminution or interruption of blood flow. Excessive contraction is opposed by the innervation of only the outer layer of smooth muscle cells and by a thick internal elastic lamina, a fenestrated cylinder of elastin; these are not always successful in preventing ischaemia due to spasm.

Veins contain blood at low or even negative pressure (Figure 6.2), act as capacitance vessels and as the reservoir of the circulation they have a large lumen and thin walls. Veins have a rich innervation throughout all layers of their walls

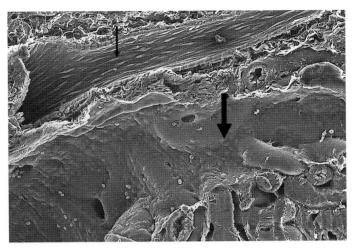

FIGURE 6.2 A scanning electron microscope view of an artery and vein. The artery (above – small arrow) has a smaller lumen and endothelium that is aligned to the direction of the rapid flow. In contrast, the vein (below – large arrow) has a large capacitance and polygonal endothelial cells.

and can contract more than arteries; during haemorrhage from the circulation shrinking the reservoir by intense vasoconstriction of veins may be life-saving by facilitating the flow of blood back to the heart.

Altered Pressure and Flow

Hyperaemia is increased blood flow and is due to dilatation of arteries and arterioles. It occurs, for example, in skeletal muscle during exercise as a physiological response. 'Reactive hyperaemia' follows diminution of blood flow, and local hyperaemia is one of the cardinal features of inflammation (see Chapter 4). In congestion there is more blood in the tissue, but flow is slow and therefore the tissue is hypoxic. Congested tissues contain increased haemoglobin with reduced oxygen saturation and are therefore bluish-purple in colour.

Hypertension is raised blood pressure and the term is applied to both the arterial and venous circulations – arterial hypertension and venous hypertension. Hypotension, low blood pressure in the systemic arterial circulation, can cause damage if blood flow is also low. Ischaemia is insufficient blood flow for the needs of the tissue. It may be caused by a fall in blood pressure but arterial narrowing is the commonest cause. Chronic ischaemia causes atrophy of specialized cells, sometimes with replacement fibrosis. Infarction is tissue necrosis caused by acute ischaemia, and the area of dead tissue is an infarct. The susceptibility of cells to ischaemia is governed by their metabolic needs and the anatomy of the supplying arteries.

Collateral Circulation

Tissues that have more than one arterial supply are said to have a collateral blood supply. Some organs such as the lung and liver are protected from ischaemia by a double blood supply. In other organs arterial anastomoses provide a collateral blood supply; for example, the circle of Willis may protect the brain from occlusion of a neck artery. In contrast, the deep penetrating cerebral arteries and arteries in the heart, kidney or spleen are end arteries whose territories do not overlap and sudden arterial occlusion will usually cause a regional infarct. Longstanding narrowing of some end arteries such as the coronary arteries may induce anastomoses between two arterial territories. This acquired collateral blood supply may reduce the size of an infarct following arterial occlusion.

Infarction

Most infarcts are due to sudden blockage (occlusion) of an artery and infarction occurs in the territory supplied (regional infarction). When the arteries are rigid due to atherosclerosis and/or arteriosclerosis (p. 109), a fall in blood pressure below the limit of autoregulation can cause infarction in the watershed or boundary zones between artery territories (boundary zone infarction). In organs such as the adrenal gland and kidney with a single draining vein, venous thrombosis may also cause infarction (venous infarction). The size of an infarct depends on the size of the occluded vessel, the severity and duration of ischaemia, the tissue susceptibility and the prevailing oxygen tension of the blood.

General Features of Infarcts

The necrosis may be coagulative or, in the case of the central nervous system, colliquative (p. 290) and, depending on the anatomy of the blood supply, the infarct may be pale or haemorrhagic. Pale infarcts occur in the heart (Figure 6.3), kidney and spleen, while haemorhagic infarcts typically affect the lung, due to the dual blood supply, and the bowel where there is rich arterial anastomosis. Venous infarcts are always haemorrhagic. Infarction triggers acute inflammation (p. 54). Infarcts heal by organization from the margins until they are replaced a fibrous scar (Figure 6.4).

Reflow of Blood and Reperfusion Injury

After acute ischaemia, restoration of flow may cause a paradoxical increase in cell injury. The highly reduced state of the mitochondrial electron transport systems and the action of enzymes such as xanthine oxidase create highly reactive free radicals and superoxide. The formation of free radicals may be dramatically increased when restoration of blood flow supplies oxygen to cells that have raised levels of nicotinamide adenosine dinucleotide (NADH) and hypoxanthine. Free radicals oxidize lipids and membrane proteins. Rupture of capillaries by a burst of free radical generation is responsible for the haemorrhage into some cerebral and myocardial infarcts. Early restoration of flow in a thrombosed coronary artery by thrombolysis or by angioplasty improves the overall survival (p. 154) at the expense of a few who die from reperfusion injury.

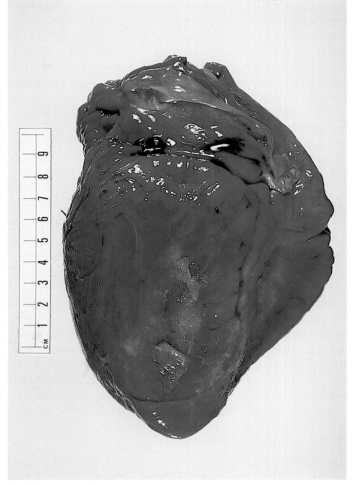

FIGURE 6.3 **The anterior surface of the heart has a yellowish area, which is a full-thickness infarct of the left ventricle. It lies in the territory of the left anterior descending coronary artery which is occluded by thrombosis. There is surrounding inflammation and a fibrinous exudate on the surface, a common response to tissue necrosis.**

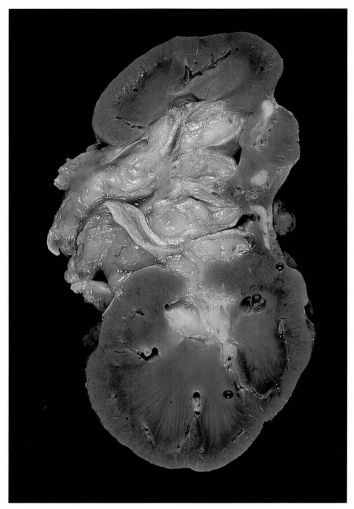

FIGURE 6.4 **A kidney with two sunken areas in its midzone. These are scars due to old healed cortical infarcts.**

The Response to Cardiovascular Injury

Minor endothelial defects are quickly sealed by adhesion of platelets, which form a platelet plug. In more severe injuries, blood coagulates within the lumen, a process termed thrombosis. Solidification of the blood outside the circulation, or within the vascular tree after death, is due to the activation of the clotting cascade and is referred to as clotting.

Thrombi

Composition of Thrombi

In rapidly flowing arterial blood, pale thrombus grows slowly by accretion of aggregated platelets and fibrin. In the region of an occlusion, stationary blood on either side coagulates rapidly, traps red cells and forms red thrombus. This extends as far as the next branch where flowing blood will deposit pale thrombus which may lead to further occlusion. This process is termed propagation (Figure 6.5).

The Fate of Thrombi

Occlusive thrombi are mainly attached to the vessel wall by the areas of white thrombus and at sites of organization. Red thrombus retracts from the vessel walls and digestion by the local action of plasmin, macrophages and neutrophil enzymes leads to the formation of spaces. Endothelial cells proliferate and migrate to line the spaces thus forming channels and branching capillary networks, which eventually anastomose. The outcome may be restoration of a lumen – recanalization – containing flowing blood. Thrombi, especially those recently formed, may become detached from the vessel wall and be carried by the blood flow to impact in a downstream vessel (embolism).

Embolism

In embolism, abnormal material is carried by the blood flow and impacts in a downstream vessel, sometimes with

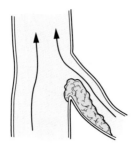

Pale thrombus

Platelets adhere to endothelium and undergo 'activation'. Coagulation cascade generates fibrin strands

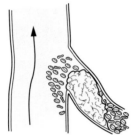

Red thrombus

Occlusion of the lumen by the thrombus causes slow or no flow which allows red blood cells to adhere to the surface

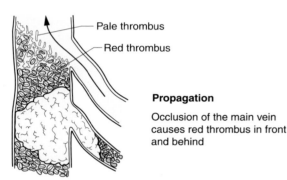

Pale thrombus

Red thrombus

Propagation

Occlusion of the main vein causes red thrombus in front and behind

FIGURE 6.5 Propagation of thrombus in a vein.

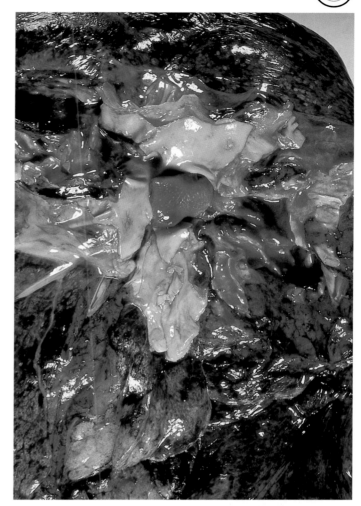

FIGURE 6.6 The hilum of a lung showing pulmonary arteries containing large red thromboemboli derived from the leg veins.

disastrous consequences, such as a stroke. The commonest embolus is thrombus – 'thromboembolism'. In the systemic arterial system emboli are usually dislodged from the heart or large arteries. Pulmonary embolism may follow systemic venous thrombosis (Figure 6.6) and is discussed on p. 180.

Major Causes of Embolism

- Systemic arterial embolism.
- Athero-embolism.
- Fat embolism.
- Air embolism.
- Septic embolism.
- Amniotic fluid embolism.
- Pulmonary thromboembolism (p. 180).
- Paradoxical embolism (p. 157).

Systemic Embolism

The commonest source of systemic thromboembolism is the left side of the heart; a stroke or intestinal infarction may be the first sign of cardiac disease (Figure 6.7); common predisposing disorders are atrial fibrillation, myocardial

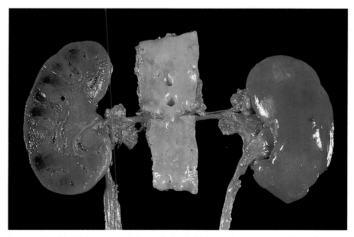

FIGURE 6.7 Multiple recent infarcts in both kidneys in a patient with atrial fibrillation, atrial thrombosis and systemic embolism.

infarction and any cause of heart failure. However, thrombi formed on ulcerated atherosclerosis (p. 110) may also embolize and block a major artery.

Athero-embolism

This is caused when the contents of a disrupted plaque are discharged into the blood, and can be identified histologically as cholesterol crystals impacted in the distal arteries (Figure 6.8). Athero-emboli may be dislodged by arterial catheterization or by angioplasty. Although usually asymptomatic, showers of athero-emboli may cause abdominal pain, hypertension or renal failure. Athero-embolism probably accounts for the common ischaemic scars in the kidneys of old persons, and contributes to the nephron loss which accompanies old age and hypertension. Loose aggregates of platelets form when blood flows over ulcerated atherosclerosis; impaction of these may cause vasospasm, which may be responsible for transient cerebral ischaemic attacks in the elderly (p. 289) and in episodes of myocardial ischaemia.

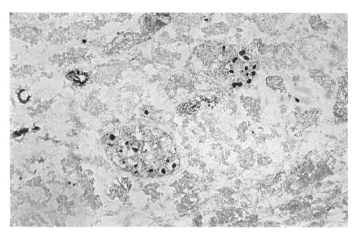

FIGURE 6.9 A section of kidney tissue from a patient who died after multiple long-bone fractures. It shows two renal glomeruli stained to reveal fat (red). The glomerular capillaries are plugged with fat globules which, being fluid at body temperature, have passed through the pulmonary capillaries.

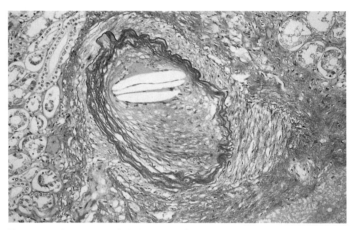

FIGURE 6.8 An artery occluded by loose fibrous tissue within which there are slits formed by crystals of cholesterol derived from an atheromatous plaque. This shows that that the occlusion is due to organized athero-embolism.

Fat Embolism

Severe injuries, usually major long-bone fractures, may be complicated by the fat embolism syndrome. The clinical features include dyspnoea, tachycardia, confusion, fever, blood-stained sputum and a petechial rash on the upper trunk. Cyanosis, coma and death occur in 10% of patients, usually in those with brain involvement. Non-traumatic causes of fat embolism include acute pancreatitis and cardiopulmonary bypass. Release of free fatty acids may damage pulmonary capillaries, and cause adult respiratory distress syndrome (p. 169), and disseminated intravascular coagulation (p. 128). Fat passes through pulmonary capillaries and then embolizes systemic capillaries (Figure 6.9); fat globules appear in the urine and sputum.

Air Embolism

Air embolism is caused by air entering the circulation via neck wounds, during cardiothoracic surgery or through intravenous infusions. Small volumes are asymptomatic, but over 100 mL may cause distress and 300 mL or more may be fatal. Large volumes of air become churned with blood in the right side of the heart and froth blocks the pulmonary circulation.

Decompression sickness is a hazard when breathing air at more than atmospheric pressure. Inhaled gases dissolve in blood and tissue fluids in proportion to the pressure. Following a rapid fall in pressure, as when a diver surfaces too quickly, or when an aircraft depressurizes at altitude, gases come out of solution (as champagne effervesces on opening the bottle). The commonest symptoms are muscle cramps (the 'bends'), cough (the 'chokes') and dyspnoea. Paraplegia may result and blockage of cerebral vessels leads to coma or death. Recompression and slow decompression is the only treatment. In chronic decompression sickness (Caisson's disease) intra-articular bone necrosis causes collapse of joints, most often the shoulder or hip.

Septic Embolism

Septic emboli may derive from thrombus forming in a vein draining a suppurating infection or from vegetations on infected heart valves. The resulting infarct may progress to abscess formation, for example in lung, brain or liver.

Amniotic Fluid Embolism

Amniotic fluid embolism is a rare complication of vaginal and caesarean delivery and has a mortality of over 80%. Due to premature placental detachment the contracting uterus may force amniotic fluid into the uterine veins. The mother becomes cyanosed, dyspnoeic and shocked and a few hours later develops pulmonary oedema with diffuse alveolar injury similar to that seen in adult respiratory distress syndrome (p. 169). Fetal squames obstruct the pulmonary circulation and cause disseminated intravascular coagulation (p. 128). Humoral factors in the amniotic fluid may also cause pulmonary vasoconstriction and impair cardiac contractility.

DISEASES OF ARTERIES

Age Changes

The structure of arteries changes with age, a process known as arteriosclerosis (hardening of the arteries). The intima becomes thickened and fibrosed and the medial smooth muscle and elastic fibres are partly replaced by collagen and other matrix proteins (Figure 6.10). Arteriosclerosis results in increased rigidity and tortuosity of arteries, often seen clinically as prominent temporal arteries of elderly people and in chest radiographs as stretching ('unfolding') of the aorta. Plasma proteins accumulate in the walls of arterioles, so-called plasmatic vasculosus, giving a histological appearance termed hyaline arteriolosclerosis (from the Greek *hyalos* meaning glass; hyaline is applied to homogeneous, refractile [glassy], usually eosinophilic material on light microscopy; see Figure 6.11).

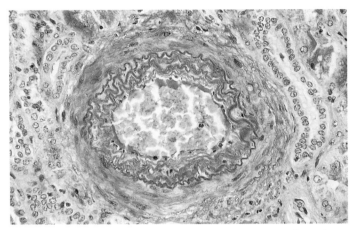

FIGURE 6.10 A medium-sized artery from a middle-aged man showing early arteriosclerosis. The intima is thickened and there is reduplication of the internal elastic lamina. This has caused thinning of the media: compare with Figure 6.1.

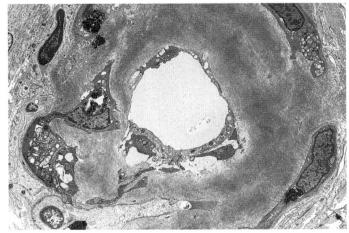

FIGURE 6.11 An electron micrograph of a renal arteriole showing advanced arteriolosclerosis. The medial smooth muscle cells are largely replaced by amorphous proteinaceous material. This is derived from retention of plasma proteins combined with some basement membrane-type proteins synthesized *in situ*.

Severe arteriosclerosis also complicates hypertension (p. 116) and diabetes mellitus (p. 471), but at an earlier age.

The increased arterial rigidity of arteriosclerosis contributes to the age-related increase in systolic and pulse pressures. The overall decrease in compliance of the arterial tree affects autoregulation in the circulation by shifting the autoregulatory curve to the right (Figure 6.12). The beneficial effect is decreased susceptibility of the elderly and chronically hypertensive to malignant hypertension (p. 118); however, the greatly increased susceptibility to hypotension accounts for the increased mortality of elderly and hypertensive patients to shock (Table 6.7 on p. 129).

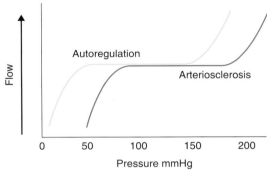

FIGURE 6.12 Autoregulation allows the cardiac, cerebral and renal circulations to maintain constant flow over a wide range of pressure. Arteriosclerosis due to age and hypertension shifts this curve to the right and renders tissues susceptible to ischaemia if blood pressure falls. Conversely, malignant hypertension is rare in the elderly and in those with longstanding hypertension.

Atherosclerosis

Key Points

- Atherosclerosis is a focal accumulation of fat with chronic inflammation and fibrosis in arteries down to 2 mm in diameter.
- This causes arterial narrowing and chronic ischaemia.
- Thrombosis of narrowed segments causes infarction.
- Ischaemic heart disease, stroke and arterial diseases are the main causes of death and disability in Western populations.

Atherosclerosis, by far the most important arterial disease in Western populations, causes more deaths and disability than any other disease. Atherosclerosis weakens and narrows arteries leading to ischaemia. When complicated by occlusive thrombosis, it causes sudden death and myocardial infarction, stroke and acute ischaemia of the legs and abdominal organs. Ischaemic heart disease and stroke together cause about a third of all deaths in the UK.

Macroscopic Appearances

Atherosclerosis is a patchy accumulation of fat in artery walls. It forms plaques, which have a soft lipid-rich centre and a fibrous (sclerotic) reaction. In large arteries early plaques are raised yellow or white patches of thickened intima which may become confluent (Figure 6.13). They may crack or ulcerate, especially if the surface collagenous cap is thin, leading to deposition of thrombus on the surface; this may produce great irregularity of the luminal surface of the aorta (Figure 6.14). There is often calcification of the wall. Erosion into the media weakens the wall, which may form a bulge or aneurysm (p. 120). This often ruptures. Plaques at the origins of the mesenteric, renal or other arteries may cause narrowing and consequently ischaemia (Figure 6.15). In smaller arteries the lumen may be narrowed to a pinhole and may be eccentric or concentric (Figure 6.16); the functional significance of this is discussed on p. 112.

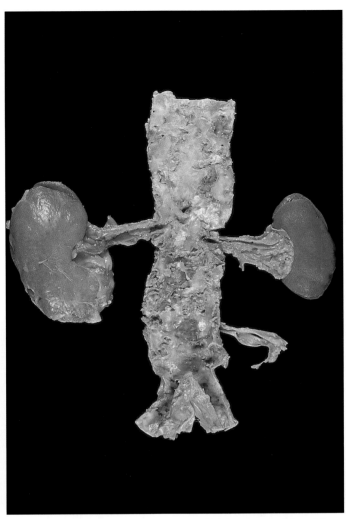

FIGURE 6.15 An aorta with severe atheroma which has narrowed the origins of one renal artery. The diminished blood flow has caused shrinkage of the kidney on that side due to ischaemic atrophy.

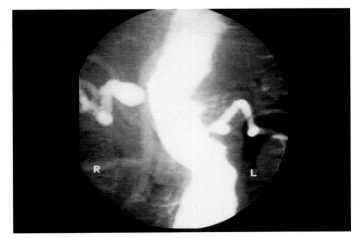

FIGURE 6.13 A piece of aorta opened out to show that the smooth endothelial surface is largely replaced by ulcerated confluent atheromatous plaques with adherent thrombus.

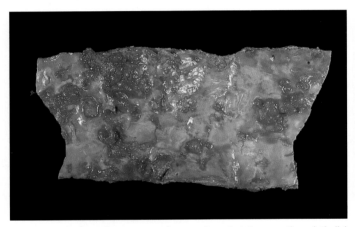

FIGURE 6.14 An aortogram showing a tortuous aorta with an irregular outline due to severe atheroma, which has also caused narrowing of the renal arteries.

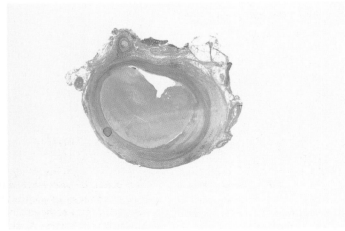

FIGURE 6.16 A histological section of iliac artery showing extreme narrowing due to a large atheromatous plaque.

Microscopic Appearances

Initially, most of the lipid is intracellular and the early plaque consists of an accumulation of macrophages, lymphocytes and smooth muscle cells in the intima. Lipid accumulates in 'foam cells' whose cytoplasm is swollen with lipid globules (Figure 6.17). Most are macrophage derived; the remainder are medial smooth muscle cells, which proliferate and migrate into the intima through the internal elastic lamina. Eventually the foam cells die and release their lipid content; extracellular lipids accumulate deep in the intima at the internal elastic lamina. There is an inflammatory response and proteoglycans, collagen and other matrix proteins are laid down in the course of surrounding fibrosis. The enlarging plaque erodes through the internal elastic lamina into the media, which is thinned. Small blood vessels grow into the plaque from the vasa vasorum and also from the lumen.

If the fibrous cap is thin it may rupture or crack leading to haemorrhage into the plaque and to luminal thrombosis, which may occlude the artery. This process is crucial to the various coronary syndromes (p. 135). Plaque development is shown diagrammatically in Figures 6.18 and 6.19.

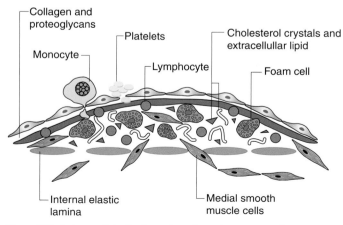

FIGURE 6.17 A histological section through an atheromatous plaque stained to show lipid as red. Beneath the lumen (right) there is a pale collagenous fibrous cap beneath which the media is replaced by a lipid rich atheromatous plaque around which there is some fibrosis and chronic inflammation.

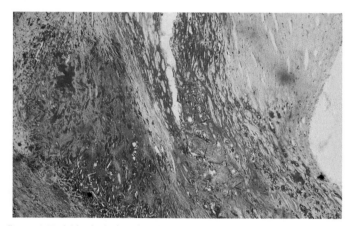

Early atheromatous plaque

FIGURE 6.18 Early events in the formation of an atheromatous plaque.

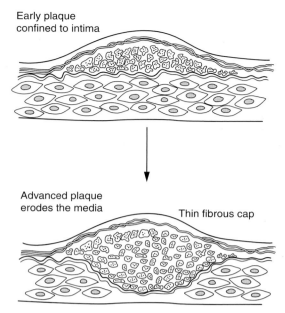

Early plaque confined to intima

Advanced plaque erodes the media

Thin fibrous cap

RBC

Complicated plaque with superimposed thrombi

Ulceration of thin cap causes thrombosis

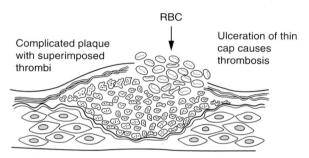

FIGURE 6.19 Stages in the development of an atheromatous plaque. It is believed that those with a thin overlying collagenous cap are more likely to crack and ulcerate and trigger thrombosis.

Distribution

Atherosclerosis affects systemic arteries down to approximately 2 mm diameter. In the aorta, it begins in the lower abdominal portion; the thoracic aorta tends to be less severely affected. The coronary, mesenteric, leg, renal and cerebral arteries are typically affected, but the distribution varies. The coronary arteries are more often involved at an early age than any other vessels, whereas severe atheroma of the cerebral arteries mainly affects the elderly. The main clinical syndromes caused by atherosclerosis are:

- ischaemic heart disease
  - sudden death
  - myocardial infarction
  - heart failure
- cerebrovascular disease
  - cerebral infarction
  - transient cerebral ischaemic attacks
  - dementia (arteriopathic)
- peripheral vascular disease
  - intermittent claudication
  - gangrene

- mesenteric vascular disease
  - mesenteric claudication
  - intestinal infarction
- renovascular disease
  - hypertension
  - renal failure
- aneurysms
  - aortic aneurysm.

The most important clinical syndromes are due to atherosclerosis of medium-sized and small arteries. Gradual narrowing causes chronic ischaemia and sudden occlusion by thrombosis causes infarction. Atherosclerosis causes almost all cases of ischaemic heart disease, the largest single cause of death and heart failure in developed countries. Most cerebrovascular disease is due to atheroma of the carotid, vertebral and intracerebral arteries. Abdominal aortic aneurysms (p. 123) are common, especially in elderly hypertensive male smokers. Aneurysms seldom occur in the smaller arteries, except occasionally in the basilar artery. Renal artery stenosis (p. 119) causes renovascular hypertension, and, especially in the elderly, bilateral disease causes renal failure. Most mesenteric vascular disease is due to atherosclerosis at the origin of the superior mesenteric artery. The leg arteries are often severely affected, especially in diabetic people and in cigarette smokers, causing peripheral vascular disease. Although a collateral circulation eventually develops, exercise-induced muscle ischaemia causes leg pain that is relieved by rest – intermittent claudication. In time, increasing ischaemia causes

gangrene, which starts in the toes and spreads proximally. Thrombi and atheromatous debris from ulcerated plaques embolize to arteries in the legs and gut, kidneys and spleen and cause infarction (pp. 107–108).

Aetiology and Risk Factors

The incidence of ischaemic heart disease (IHD) is an indicator of the extent of atheroma in a community. Epidemiological studies have identified risk factors associated with an increased or decreased risk of developing IHD. We shall deal with only the major independent ones. Age, sex and heredity are all important, but hyperlipidaemia, hypertension, cigarette smoking and diabetes are the most important because they are modifiable (Table 6.1).

Age and Sex

Ischaemic heart disease begins in men in the fourth decade and increases in incidence thereafter. It is uncommon in women before the menopause, probably due to a hormonal basis. Post-menopausal hormone replacement increases the risk slightly.

Hyperlipidaemia

Accumulation of lipid in arteries is central to the pathogenesis of atheroma and hyperlipidaemia often predisposes to IHD. Insoluble cholesterol and other lipids circulate within the centre of lipoprotein particles, whose hydrophobic lipid core is surrounded by an outer hydrophilic layer of phospholipid and apolipoproteins. Apolipoproteins are protein ligands that bind to receptors on cells. They are divided into groups labelled alphabetically (Apo-A, B, C, etc.), within which subclasses are labelled numerically (Apo-A1, Apo-A2, etc.). Decreasing particle size is associated with increasing density. They range from large chylomicrons through very low density lipoproteins (VLDL) and low density lipoprotein (LDL) to high density lipoprotein (HDL) (Table 6.2 and Figure 6.20). Lipoproteins bound to membrane receptors are internalized by endocytosis and metabolized, or modified by lipase enzymes on the cell surface (Figure 6.21). The endothelium is permeable to lipoprotein, some of which binds to the extracellular matrix and some is taken up by cells in the vessel wall.

TABLE 6.1 Risk factors for ischaemic heart disease

Modifiable	Non-modifiable
Cigarette smoking	Age
Hyperlipidaemias	Male sex
Hypertension	Family history
Diabetes	Personality type
High density lipoprotein levels	
Obesity	
Exercise level	

TABLE 6.2 Properties of the main lipoprotein particles

Particle	Diameter (nm)	Apolipoprotein	Cholesterol content (%)
Chylomicron	80–1200	A-1, A-2, A-4, B-48 and C	<5
Very low density lipoprotein (VLDL)	30–80	B-48, C, E	25
Intermediate density lipoprotein (IDL)	25–35	B-100, E	40
Low density lipoprotein (LDL)	15–25	B-100	65
High density lipoprotein (HDL)	5–15	A-1, A-2, C	<20

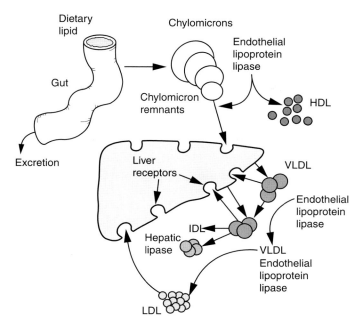

FIGURE 6.20 Schematic diagram of lipoprotein pathways. VLDL = very low density lipoprotein; IDL = intermediate density lipoprotein; LDL = low density lipoprotein; HDL = high density lipoprotein.

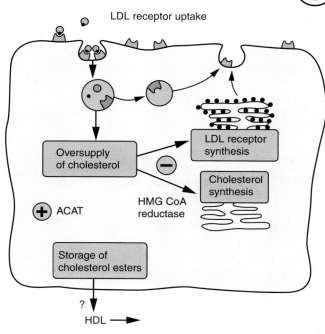

FIGURE 6.21 Intracellular cholesterol metabolism. ACAT = Acyl-CoA: Cholesterol acyltransferase; LDL = low density lipoprotein.

○ 6.1 SPECIAL STUDY TOPIC

CHOLESTEROL METABOLISM AND LIPID LEVELS AS RISK FACTORS

Low-density lipoprotein carries 70% of blood cholesterol. All cells possess LDL receptors, but the liver possesses by far the most and 75% of plasma LDL is removed by hepatocytes, which therefore control blood cholesterol levels. The number of LDL receptors on each hepatocyte is regulated by the intracellular cholesterol level. Increasing hepatocyte cholesterol content switches off LDL receptor synthesis, and plasma LDL levels rise. Thus a low cholesterol diet can lower blood cholesterol levels via hepatocyte LDL receptors. Lowering intestinal reabsorption of bile acids increases the conversion of cholesterol to bile acids in the hepatocyte; this fall in intracellular cholesterol lowers blood cholesterol. This knowledge is important in devising strategies to treat hyperlipidaemia.

High-density lipoprotein is synthesized mainly in the small intestine and in hepatocytes. It is believed to take up cholesterol from cells and from other lipoproteins and transport it to the liver. In different communities mean adult levels of total plasma cholesterol (TC) vary from about 3.9 mmol/L (150 mg/dL) to over 7 mmol/L (275 mg/dL). In countries with a mean TC level below 4 mmol/L ischaemic heart disease (IHD) is rare, whereas communities with mean TC levels of 5.2 or more invariably have high IHD rates. In prospective studies TC levels predict the risk of developing IHD, in communities with both high and low TC levels.

Blood levels of lipoprotein-A, which contains a unique apolipoprotein-A is an independent risk factor for IHD in that raised levels confer a high risk of IHD, even when LDL and other lipids are normal. By contrast, plasma levels of HDL are related inversely to the risk of IHD; HDL levels may be of greater predictive value than TC or LDL levels within communities.

Hyperlipidaemias, which are grouped according to the class of lipid that is in excess, may be inherited or result from another disorder. Multiple unknown genes influence blood lipid levels, and the commonest hyperlipidaemia is the polygenic form. The commonest monogenic hyperlipidaemia is LDL receptor deficiency. Low hepatocyte LDL receptors are due to mutation of one of the many genes that regulate the synthesis and transport of receptors; 1/500 live births are heterozygotes who possess 50% of normal LDL receptors. This results in plasma LDL levels that are two to four times normal. This increases the risk of IHD, which develops in early adulthood. Homozygotes constitute 1/1 000 000 live births and usually die of IHD in childhood. Sufferers are treated aggressively with lipid lowering stratagies.

Cigarette Smoking

Smoking is one of the most powerful risk factors for IHD, is dose related, and is an especially potent risk factor in young men. On cessation, the risk falls over several years to that of matched non-smokers. Smoking affects the coagulation system: it decreases endothelial prostaglandin I_2 (PGI_2) and nitric oxide synthesis, and increases platelet stickiness and blood fibrinogen levels.

Hypertension

Increased blood pressure (both systolic and diastolic) is associated with increased risk of IHD. In some community studies the risk in the 20% of the population with the highest pressure was four times that for the 20% with the lowest pressures. Lowering blood pressure decreases the risk of ischaemic heart disease, especially in the elderly, but the effect is not as marked as the reduction in stroke (p. 293).

Diabetes Mellitus

Diabetes doubles the risk of IHD and 20% of people with type II diabetes have evidence of vascular disease at presentation. Diabetic people also tend to develop cerebrovascular and peripheral vascular disease. The complex mechanisms are linked to the 'endothelial dysfunction', hypertension, hyperlipidaemia and obesity that occur in insulin resistance (p. 468). Good metabolic control lowers the risk.

Other Risk Factors

Diet

Diets rich in saturated fats and cholesterol are associated with high mean plasma levels of TC, LDL and VLDL. Prospective studies have demonstrated that the risk of IHD is related directly to: (i) the percentage of calories derived from saturated fats; (ii) high ratios of saturated/polyunsaturated dietary fats; and (iii) dietary intake of cholesterol. The risk of IHD is inversely related to the amount of dietary fibre and polyunsaturated fats. Consumption of fish oils and fruit high in natural antioxidants may be protective, but dietary supplements of the antioxidant vitamin E and β-carotene are not.

Alcohol Consumption

Alcohol consumption of more than 5 units (50 mg) daily is an independent risk factor for IHD; heavy drinking is associated with hypertension (p. 119) but the mechanisms are unclear. However, consumption of fewer than 2–3 units per day confers a lower risk of IHD than abstainers.

Regular Exercise

This lowers the risk of IHD. Exercise lowers weight and blood pressure, raises blood HDL levels and upregulates endothelial nitric oxide synthase. *Obesity* raises blood pressure, blood lipids and insulin resistance, but in addition, is an independent risk factor. Abdominal obesity, the predominant male pattern, is believed to be especially harmful.

Oral Contraceptives

These raise blood pressure and lipids and increase the risk of thrombosis. This slight risk is increased by age, smoking and obesity.

Behavioural Patterns and Stress

Stress is an undoubted risk factor especially when associated with a poor diet and poverty. Epidemiological studies show that low birth weight is a risk factor for IHD as well as hypertension (p. 119). This effect appears to be separate from social factors but the mechanisms are unknown.

The above risk factors are synergistic (Figure 6.22), each adding to the risk of developing IHD. They also contribute to the risk of the other major complications of atherosclerosis.

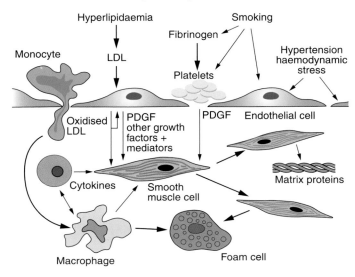

FIGURE 6.22 Interaction between risk factors and cells. LDL = low density lipoprotein; PDGF = platelet-derived growth factor.

Genetic Predisposition

Environmental risk factors probably account for most of the differences in the IHD rates between communities, but they do not predict accurately within a community who will develop IHD. Genetic influences clearly determine very important risk factors and protective mechanisms that at present remain unknown.

Some Pathogenetic Factors

Lipids in the Vessel Wall

The net influx of lipoproteins into the artery wall is proportional to plasma levels. Lipid influx is greater around the ostia of branches where the endothelium is more permeable. In the vessel wall LDL is immobilized by binding to proteoglycans where it can be oxidized by endothelial cells, by macrophages and by exposure to chemical factors and free radicals generated by platelets and leucocytes in the vessel wall. Receptor-mediated endocytosis of native LDL is regulated by negative feedback from the levels of intracellular cholesterol. However, foam cells gorge on oxidized LDL because it is absorbed via an unregulated pathway. Oxidized LDL is also antigenic and autoantibodies to oxidized LDL increase with the severity of atherosclerosis. LDL–antibody complexes are also taken up by macrophages via Fc receptors.

Oxidized LDL is toxic to endothelial cells and causes endothelial dysfunction. This leads to increased stiffness of large arteries and raises blood pressure by deficient nitric oxide release. Endothelial function is improved by administration of antioxidants. Oxidized LDL is chemotactic for monocytes and their recruitment could contribute to plaque growth. There is therefore substantial evidence that in the vessel wall oxidized LDL mediates some of the atherogenicity of raised blood LDL.

HDL provides a theoretical clearance system for cellular cholesterol. HDL may also prevent the chemical and physical changes such as oxidation, which promote the uptake of LDL. Although there is little *in vivo* evidence, these notions accord with the beneficial effect of raised plasma levels of HDL.

Haemodynamic Factors

Atherosclerosis is increased by haemodynamic stress; for example, the pulse pressure is greater in the lower aorta and legs than in the arms. In addition, hypertension and age aggravate atherosclerosis. Plaques occur on the outer aspects of branching points and at the ostia of branches. These are areas of low shear stress where the endothelial cells are more permeable to lipoproteins and have a more prothrombotic surface.

Blood Coagulation

Platelets and fibrin form a fine layer on the surface of plaques and their products are detectable within the plaque itself. Incorporation of thrombus could therefore play a role in the growth of plaques. Endothelial dysfunction renders the endothelial surface prothrombotic. It is therefore likely that thrombosis, which has a crucial role in myocardial infarction and the other acute complications of atherosclerosis, also contributes to plaque growth.

Inflammation

Most inflammatory cells probably enter the plaque via the small vessels derived from the vasa vasorum rather than from the lumen. Macrophages and activated T lymphocytes are universal. In some instances neutrophil polymorphs are plentiful. Acute inflammation has been implicated in plaque rupture, which precedes occlusive thrombosis and lytic enzymes released from leucocytes have been implicated in this. Infection by herpesvirus and *Chlamydia pneumoniae* has been implicated in coronary heart disease. This could explain the acute inflammation associated with plaque rupture. An infectious component in atherosclerosis is an important and intriguing possibility, but the evidence remains inconclusive.

The cellular and cytokine mechanisms in atherogenesis are similar to chronic inflammation and healing elsewhere (p. 61). Cytokines released from inflammatory cells may also activate endothelial cells and alter endothelial function as well as influence the growth and differentiation of various cell types in the vessel wall (Figures 6.18 and 6.22). In addition, continuing inflammation may result in fibrous thickening of the vessel wall and of the adjacent tissues – if severe, it is called periarteritis.

Precursor Lesions

Fatty streaks are the earliest arterial lipid deposits; they occur in the intima of large arteries in childhood. These yellow, slightly raised spots on the aortic intima enlarge and coalesce to form irregular yellow streaks. They consist of foam cells and some extracellular lipid (Figure 6.23), and some of them represent an early stage of this disease. In societies with a high prevalence of IHD, intimal thickenings occur in the coronary and in other arteries in some young children; they may even be present at birth. They are the putative precursors of 'premature' coronary atherosclerosis, which occurs in some young men. Intimal thickenings (intimal cushions) are normal features of arterial branching points, and diffuse intimal thickening of age-related or hypertensive arteriosclerosis (p. 109) are the substrates for development of 'normal' late-onset atherosclerosis. Thus, all of the putative precursors of atheroma have in common intimal thickening due to accumulation of cells and matrix.

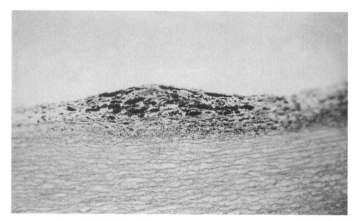

FIGURE 6.23 A histological section through a fatty streak in the aorta of a child stained to show fat red. The fatty streak consists mainly of groups of lipid-containing foam cells in the intima.

Cellular Interactions in Atherogenesis

It is likely that intimal thickening is orchestrated by the endothelial cell. However, the focal distribution of atheroma is determined by haemodynamic factors, of which haemodynamic stress and shear stress are the most important. Haemodynamic stress modulates endothelial cell function. Endothelial cells modulate haemostasis and platelet and leucocyte adherence. The latter release growth factors and cytokines, which stimulate the migration and proliferation of subendothelial smooth muscle cells which transform into myofibroblasts. As in wound healing these myofibroblasts synthesize extracellular matrix proteins and proteoglycans that contribute to the bulk of the plaque, affect cell growth and differentiation and bind lipoproteins.

Future Trends

In developed countries conscious of risk factors, the epidemic of IHD that developed over the first half of past century is on the wane, the incidence of IHD has fallen, in some countries by 50%. Lifestyle changes are believed to be responsible. Lipid-lowering drugs such as HMG CoA reductase inhibitors decrease mortality both in patients with complications of atherosclerosis and in healthy adults. Recent studies using quantitative imaging have shown that lowering risk factors and aggressive therapeutic reduction of serum cholesterol levels can induce regression of individual lesions. Ischaemic heart disease has now become the fate of the poor who are stressed, smoke and have a poor diet. It is increasing rapidly in eastern Europe and increasing affluence and adoption of a westernized lifestyle is producing new epidemics of the complications of atherosclerosis in developing nations. Prevention strategies are aimed at lifestyle modification for whole populations to which are added lipid-lowering therapies for high-risk individuals with hyperlipidaemia, low blood HDL levels, hypertension and diabetes.

HYPERTENSION

Key Points

- Hypertension is raised pressure in any vascular bed, for example pulmonary hypertension (p. 180), portal hypertension (p. 271).
- Without qualification, hypertension is usually synonymous with systemic arterial hypertension.
- Its main clinical importance is as a major risk factor in the cardiovascular diseases due to atherosclerosis.

Variation in Blood Pressure and the Definition of Hypertension

Within any population the distribution of blood pressure is a unimodal bell-shaped curve skewed to the right. The risk of cardiovascular disease increases with blood pressure, even within the normal range. The definition of hypertension is therefore arbitrary. Taking a cut-off point of 140/90 mmHg, single measurements of blood pressure suggest a prevalence of 4% in the third decade of life and over 60% in the eighth decade. In the UK and many western countries the overall prevalence of hypertension in adults reaches 20%.

In individuals, blood pressure shows a diurnal variation. The lowest levels occur during sleep. Blood pressure rises on standing up, during exercise and on exposure to cold and emotion. Individuals with a larger than normal pressure rise in response to these stimuli have an increased risk of permanent hypertension and are said to have labile hypertension. A single blood pressure reading should therefore be interpreted with caution and additional information can be obtained from 24-hour recording.

Normally, blood pressure rises through childhood and adolescence and reaches adult levels in the third decade. Those children and adolescents with highest blood pressures become adults with highest pressure – the hypertensive population. This phenomenon of 'tracking' of blood pressure has implications for early detection and treatment of hypertension.

Classification and Causes of Hypertension

In 95% of cases of hypertension there is no detectable cause; such patients are said to have primary or essential hypertension. In the remaining cases, hypertension is secondary to an underlying condition, often renal disease, alcohol misuse or occasionally, an endocrine disorder (Table 6.3).

TABLE 6.3 Classification of systemic hypertension

Type	Benign/Malignant	Causes
Essential (95%)	90% Benign 10% Malignant	

Secondary (5%)	80% Benign
	20% Malignant
		(a) Renal artery stenosis
		(b) Renal parenchymal disease, e.g.:
		    End stage renal failure
		    Glomerulonephritis
		    Reflux nephropathy
		    Diabetic nephropathy
		    Adult polycystic disease
		(c) Coarctation of the aorta
		(d) Endocrine causes, e.g.:
		    Cushing's syndrome
		    Conn's syndrome
		    Phaeochromocytoma
		    Acromegaly
		(e) Others, e.g.:
		    Pre-eclampsia
		    Alcohol abuse

The prognosis of hypertension is related both to the height and the rate of rise of pressure. Hypertension has been classified into a 'benign' form in which the prognosis is measured in decades, and a 'malignant' or accelerated form, which, if untreated, is universally fatal within 2 years.

Clinical features

Benign Hypertension

Benign hypertension causes:

- IHD
- heart failure
- stroke
- acceleration of renal disease
- malignant hypertension.

Benign hypertension is usually asymptomatic and most cases are discovered when pressure is measured at a routine medical examination, often in middle age. Blood pressure rises slowly over many years, usually only to moderately high levels, for example 180/100 mmHg. The elderly may develop a form with disproportionately high systolic pressure, systolic hypertension that is probably due to arterial disease.

Benign hypertension affects the heart and arteries of all sizes (Figure 6.24). The main target organs are the heart, brain and kidneys. The commonest complication is IHD including heart failure, accounting for about 60% of deaths, and another 30% die of stroke. Benign hypertension causes changes in the kidney, and hypertension is a major aggravating factor in patients with renal diseases. However, renal failure is uncommon and only affects those at the most severe end of the spectrum.

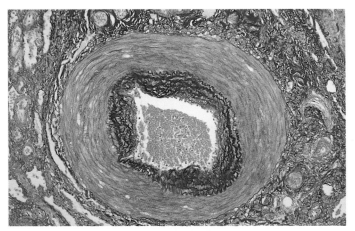

FIGURE 6.24 A renal interlobar artery in early established hypertension. There is intimal thickening but the predominant feature is hypertrophy of the muscular media causing increased wall to lumen ratio. This causes increased response to prevailing pressor stimuli – the 'vascular amplifier'.

Cardiovascular System

Increased pressure load causes hypertrophy of arteries and the heart. The muscle hypertrophy normalizes the workload of individual cardiac myocytes and arterial smooth muscle cells, but also has adverse effects on both the heart and on the arteries. The arterial geometry changes such that the resistance arteries have thicker walls and narrower lumina (Figure 6.25).

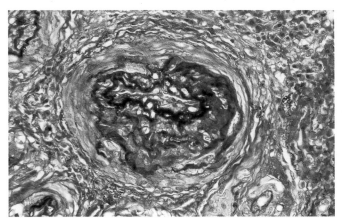

FIGURE 6.25 Advanced arteriosclerosis in a renal radial artery in an elderly subject with longstanding benign hypertension. The intima is grossly thickened by excess matrix proteins including collagen and elastic tissue. There has been almost complete loss of the medial smooth muscle, presumably due to atrophy.

The changes of arteriosclerosis which ensue are more severe and occur earlier than the age changes described on p. 109. These permanent structural changes in the arterial tree perpetuate hypertension regardless of its aetiology. The longitudinal and circumferential stretching of arteries, if severe, may cause dilatation of the aortic root and rarely, leakage (incompetence) of the aortic valve (p. 148). Longstanding hypertension aggravates atherosclerosis and contributes to the development and rupture of aneurysms and dissections (p. 123).

Heart

In the heart, left ventricular hypertrophy (Figure 6.26) impairs diastolic function; the thickened ventricle is stiffer due to both increased muscle mass and interstitial fibrosis. As the ventricle is only perfused during diastole, coronary artery

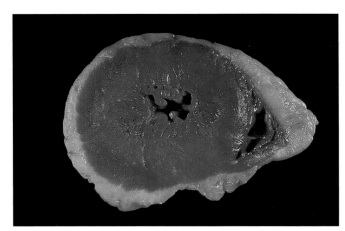

FIGURE 6.26 This transverse slice of the left ventricle shows gross hypertrophy that is present in some hypertensive patients.

perfusion is poor. In addition, people with hypertension are likely to have coronary atherosclerosis. In addition, the increased oxygen demand of the hypertrophied left ventricle contributes to ischaemia, even at rest. Thus, left ventricular hypertrophy causes increased mortality, proportional to the degree of hypertrophy, from cardiac arrhythmias and myocardial infarction.

Brain

In addition to arteriosclerosis and atherosclerosis of the cerebral arteries, hypertension causes multiple tiny aneurysms in the deep penetrating arteries supplying the basal ganglia, pons and cerebellum. These aneurysms rupture and cause hypertensive cerebral haemorrhages (p. 249). Hyper-tension also predisposes to regional and watershed zone cerebral infarction. In addition, over-enthusiastic treatment of hypertension in the elderly can cause boundary zone infarction of the brain due to the rightward shift in the cerebral autoregulatory curve (Figure 6.12 on p. 109).

Kidney

Arteriosclerosis affects the afferent arterioles and to a lesser extent the glomeruli and efferent arterioles. This accelerates the normal age-related loss of nephrons and diminishes the functional reserve of the kidneys. Hypertension is an important aggravating factor for renal diseases (Chapter 13), but only in the most severe cases does benign hypertension cause renal failure.

Malignant Hypertension

Malignant hypertension is defined clinically as hypertension (diastolic blood pressure >130 mmHg) together with retinal changes of bilateral flame-shaped haemorrhages and/or papilloedema. In about 50% of cases malignant hypertension develops without a preceding history of hypertension; fewer than 5% of patients with benign essential hypertension develop the malignant phase. It is commoner in the black races and in those with secondary hypertension, especially if caused by renovascular disease. Malignant hypertension usually affects younger hypertensives; *de novo* cases usually present at 30–40 years.

Patients with malignant hypertension are ill. If they survive the usual complications of raised blood pressure – heart failure and cerebral haemorrhage – renal failure becomes universal and is the commonest cause of death in untreated cases. Occasionally 'hypertensive encephalopathy' occurs, a syndrome characterized by altered consciousness, fits and transient paralyses. The renal damage and encephalopathy are due to failure of autoregulation when the resistance vessels cease to protect the microcirculation from the increased pressure. This is rare in the elderly because the cerebral autoregulatory curve is shifted to the right (Figure 6.12 on p. 109), but is commoner in the young and especially in children whose arteries are unprotected by arteriosclerosis. Malignant hypertension causes:

- renal failure
- heart failure
- stroke
- hypertensive encephalopathy
- microangiopathic haemolytic anaemia.

Pathology and Pathogenesis of the Arterial Lesions

Failure of autoregulation in the kidney transmits increased pressure to glomeruli causing fibrinoid necrosis and microaneurysms of glomerular capillaries. The pressure also causes fibrinoid necrosis of afferent glomerular arterioles (Figure 6.27) which may rupture (Figure 6.28) or be associated with luminal thrombosis resulting in small infarcts. Thrombosis causes damage to red blood corpuscles – microangiopathic haemolytic anaemia (Figure 6.29). Ischaemia of the juxtaglomerular apparatus leads to

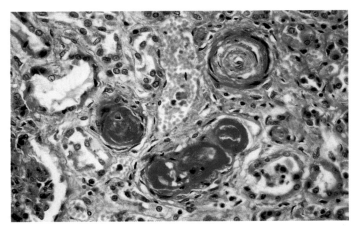

FIGURE 6.27 A section of kidney showing fibrinoid necrosis and thrombosis of arterioles (stained red). A small radial artery shows intimal proliferation probably due to a healing response which causes extreme narrowing.

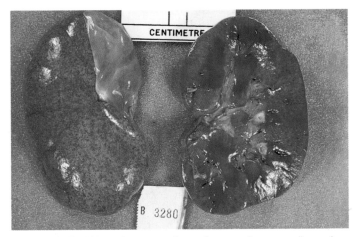

FIGURE 6.28 The kidneys in acute malignant hypertension are swollen and their surfaces show small haemorrhages.

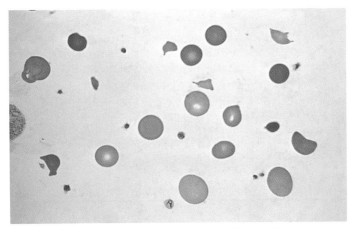

FIGURE 6.29 A peripheral blood smear showing red blood cells fragmented due to intravascular thrombosis in malignant hypertension.

increased secretion of renin, which further increases blood pressure leading to a vicious circle. Together, these effects give rise to proteinuria and haematuria. Similar changes occur in the brain in hypertensive encephalopathy. The circulation in the heart is, however, protected from the brunt of the pressure by systolic contraction of the cardiac muscle and other organs are usually spared.

Healing arterial damage results in intimal proliferation. This may cause chronic renal failure due to ischaemia and may require dialysis and renal transplantation a few years after successful treatment. With better detection and treatment of benign hypertension the incidence of malignant hypertension has fallen steeply in countries with adequate medical care. By contrast, malignant hypertension is still the commonest reason for acute renal failure in black races in some African countries.

Aetiology of Essential Hypertension

Key Points

- Hypertension is due to an interplay of genetic and environmental factors.
- Blood pressure has a polygenic inheritance.
- The most important environmental factors are stress, diet and the intrauterine environment.

Genetic and Racial Factors

A polygenic inheritance has been established. The candidate genes include those encoding angiotensinogen, which is estimated to account for 6% of blood pressure variation in humans, renin and atrial natriuretic peptide receptor genes.

Black people are more susceptible to hypertension than white people; in the USA the black population has twice the incidence of hypertension and six times the mortality. Females have a higher incidence of hypertension, but mortality in males is 1.5–2 times the mortality of females

with the same levels of blood pressure, probably because of increased atherosclerosis.

Environmental Factors

City dwellers have higher blood pressures than rural populations and migration studies suggest environmental influences. Although difficult to quantify, stress seems to be the important factor and animal experiments support this notion. Epidemiological, clinical and animal studies implicate sodium intake, which is excessive in most westernized countries. Diets high in salt are often also high in animal fats, and low in dietary potassium, which can lower blood pressure.

There is a linear relationship between alcohol intake and blood pressure. The oestrogen containing contraceptive pill increases the blood pressure by a few mmHg in most women who take it. This will therefore tip some women into clinical hypertension. Regular exercise lowers blood pressure, probably because of induction of endothelial nitric oxide synthase (p. 67). Smoking only aggravates the complications of hypertension. The effects of the intrauterine environment are of current interest. Babies with low birth weight have an increased incidence of hypertension and other cardiovascular disorders in adult life. It is likely that the renin system is involved.

Secondary Hypertension

Renal disease is 10 times commoner than all other causes together. Hypertension is caused by disorders of the renal blood vessels (renovascular hypertension), many renal diseases (renal parenchymal hypertension) or simply to loss of nephrons in renal failure.

Renovascular Hypertension

In the community, 3% of the hypertensive population have renovascular hypertension. Any narrowing of renal arteries causes hypertension because of activation of the renin–angiotensin system. The commonest is renal artery stenosis, which may be unilateral or bilateral. Over 50 years of age this is usually due to atherosclerosis while in younger patients fibromuscular dysplasia is usually the cause. This may present in childhood but is more common in women about 40 years of age.

In renal artery stenosis the pathogenesis of hypertension has three phases. In the first phase, hypertension is maintained by high blood angiotensin II through a direct pressor effect due to vasoconstriction combined with a 'slow pressor effect' probably due to vascular smooth muscle cell growth. In the second phase, renin and angiotensin levels fall, but the blood pressure is still dependent on renin. In the third phase renin and angiotensin levels may be normal but, as in hypertension due to any cause, the blood pressure is sustained by permanent changes in the vascular tree. Surgical treatment of the stenosis at this stage is therefore disappointing. At any time during this sequence of events, malignant hypertension may be triggered.

Restoration of blood flow to the ischaemic kidney can cure the hypertension in selected cases, and can restore normal function to the atrophied kidney, which is protected from the effects of hypertension by the narrowed artery.

Renal Parenchymal Hypertension

End-stage renal failure is always accompanied by hypertension due to sodium and water retention. Hypertension is also common in the early stages of glomerulonephritis. In children reflux nephropathy is the commonest cause of secondary hypertension. The reason for increased renin secretion by the damaged kidney is unclear.

Coarctation of the Aorta

Hypertension in the upper half of the body, mainly due to renal underperfusion and hyper-reninism, is a feature of this congenital disorder (p. 158).

Adrenal Hypertension

Hypertension occurs in several adrenal disorders:

- primary aldosteronism
- cushing's syndrome
- phaeochromocytoma
- congenital adrenal hyperplasia.

These are discussed in Chapter 17.

Other Endocrine Diseases

Hyperparathyroidism, acromegaly and both hypo- and hyperthyroidism may be complicated by hypertension, but the mechanisms are poorly understood. Gestational hypertension is usually caused by pre-eclampsia, a disease characterized by hypertension, proteinuria and oedema, which complicates 3–5% of pregnancies. In some cases essential hypertension may present in pregnancy.

VASCULITIS (ANGIITIS)

Key Points

- In vasculitis there is focal inflammation of blood vessels.

- Involvement of arteries or arterioles is often termed arteritis; when veins and capillaries are also affected, the terms vasculitis or angiitis are preferred.
- In some types of arteritis necrosis of an artery wall (necrotizing arteritis) may cause occlusive thrombosis and infarction, aneurysm formation or rupture with haemorrhage.
- Intimal proliferation in the healing phase often narrows the lumen, and chronic ischaemia ensues.

Aetiology and Pathogenesis

The aetiology of most types of vasculitis is unknown. In serum sickness and in the vasculitis that occurs in systemic lupus erythematosus and rheumatoid arthritis there is immune complex deposition. In some cases of polyarteritis nodosa the complexes contain hepatitis B surface antigens; other viruses and streptococci have also been implicated as antigens. Some types of vasculitis are caused by infection by microorganisms (see below). Vasculitis may follow the administration of drugs, for example penicillin, sulphonamides, gold salts and amphetamines, which may cause immune complex deposition or induce a hypersensitivity reaction to endothelial cells by binding to their surface. Circulating antiendothelial cell antibodies in some cases imply a type II hypersensitivity reaction. These autoantibodies may be useful in monitoring disease activity but their role in pathogenesis is dubious. Antineutrophil antibodies occur in some cases. The pattern of staining, whether cytoplasmic or perinuclear has some diagnostic value (Table 6.4). Types of vasculitis are discussed in Special Study Topic 6.2.

ANEURYSMS

An aneurysm is an abnormal localized dilatation of a blood vessel. Aneurysms occur in vessels of any sizes ranging from the aorta to capillaries (Table 6.6); some types may also affect veins. Symmetrical stretching of the whole circumference produces a fusiform aneurysm, while segmental stretching of part of the circumference causes an asymmetrical bulge known as a saccular aneurysm. Local weakening causes the wall of a blood vessel to stretch under the distending force of the blood pressure. Stretching causes thinning of the wall and further weakening, so that once an aneurysm has formed it tends to expand, and eventually rupture.

TABLE 6.4 Patterns of ANCA staining and their associations

ANCA	Antigen	Associated vasculitis
cANCA	Proteinase 3	Wegener's granulomatosis (90%), occasionally, Churg–Strauss syndrome; polyarteritis, classical and microscopic
pANCA	Myeloperoxidase, elastase, lysozyme, cathepsin G	Microscopic polyarteritis, rheumatic and collagen vascular diseases

cANCA = cytoplasmic antineutrophil cytoplasmic antigen; pANCA = perinuclear antineutrophil cytoplasmic antigen.

6.2   SPECIAL STUDY TOPIC

TYPES OF VASCULITIS

Vasculitis is diagnosed by a combination of clinical and histological features. The histological features vary, but always include inflammation of the vessel wall. There is neither a satisfactory aetiological or morphological classification. The pattern of vessel involvement is helpful in making a diagnosis and Table 6.5 combines a list of the vasculitis syndromes and their distribution.

TABLE 6.5   Vessels involved in the various vasculitis syndromes

Large and medium-sized arteries
Giant cell arteritis, Takayasu's disease, rheumatic disease, syphilis and other infections

Medium-sized arteries
Polyarteritis nodosa, Kawasaki's disease, Wegener's granulomatosis, Churg–Strauss syndrome, collagen vascular diseases, Behçet's disease, Buerger's disease, Takayasu's disease and fungal infections

Arterioles, capillaries and venules
Henoch–Schönlein purpura, microscopic polyarteritis, serum sickness, drug-induced vasculitis, Wegener's granulomatosis, Churg–Strauss syndrome, cryoglobulinaemia, hypocomplementaemia, Goodpasture's syndrome, inflammatory bowel disease and malignancy associated

Giant Cell Arteritis (Cranial Arteritis, Temporal Arteritis)

Giant cell arteritis is commonest in cranial arteries and may be diagnosed by temporal artery biopsy. Giant cell arteritis affects mostly the elderly of both sexes. Uncommonly, it is widespread and the aortic arch and its major branches may be involved.

Full thickness granulomatous inflammation causes multiple focal lesions along the artery's length. Lymphocytes, macrophages and multinucleated giant cells accumulate around fragments of internal elastic lamina (see Figure 6.10). This causes localized reddening, tenderness, pain or nodularity of the arteries. There may be headache, facial pain and visual disturbances; a very high erythrocyte sedimentation rate (ESR) is typical. The most severe complications are blindness (from involvement of the retinal arteries) and cerebral infarction. The disease is sometimes associated with polymyalgia rheumatica. It is of unknown aetiology, but the histological features suggest a Type IV hypersensitivity reaction. There is good clinical response to steroids.

Takayasu's Disease

In this rare condition, which affects mainly young women (male:female ratio 1:4), the aorta and its branches are affected by a necrotizing granulomatous arteritis. This causes narrowing or occlusion of the subclavian, carotid and innominate arteries (hence the term pulseless disease). Ischaemia of the limbs is accompanied by visual and neurological defects, which may extend to total blindness and hemiparesis. Involvement of the coronary, renal and other visceral arteries occasionally occurs with consequent ischaemia. The aetiology is unknown.

Polyarteritis Nodosa

Polyarteritis nodosa affects a wide age range, but is commonest between 20 and 40 years and affects men more often than women. Any part of the body may be affected, but the lesions predominate in kidney, heart, skeletal muscle, gut and nervous system. The walls of medium-sized and small arteries show focal and segmental inflammation. Early lesions consist of fibrinoid necrosis of the intima and media of an artery accompanied by acute inflammation of the whole thickness of the vessel wall. Lesions affect the whole circumference of smaller arteries, but often only a segment of larger vessels. In the acute stage, the main complications are occlusive thrombosis with infarction and artery rupture with severe haemorrhage. Bulging of the weakened wall may form an aneurysm (p. 120). In severe cases there is fever, prostration, neutrophil (and sometimes eosinophilic) leucocytosis and a very high ESR; such cases are often rapidly fatal. The acute changes resolve with chronic inflammation and fibrosis and the main late complications are due to chronic ischaemia. Angina, cardiac failure, renal failure and hypertension are among the commoner manifestations, but infarction of the gut or the brain can also occur. Lesions in the small arteries of peripheral nerves result in peripheral neuropathy. In some cases arteriography showing multiple aneurysms is diagnostic; in others, vasculitis can be confirmed by biopsy.

The relapsing clinical course extends over some years, often complicated by hypertension due to renal ischaemia.

Microscopic Polyarteritis

This vasculitis affects small arteries, arterioles and capillaries (Figure 6.30) and the lesions predominate in the skin, kidney, gut, skeletal muscles and heart. In addition to the vessel involvement, glomerulonephritis is seen in many cases (Chapter 13). Antineutrophil cytoplasmic antibodies (cANCA) are present in the serum of over 90% of patients.

SPECIAL STUDY TOPIC CONTINUED . . .

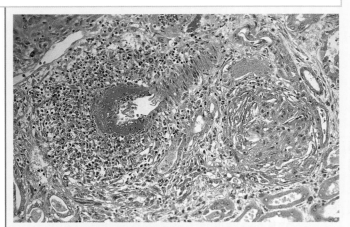

FIGURE 6.30 **A section of kidney from a case of polyarteritis showing a damaged glomerulus and a radial artery which in its lower part shows fibrinoid necrosis. There is intense surrounding inflammation.**

Kawasaki's Disease (Mucocutaneous Lymph Node Syndrome)

This febrile illness is characterized by skin rashes, inflammation of the conjunctival and buccal mucosae, generalized lymphadenopathy and sometimes arthritis. It affects mainly children and is likely to have a viral aetiology. There is an arteritis resembling polyarteritis nodosa associated with circulating antibodies to endothelial cells, but most patients recover spontaneously after 3–6 weeks. Coronary arteritis develops in approximately 2% of cases and sometimes is fatal.

Wegener's Granulomatosis

In this disease vasculitis and necrotizing granulomatous inflammation affect the upper respiratory tract, lungs (p. 182) and kidneys in various combinations. Males are affected twice as commonly as females. There may be accompanying skin rashes, polyarthritis and polyneuritis. Cytotoxic drugs such as cyclophosphamide cure 90% of patients.

Churg–Strauss Syndrome (Eosinophilic Granulomatous Vasculitis)

This is characterized by asthma, vasculitis of small arteries and veins and extravascular granulomatous inflammation with necrosis and intense eosinophil infiltration in the surrounding tissues. The lungs are most commonly affected although other organs such as spleen, skin and peripheral nerves may also be involved.

Buerger's Disease (Thromboangiitis Obliterans)

Buerger's disease is a vasculitis of medium-sized and small arteries and veins, with thrombosis, organization and recanalization of the affected vessels. It occurs predominantly in males, affects mainly the legs, and gives rise to severe pain and progressive ischaemic changes that may progress to gangrene. The inflammatory changes may involve the entire neurovascular bundle explaining the characteristic severity of the pain. The disease is practically confined to heavy smokers; its progress is arrested or diminished by cessation and resumption of smoking produces an exacerbation. An increased prevalence of human leucocyte antigen (HLA) A9 and B5 suggests a genetic predisposition.

Vasculitis in Other Diseases

Arteritis with lesions indistinguishable from polyarteritis nodosa occurs in a number of diseases (Table 6.5) especially connective tissue diseases, notably systemic lupus erythematosus and rheumatoid arthritis. Henoch–Schönlein purpura, which may sometimes follow streptococcal or viral infections, affects the skin and gut and may cause glomerulonephritis (p. 392). Vasculitis is also associated with haematological malignancies.

Infective Vasculitis

Arteries are relatively resistant to bacterial invasion and are usually spared in acute infections unless suppuration or gangrene occur. Infected emboli, for example from infective endocarditis (p. 149), may cause an acute arteritis resulting in necrosis and rupture or the development of a mycotic aneurysm. The purpuric rash of meningococcal septicaemia is caused by an acute meningococcal vasculitis affecting the cutaneous capillaries.

A vasculitis can result from widespread invasion of arterioles, capillaries and venules by microorganisms such as rickettsia, for example typhus and Rocky Mountain spotted fever. In immunosuppressed patients and drug addicts fungi such as aspergillus and mucor invade veins and arteries, causing thrombosis and infarction.

TABLE 6.6 Key features of the main types of aneurysm

Type of aneurysm	Main location	Comments
Atherosclerotic aneurysm	Abdominal aorta, iliac arteries, popliteal and cerebral arteries	Asymptomatic or presents with abdominal pain and shock
Syphilitic aneurysm	Thoracic aorta	Prominent pressure symptoms
Dissecting aneurysm	Thoracic aorta	Acute chest pain with hypertension or shock. Sometimes associated with Marfan's syndrome
Traumatic aneurysm	Scalp or anywhere	Also causes false aneurysm
Berry aneurysm	Branching points of circle of Willis and cerebral arteries	Causes subarachnoid haemorrhage
Microaneurysm	Penetrating branches of cerebral arteries	Cause hypertensive cerebral haemorrhages
Mycotic aneurysm (infective)	Aorta and elsewhere, especially cerebral and mesenteric arteries	Embolism from bacterial endocarditis is commonest cause

Aortic Aneurysms

Atherosclerosis is the commonest cause of aortic aneurysms which usually occur after the age of 60 and are much commoner in males, especially hypertensive smokers. The aneurysms complicate severe atheroma because of erosion of the media by advanced plaques. They may be fusiform or saccular (Figure 6.31) and occur in the lower abdominal aorta, usually distal to the renal arteries, occasionally in the thoracic aorta, but seldom in the ascending aorta. When the thoracic aorta is affected, the abdominal aorta is still more severely affected and the whole aorta may be dilated (Figure 6.32). Abdominal aneurysms may extend into the iliac arteries. Atherosclerotic aneurysms occur much less commonly in the popliteal artery and cerebral, splenic, renal and other visceral arteries.

Abdominal aneurysms are often incidental findings during medical or radiological examination but may cause pain due to pressure effects or stretching. Large aneurysms are liable to rupture with massive retroperitoneal, and occasionally intraperitoneal, haemorrhage that is frequently fatal. The larger the aneurysm, the greater the risk of rupture: 5% of those more than 5 cm in diameter rupture yearly, and thus are treated by insertion of a prosthetic graft. Mural thrombus frequently forms over ulcerated plaques and may form thick layers filling the whole sac; embolism may occur and occlude leg arteries. Extension of the aneurysm or the thrombus to the origins of the renal or mesenteric arteries may cause visceral ischaemia.

Aortic Dissection (Dissecting Aortic Aneurysm)

Arterial dissection is commonest in the aorta but can affect other arteries. Aortic dissection is three times commoner in males. Patients develop a tearing pain in the chest; shock and death may occur at any time from haemorrhage or from compression of the coronary arteries or other vessels. Untreated,

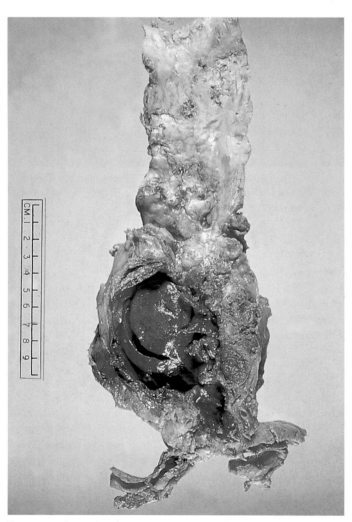

FIGURE 6.31 A saccular atheromatous aneurysm of the descending aorta in the typical position above the iliac arteries. Its lumen contains abundant soft thrombus.

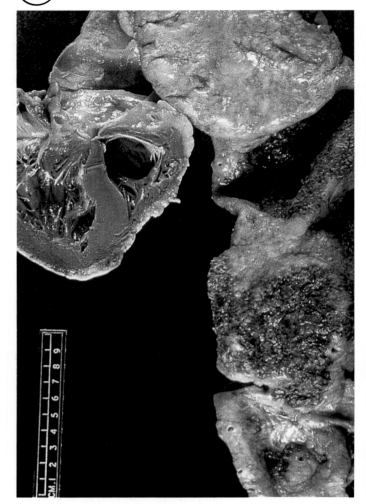

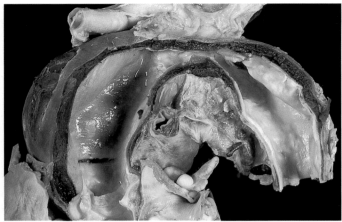

FIGURE 6.33 The ascending arch and descending aorta from a 26-year-old man, who died of a dissecting aneurysm. The transverse intimal tear is just above the aortic valve and the cause is the narrowing (coarctation) at the aortic arch (p. 158).

FIGURE 6.32 The heart is enlarged due to longstanding hypertension and the aorta is diffusely affected by severe atheroma and arteriosclerosis. It is dilated due to an aneurysm and elongated.

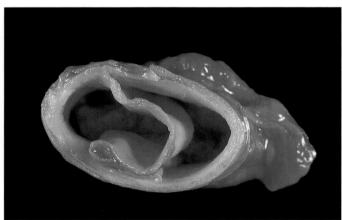

FIGURE 6.34 Another case showing that the haematoma is within the layers of the aorta.

90% of cases die within a few days, but early diagnosis and prompt surgical treatment have improved the immediate prognosis. Most aortic dissections are spontaneous but may also be precipitated by blunt chest injury, arterial catheterization and surgery.

Pathology

Blood enters a tear, usually transverse, in the intima; in 60% of cases it occurs in the ascending aorta (Figure 6.33), and in 30% at the start of the descending aorta. It is usually less than 3 cm in length but may involve the whole circumference. The blood dissects the artery wall into inner and outer layers (Figure 6.34), the plane is usually between the inner two-thirds and the outer one third of the media, so external rupture is common. The blood may rupture the artery wall almost immediately, with little dissection. Usually, however, blood tracks proximally and distally in the media. At the aortic valve ring, the dissection may cause prolapse of one or more valve cusps causing aortic incompetence. More often it ruptures into the pericardial sac causing fatal cardiac tamponade. Tears in the ascending aorta therefore have a worse prognosis than more distal dissections. The dissection may also track distally into the abdominal aorta. Sites of rupture include the mediastinum, pleura, retroperitoneum or peritoneal cavity. The blood in the media can compress any of the branches of the aorta and can track along them, causing acute ischaemia: if the coronary arteries are affected, myocardial infarction can result. Occasionally, the dissection remains localized and the medial haematoma may heal by organization leaving a scar. Occasionally, a second intimal tear sometimes in an atheromatous patch permits flow to re-enter the lumen. If the patient survives, the channel formed in the media becomes lined by endothelium, giving a 'double-barrelled' aorta.

The two important factors in the pathogenesis of aortic dissection are the blood pressure and medial weakness. During ventricular systole the frictional force of the blood

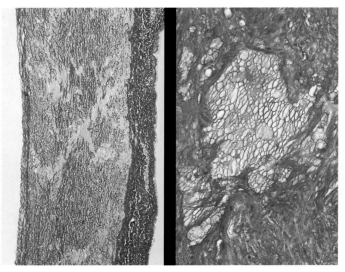

FIGURE 6.35 The low power view (left) shows that the elastic fibres (stained black) have fragmented and the higher power view (right) shows that the spaces are filled with connective tissue mucins (stained blue).

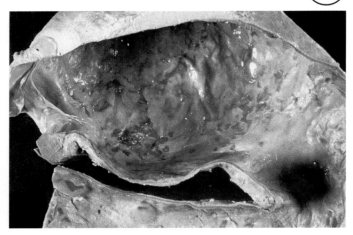

FIGURE 6.36 The ascending aorta severely dilated due to a syphilitic aneurysm. The intimal surface is covered by white thickenings that give rise to a 'tree bark' appearance.

stretches the intima downstream. Degeneration of the media allows increased stretching of the inner part of the wall, which eventually tears. Weakness in the media then facilitates arterial dissection by the haematoma. The more important factor is hypertension; 70% of patients are hypertensive. The weakness of the media is due to myxoid degeneration with patchy loss of elastic fibres and replacement of the musculo-elastic tissue by proteoglycan-rich extracellular matrix (Figure 6.35). The cause of myxoid degeneration is unknown. There is a high incidence of severe myxoid degeneration and aortic dilatation and dissection in Marfan syndrome an autosomal dominant mutation in the gene for fibrillin a protein necessary for the deposition of elastic fibres.

Syphilitic Aneurysm

The large aneurysms of the thoracic aortic arch due to syphilis are now seldom seen. Syphilitic mesaortitis develops 20 or more years after primary infection. Arteritis of the vasa vasorum causes ischaemia in the media and patchy loss of musculo-elastic laminae which coalesce to involve the whole thickness of the media. The weakened areas stretch, and fibrous intimal thickening is seen as smooth grey-white areas which extend, fuse and become irregularly contracted to produce a wrinkled 'tree-bark' appearance (Figure 6.36). The intimal thickening predisposes to severe atherosclerosis.

Pressure effects include superior mediastinal compression, dysphagia, bronchial obstruction with pneumonia, left recurrent laryngeal nerve palsy and painful vertebral or sternal erosion. Mesaortitis may cause dilatation of the aortic root and aortic valve incompetence, and involvement of the ostia of the coronary arteries may cause myocardial ischaemia. Rupture results in massive fatal haemorrhage.

Trauma

Arterial injury by blunt trauma, a penetrating wound or angiography may cause a traumatic aneurysm or an arterial dissection (see below). Penetration of an artery may cause a false aneurysm in which the sac is the fibrous wall of an organized haematoma that communicates with the lumen. Injury of an adjacent artery and vein may cause an arteriovenous fistula.

Miscellaneous Aneurysms

Infective (mycotic) aneurysms are due to infection of the vessel wall either from an infected embolus for example in infective endocarditis, or from an adjacent local inflammation such as tuberculosis. Berry aneurysms are small saccular aneurysms in the intracranial arteries. They arise because of congenital weaknesses at artery bifurcations; some may be acquired as a result of atheroma; they are discussed fully on pp. 293–294. Microaneurysms of the deep penetrating cerebral arteries which occur in the elderly and in hypertension may rupture causing intracerebral haemorrhage (p. 293). Capillary aneurysms are seen in the fundi in diabetic retinopathy (p. 325) and also occur in the glomerular capillaries. Cardiac aneurysm is usually a complication of myocardial infarction.

Other Arterial Diseases

Raynaud's Disease

This is intermittent abnormal vasoconstriction of the extremities on exposure to cold. It occurs mainly in young women, usually starting in adolescence. It affects the fingers symmetrically and occasionally the tip of the nose, ears and toes. Trophic changes may eventually occur, but ulceration and gangrene seldom occur. There are no histological abnormalities in the vessels. The mechanisms causing vasoconstriction are not known, but may include local dysfunction of peptidergic innervation of the digital vessels.

In Raynaud's phenomenon similar symptoms occur secondary to other diseases, including connective tissue diseases such as systemic lupus erythematosus. Raynaud's phenomenon may be an early manifestation of progressive systemic sclerosis; the combination of calcinosis, Raynaud's phenomenon, erythema, oesophageal involvement, sclerodactyly and telangiectasia constitute the CREST syndrome. Buerger's disease; trauma from the use of vibratory power tools, drugs or toxins (ergot, α-adrenergic blockers and polyvinyl chloride monomer); and hyperviscosity syndromes such as cryoglobulinaemia are also sometimes responsible. In Raynaud's phenomenon trophic changes, ulceration and gangrene may occur.

Mönckeberg's Arteriosclerosis (Medial Calcification)

In this disease dystrophic calcification occurs in the circular medial muscle layer of arteries in elderly people. The radiological appearance is striking but there is no arterial narrowing and the only clinical effects are those of arteriosclerosis.

Fibromuscular Dysplasia

This disease affects medium-sized arteries mainly in middle-aged women. There are various types; but in all of them the artery wall is focally abnormal. Fibrous or fibromuscular thickening of the wall causes stenosis. As the renal arteries are most commonly affected the commonest clinical problem is hypertension. The carotid, vertebral and splanchnic arteries may also be involved. Thrombosis may occur and the abnormal structure of the media also leads to the formation of true aneurysms or dissections.

Disorders of Endothelium and the Microcirculation

The microcirculation is the capillaries, the arterioles that supply them and the venules that drain the blood from the capillary bed. A capillary consists of a single endothelial cell encircling a lumen that only just admits the passage of red blood cells. Intercellular junctions join adjacent endothelial cells. The microcirculation is adapted to each organ and tissue. Thus the liver sinusoids and kidney have a highly permeable fenestrated endothelium (Figure 6.37), while the capillaries in the brain are watertight and contribute to the blood–brain barrier (Figure 6.38). Capillary endothelial cells are surrounded by pericytes, which support them, synthesize basement membrane and which can differentiate into a variety of cell types including vascular smooth muscle cells. Capillaries act as a semipermeable membrane. They retain most of the protein but permit free exchange of fluid.

The flow of interstitial fluid is governed by the balance between the hydrostatic and plasma oncotic pressures in the microcirculation and by the endothelial permeability (p. 55). Interstitial fluid, rich in oxygen and nutrients, is

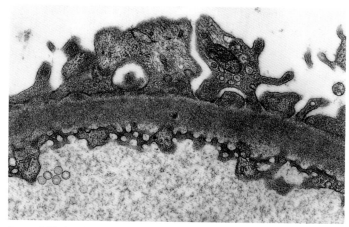

FIGURE 6.37 An electron micrograph showing a renal glomerular capillary with the endothelial cell cut tangentially to reveal the presence of round pores which give rise to a highly permeable fenestrated endothelium.

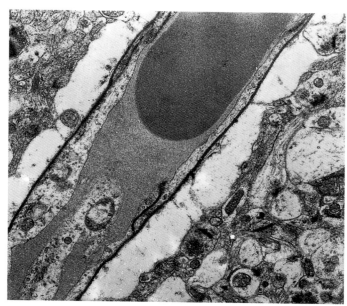

FIGURE 6.38 An electron micrograph showing a capillary in the cerebral cortex. It contains a red blood cell. There are two endothelial cells whose cytoplasm is non-fenestrated. The endothelial cells overlap and there is a tight junction between the cells seen as a black line. This is characteristic of a less permeable endothelium.

formed by egress of fluid from the arterial end of capillaries where blood pressure exceeds plasma oncotic pressure. At the venous end of the capillary, plasma oncotic pressure exceeds blood pressure, and interstitial fluid re-enters the circulation, carrying with it carbon dioxide, urea and other metabolic waste products.

The endothelium controls the permeability of the circulation. Endothelial cells increase their permeability in response to mediators of inflammation (p. 55), to direct injury, and to secretion of endothelial permeability factor (vascular endothelial growth factor [VEGF]). When injured, endothelial cells contract opening gaps between them; this dramatic rise in the permeability increases the volume and flow of interstitial fluid. Widespread endothelial injury by bacterial toxins, leucocyte enzymes or hypoxia may cause disseminated intravascular coagulation and contributes to the syndrome of shock.

Oedema

> **Key Points**
>
> - Oedema is an abnormal increase in the volume of interstitial fluid.
> - There are three main pathogenic mechanisms: increased hydrostatic pressure in the microcirculation, decreased plasma oncotic pressure and lymphatic obstruction.
> - Oedema is either localized or generalized.

Localized Oedema

Pulmonary oedema and cerebral oedema, both of which may be fatal, are the most important forms of localized oedema. Normally oedema fluid has a low protein content – a 'transudate'. However, because of the increased permeability of the microcirculation in inflammation, inflammatory oedema is protein rich and constitutes an 'exudate' (p. 56).

The most important causes of localized oedema are:

- left heart failure (pulmonary oedema)
- inflammation
- venous hypertension
- lymphatic obstruction.

Pulmonary oedema

The osmotic pressure of the plasma (25 mmHg; 3.32 kPa) is greater than the normal hydrostatic pressure in the pulmonary capillaries (8–10 mmHg; 1.06–1.33 kPa). This maintains the dryness of the alveoli and facilitates gas exchange. In left heart failure increased pressure in the pulmonary veins (pulmonary venous hypertension) increases the capillary hydrostatic pressure and oedema ensues. Overloading the circulation by rapid transfusion of blood or fluids produces pulmonary oedema, especially in the elderly. Oedema occurs first in the interstitium – 'interstitial oedema' which gives rise to characteristic streaky opacities on chest radiographs. The oedema fluid then escapes into the alveoli and fills the lung (p. 181).

Pulmonary oedema is seen in other circumstances. It is pronounced in influenza and in lobar pneumonia. It may be part of generalized oedema, for example in renal disease. Pulmonary oedema also complicates raised intracranial pressure, probably due to neuroendocrine activation.

Local venous hypertension

Prolonged sitting causes temporary oedema of the feet and ankles. Thrombosis of the deep leg veins is an important cause of local venous hypertension and oedema.

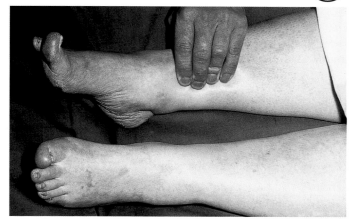

FIGURE 6.39 'Pitting' oedema of the lower legs demonstrated clinically.

Pitting oedema of the lower legs is a useful sign of right heart failure (Figure 6.39).

Chronic lymphatic obstruction (lymphoedema)

In this form of oedema the fluid is protein-rich because normal lymph contains protein. In time, growth of connective tissue renders the tissues firm and they do not 'pit' on pressure. Lymphoedema may be due to lymphatic permeation by cancer cells, or following lymph node dissection, for example for breast cancer. Lymphatics can also be obstructed by chronic inflammation, for example in filariasis, which causes elephantiasis.

Generalized Oedema

In generalized oedema, fluid also accumulates in serous cavities; ascites within the peritoneum, hydrothorax or pleural effusion and pericardial effusion. Generalized oedema is only detected clinically when the accumulated fluid exceeds 5 L. The most important causes of generalized oedema are:

- total heart failure
- hypoproteinaemia
- nutritional oedema.

The principal mechanisms of development of generalized oedema are discussed below.

Hydrostatic factors

In heart failure venous hypertension results in increased hydrostatic pressure in the microcirculation. Also, a fall in cardiac output and in arterial blood flow stimulates arginine vasopressin and renin secretion, and secondary aldosteronism leads to sodium and water retention. However, secondary aldosteronism is present in only 50% of patients with cardiac failure and renal sodium and water retention occurs for other reasons.

Hypoproteinaemia

Plasma oncotic pressure is governed largely by the concentration of albumin, and oedema occurs when the serum albumin level falls below 25 g/L. Hypoalbuminaemia may be due to leakage into the urine in the nephrotic syndrome and other renal diseases, into the gut in protein-losing enteropathies or to insufficient synthesis in liver failure and in malnutrition.

Nutritional oedema

In severe malnutrition, notably kwashiorkor, a combination of low plasma protein, a poorly understood increased vascular permeability and deficiencies in vitamins and other essential dietary components is responsible.

Disseminated Intravascular Coagulation

In disseminated intravascular coagulation (DIC) there is thrombosis throughout the microcirculation which lowers the platelet count and circulating levels of coagulation factors; thus the other term for DIC is 'consumptive coagulopathy'.

Pathogenesis

In DIC excessive activation of coagulation is usually due to diffuse endothelial injury. Massive or prolonged release of soluble tissue factors and/or endothelial-derived thromboplastins into the circulation causes generalized activation of the coagulation system. Damaged endothelium also synthesizes less of the natural anticoagulants nitric oxide, prostacyclin and protein S; and severe damage exposes procoagulant subendothelial collagen, which activates the coagulation system. Widespread thrombosis throughout the microcirculation causes thrombocytopenia due to widespread platelet aggregation by thrombin. Consumption of coagulation factors reduces circulating levels of coagulation inhibitors (antithrombin, protein C), which are consumed by the activated clotting factors. Plasminogen activators released from damaged endothelial cells, platelets or tissue cells convert plasminogen to plasmin, which degrades fibrin so that fibrin degradation products (FDPs) appear in the blood and urine. However, plasmin also digests fibrinogen, factor V and factor VIII, further reducing the levels of coagulation factors in the blood. In the chronic form of DIC, some tumours release tissue factors as a result of necrosis or production of thromboplastins.

Aetiology

Disseminated intravascular coagulation may be acute or chronic but is always secondary. Approximately 50% of acute cases are due to obstetric conditions such as placental abruption (retroplacental haemorrhage) or rarely, to amniotic fluid embolism. In neonates, severe hypoxia also causes acute DIC due to endothelial injury. The other conditions most often associated with DIC are sepsis and shock in which there is widespread endothelial damage by hypoxia and by other factors.

Chronic DIC accompanies some malignant tumours, particularly adenocarcinomas of the pancreas, lungs or stomach and acute myeloid leukaemia. Some of these tumours secrete thromboplastins.

Causes of Disseminated Intravascular Coagulation

- Acute
  - shock
  - sepsis
  - placental abruption
  - severe trauma and burns
  - severe hypoxia
  - acute pancreatitis
  - fat embolism
  - intravascular haemolysis.
- Chronic
  - adenocarcinomas
  - acute myeloid leukaemia
  - malignant hypertension.

Clinical Features

Widespread petechiae and ecchymoses are often accompanied by epistaxis, and bleeding from the gums or from venepuncture sites. Massive gastrointestinal or pulmonary bleeding (Figure 6.40), or intracranial haemorrhage, both subdural and intracerebral, are common causes of death. Thrombosis of small blood vessels may cause ischaemia of distal digits and a spreading, haemorrhagic necrotic, gangrenous rash (purpura fulminans) may develop. Peritubular and glomerular capillaries and the renal arterioles may all be occluded, causing or aggravating acute renal failure.

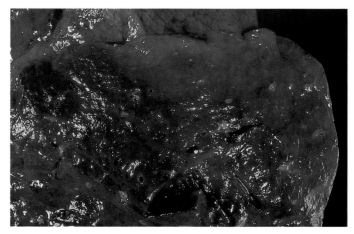

FIGURE 6.40 A sectioned lung showing spontaneous pulmonary haemorrhage in disseminated intravascular coagulation.

Shock

Shock is a complex syndrome with a variety of aetiologies (Table 6.7). All causes culminate in acute circulatory failure with hypotension and inadequate tissue perfusion. A large component of the syndrome, whatever the aetiology, is failure of the microcirculation. If not quickly reversed, death occurs due to multiorgan failure. The major types of shock are:

- hypovolaemic shock – due to reduced blood volume
- cardiogenic shock – due to an acute severe fall in cardiac output

TABLE 6.7 Types of shock

Types of shock	Clinical examples	Chief mechanisms
Hypovolaemic	Haemorrhage – internal/external; burns/scalds; vomiting/diarrhoea	Insufficient circulating volume
Septic	Endotoxaemia; Gram-negative septicaemia; Gram-positive septicaemia; overwhelming infection with any microorganism	Fixed peripheral vasodilatation and pooling of blood in the microcirculation due to nitric oxide release; endothelial cell and leucocyte activation by cytokines; activation of plasma enzyme cascades
Cardiogenic	Massive myocardial infarction; cardiac tamponade; ventricular arrhythmia; massive pulmonary embolism	Pump failure
Anaphylactic	Acute hypersensitivity reaction	Massive mast cell degranulation causes release of vasodilators and permeability factors

- septic shock – due to infection
- anaphylactic shock – due to an acute hypersensitivity reaction causing massive degranulation of mast cells and eosinophils.

Some causes of shock do not fall into these main categories. Acute peritonitis due to escape of gastric juice into the peritoneal cavity from a perforated peptic ulcer; acute pancreatitis (p. 275) and poisoning can all cause severe 'chemical' shock. So-called neurogenic shock may complicate anaesthesia or spinal cord injury. Severe shock develops when incompatible blood is transfused accidentally. Although they differ in aetiology, and in early aspects of their pathogenesis, the end results, namely acute circulatory failure and its complications, are similar in all types of shock.

In the early stages of shock, compensatory mechanisms maintain the blood flow to the vital organs – the central nervous system, the kidneys and the heart. However, the compensation is achieved at the expense of reduced perfusion of other tissues. Initially, the shocked patient is restless and confused, with a pale, cold, sweaty skin, often with peripheral cyanosis, a rapid weak pulse, a low blood pressure, increased rate and depth of respiration; eventually they may become drowsy and finally comatose. Unless tissue perfusion is urgently restored, ischaemia causes multi-organ failure and death. The altered haemodynamics have been best studied in hypovolaemic shock which will be used as an example.

Hypovolaemic Shock

Trauma is one of the commonest causes of death in young adults and many die of severe haemorrhage. In burns, plasma leakage from the damaged microcirculation causes hypovolaemia; hence the mortality of burns is related to their surface area. Severe vomiting and/or diarrhoea can also cause hypovolaemic shock. In a normal healthy adult a 500 mL blood loss, (about 10% of the blood volume), is asymptomatic. The blood volume is restored within a few hours by absorption of fluid from the extravascular compartment. Plasma protein replacement takes a day or two and restoration of red cells takes weeks. Loss of one third of the blood volume (about 1250 mL) results in significant hypovolaemia over the subsequent 36 hours, while a rapid loss of half of the blood volume results in coma and death. Elderly and hypertensive patients tolerate blood loss much less well due to structural changes, in their arterial tree.

Early Compensatory Changes

Acute hypovolaemia lowers central (systemic) venous pressure and a diminished venous return decreases cardiac filling with a fall in stroke volume, cardiac output and arterial blood pressure. These changes trigger peripheral and central baroreceptors with intense sympathico-adrenal stimulation, and activation of the renin–angiotensin–aldosterone system and vasopressin release. This stimulates the cardiovascular system and augments fluid retention. The heart rate increases to restore cardiac output and widespread arteriolar and venular constriction reduce tissue perfusion.

The beneficial effects are sodium retention and increased systemic venous tone, which increases central venous pressure, venous return to the heart and cardiac output. Thus, even without treatment, the blood pressure may be partially or fully restored, although tissue perfusion is reduced. The central nervous system, heart and kidneys are protected because they autoregulate their own perfusion. In young persons cerebral and coronary blood flow are maintained close to normal levels at blood pressures down to about 50 mmHg. At this pressure, however, arteriolar relaxation is maximal and perfusion rapidly declines at lower pressures. In older patients with arteriosclerosis or in those with hypertension the lower limit of autoregulation may be 80–90 mmHg. These groups are susceptible to circulatory disturbances.

The compensatory mechanisms can cope with loss of up to 25% of the blood volume. Arterioles constrict more than the venules, thereby lowering the hydrostatic pressure in the capillaries. Also, circulating cytokines cause capillary leakage (see below) and extravascular fluid enters the intravascular compartment. Tissue perfusion is, nevertheless, precarious and it is important to restore the blood volume by prompt intravenous administration of fluid. Macromolecular solutions, such as plasma or dextrans, maintain plasma osmotic pressure and retain fluid in the circulation. Blood transfusion is required when the loss exceeds 25% of blood volume. Blood pressure, haemoglobin and haematocrit levels are poor indicators of the degree of hypovolaemia during the first 36 hours. Central venous pressure gives a more accurate indication and should be monitored in all cases of severe shock.

Established Shock

In advanced shock, hypovolaemia is complicated by cardiorespiratory failure and bacterial infection. If shock persists, the widespread arteriolar constriction gradually passes off, and peripheral vasodilation causes hypotension. After 2 hours, cytokine-mediated increased capillary permeability leads to loss of fluid into the extravascular space and a further fall in blood volume. Capillary congestion with slowly flowing blood causes cyanosis and reduced tissue perfusion, which is aggravated by a number of factors (see Figure 3.23 on p. 64). Loss of intravascular fluid leads to sludging of red cells and rouleaux formation. Viscosity is further increased by a rise in plasma fibrinogen. Release of thromboplastin from hypoxic endothelium and tissue cells generates thrombin, which promotes platelet aggregation and DIC.

Leucocytes are important contributors to tissue damage. Neutrophil polymorphs adhere to the activated and injured endothelium of small vessels, especially in the lungs and after 12 hours there may be significant neutropenia. Activated leucocytes and hypoxic cells release cytokines, especially tumour necrosis factor α (TNFα) and interleukin 4 (IL4) into the blood. This causes increased endothelial output of nitric oxide. They also release proteolytic enzymes which activate the kinin and complement systems and the circulation is further embarrassed by vasodilatation and increased permeability. Metabolic acidosis directly depresses cardiac myocytes, and a myocardial depressant factor is released from the ischaemic pancreas.

Cardiogenic Shock

Cardiogenic shock is caused by severe acute reduction in cardiac output because of pump failure; most often this is due to cardiac catastrophes such as massive myocardial infarction, rupture of a valve cusp, or cardiac tamponade due to haemopericardium. The main metabolic and circulating effects are summarized in Figure 6.41. Unlike other forms of shock both the central venous pressure and the ventricular end-diastolic pressures are raised. The haemodynamic changes are otherwise similar to hypovolaemic shock and are triggered by the fall in blood pressure and the reduced tissue perfusion. Mortality approaches 80%. Surgical intervention is sometimes appropriate and aortic pumps can support the circulation prior to surgery.

Septic Shock

Septicaemia or localized infections may cause shock. This important type of shock is described in detail in Chapter 19 (p. 543).

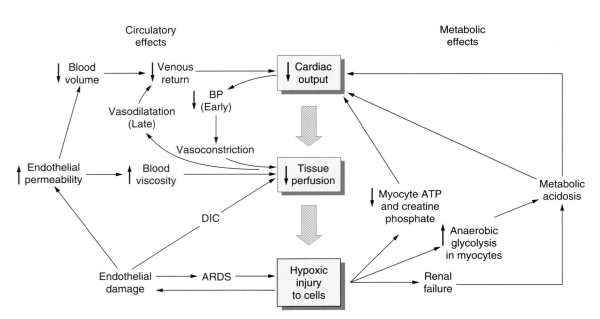

FIGURE 6.41 Metabolic and circulatory effects of cardiogenic shock. BP = blood pressure; DIC = disseminated intravascular coagulation; ARDS = acute respiratory distress syndrome.

Metabolic Consequences of Shock

Hypoxia has a profound effect on cell metabolism. It prevents the conversion of pyruvate into acetyl CoA and blocks the citric acid cycle; conversion of pyruvate to lactate causes accumulation of lactic acid and contributes to the metabolic acidosis. In this case, each molecule of glucose yields only two molecules of ATP; whereas in the presence of oxygen complete oxidation of one molecule of glucose via the citric acid cycle and the electron carrier chain yields about 38 ATP molecules for each glucose molecule. Because of insufficient ATP, energy dependent cell functions run down. Slowing of the membrane ATP-ase ion pumps causes potassium to leak from cells and the entry of sodium and water causes cell swelling. Hypoxic cells also leak glucose leading to insulin-resistant hyperglycaemia and increased glycogenolysis. These metabolic disturbances, together with high levels of catecholamines, raise the blood levels of fatty acids and amino acids. These effects are sometimes termed the 'sick cell syndrome' (Figure 6.42).

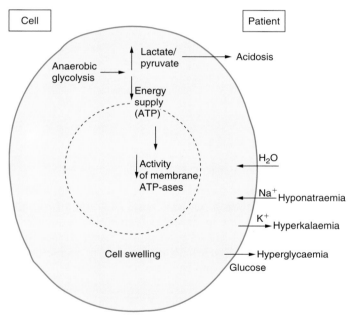

FIGURE 6.42 Some effects of hypoxia.

Tissue Pathology in Shock

All organs are affected in severe shock. The typical histological findings are haemorrhages, microthrombi and necroses; however, morphological changes are often inconspicuous. Failure of autoregulation may cause acute tubular necrosis in the kidney, boundary zone infarction of the brain, selective neuronal necrosis and subendocardial infarction of the heart.

Acute heart failure, first of the left and then of both ventricles, may develop in severe cardiogenic, hypovolaemic or septic shock and is particularly common in older patients with hypertension or coronary artery disease. Inadequate myocardial perfusion produces focal necrosis or global infarction. Tachypnoea is produced by metabolic acidosis.

In established shock, progressive reduction in gas exchange is due to a combination of causes – pulmonary oedema, alveolar collapse, intravascular and intra-alveolar fibrin formation, haemorrhage and infection. These features, known collectively as shock lung or adult respiratory distress syndrome (ARDS) are discussed in detail on p. 169.

Below the lower level of autoregulation, perfusion of the kidneys is directly proportional to the blood pressure. Production of urine ceases at about 50 mmHg and if the pressure remains low for some hours, hypoxic injury leads to renal failure with acute tubular necrosis. The kidneys usually show cortical pallor and swelling; in more severe shock often complicating obstetrical catastrophes or septic shock, complete necrosis of the whole renal cortex may occur, giving rise to acute cortical necrosis which is irrecoverable (p. 389).

There may be gastrointestinal haemorrhage and, in DIC, more widespread small haemorrhages affect mucosal and serosal surfaces (Figure 6.43). Ischaemic necrosis of perivenular liver cells may be noted at autopsy and are responsible for raised serum transaminase levels, and cholestatic liver injury also occurs. Hypotension may also precipitate acute pancreatitis, which will aggravate shock. The adrenals occasionally show a combination of haemorrhage and necrosis (Waterhouse–Friderichsen syndrome), particularly in septic shock associated with meningococcal septicaemia (p. 295).

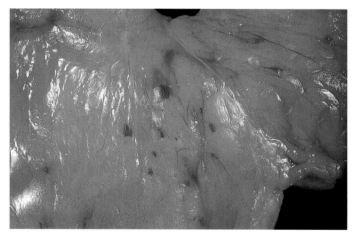

FIGURE 6.43 Spontaneous serosal haemorrhages in a case of meningococcal shock with DIC.

The most severely affected organs are the heart, lungs, kidneys and brain. These patients require intensive care in specialized units. In young patients with hypovolaemic shock the mortality may be as low as 20%. However septic (mortality 60%) and cardiogenic shock (mortality 80%) are more difficult to treat. Because renal failure and cardiac failure are both treatable, respiratory failure is the commonest late organ failure; residual brain damage may also affect some patients who recover.

Diseases of Veins

Venous Thrombosis

Veins readily thrombose because flow is slow. Thrombosis of the leg or pelvic veins is common and may lead to potentially fatal pulmonary embolism. Thrombosis of leg veins usually starts in deep veins within the calf muscles and may extend progressively (propagate) to the popliteal, femoral and iliac veins and occasionally into the inferior vena cava. Risk factors for deep venous thrombosis include:

- trauma, surgery
- immobilization, for example in bed, on long haul flights
- heart failure
- old age
- obesity
- pregnancy and puerperium
- familial thrombophilia
- contraceptive pill.

Deep venous thrombosis starts during or shortly after surgical operations. The coagulability of blood increases as part of the metabolic response to trauma. Normal venous return is aided by the pumping action created by contraction of the leg muscles and by abdominal breathing; inhibition of movement and breathing by postoperative pain contributes to venous thrombosis. Deep venous thrombosis may cause swelling and tenderness of the calf muscles, but in most patients the condition is undiagnosed. The incidence is reduced by subcutaneous low-dose heparin and by early mobilization of patients after operation, myocardial infarction and childbirth.

Pulmonary Thromboembolism

Thromboemboli usually originate in the leg veins where recently propagated thrombi are poorly anchored by retraction from the vein wall; less commonly, thromboemboli arise in the pelvic or other systemic veins or the right side of the heart. The effects depend on both the size of the embolus and the state of the pulmonary circulation. A large embolus, for example one derived from thrombosis of the femoral or iliac vein, may become detached and impact in the outflow tract of the right ventricle or the main pulmonary trunk (see Figure 6.6). When it coils up blockage of the pulmonary circulation causes sudden death by circulatory arrest. Occlusion of more than half the pulmonary arterial tree in previously healthy individuals, causes pulmonary hypertension and acute right ventricular failure. Occlusion of medium-sized or small pulmonary arteries only causes pulmonary hypertension if many vessels are occluded by showers of small emboli or by recurrent embolism over of months or years. Obstruction of medium-sized pulmonary arteries does not cause infarction in a normal pulmonary circulation because thromboemboli are rapidly removed by fibrinolysis. Because of the double circulation, lung infarction usually occurs only in cardiac failure.

Outcomes of Venous Thrombosis (Figure 6.44)

- Massive pulmonary embolism and sudden death.
- Asymptomatic pulmonary embolism.
- Pulmonary infarction.
- Showers of pulmonary emboli and pulmonary hypertension.

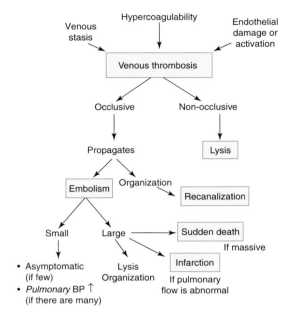

FIGURE 6.44 Outcomes of leg vein thrombosis.

Other Diseases of Veins

Thrombophlebitis is thrombosis with associated inflammation and often affects superficial veins. Migrating thrombophlebitis, where veins in different regions are sequentially affected, is often associated with cancer, particularly of the pancreas (Trousseau's sign). Veins draining pyogenic infections often thrombose and may become infected. In septic venous thrombosis, suppuration causes softening and fragments of infected thrombus may break away, giving rise to pyaemia or embolism with distant abscesses. Dystrophic calcification of thrombi in veins produces phleboliths, which are particularly common in pelvic veins.

Varicose Veins

In this common disease venous hypertension produces dilated and elongated veins (varicosities). In the legs, varicose veins occur in almost 10% of the adult population. Although familial, the risk factors include occupations requiring prolonged standing, obesity and pregnancy. It is uncertain whether dilatation of the veins causes, or is caused by failure of the valves. Haemorrhoids occur in those with venous hypertension in the pelvic and abdominal veins. Predisposing factors are constipation, obesity and pregnancy. A varicocoele is a mass formed by varicosity of the pampiniform venous plexus in the testicle. Oesophageal varices complicate portal hypertension of any cause, and profuse haemorrhage from them is a common cause of death in patients with chronic liver disease.

DISEASES OF LYMPHATICS

Lymphangitis is inflammation of lymphatic channels. Acute lymphangitis is usually caused by virulent bacteria, most commonly *Streptococcus pyogenes*, which invade and multiply in the lymphatics. This is seen clinically as subcutaneous red streaks draining an infected area. Lymphangitis is associated with lymphadenitis – inflammation of lymph nodes. Since the lymphatics drain eventually into the bloodstream, lymphangitis should be taken seriously as it may herald septicaemia. Chronic filarial lymphangitis is the cause of elephantiasis and gives rise to lymphoedema. Milroy's disease is a rare congenital form of oedema, often affecting only one limb; it is associated with gross and diffuse dilatation of lymphatics. Its aetiology is unknown.

VASCULAR TUMOURS

Vascular tumours are common. Many benign ones are debatedly true neoplasms; other endothelial proliferations are triggered by trauma or infective agents. Haemangiomas are masses of atypical blood vessels.

Capillary Haemangiomas

Capillary haemangiomas occur in most internal organs, but are commonest in the skin where they form 'birthmarks'. The 'port wine stain' is a diffuse cutaneous angioma. The juvenile capillary haemangioma, the so-called strawberry naevus of infancy, often grows rapidly for some months then usually regresses completely by 5 years of age. Large placental angiomas may cause heart failure in the fetus. The pyogenic granuloma (lobular capillary haemangioma) is a polypoid cutaneous capillary angioma that often ulcerates and bleeds. Many follow trauma, especially in pregnancy. Bacillary angiomatosis is a proliferation of capillaries associated with inflammatory cells that occurs in immunocompromised patients, especially acquired immune deficiency syndrome (AIDS). It is caused by an infection by Gram-negative bacilli of the *Bartonella* genus.

Cavernous Haemangiomas and Rarer Entities

Cavernous haemangiomas consist of large dilated thin-walled vascular channels. The most dangerous occur in the brain where they may rupture and cause haemorrhage. Vascular hamartomas consist of cavernous channels admixed with fat, smooth muscle and fibrous tissue. They occur often in muscles and cause pain due to thrombosis. Multiple angiomas form part of several syndromes. These include: von-Hippel Lindau disease, Osler Weber-Rendu disease and Sturge-Weber syndrome. The lesions of epithelioid haemangioma consist of clusters of vessels lined by plump (epithelioid) endothelial cells surrounded by chronically inflamed fibrous tissue containing eosinophils. Glomus tumour (glomangioma) arises from the glomus bodies of the skin. It is therefore found mainly in the extremities, especially the digits. They form small nodules that are exquisitely tender because of the tumour's dense innervation. In other tumours glomus cells are associated with larger channels, occur more on the proximal limbs and trunk and are less often tender; these are called glomangiomas.

Malignant Vascular Tumours

These tumours are rare. There is a spectrum of malignancy ranging from low grade, slow-growing haemangioendotheliomas to highly malignant angiosarcomas. Epithelioid haemangioendotheliomas occur in large vessels, usually a vein, but may occur in soft tissues, liver, lung and other organs. The tumour cells show primitive endothelial differentiation. These tumours are often multifocal so that many patients eventually die of their disease. Angiosarcomas occur most often in the skin, breast, soft tissues and liver. Those in the skin arise at sites of chronic sun exposure; those in the liver have in the past been associated with industrial exposure to vinyl chloride monomer in the plastics industry. The commonest aggressive endothelial tumour is Kaposi's sarcoma. This is discussed on p. 504 and its relationship with human immunodeficiency virus (HIV) infection on p. 517.

Tumours of Lymphatic Endothelium

Lymphangiomas, like haemangiomas, are often congenital and may be composed of ramifying small channels of large cavernous spaces. They may form a large mass, a 'cystic hygroma' especially in the neck. Occasionally, a single large cyst lined by lymphatic endothelium forms a lymphatic cyst. Lymphangiomas are commonest in the retroperitoneum and mediastinum.

THE HEART

The Work of the Heart

Assuming a resting stroke volume of 70 mL from the left ventricle beating at 70/min, the cardiac output is about 5 L/min amounting to a daily output of 7200 L (about 7.5 tons). The normal heart has great reserve power which can be substantially increased by physical training. During exertion, there is a greater venous return with consequent increase in diastolic filling and stretching of the muscle fibres; the response is a more vigorous contraction (Starling's law) and a greatly increased stroke volume. The heart rate also increases during exertion. These two factors together can raise the cardiac output to about seven times that of the resting state. This physiological performance can be maintained only if the myocardium is healthy, the valves function efficiently, the conducting system of the heart coordinates contraction of the chambers, and peripheral resistance to blood flow is not raised. Disturbance of any of these components can cause heart failure.

Heart Failure

In heart failure impaired cardiac function fails to maintain a circulation adequate for the metabolic needs of the body despite an adequate blood volume. Inadequate tissue perfusion leads ultimately to a complex syndrome of clinical features (typically breathlessness, fatigue, peripheral and pulmonary oedema) and multiorgan involvement (renal impairment, skeletal muscle dysfunction, impaired pulmonary and peripheral gas exchange, and hepatic dysfunction). Heart failure has a high morbidity and mortality (impaired effort capacity and quality of life, recurrent hospitalization, and death within 1–10 years depending on severity). As Western populations age, the incidence of heart failure increases, and it is now a major public health problem.

The clinical spectrum ranges from asymptomatic cardiac dysfunction through reduced exercise tolerance, in which compensatory mechanisms (ventricular hypertrophy, peripheral vasoconstriction, salt and water retention) maintain tissue perfusion, to a stage in which these mechanisms are exhausted and symptoms and signs of heart failure occur at rest.

Causes of Heart Failure

The main causes of heart failure are summarized in Table 6.8. They are due to excessive load on the myocardium, poor myocardial function (contraction or relaxation) or a combination of both mechanisms. The major causes of heart failure vary geographically. In Western countries, ischaemic heart disease and hypertension are by far the most common causes while, in developing countries, valve disease or myocardial infections are more important. Intrinsic heart muscle disease (cardiomyopathy) is an uncommon cause of heart failure.

Manifestations of Heart Failure

Heart failure may be acute or chronic, and may affect the left ventricle, right ventricle or both. Acute heart failure occurs most frequently in myocardial infarction and arrhythmias; less frequent causes are gross pulmonary embolism, myocarditis or rupture of a valve cusp. In severe acute heart failure, the marked fall in cardiac output is accompanied by peripheral vasoconstriction and cardiogenic shock develops. Chronic heart failure occurs when the causal factors develop slowly. It is most commonly due to IHD, systemic arterial hypertension, chronic valvular dysfunction or diseases of the lungs with pulmonary hypertension. Two-thirds of patients with chronic heart failure die from progressive pump failure; the other third die suddenly due to an arrhythmia.

Left Ventricular Failure

Left ventricular failure is most commonly due to ischaemic heart disease, particularly myocardial infarction, but also to systemic hypertension and aortic and mitral valve disease. The failing ventricle dilates which further impairs contraction as described earlier. The main clinical features are dyspnoea and cough due to pulmonary venous hypertension and pulmonary oedema. Increased venous return in the recumbent position and increased blood reabsorption of fluid from the extravascular space cause acute exacerbations of left ventricular failure, commonly during the night (paroxysmal nocturnal dyspnoea). In acute left ventricular failure, death may occur rapidly from acute pulmonary oedema, which may be complicated by cardiogenic shock.

Right Ventricular Failure

Right ventricular failure is usually secondary to left ventricular failure. When the left ventricle fails increased pressure in the left atrium and pulmonary veins leads to pulmonary arteriolar vasoconstriction and resultant pulmonary artery hypertension. Persistent pulmonary hypertension causes right ventricular hypertrophy and eventually failure. Isolated

TABLE 6.8 Causes of heart failure

Left ventricle	Right ventricle
Myocardial injury	Increased workload
Ischaemia/infarction	Pulmonary hypertension due to:
Myocarditis	left ventricle failure
Cardiomyopathy	chronic lung disease
	left-to-right shunting with increased blood flow
	pulmonary thromboembolism
	pulmonary and tricuspid valve disease
Increased workload	Myocardial injury
Systemic hypertension	Ischaemia/infarction
Aortic and mitral valve disease	Myocarditis
Coarctation of the aorta	Cardiomyopathy
Increased cardiac output:	
anaemia	
thyrotoxicosis	

right ventricular failure is usually due to chronic obstructive pulmonary disease (COPD) and less often pulmonary embolism. When the right ventricle fails, it dilates; stretching of the tricuspid ring results in valve incompetence and dilatation of the right atrium. Raised central venous pressure gives rise to systemic venous congestion and dependent peripheral oedema.

High Output Failure

High output failure results from increased workload on both ventricles. Causes include thyrotoxicosis, anaemia and arteriovenous fistulae. The onset of heart failure is associated with a fall in cardiac output but because of the previously abnormally high output, even in failure, the absolute output may be normal or even increased.

Ischaemic Heart Disease

Ischaemic heart disease is the largest cause of cardiac morbidity and mortality in the developed world. In many industrialized countries, including the UK, death rates due to IHD have been falling for both men and women especially in the higher socio-economic groups who have undertaken lifestyle changes including cessation of smoking. This contrasts with a rising death rate in developing countries. Most deaths occur over the age of 40 and death rates are higher for men than women. The risk factors for IHD are considered on p. 112.

Syndromes of Ischaemic Heart Disease (Table 6.9)

- Stable angina.
- Unstable angina.
- Myocardial infarction.
- Sudden death.
- Heart failure.

Angina

Angina is episodic chest pain, often crushing, usually retrosternal and commonly radiating to the arms, neck and jaw. It is induced by increased workload on the heart such as exercise, cold exposure, emotional upset or a heavy meal. Stable angina is provoked predictably by increased cardiac work. It is caused by stenosis of one or more coronary artery segments to at least 50% diameter (75% cross-sectional area). At the site of the stenosis the plaques may be eccentric or less commonly concentric (Figure 6.45). Eccentric plaques allow retention of an arc of functional medial smooth muscle which responds to vasomotor stimuli and so could further reduce the calibre of the stenosis; concentric plaques cause circumferential atrophy of the underlying media and so loss of vasomotor responsiveness. Plaques can therefore produce a fixed stenosis or segments that can vary in luminal calibre.

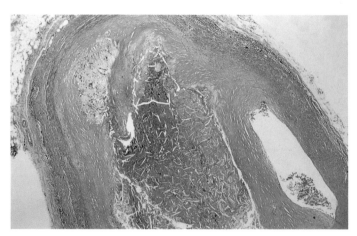

FIGURE 6.45 A histological section of a coronary artery from a case of stable angina. The residual lumen is an eccentric tiny slit. The artery is severely narrowed by an atheromatous plaque filled with amorphous lipid material. It is surrounded by collagen (stained green).

Unstable angina is unpredictable onset of chest pain that is unrelated to exercise, sometimes with increasing severity or frequency. There are two pathogenetic mechanisms: most cases are due to fluctuating luminal thrombosis on an eccentric ulcerated coronary artery stenosis with resultant further reduction in luminal calibre or even occlusion. Secondly, an abnormal vasomotor tone may cause coronary artery spasm and further reduction in luminal diameter in the area of an eccentric atheromatous plaque. Unstable angina may progress to myocardial infarction or sudden death.

Myocardial Infarction

There are two main types of myocardial infarction. Most are regional infarcts in the distribution of a coronary artery. Regional infarcts are most commonly transmural (Figure 6.46) with full thickness necrosis of the ventricular wall. In over 90% of cases, a thrombus occludes the coronary artery supplying the infarcted region. Underlying the thrombus there is cracking or ulceration of the underlying atheromatous plaque in 75% of cases. The usual sequence of events in regional myocardial infarction is shown in Figure 6.47. A similar sequence occurs in unstable angina, but without luminal

TABLE 6.9 How atheroma causes ischaemic heart disease

Event in plaque	Clinical syndrome
Atheromatous plaque with luminal stenosis	Stable angina
↓	
Plaque rupture	
↓	
Penetration of blood into plaque	Unstable angina or sudden death
↓	
Acute plaque enlargement with luminal thrombosis	Acute infarction or sudden death
↓	
Occlusion of lumen	

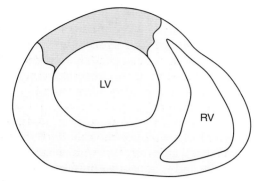

FIGURE 6.46 A transverse section through the long axis of the heart showing transmural myocardial infarction. The recently infarcted tissue is the shaded area.

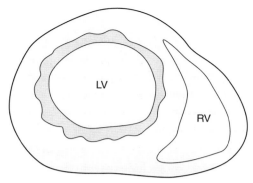

FIGURE 6.48 Global subendocardial myocardial infarction. The recently infarcted tissue is the shaded area.

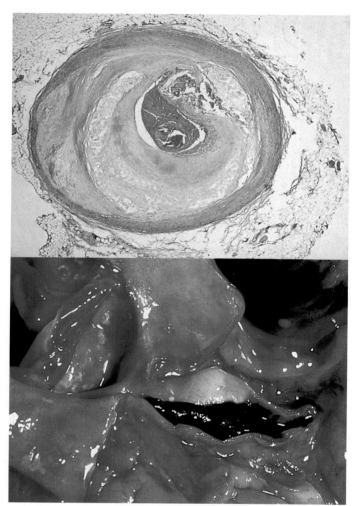

FIGURE 6.47 The top panel shows a histological section depicting a ruptured atheromatous plaque which has precipitated luminal thrombosis. The bottom panel shows the propagated thrombus it has caused.

implicated. In the 25% of cases without detectable plaque rupture, occlusive thrombi may be due to more superficial plaque injury with endothelial denudation and exposure of underlying prothrombotic basement membrane.

Subendocardial infarction affects the inner half or one-third of the ventricular wall (Figure 6.48). When most or all of its circumference is affected this is known as global subendocardial infarction. All three major coronary arteries are usually severely stenosed but no thrombus is found in 75% of cases at autopsy. The subendocardial zone is prone to ischaemic damage particularly in the presence of left ventricular hypertrophy; the cause of subendocardial infarction is therefore failure of perfusion due to a fall in blood pressure, sometimes shock. Subendocardial infarction may occur in the absence of coronary artery disease particularly when marked left ventricular hypertrophy has resulted from aortic stenosis. Transmural infarction may be combined with subendocardial infarction.

Pathology of Myocardial Infarction

The distribution of regional myocardial infarcts is as follows:

- In 40–45% of cases, anterior infarcts extend up the anterior wall of the left ventricle from the apex and can include the anterior portion of interventricular septum or the adjacent anterior wall of the right ventricle. An anterior infarct is usually due to thrombosis of the anterior descending branch of the left coronary artery.
- Right coronary artery thrombosis (30–40% of cases) often leads to an inferior (or posterior) myocardial infarct which extends from the apex of the heart up the inferior wall of the left ventricle. It can involve the posterior aspect of the interventricular septum and the inferior (posterior) aspect of the right ventricle.
- In approximately 15% of cases, occlusion of the circumflex branch of the left coronary artery leads to infarction of the lateral wall of the left ventricle.

Left main coronary artery thrombosis or thrombosis of two major coronary arteries are less common, and are associated with more extensive damage and cardiogenic shock.

occlusion. It is easy to appreciate the potential for unstable angina to progress to infarction. The cause of plaque disruption leading to thrombotic occlusion is uncertain. Sheer stress, surges in blood pressure, production of lytic enzymes by inflammatory cells and local vasospasm have all been

Gross and Microscopic Appearances of Myocardial Infarcts

- Irreversible myocyte damage follows 20 minutes total ischaemia.
- Naked eye changes begin around 15 hours and microscopic changes at 8–12 hours.
- Gradual removal of necrotic myocardium by organization during next 1–2 months.
- Maximal fibrous scar formation at 2–3 months.

Irreversible cardiac myocyte damage occurs after approximately 20 minutes of total ischaemia, although initially the infarcted muscle appears grossly and microscopically normal. The earliest naked eye changes occur around 15 hours, when the affected muscle appears pale and swollen. By 24–48 hours there is softening and the colour changes from dark red to brown to yellow (Figure 6.49); sometimes there is focal haemorrhage, particularly at the margins. After 3–4 days the infarct is more sharply defined by the development of a peripheral red zone of granulation tissue (Figure 6.50). Removal of dead myocytes by phagocytosis and organization proceeds with variable thinning of the infarcted area at 3 weeks and some fibrosis. By 3 months the scar tissue appears white. A fibrinous or haemorrhagic pericarditis is common in transmural infarction. Under the endocardium, a thin surviving subendocardial band of myocytes is almost invariable, these cells being nourished by blood in the ventricular lumen. After several days, mural thrombus often forms on the endocardial surface overlying the infarct.

Microscopically the infarcted tissue shows the changes of coagulative necrosis after 8–12 hours (Figure 6.51). By 24 hours, invasion by polymorphs has begun and after a few days digestion by macrophages and organization with granulation tissue formation occurs at the periphery. Over the next 2–3 months the infarcted myocardium is eventually replaced by a fibrous scar. Hypertrophy of the non-infarcted myocardium with chamber enlargement then compensate for loss of contractility caused by the healed infarct. This is known as ventricular remodelling. In up to a third of regional transmural infarcts, stretching of the infarcted zone occurs; when extreme, this forms an aneurysm in 15% of cases (Figure 6.52).

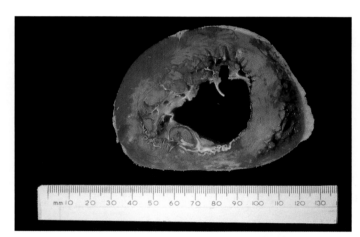

FIGURE 6.49 A transverse section through the heart showing global subendocardial infarction. In addition the anterior portion also shows a transmural regional myocardial infarction.

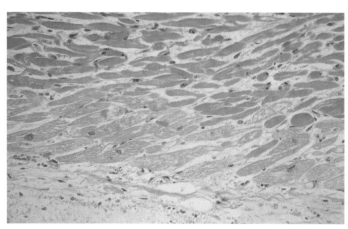

FIGURE 6.51 A histological section showing a zone of dark red myocytes with coagulative necrosis next to a zone of pale staining viable myocytes that have retained their nuclei and cytoplasmic striations.

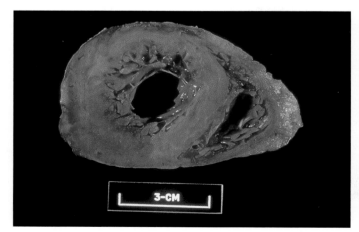

FIGURE 6.50 A large myocardial infarct at 5 days showing the colour changes associated with coagulative necrosis.

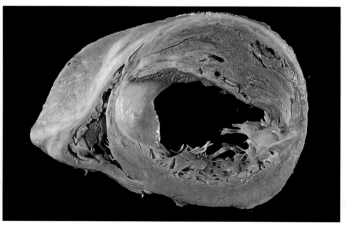

FIGURE 6.52 A heart with a previous myocardial infarct that has stretched to form an aneurysm which contains mural thrombus.

Clinical Features, Course and Outcome

Severe retrosternal chest pain not relieved by rest or vasodilators and often persisting for several hours is the dominant symptom. Nausea, vomiting, sweating, weakness and prostration are frequent accompaniments. However, a silent myocardial infarct with little or no constitutional upset is well recognized. Ambulatory electrocardiogram (ECG) recordings suggest that 20% of ischaemic episodes are painless. Myocardial infarction may be confirmed by characteristic ECG changes including pathological Q waves and elevated serum levels of cardiac myocyte specific enzymes such as creatine phosphokinase MB, lactate dehydrogenase 5 and troponin T which are released into the serum from necrotic cells.

Up to half of patients with acute myocardial infarction die in the first week, particularly from ventricular fibrillation during the first 48 hours. After this, mortality in the first year is approximately 10%, and 5% per annum in succeeding years. Rapid thrombolytic therapy, particularly if carried out within an hour, and low-dose aspirin and β-blocker therapy have substantially reduced post-infarct mortality. Infarct size is also directly related to mortality.

Complications

- Sudden ischaemic cardiac death.
- Arrhythmias.
- Heart failure and cardiogenic shock.
- Ventricular rupture.
- Mural thrombosis and thromboembolism.
- Venous thrombosis.
- Ventricular aneurysm.

Sudden Ischaemic Cardiac Death

Sudden cardiac death is not synonymous with death from early myocardial infarction since only 25–50% of resuscitated victims develop a clinically demonstrable infarct. However, ischaemic heart disease is the commonest cause of sudden cardiac death, usually due to the onset of ventricular fibrillation. Pathological studies usually show two groups of patients: those with an acute arterial lesion, usually a ruptured atheromatous plaque with resultant overlying thrombus which may occlude the artery; those with severe coronary artery disease with myocardial scarring and left ventricular hypertrophy but no acute coronary thrombotic event.

Arrhythmias

Arrhythmias occur in up to 80% of patients with acute myocardial infarction and are the commonest cause of death. Early ventricular fibrillation, especially in the first hour, is responsible for most sudden cardiac deaths. Ventricular fibrillation occurring days after infarction complicates extensive infarcts and is associated with reduced short- and long-term survival. Heart block is associated with increased mortality; both bundle branches of the conducting system may be damaged in anterior infarcts. In a posterior infarct, atrioventricular (AV) node block may be induced but most patients who survive revert to sinus rhythm.

Heart Failure and Cardiogenic Shock

Acute heart failure is caused by large infarcts, usually involving more than 20% of the ventricular muscle mass while necrosis of more than 40% causes cardiogenic shock. Chronic heart failure may also develop at any time after an infarct.

Ventricular Rupture

Rupture of the left ventricle is a complication of transmural infarction and usually occurs during the first 10 days with resulting haemopericardium and death from cardiac tamponade (Figure 6.53). After ventricular arrhythmias and cardiogenic shock, it is the commonest cause of death. Rupture of either the interventricular septum causing an acquired septal defect or a mitral valve papillary muscle (see case history) may also occur thereby precipitating or worsening acute heart failure.

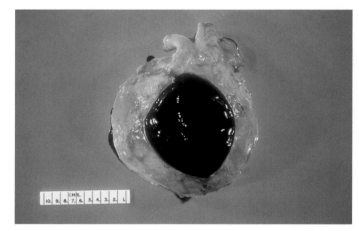

FIGURE 6.53 Cardiac tamponade which shows gross distension of the pericardial sac by blood. The pericardium has been incised to reveal a mass of fresh blood clot.

Mural Thrombosis and Thromboembolism

Endocardial damage, release of tissue thromboplastins and low sheer stress in a non-contractile segment all predispose to mural thrombosis following acute myocardial infarction. Left ventricular thrombus may cause systemic thromboembolism, the peak incidence being between the second and third week post infarct. Eventually, mural thrombus will become organized. Thromboembolism may originate from ventricular aneurysms (see Figure 6.52) and from the atrial appendages particularly in atrial fibrillation. Occasionally a thromboembolic event may be the first clinical manifestation of myocardial infarction. Systemic venous thrombosis, usually in the leg veins, occurs in up to 30% of patients following a myocardial infarct. This has led to the modern trend of early mobilization. Fatal pulmonary thromboembolism is, however, an uncommon cause of death.

Ventricular aneurysms resulting from stretching of the infarcted area with fibrous replacement occur in up to 20% of long-term survivors of transmural myocardial infarction. Laminated thrombus may be a source of emboli, while cardiac failure and persistent ventricular arrhythmias are other sequelae. Surgical excision of the aneurysm may correct the problems.

Post-infarction (Dressler's) syndrome is characterized by fever, increased erythrocyte sedimentation rate, leucocytosis and pericardial/pleural effusions and usually starts 10 weeks following infarction, although occasionally longer. An autoimmune aetiology is likely.

Rare Causes of Ischaemic Heart Disease and Myocardial Infarction

These include congenital anomalies of the coronary arteries, aortic dissection, coronary arteritis, embolism from the vegetations of infective endocarditis and therapeutic irradiation resulting in coronary artery damage. In up to 3% of patients with a proven myocardial infarct the coronary arteries are angiographically normal. These patients tend to be young, are more commonly women and lack the usual risk factors for atheroma except smoking. In some cases thrombosis occurs in arteries with no evidence of atheroma, the aetiology being uncertain. In some cases a diagnosis of coronary artery spasm is made. Cocaine and sympathomimetic drug ingestion should always be considered.

6.1 CASE HISTORY

A 53-year-old woman developed crushing chest pain radiating into her neck. This was associated with shortness of breath. She was admitted to hospital and an ECG suggested acute myocardial infarction. She was given opioids for pain, aspirin and a β-blocker, then thrombolysis was achieved by intravenous streptokinase. Her condition stabilized, and over the next few days serial plasma enzyme studies confirmed that she had had a myocardial infarction. On the sixth day she developed sudden breathlessness with associated tachypnoea. Auscultation revealed crepitations and a loud pan-systolic murmur. The chest X-ray (Figure 6.54) showed fine streaky mottling in the lung fields. This was diagnosed as acute pulmonary oedema due to left ventricular failure. In spite of prompt treatment with morphine, aminophylline and diuretics her condition deteriorated rapidly and she died just after emergency echocardiography was carried out. Figure 6.55

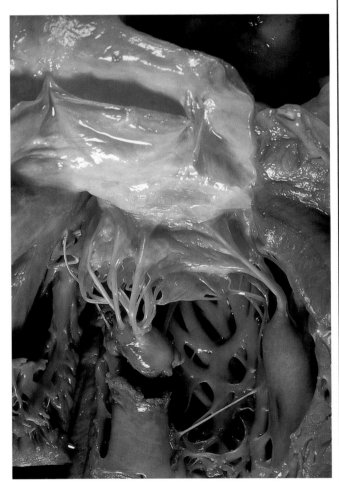

FIGURE 6.55 The interior of the left ventricle showing the aortic valve at the top and the posterior surface of the anterior mitral valve leaflet. The head of the infarcted papillary muscle has been ruptured and avulsion of the attached chordae tendineae caused mitral incompetence.

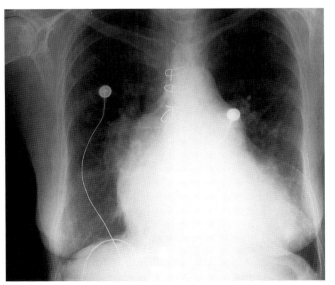

FIGURE 6.54 A chest X-ray showing enlargement of the heart cause by heart failure. There are streaky opacities in both lung fields due to pulmonary oedema due to left ventricular failure. ECG leads are also visible.

shows the interior of her left ventricle at autopsy. It shows complete rupture and avulsion of the head of a papillary muscle.

In summary, this woman had a myocardial infarction. In spite of appropriate treatment she then developed rapidly fatal acute left ventricular failure due to sudden mitral valve incompetence. This was due to papillary muscle rupture. There are three sites of rupture: free wall rupture causes cardiac tamponade, septal rupture causes an acquired ventricular septal defect that can be operatively patched, and papillary muscle rupture.

Avulsion of the head of a papillary muscle causes acute left ventricular failure due to sudden mitral incompetence from leakage via the unsupported part of the cusp. Rupture of the body of a papillary muscle causes cardiogenic shock because an unsupported whole mitral cusp abolishes mitral valve function.

Myocarditis

Key Points

- There is inflammation and damage to myocardium.
- Many causes: viral infection commonest.
- It usually resolves completely.
- Rarely it progresses to dilated cardiomyopathy.

Myocarditis is defined as inflammation of the myocardium, excluding the acute inflammatory reaction to myocardial infarction. The main causes include: infection; toxins and drugs; hypersensitivity reaction. A list of the main causes under these three categories is shown in Table 6.10. Some cases are idiopathic. The clinical diagnosis is made on a history of sudden onset of flu-like symptoms, fever, pulse rate disproportionate to temperature, rapidly progressive heart failure and arrhythmias in a previously fit individual with no evidence of other disease especially pneumonia. The diagnosis may be confirmed by cardiac biopsy demonstrating an inflammatory infiltrate within the myocardium causing myocyte damage.

TABLE 6.10 **Causes of myocarditis**

Infective	*Viruses*	
	Coxsackie A and B	Viruses causing myocarditis alone or as the main clinical feature
	Echoviruses	
	Influenza A and B	
	Epstein–Barr virus	
	Cytomegalovirus	
	Herpes simplex	Viruses more commonly causing systemic disease with myocarditis as a possible component
	Varicella zoster	
	Mumps	
	Measles	
	Respiratory syncytial virus	
	Polio virus	
	Hepatitis A virus	
	Bacteria	
	Staphylococcus aureus	
	Streptococcus pyogenes	
	Other organisms	
	Trypanosoma cruzi (Chagas' disease)	
	Toxoplasma gondii	
	Borrelia burgdorferi (Lyme disease)	
	Weil's disease	
	Trichinella spiralis	
	Fungi	
	Bacterial exotoxins	
	Diphtheria	
	Typhoid	

(*Continued*)

TABLE 6.10 (Continued)

Toxic drugs	Fluorouracil
	Arsenic
	Antimony
	Lithium
	Phenothiazines
Drug hypersensitivity reaction	Penicillin
	Methyldopa
	Streptomycin
	Sulphonylureas
	Tetracycline
Miscellaneous	Acute rheumatic fever
	Connective tissue diseases	Systemic lupus erythematosus, rheumatoid arthritis
	Cardiac allograft rejection
Idiopathic	Sarcoidosis (granulomatous myocarditis)
	Giant cell myocarditis (Fiedler's myocarditis)

 6.3   SPECIAL STUDY TOPIC

TYPES OF MYOCARDITIS

Viral Myocarditis

The most commonly implicated virus is Coxsackie B, however, the exact number of cases it causes is still controversial. As shown in Table 6.10, many viral diseases may be associated with myocarditis, which is usually a minor component of the illness with complete recovery being the rule. However, a few cases produce severe damage and fatal cardiac failure. Young adults, especially males, are most commonly affected although no age group is exempt, including infants. A history suggestive of viral myocarditis may be elicited from some patients who develop dilated cardiomyopathy. Immunosuppressed patients are predisposed to cytomegalovirus myocarditis. Histologically there is mononuclear cell infiltration of the myocardium (Figure 6.56) with a predominance of lymphocytes and macrophages along with myocyte damage in the absence of fibrosis or hypertrophy of surviving myocytes. Characteristic intracellular inclusions may be seen in cytomegalovirus myocarditis (see Chapter 19).

Suppurative Myocarditis

Septicaemia or pyaemia due to *Staphylococcus aureus* or *Streptococcus pyogenes* can result in abscess formation or spreading infection with necrosis respectively. Infective endocarditis causes myocardial abscesses in two ways: fragments of infected vegetations can embolize into

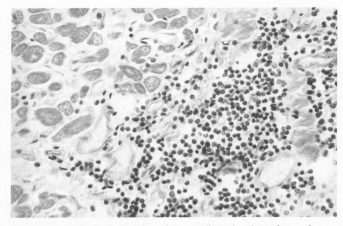

FIGURE 6.56 A histological section of myocardium showing a focus of lymphocytic myocarditis.

the coronary arteries or, infection by a virulent organism can spread directly into the myocardium from the valve lesions.

Protozoal Myocarditis

Trypanosoma cruzi may cause acute myocarditis (Chagas' disease) and is a major cause of cardiac morbidity and mortality in South America. Chronic infection results in enlargement of the heart, ventricular scarring and worsening cardiac failure often with heart block. *Toxoplasma gondii* is found worldwide but causes clinically significant myocardial involvement only in the immunosuppressed.

SPECIAL STUDY TOPIC CONTINUED . . .

Toxic Myocarditis

The agents listed in Table 6.10 act directly on the myocardium to produce focal myocyte death with a secondary inflammatory response consisting mainly of macrophages with polymorphs and some lymphocytes. The degree of drug-induced toxic damage is dose related and cumulative. If the individual survives, healing and focal scarring result. Occasionally dilated cardiomyopathy may develop, especially with anthracyclines. Diphtheria now rarely causes toxic myocarditis in developed countries because of well-established immunization programmes.

Hypersensitivity Myocarditis

In drug-induced hypersensitivity myocarditis, myocardial inflammation occurs soon after the drug is administered. The inflammatory response is often rich in eosinophils but in contrast to toxic myocarditis, myocyte damage is scanty. There may be inflammation of the walls of intramyocardial blood vessels. The myocarditis usually resolves rapidly with minimal fibrosis on withdrawal of the offending drug. Myocarditis may also complicate rheumatoid arthritis and systemic lupus erythematosus but seldom produces severe clinical disease. Acute rheumatic fever is dealt with below (p. 144).

Idiopathic Myocarditis

Granulomas and giant cells occur in the myocardium in sarcoidosis and idiopathic giant cell myocarditis. In sarcoidosis less than 5% of patients have clinically diagnosed cardiac involvement, however, granulomas can be found in the heart at autopsy in up to 58% of patients. Myocardial involvement usually results in ventricular scarring adjacent to granuloma formation. Giant cell myocarditis results in areas of necrosis with an associated inflammatory reaction comprising macrophages, eosinophils and giant cells which are macrophage in origin. Heart failure and sudden death may result. The aetiology of giant cell myocarditis is unknown.

Cardiomyopathies

The cardiomyopathies are a group of conditions in which the primary abnormality is chronic myocardial disease and dysfunction that is due neither to pressure and volume overload (thereby excluding hypertensive, valvular and congenital heart disease) nor to ischaemic heart disease. The most widely accepted classification is based on the type of abnormality of ventricular structure and function observed clinically, namely dilated cardiomyopathy, hypertrophic cardiomyopathy and restrictive cardiomyopathy.

Dilated Cardiomyopathy

> **Key Points**
>
> - Four-chamber dilatation of total heart failure.
> - There is poor systolic function.
> - DCM is the end stage of many insults to the myocardium.
> - Pathology: myocyte stretching and hypertrophy, myocyte damage, diffuse fibrosis.

TABLE 6.11 Causes of dilated cardiomyopathy

Idiopathic	
Post-inflammatory (myocarditic)	Most commonly viral but includes protozoal and bacterial
Genetic	With or without skeletal muscle myopathy
	Associated with inborn errors of metabolism, e.g. carnitine deficiency or haemochromatosis
	Sex-linked
Nutritional	Severe protein malnutrition
	Selenium or thiamine deficiency
Metabolic	Endocrine disease, e.g. diabetes, hypoparathyroidism, phaeochromocytoma
	Uraemia
Toxic	Alcohol, drugs, e.g. chemotherapeutic agents especially doxo-rubicin
	Heavy metals, e.g. lead, cobalt, arsenic
Peripartum	

All four heart chambers are dilated (Figures 6.57 and 6.58), the ventricular wall is usually thinned and the ventricles often contain mural thrombus. There is severe global impairment of contraction. Dilated cardiomyopathy (DCM) is the end stage of a variety of insults to the myocardium (Table 6.11). Most cases belong to the idiopathic group, which will diminish as the aetiology of DCM is better defined in individual patients. An unknown proportion follows chronic viral myocarditis. There are many genetic causes for the fifth of cases that are inherited; skeletal muscle myopathies such as myotonic dystrophy and Duchenne's/Becker's dystrophy are established causes of DCM. Gene mutations involving the mitochondrial respiratory chain are being increasingly recognized in DCM.

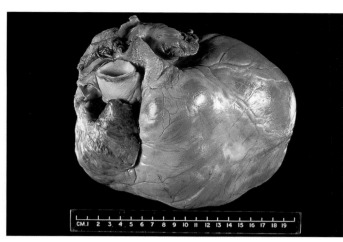

FIGURE 6.57 A grossly enlarged heart showing a marked globular shape in dilated cardiomyopathy.

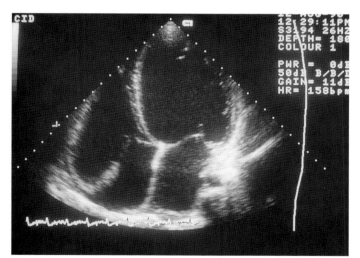

FIGURE 6.58 An echocardiogram shows that all four chambers are dilated with thin walls.

Microscopically, myocyte hypertrophy, vacuolation and myofibrillary loss with diffuse interstitial fibrosis and focal chronic inflammation may all be seen in varying proportions but these changes are not specific for DCM (Figure 6.59).

Hypertrophic Cardiomyopathy

Key Points

- It causes sudden death.
- There is left ventricular hypertrophy (usually asymmetrical) especially involving the interventricular septum.
- There is diastolic and systolic dysfunction.
- Many cases are due to myocyte contractile protein gene mutations, especially myosin heavy chain.
- Pathology: myocyte hypertrophy and disarray, variable diffuse fibrosis.

Hypertrophic cardiomyopathy commonly causes sudden death in young adults but may present at any age with syncopal attacks, angina or dyspnoea. Some cases present in athletes. It is usually diagnosed by echocardiography. The main feature is left ventricular hypertrophy without dilatation of the cavity. The hypertrophy may be symmetrical or asymmetrical (Figure 6.60) and the latter often predominates in the interventricular septum. The right ventricle, particularly the anterior wall of the outflow tract, is also involved in many cases. Resulting functional abnormalities include: diastolic dysfunction characterized by reduced ventricular compliance and diastolic filling; variable obstruction to the left ventricular outflow tract due to contact between the anterior cusp of the mitral valve and the hypertrophied interventricular septum during systole; mitral valve dysfunction including regurgitation.

The disease is due to inherited or spontaneous mutations in genes that code for myocyte contractile filament proteins, approximately 50% of cases having abnormalities in the

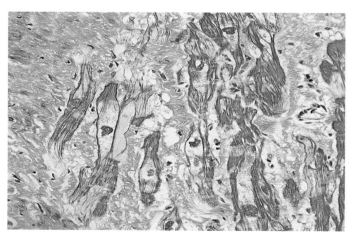

FIGURE 6.59 The myocardium in dilated cardiomyopathy shows vacuolation of myocytes and diffuse fibrosis.

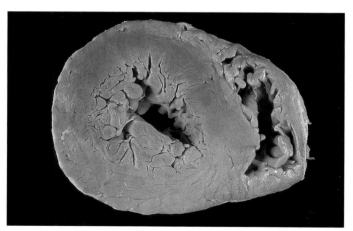

FIGURE 6.60 A grossly hypertrophied left ventricle in hypertrophic cardiomyopathy with some asymmetrical hypertrophy.

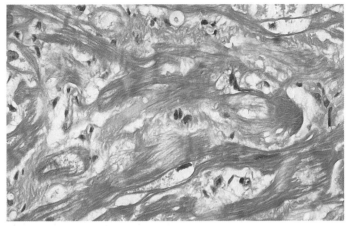

FIGURE 6.61 A focus of abnormal hypertrophied myocytes in hypertrophic cardiomyopathy. There is an irregular arrangement showing disarray and this is associated with interstitial fibrosis.

gene on chromosome 14 encoding the β-heavy chain of cardiac myosin. Myosin mutations that produce the greatest change in molecular charge cause more severe clinical manifestations; others appear relatively benign and are associated with a normal lifespan. Within a single kindred, with an identical mutation, there is often marked difference in phenotype, therefore other genes, such as the polymorphic angiotensin converting enzyme genes also influence the myocyte hypertrophy. Mutations in the genes for troponin T and tropomyosin, both of which are myocyte sarcomere fibrillary proteins, have also been shown to produce hypertrophic cardiomyopathy.

Microscopy shows myocyte hypertrophy and a whorled arrangement of the myocytes, known as disarray (Figure 6.61), attributable to their content of abnormal contractile filaments. There are variable degrees of myocardial scarring.

Restrictive Cardiomyopathy

Restrictive cardiomyopathy is the least common form of cardiomyopathy. The two main subtypes are endomyocardial fibrosis and endocardial fibroelastosis. In both, fibrosis produces abnormal diastolic relaxation with resultant impaired diastolic filling and progressive diastolic dysfunction. Variable systolic dysfunction also occurs.

In endomyocardial fibrosis there is fibrosis of the endocardium and underlying myocardium of the inflow tracts of either or both ventricles which restricts ventricular contraction. The fibrosis also involves the papillary muscles and chordae tendineae, causing incompetence of the mitral and/or tricuspid valves. Mural thrombus may embolize. It occurs in the tropics and temperate zones of the world. Marked eosinophilia is a common accompaniment and it is thought that endomyocardial fibrosis is due to endomyocardial damage caused by circulating activated eosinophils releasing eosinophilic granule basic proteins.

Endomyocardial fibroelastosis is an uncommon cause of progressive heart failure in infants and young children. A diffuse layer of dense, white tissue composed largely of parallel arrays of elastic fibres develops in the endocardium, usually of the left atrium and ventricle. It may occur in association with congenital heart abnormalities such as congenital aortic or mitral stenosis. It has been suggested that endomyocardial fibroelastosis simply represents a reaction to other heart diseases in early childhood rather than a separate disease.

Amyloid Heart Disease

All known types of amyloid may be deposited within the myocardium and cause restrictive heart dysfunction. The left ventricle may remain small or become enlarged. Amyloid deposited in the interstitium surrounding the myocytes causes atrophy and progressive myocyte loss with deterioration of ventricular function. Intramyocardial vessels may also be involved. Amyloid deposition becomes increasingly common over the age of 70; this 'senile' cardiac amyloid may be confined to the atria or involve atria and ventricles.

Rheumatic Heart Disease

Acute Rheumatic Fever

This is an acute multisystem illness in which the major lesions occur in the heart, the joints and the subcutaneous tissues. It develops 2–4 weeks after an attack of streptococcal pharyngitis with a peak age incidence of 5–15 years. Symptoms may be mild but there is usually fever, tachycardia, malaise and flitting arthralgia; the affected joints may be swollen. There is no specific test for rheumatic fever but a raised ESR, anaemia, slight leucocytosis and raised titres of streptococcal antibodies such as anti-streptolysin O (ASO) are usually present. The incidence has fallen greatly in developed countries probably as a result of improved living conditions and the use of antibiotics. However, it is still common in parts of Africa, India, the Middle East and South America.

Rheumatic fever causes a pancarditis. Diffuse myocardial injury may cause heart failure during the acute illness and is occasionally fatal, but in most cases myocardial function recovers completely. Valvular lesions are clinically undetectable in the acute stage of the illness, although there may be evidence of secondary mitral incompetence due to dilatation of the left ventricle. Subsequent disability is due to chronic injury to the cardiac valves. The scarring results in permanent distortion which takes a minimum of 10 years after the first attack and often leads to chronic heart failure. Rheumatic fever tends to recur after subsequent attacks of streptococcal pharyngitis and each recurrence increases the risk of serious valvular disease.

Pathology of Acute Rheumatic Fever

Key Points

- Pancarditis: endocarditis, myocarditis and pericarditis.

- Chronic endocarditis may lead to chronic rheumatic valve disease.
- Myocarditis can cause arrhythmias, heart failure and rarely death.
- Acute fibrinous pericarditis usually causes no significant long-term effects.

The endocarditis comprises diffuse oedema and a mild inflammatory infiltrate. Most importantly, small thrombotic vegetations form along the apposition lines of the valve cusps, particularly on the mitral valve; vegetations also form on the chordae tendineae. The vegetations are sessile, consist mainly of platelets and do not lead to systemic emboli. These acute changes are followed by organization of the vegetations with resulting fibrous thickening and vascularization of the cusps. Fibrous union between adjacent cusp margins starts at the commissures and there is thickening, shortening and fusion of the chordae tendineae. With recurrent acute attacks, valve injury becomes more severe with progressive fibrosis and deformity.

The myocarditis is characterized by the formation of small giant cell granulomas, called Aschoff's bodies, in the connective tissue of the myocardium especially in the left atrium and ventricle. In time these heal to leave tiny, focal scars. The acute fibrinous pericarditis is often accompanied by a serous effusion. It is usually transitory and, while it may result in pericardial fibrosis or adhesions, there are usually no serious long-term sequelae.

Changes in Other Tissues

- Synovitis.
- Subcutaneous nodules.
- Skin rashes.
- Encephalitis and chorea.

The joints show mild synovitis sometimes accompanied by effusions. Subcutaneous nodules develop over bony prominences of the arms and legs, most commonly on the extensive surface of the elbow. The nodules are usually 1–2 cm in diameter, are painless and they resemble large Aschoff's bodies. Various erythematous skin rashes may occur, the commonest being erythema marginatum. In some cases there may be a mild encephalitis causing chorea. These manifestations may develop during or apart from the acute attack of rheumatic fever.

Pathogenesis

Acute rheumatic fever occurs following pharyngeal infection with Lancefield group A *Streptococcus pyogenes* in approximately 3% of affected individuals. The organism is not found in the heart in fatal cases and the pancarditis is not caused by streptococcal toxins. Acute rheumatic fever is an immune reaction involving both cell-mediated immunity and antibodies to streptococcal antigen crossreacting with myocardial antigens.

Chronic Rheumatic Valve Disease

Key Points

- It causes valve cusp commissural fusion, cusp fibrosis and cusp calcification.
- There is valve stenosis and/or regurgitation.
- Mitral and aortic valves are most commonly involved.
- It predisposes to infective endocarditis.

Chronic valve disease develops up to 30 years after acute rheumatic fever; there is a higher risk of chronic valve disease after childhood rheumatic fever and repeated attacks. In severe cases valve disease may occur in late childhood, especially in developing countries. In up to 30% of patients with acute rheumatic fever, the chronic valve lesions lead to heart failure.

The pathological features of chronic rheumatic valve disease are commissural fusion, cusp fibrosis with retraction thereby reducing cusp area, and cusp calcification; these changes result in all permutations of valve stenosis and/or regurgitation (Figure 6.62). Characteristically, more than one valve is involved with a mixture of functional abnormalities. Mitral and aortic involvement is seen in about 50% of cases (see Figure 6.67 on p. 150) and mitral involvement alone in about 25%; involvement of all valves is seen in approximately 15% of cases. The greater degree of haemodynamic stress probably accounts for the susceptibility of the mitral and aortic valves. Right-sided valves are seldom affected alone. Chronic rheumatic valve disease predisposes to infective endocarditis (p. 149).

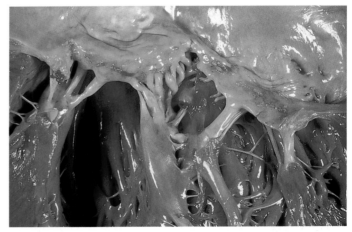

FIGURE 6.62 A mitral valve with severe shortening and thickening of the cusps and shortening and fusion of the chordae tendineae.

Valvular Heart Disease

Abnormalities of cardiac valves may be congenital or acquired. In many developing countries acute rheumatic fever remains the major cause of acquired valvular heart disease, but in most industrialized countries other valve lesions have increased in importance as acute rheumatic fever has virtually disappeared. Chronic rheumatic valve disease is now seen mostly in the older age groups. Any abnormality of the cardiac valves increases the risk of infective endocarditis.

Serious reduction of the size of the valve orifice (stenosis) increases the pressure load on the preceding chamber. Failure to close completely (incompetence) results in regurgitation of blood which increases the volume load on both sides of the valve. Either defect, if severe, is likely to cause cardiac failure. Diagnosis and assessment of valve lesions is mainly carried out by echocardiography and Doppler ultrasound. Surgical repair or replacement produces good results in suitable patients.

Pathology of Individual Heart Valves

Mitral Valve

Normal mitral valve function depends on the mechanical efficiency of its cusps, chordae and papillary muscles, on the pliability and size of the fibrous valve ring or annulus, and on the adequacy of left ventricular contraction which normally halves the area of the orifice during systole. Each cusp consists of a central fibrous plate (fibrosa) covered on either side by loose subendothelial connective tissue. The cusps are normally avascular.

Mitral stenosis (Figures 6.62 and 6.63)

Key Points

- This is almost always due to rheumatic fever.
- There is atrial dilatation, atrial fibrillation and atrial thrombosis.
- It leads to pulmonary venous hypertension and oedema.
- Pulmonary arterial hypertension causes right ventricular hypertrophy and failure.

Rheumatic heart disease is the cause of almost all cases of mitral stenosis; similar lesions are seen occasionally in

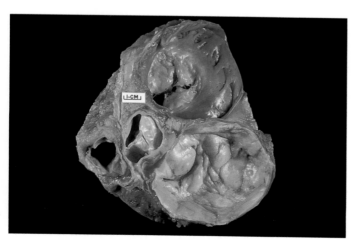

FIGURE 6.63 The mitral, aortic and tricuspid valves visualized through the atria. There is mitral stenosis and severe aortic stenosis.

patients with systemic lupus erythematosus (pp. 26–27). In chronic rheumatic disease the changes described above lead to cusp fusion thus forming a fibrous diaphragm with a central slit-shaped or oval orifice whose area depends on the extent of fusion of the cusps and on their rigidity. Pure stenosis results when the diaphragm is thin and pliable. Greater thickening and rigidity usually results in a combination of stenosis and incompetence.

Mitral stenosis results in atrial hypertrophy and dilatation often accompanied by atrial fibrillation. Thrombosis frequently occurs in the left atrium, beginning in its appendage. This may cause systemic embolism, for example with cerebral infarction. Pulmonary venous hypertension and oedema cause dyspnoea and persistent cough. Attacks of acute pulmonary oedema are brought on by exercise and paroxysmal nocturnal dyspnoea occurs. Mild haemoptysis occurs due to haemorrhage from engorged pulmonary capillaries. Pulmonary venous hypertension leads to increased tone and hypertrophy of the pulmonary arterial tree causing pulmonary hypertension, right ventricular hypertrophy and right heart failure. In pure mitral stenosis, the left ventricle is normal or small in size.

Mitral incompetence

Key Points

- Its causes include post-rheumatic, infective endocarditis, floppy mitral valve, papillary muscle pathology, valve ring dilatation.
- It results in compensatory left ventricular hypertrophy.
- There is impaired left ventricular function and failure.

The main causes of mitral incompetence are shown in Table 6.12. These can be divided into three main groups.

Lesions of the valve cusps and chordae

Post-inflammatory scarring of the mitral valve may follow rheumatic or infective endocarditis, and if severe, may hold the cusps in a partly opened position. Increased rigidity and fusion of the cusps often results in a combination of stenosis and incompetence; pure incompetence is unusual. Sudden mitral incompetence may develop in infective endocarditis as a result of perforation of cusps or rupture of chordae.

The floppy mitral valve or mitral valve cusp prolapse syndrome is increasing in importance as the incidence of rheumatic heart disease has declined. Minor degrees occur in up to 15% of women and up to 3% of men with an increase in old age. The valve cusps and chordae stretch and the latter may rupture due to myxoid degeneration of the dense fibrous tissue core. During ventricular systole, the slack in the valve cusps is taken up and the chordae are jerked taut, giving an audible systolic click. Part or all of one or both cusps bulges into the atrium. A systolic murmur follows the click due to regurgitation. At autopsy the cusps appear dome shaped,

TABLE 6.12 **Causes of mitral incompetence**

Cusp pathology	
Fibrosis and contraction	Rheumatic disease, systemic lupus erythematosus (rare)
Stretching	Floppy mitral valve, Marfan syndrome
Perforation	Infective endocarditis
Chordal pathology	
Shortening or fusion	Rheumatic disease
Elongation	Floppy mitral valve, Marfan syndrome
Rupture	Floppy mitral valve, infective endocarditis
Papillary muscle pathology	
Infarction and rupture	Ischaemic heart disease
Scarring	Ischaemic heart disease
Valve ring pathology	
Dilation	Failing dilated left ventricle, Marfan syndrome, floppy mitral valve
Calcification	Advancing age

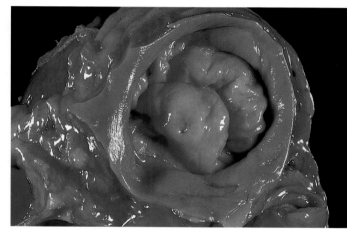

FIGURE 6.64 **A floppy mitral valve viewed through the atrium showing soft thickened and stretched cusps bulging into the atrium.**

bulging towards the atrium (Figure 6.64). Incompetence is usually slight unless one or more of the chordae rupture. Floppy mitral valve may complicate Marfan syndrome, osteogenesis imperfecta or pseudoxanthoma elasticum. When severe, the aortic valve is also affected.

Papillary muscle ischaemia

Loss of contractility of a papillary muscle as a result of ischaemia causes mitral incompetence by allowing the related cusp to prolapse into the atrium. Following myocardial infarction, rupture of an infarcted papillary muscle may cause sudden and severe incompetence with rapidly fatal left ventricular failure. Ischaemic damage can also lead to scarring and papillary muscle dysfunction.

Dilatation of the mitral ring is usually caused by dilatation of a failing left ventricle

It may occur rarely as a primary event, for example in Marfan syndrome.

Incompetence of the mitral valve allows regurgitation of blood into the left atrium during ventricular systole so that the left atrium distends. The additional volume of blood returns freely into the left ventricle during ventricular diastole and stretching of the left ventricle by the extra volume load results in more forcible contraction. When mitral incompetence develops gradually there is time for the left ventricle to undergo hypertrophy and unless the leakage is severe this enables it to eject the normal amount of blood into the aorta. However, maximal effective stroke volume is reduced, exercise tolerance is diminished and fatigue and weakness are often the presenting symptoms. Attacks of acute pulmonary oedema with exertional and nocturnal dyspnoea are much less common than in mitral stenosis. Although atrial fibrillation is common, left atrial thrombosis and embolic phenomena occur less often than in mitral stenosis. Eventually the increased volume load leads to left ventricular failure. As its contractions weaken and residual blood accumulates, the pressure in the left atrium rises and pulmonary venous hypertension and oedema develop. Death may result from left ventricular failure but in some cases pulmonary venous hypertension leads to pulmonary artery hypertension, right ventricular hypertrophy and failure.

In acute mitral incompetence, the left ventricle is unable to compensate and quickly fails. The left atrium cannot dilate rapidly to accommodate the additional volume of blood entering it and so the left atrial pressure rises quickly, leading to severe pulmonary venous hypertension and oedema.

Aortic Valve

Aortic stenosis

> **Key Points**
> - Main causes are idiopathic calcific aortic stenosis and rheumatic heart disease.
> - There is concentric left ventricular hypertrophy.
> - Inadequate coronary perfusion causes syncope and angina.
> - There is a significant risk of sudden cardiac death.
> - Eventually left ventricular failure develops.

In the UK, approximately two-thirds of cases are due to calcific aortic stenosis and in patients under 70 years of age most are calcified congenitally bicuspid valves (Figure 6.65). Rheumatic endocarditis accounts for approximately 20% of cases, 5% are due to other congenital abnormalities and the remaining 10% have no identifiable cause.

In post-rheumatic aortic valve disease, the cusps are thickened, vascularized, rigid and partially fused. Stenosis is usually combined with incompetence. In over 90% of cases the mitral valve is also affected. In contrast, calcific aortic stenosis is usually associated with a normal mitral valve and presents as

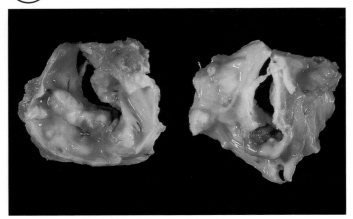

FIGURE 6.65 Two aortic valves surgically removed for calcific aortic stenosis. This occurred prematurely because the valves were congenitally bicuspid.

TABLE 6.13 Causes of aortic incompetence

Cusp pathology	
Fibrosis, calcification and contraction	Rheumatic disease, senile calcific aortic stenosis, bicuspid valve
Stretching	Myxoid change
Perforation	Infective endocarditis
Aortic sleeve pathology	
Inflammatory dilatation	Syphilis, HLA-B27 associated disease (especially ankylosing spondylitis), rheumatoid arthritis, giant cell aortitis
Non-inflammatory dilatation	Marfan syndrome, idiopathic cystic medial necrosis, advanced age
Disruption of aortic wall	Dissection, Marfan syndrome, trauma causing loss of cusp support

stenosis usually without serious incompetence. The changes in calcific aortic stenosis are an exaggeration of those seen in old age when the cusps become thickened and fibrotic with irregular nodules of dystrophic calcification; these usually begin at the base of the cusps and extend towards the free margin. Resulting cusp rigidity converts the orifice to a narrow slit. Calcific aortic stenosis in a congenitally bicuspid aortic valve develops in a younger age group, usually becoming apparent between 40 and 60 years of age. In congenital aortic valve stenosis, the cusps are usually fused to form a diaphragm with a central eccentric orifice.

Reduction of the area of the aortic valve orifice by over 50% significantly increases the resistance to ejection of blood into the aorta and there is compensatory left ventricular hypertrophy. In most patients this maintains an adequate cardiac output for many years, but to achieve this compensated state the left ventricle must generate a considerable pressure, sometimes over 250 mmHg. As the pressure in the aorta is not increased and may fall below normal during ventricular diastole, coronary perfusion pressure is diminished. This, with left ventricular failure, predisposes to angina pectoris, which can occur in the absence of coronary atheroma. Fainting is common, perhaps due to transient arrhythmias and up to 15% of people with aortic stenosis die suddenly, presumably due to ventricular fibrillation. Death may also result from left heart failure.

Aortic incompetence

Key Points

- Main causes include post-rheumatic, calcific aortic stenosis, dilatation of aortic sleeve, infective endocarditis (see Table 6.13).
- It leads to collapsing pulse and left ventricular failure with dilatation.
- There is angina due to inadequate coronary perfusion.
- Eventually left ventricular failure develops.

Rheumatic heart disease is still an important cause of aortic valve incompetence due to fibrous thickening and contraction of the cusps, usually combined with aortic stenosis and in most cases the mitral valve is also diseased. Some incompetence may also be associated with calcific aortic valve stenosis, while some bicuspid valves, particularly those with grossly unequal cusps, are incompetent at birth or become so later. Infective endocarditis may erode and rupture a cusp causing acute aortic incompetence.

Dilatation of the aortic valve sleeve causes aortic incompetence. Aortitis may be due to syphilis (Figure 6.66) or associated with seronegative arthritis such as ankylosing spondylitis and Reiter's syndrome. Non-inflammatory stretching of the aortic valve sleeve occurs in Marfan syndrome and other rare genetic syndromes causing a defect in connective tissue synthesis. It is a rare complication of extreme arteriosclerosis in advanced age. Proximal aortic dissection may involve the aortic valve sleeve and cause one or more cusps to prolapse because of loss of their attachment leading to acute aortic incompetence.

The left ventricle hypertrophies and dilates in response to the increased volume and pressure loads. This results in a raised systolic blood pressure; during diastole the regurgitation of blood results in a rapid fall to abnormally low aortic pressure. The pulse pressure is thus increased, giving a collapsing (water-hammer) pulse. A compensated state may last for many years. However, coronary blood flow, compromised by the reduced diastolic pressure, may not meet the demands of the hypertrophied left ventricle and so, as in aortic stenosis, angina pectoris is often a feature. While arrhythmias and sudden death are less common than in aortic stenosis, the left ventricle eventually fails with a fatal outcome.

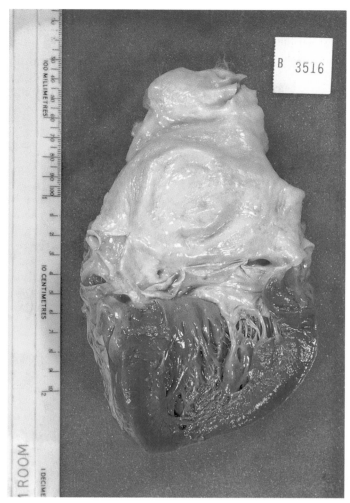

FIGURE 6.66 Syphilitic aortitis causing thickening and stretching of the aortic root and aortic incompetence.

Tricuspid Valve

The commonest cause of primary tricuspid valve disease is infective endocarditis due to intravenous drug misuse. Together with the mitral and aortic valves, the tricuspid valve is affected in approximately 15% of cases of post-rheumatic valvular disease. Tricuspid valve changes are similar to those in the mitral valve but are less severe and give rise to stenosis or stenosis/incompetence. The carcinoid syndrome (p. 256) may cause tricuspid stenosis, either pure or combined with incompetence. Stenosis may also result from congenital malformations of the valve. Pure incompetence due to dilatation of the valve ring is a feature of right ventricular failure.

Tricuspid stenosis or incompetence or a combination of the two have similar effects. Pressure rises in the right atrium which dilates, the central venous pressure increases and systemic venous hypertension results in peripheral oedema. If mitral stenosis or left ventricular failure co-exist, the tricuspid lesions tend to reduce the degree of pulmonary venous hypertension by limiting the volume of blood reaching the left side of the heart.

Pulmonary Valve

Pulmonary stenosis is most commonly congenital, and is also a feature of the carcinoid syndrome. Right ventricular hypertrophy and right ventricular failure result. Pulmonary incompetence is most commonly secondary to pulmonary hypertension with dilatation of the pulmonary artery and valve ring. It also occurs in the carcinoid syndrome or as a congenital malformation and rarely infective endocarditis. The effects are not serious unless there is pulmonary hypertension and indeed the valve may be excised in patients with refractory infective endocarditis involving the valve without greatly impairing cardiac function.

INFECTIVE ENDOCARDITIS

Key Points

- There is infection of the valve with formation of thrombotic vegetations.
- The virulence of the organisms dictates severity of infection and degree of valve damage.
- Pre-existing valve disease, immunosuppression and bacteraemia are all predisposing factors.
- Complications are: valve damage, heart failure, septic embolism, toxaemia, glomerulonephritis.

Microorganisms entering the bloodstream are usually rapidly eliminated. However, in some circumstances they may infect the endocardial surface, usually of the valve cusps. The endocardial damage leads to formation of thrombi known as vegetations within which the organism proliferates. Infective endocarditis is characterized by fever, toxaemia, embolic phenomena, heart failure and sometimes glomerulonephritis. Traditionally, infective endocarditis is classified into acute and subacute types. The former affects a normal heart and is rapidly fatal because it is due to microorganisms of high virulence. Subacute endocarditis affects a damaged heart, gives rise to a more prolonged illness and is due to less virulent organisms. The distinction is valuable but many patients present with features intermediate between these two extremes and so it is best to regard infective endocarditis as a spectrum of disease.

Everyone develops transient bacteraemia due to, for example, hard chewing and vigorous use of a toothbrush. Boils, pneumonia, and infection of the urinary, gastrointestinal and biliary tracts are also associated with bacteraemia. Intravenous drug misuse is an increasingly important cause of tricuspid and pulmonary valve infection. Surgery and even minor procedures such as dental treatment, urethral catheterization, cystoscopy and sigmoidoscopy also cause transient bacteraemia. These procedures do not carry a significant risk of infective endocarditis unless there is predisposing valve disease or depression of host defence mechanisms. Up to 10% of patients with endocarditis have no obvious portal of entry for the organism.

Distortion of the heart valves predisposes to infective endocarditis: chronic rheumatic disease, calcific aortic stenosis, floppy mitral valve, congenital bicuspid aortic valve and age-related changes. In children, congenital heart lesions predispose to infection. Other predisposing factors are valve prostheses, intracardiac catheters and pacemakers. Distorted valve surfaces encourage formation of small thrombi in which entrapped microorganisms, protected from circulating host defences, multiply and invade the underlying valve.

Immunodeficiency and impaired function of phago-cytes, whether caused by natural disease or cytotoxic therapy, predispose to infective endocarditis. The increasing incidence in the elderly may in part be associated with decline in immune function.

Subacute Infective Endocarditis

Subacute infective endocarditis is usually caused by bacteria of low virulence, most commonly the 'viridans' group of α-haemolytic streptococci which form part of the normal flora of the mouth and pharynx and are important in periodontal infection. Group D streptococci, gut commensals, and *Staphylococcus epidermidis*, a skin commensal which infects indwelling venous catheters and pacemaker wires, are also important. Other Gram-negative bacilli, *Coxiella*, mycoplasma and fungi are less commonly seen. Endocarditis due to fungi and yeasts tends to occur in intravenous drug misusers; in immunosuppressed patients, infection with *Candida* and *Aspergillus* is most common.

Pathology

The valvular vegetations consist of friable, soft thrombi ranging in size from a few millimetres to a few centimetres in diameter. They usually develop on and project from the contact surface of a cusp (Figure 6.67). The microorganisms eventually invade the cusp and may cause necrosis and cusp rupture. Involvement of the chordae is more frequent and severe in acute infective endocarditis. Infection may extend from the base of the valve cusp into the adjacent myocardium or aortic root. The vegetations consist mostly of fibrin, platelets, colonies of microorganisms and often scanty polymorphs. The underlying cusp is inflamed and may be focally necrotic.

Clinical Features and Course

Subacute infective endocarditis starts insidiously with fever, malaise and mild anaemia. Petechiae may occur in the skin, mucous membranes and retina and 'splinter' haemorrhages are seen under the nails. Some of these changes are probably embolic in origin. The spleen is usually enlarged and palpable (Figure 6.68). Cardiac murmurs may be a result of previous heart disease or may develop and change in quality as the vegetations progress. As vegetations grow and disintegrate, emboli may cause infarction of the brain, myocardium, spleen (see Figure 6.68) and kidneys. Gross or microscopic haematuria may result from either renal infarction or

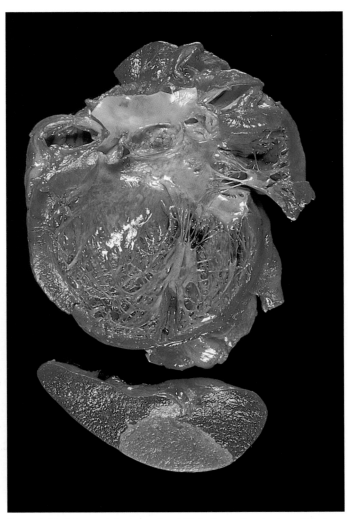

FIGURE 6.68 Subacute infective endocarditis in the aortic valve in a dilated heart. The spleen is also enlarged and shows an infarct due to embolism.

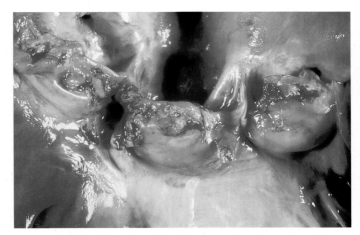

FIGURE 6.67 Vegetations on an infected aortic valve in subacute bacterial endocarditis. The valve is thickened, scarred and fused at the commissures due to previous rheumatic damage.

glomerulonephritis, the latter being mediated by immune complex deposition (p. 377). Untreated subacute infective endocarditis is invariably fatal within a few months from heart failure, embolic phenomena or renal failure. Blood cultures and echocardiography to visualize the valves are mandatory investigations. Appropriate antimicrobial therapy reduces the mortality, which still remains high even when the infecting organism is identified.

Acute Infective Endocarditis

Acute infective endocarditis is a severe acute bacterial infection. The mitral and aortic valves are usually involved, but the tricuspid valve is often infected in intravenous drug misusers. *Staphylococcus aureus*, *Streptococcus pyogenes* and enterococci are most often responsible. Blood culture is nearly always positive. Rapidly changing cardiac murmurs occur as valve cusps are destroyed. Septicaemia and embolic phenomena occur and without treatment the condition is rapidly fatal due to overwhelming infection or acute heart failure. Mortality is over 50%, even with intensive treatment. Early surgery may be beneficial in selected patients.

Pathological Features

Compared with subacute endocarditis, the vegetations are larger and more localized to one part of the valve. They consist mainly of fibrin containing large clusters of organisms surrounded by neutrophil polymorphs. Rapid cusp invasion causes necrosis, suppuration and often complete rupture. Infection and rupture of chordae tendineae are common. Local invasion into the myocardium or adjacent aorta causes abscess formation.

Lesions Simulating Infective Endocarditis

Non-bacterial Thrombotic Endocarditis

Non-bacterial thrombotic endocarditis (marantic or terminal endocarditis) consists of small thrombi on the heart valves, usually in a patchy fashion along the lines of cusp closure of the mitral and aortic valves. They are probably caused by a hypercoagulable state since identical lesions occur in any patient with acute DIC. They are usually asymptomatic but both systemic embolism and secondary infection of the thrombi are recognized complications. Characteristically, this condition occurs in patients with a debilitating illness such as cancer or tuberculosis.

Libman–Sacks Endocarditis

This may develop in patients with systemic lupus erythematosus and can involve the mitral, aortic, or tricuspid valves. The vegetations are sterile, platelet-rich and rarely exceed 2 mm in size. Fibrinoid necrosis is a characteristic feature.

6.2 CASE HISTORY

A 56-year-old woman complained of fatigue and diminished exercise tolerance. She developed a left hemiplegia and on admission auscultation revealed a rumbling mid-diastolic murmur and a pan-systolic murmur suggestive of mitral stenosis and incompetence. Chest X-rays showed some streaky shadowing in the lung fields which did not resolve despite diuretic therapy. A diagnosis of atrial fibrillation and cerebral embolism due to long-standing rheumatic heart disease with mitral stenosis and incompetence was made. This was confirmed by an echocardiogram (see Figure 6.69).

When recuperating, she became unwell with a pyrexial illness. There was no obvious site of infection until echocardiography revealed a vegetation on the mitral valve. Blood cultures grew no pathogens and she was treated with intravenous antibiotics for several weeks without response. As she was deteriorating clinically a mitral valve replacement was undertaken. Figure 6.70 shows the valve removed at operation. A year later she became more breathless and had a pansystolic murmur of mitral incompetence and the prosthetic valve was removed (Figure 6.71) and replaced. This effected a symptomatic cure and she remains well.

In summary, this woman had chronic rheumatic heart disease due to recurrent subclinical rheumatic fever. Her mitral stenosis and incompetence was complicated by atrial

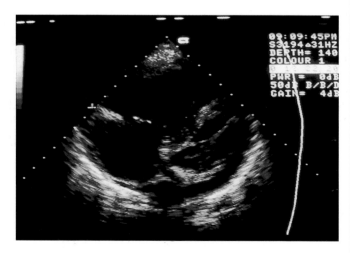

FIGURE 6.69 Echocardiogram showing the heart in ventricular systole. The thickened and scarred cusps and chordae tendineae are visible. The mitral valve remains open during systole indicating regurgitation which was confirmed by colour Doppler studies.

fibrillation. This has a high risk of thrombus formation and she had a stroke due to cerebral infarction from thromboembolism. She developed subacute infective endocarditis that was resistant to treatment and only cured by mitral valve replacement. The flap valve prosthesis failed because it became blocked by the formation of adherent thrombus.

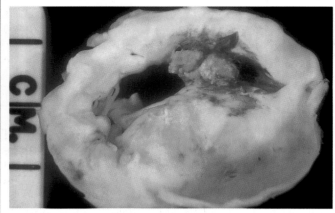

FIGURE 6.70 A mitral valve removed at operation. It is thickened, calcified and the orifice is reduced to a slit by fusion of the commissures due to rheumatic scarring. It is rigid and can neither open or close. A large friable vegetation protrudes into the orifice.

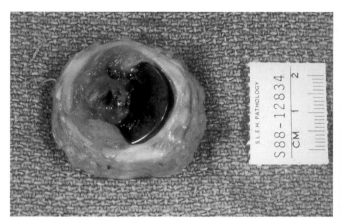

FIGURE 6.71 The valve flap of the prosthetic mitral valve replacement is jammed with thrombus. It can neither open nor close fully.

DISORDERS OF THE CONDUCTION SYSTEM

The conducting system consists of specialized cardiac myocytes which initiate the heartbeat in the sinoatrial node and conduct the impulse through the AV node and then through the common AV bundles (bundles of His) and the left and right bundle branches to the apex of the ventricles, which is the first region to contract. Disturbances of rhythm complicate many types of heart disease: some are due to damage to the conducting system, its most vulnerable regions being the AV bundle and the left and right bundle branches; however, many arrhythmias, such as extra systoles, paroxysmal tachycardia and fibrillation are due to spontaneous 'impulses' or irregularities arising in the myocardium itself.

Acquired conducting system defects include ischaemic damage, inflammatory conditions such as myocarditis, sarcoidosis or connective tissue diseases, infiltrative disorders such as amyloidosis or metastatic tumour and finally surgical trauma.

DISEASES OF THE PERICARDIUM

Key Points

- Pericarditis has multiple aetiologies including infection, myocardial infarction, connective tissue diseases and uraemia.
- Pericardial effusion and haemopericardium can both cause cardiac tamponade.
- Constrictive pericarditis is due to fibrous obliteration of the pericardial cavity with resulting impaired cardiac function.
- Pericardial involvement by metastatic tumour may produce effusion, inflammation or restriction.

The pericardium is a fibrous sac which surrounds the heart, comprises visceral and parietal layers, and may become inflamed (pericarditis). A pericardial effusion is an accumulation of fluid in the pericardial sac, often due to metastatic carcinoma, but also in cardiac failure and in other types of oedema. Blood too can accumulate (haemopericardium). The pericardial sac can dilate to contain over a litre of fluid without a significant rise in pressure if the fluid accumulates slowly. If accumulation is rapid, even a small rise in fluid volume increases the pericardial pressure, interferes with cardiac filling and leads to cardiac tamponade. In the most severe form, cardiogenic shock with low cardiac output ensues. There is hypotension with a low pulse pressure, particularly during inspiration (pulsus paradoxus) and death results. Cardiac tamponade is usually due to haemopericardium caused by rupture of the heart or aortic root, but it may be caused by a tense effusion.

Pericarditis

The clinical features of acute pericarditis include fever, tachycardia and chest pain, although sometimes the condition is silent. An inflammatory exudate accumulates in the pericardial sac and fibrin is deposited on the pericardial surfaces (Figure 6.72). A fine deposit of fibrin on the pericardial surfaces undergoes lysis, but a thicker layer becomes organized with consequent fibrous thickening and adhesions between the two pericardial layers.

The main causes of pericarditis are summarized in Table 6.14. Viral and idiopathic pericarditis most commonly occurs in young adults, often after an upper respiratory tract infection, and usually subsides within 2 weeks. Coxsackie A and B viruses, echoviruses and polioviruses are most commonly implicated. Rarely, fibrosis due to repeated attacks may eventually progress to chronic constrictive pericarditis.

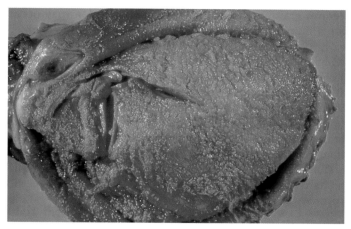

FIGURE 6.72 The anterior surface of the heart with the pericardium opened to reveal a fibrinous pericarditis.

TABLE 6.14 Aetiology of pericarditis

Infections	Viral – Coxsackie A, B, echoviruses and polioviruses
	Bacterial – pyogenic organisms, tuberculosis
	Fungal and protozoal
Malignant disease	Direct spread from carcinoma of bronchus or oesophagus
	Metastatic tumour
Myocardial infarction	
Metabolic	Uraemia
	Hypothyroidism
Immunologically mediated	Rheumatic fever
	Connective tissue diseases – rheumatoid arthritis, systemic lupus erythematosus, mixed connective tissue disease
	Post-cardiotomy or post-myocardial infarction (Dressler's syndrome)
Iatrogenic	Post-irradiation
	Drug hypersensitivity reaction
Idiopathic	

Bacterial pericarditis may complicate septicaemia or pyaemia, or arise due to direct spread from pneumonia, empyema or an ulcerating carcinoma of the bronchus or oesophagus. *Staphylococcus aureus*, *Haemophilus influenzae* and streptococci are the most common causal organisms.

Tuberculous pericarditis is due to either haematogenous spread, most commonly from the lung, or due to direct extension from the trachea, bronchi or mediastinal lymph nodes. The pericardial exudate has a high protein concentration. Later caseating granulomatous inflammation may progress to fibrous obliteration of the pericardial sac, calcification and

constrictive pericarditis. Transmural myocardial infarction may cause mild localized pericarditis in the first week. A more diffuse persistent pericarditis (Dressler's syndrome, p. 139) may follow myocardial infarction or cardiac surgery. Pericarditis commonly complicates rheumatoid arthritis, systemic lupus erythematosus and uraemia.

Constrictive Pericarditis

Constrictive pericarditis is characterized by obliteration of the pericardial sac by a thick layer of dense fibrous tissue which may become calcified. It can result from prolonged pyogenic, tuberculous or viral infection, but in many cases the aetiology is unknown. The fibrotic pericardium adheres to the heart and interferes with diastolic filling, possibly aggravated by constriction of the great veins as they enter the atria. Clinically the picture is one of progressive heart failure associated with a small heart and low stroke volume. Surgical excision of the fibrotic pericardium is an effective treatment.

TUMOURS OF THE HEART AND PERICARDIUM

Key Points

- The commonest malignant cardiac/pericardial tumour is metastatic carcinoma.
- Primary cardiac tumours are rare.
- Atrial myxoma is commonest primary tumour.
- Primary malignant cardiac/pericardial tumours are rare.

The commonest primary tumour is the cardiac myxoma (Figure 6.73) which usually occurs in adult life in the left atrium. It forms a gelatinous mass up to 6 cm in diameter which may create an intermittent ball valve obstruction of the mitral valve or present with embolic phenomena or a

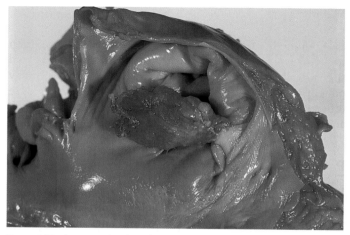

FIGURE 6.73 An opened atrium showing a myxoma as a soft ovoid gelatinous mass on a stalk which may obstruct the mitral valve or give rise to embolism.

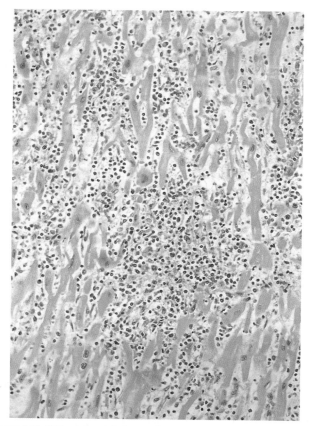

FIGURE 6.76 Diffuse chronic inflammation and myocyte damage indicate severe acute rejection of the allograft.

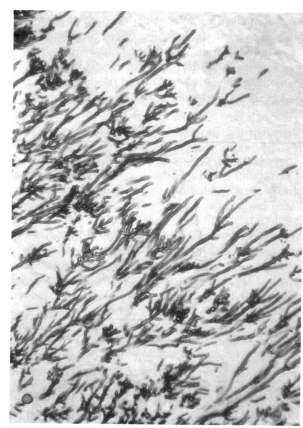

FIGURE 6.77 A methenamine silver stained preparation showing septate fungi with dichotomous branching morphologically consistent with *Aspergillus*.

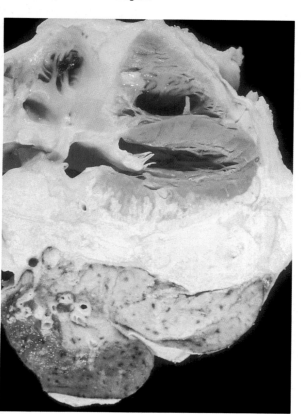

FIGURE 6.78 The heart is embedded in a white tumour mass consisting of diffuse large B-cell lymphoma occupying most of the mediastinum.

Each is divided into two by a separate septum, defects in the formation of which result in most congenital abnormalities. Important abnormalities arise in relation to the growth of the ventricular septum and the division of the aortic bulb into the aorta and pulmonary artery. The ventricular septum grows upwards from the apex of the ventricle, whereas the aortic bulb is divided into two nearly equal parts by the formation and fusion of two longitudinal folds in its wall. The two vessels formed must rotate spirally to establish their normal continuity with the ventricles. The septum of the bulb fuses with the upgrowing ventricular septum, the last portion to close being represented by the membranous part of the interventricular septum.

Congenital heart diseases can be divided into those which produce cyanosis and those which do not. The cyanosis results from admixture of venous blood with oxygenated blood leaving the heart. The lowered oxygen tension in arterial blood leads to a compensatory erythrocytosis which makes cyanosis more prominent. The cyanosis may be further aggravated by impaired oxygenation of blood by the lungs in conditions where there is pulmonary disease or when heart failure develops.

Pathology of Cyanotic Congenital Heart Disease

The commonest anomaly in this group is the tetralogy of Fallot. There is obstruction to the outflow tract of the right ventricle usually from stenosis of the pulmonary valve which results in right ventricular hypertrophy; high right ventricular pressures force unoxygenated blood into the aorta through a high interventricular septal defect. The aorta partially overrides the septal defect and receives both venous blood from the right ventricle and oxygenated blood from the left ventricle. The features of Eisenmenger's complex resemble those of Fallot's tetralogy but there is no obstruction to the outflow from the right ventricle. Initially little right to left shunting of blood occurs and there is little cyanosis, but later, with the onset of pulmonary hypertension, overt cyanosis appears partly from admixture cyanosis and partly from faulty oxygenation of the blood by the lungs.

Malformations of the aortic bulb can result in pulmonary or aortic stenosis. Most commonly pulmonary stenosis results from an unequal division of the bulb; the septum is pushed to the right producing an abnormally large aorta that arises partly from the left and partly from the right ventricle; there is usually a defect in the interventricular septum. The site of stenosis varies: sometimes the pulmonary artery is small, occasionally completely obliterated and in other cases the narrowing is at the valve where cusp fusion may form a thickened diaphragm with a reduced aperture. All these abnormalities interfere with flow of blood into the pulmonary artery and lead to varying degrees of right ventricular hypertrophy. Some of the blood from the right ventricle passes through the interventricular septal defect into the aorta. The ductus arteriosus usually remains patent after birth and the lungs receive part of

their blood supply through it. The foramen ovale also remains open and may be large.

Transposition of the great vessels results from failure of the proximal aorta and pulmonary artery to undergo the spiral rotation necessary for the establishment of their correct relationship to the ventricles. Consequently, the aorta arises from the right ventricle and the pulmonary artery from the left ventricle. In isolation this abnormality is incompatible with extrauterine life; however, persistence of the ductus arteriosus, a patent foramen ovale or a defect in the interatrial or interventricular septum may offer temporary compensation. Combinations of these defects are common. If shunting allows oxygenated blood to reach the systemic circulation, cyanosis is less marked.

In persistent truncus arteriosus the aorta and pulmonary artery arise from a common stem vessel, the truncus arising from both ventricles and overriding a ventricular septal defect. If the septum fails to develop, a single ventricular cavity results. Interatrial septal defects are also common.

Pathology of Acyanotic Congenital Heart Disease

Interatrial septal defect, the commonest congenital heart disease, usually has little effect on the circulation although the most severe cases may cause pulmonary hypertension late in life. The important defects are of three main types: persistent osteum primum, osteum secundum and persistent AV canal. In the last condition there is often fusion of the tricuspid and mitral valve to form a common atrioventricular valve. Rarely, embolizing thrombus from the venous circulation may pass from the right atrium through the interatrial defect to reach the left atrium and cause crossed or paradoxical embolism.

Interventricular septal defect may form part of another congenital anomaly such as Fallot's tetralogy where it is high in the septum. An isolated high interventricular septal defect (maladie de Roger) is not uncommon. The size and location of the defect varies. The left-to-right shunt causes pulmonary hypertension in young adults.

Aortic valve stenosis and subaortic stenosis may each occur as isolated abnormalities. So too may a bicuspid aortic valve, with an overall incidence of approximately 2%. Usually symptomless in early life, it predisposes to the development of calcific aortic stenosis and infective endocarditis.

Patent ductus arteriosus, which can coexist with many other anomalies, may be the only abnormality present, in which case closure by surgery restores the circulation to normal. Failure to close leads eventually to heart failure, and there is a risk of infective 'endocarditis' involving the ductus. If there is pulmonary hypertension, blood flow in the ductus may be reversed so that unoxygenated blood passes from the pulmonary artery into the aorta via the ductus beyond the origin of the left subclavian artery. Such a patient may thus have a cyanotic tinge in the nail beds of the toes but not in those of the hands.

Coarctation (stenosis) of the aorta (Figure 6.79) is a localized narrowing of the aorta between the left subclavian artery and the orifice of the ductus arteriosus. This abnormality is not uncommon and occurs predominantly in males and in females with XO Turner syndrome. All degrees of narrowing up to complete atresia occur. Severe narrowing causes an extensive collateral network from the carotid and subclavian arteries to link the aorta above and below the narrowed segment. Pulses in the legs are poor compared with those of the arms. Hypertension develops and death is likely to ensue from cardiac failure, cerebral haemorrhage or, less commonly, from local complications at the site of coarctation including aneurysm, dissection or infection. Surgery is curative.

Anomalies of the aortic arch are commonly associated with Fallot's tetralogy; however, as isolated anomalies they rarely cause symptoms. When a vascular ring is formed around the trachea and oesophagus by a right aortic arch and the left descending aorta together with a persistent ductus arteriosus, ligamentum arteriosum or an anomalous left subclavian artery, pressure effects mainly on the trachea may result. A double aortic arch may give similar symptoms.

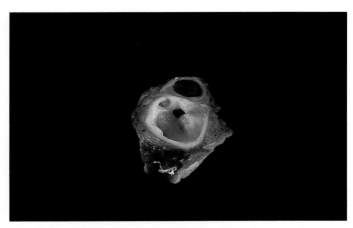

FIGURE 6.79 A surgically excised coarctation showing a tight stenosis of the aortic arch.

SUMMARY

● Ischaemia, infarction, thrombosis and embolism are the key pathogenetic mechanisms in the cardiovascular system.

● As arteries age they harden (arteriosclerosis).

● Atherosclerosis is the most important arterial disease in Western populations. It narrows arteries causing ischaemia and weakens the aorta causing aneurysms. Many factors predispose to its development.

● Hypertension (systemic arterial hypertension) damages the heart and arteries. It causes ischaemic heart disease, heart failure, stroke, renal and retinal disease. It is caused by an interplay between genetic and environmental factors.

● Disorders of the endothelium and the microcirculation result in oedema, disseminated intravascular coagulation and shock.

● Heart failure may be acute or chronic and may affect the left or right ventricle or both.

● Ischaemic heart disease is the largest cause of cardiac morbidity and mortality in the developed world. It presents with a variety of syndromes.

● Rheumatic heart disease includes acute rheumatic fever and chronic rheumatic valve disease. Other causes of chronic valve disease are becoming relatively more important in the West. Chronic valve disease predisposes to infective endocarditis.

FURTHER READING

Nkomo VT, Gardin JM, Skelton TN, *et al.* Burden of valvular heart diseases. *Lancet* 2006; **368**: 1005–1011.

Sheppard M, Davies MJ. *Practical Cardiovascular Pathology*. London: Arnold, 1998.

Tunstall-Pedoe H. *Monica Monograph and Multimedia Sourcebook. World's largest study of heart disease, stroke, risk factors and population trends 1979–2002*. Geneva: World Health Organization, 2003.

Zipes DP, Libby P, Bonow RO, Braunwald E. *Braunwald's Heart Disease. A Textbook of Cardiovascular Medicine*, 7th edn. Philadelphia: Elsevier Saunders, 2006.

Philip S Hasleton and David J Harrison

THE NORMAL RESPIRATORY TRACT

Key Points

- Upper airways conduct, warm, humidify and filter air.
- Mucociliary transport mechanism traps organisms and particulate matter.
- The lower airways are responsible for gaseous exchange.

The Nose

The nose warms, humidifies and filters air. Filtration is by the nasal hairs and conchae (turbinates), causing alteration in air flow, so particles larger than $6\,\mu m$ in diameter are trapped in nasal mucus. Sneezing, caused by nasal irritation, helps clear the nasal passages.

The inner nasal cavity sinuses, with their ostia in the lateral nasal walls are lined by ciliated, pseudostratified columnar epithelium. Goblet cells appear in the sinuses. The nasal sinuses consist of the frontal, sphenoidal, maxillary and ethmoid, which is a collection of air cells. Beneath the epithelium are seromucinous glands, which produce mucus, IgA and other immunoglobulins as defence mechanisms. These extend to the bronchial tree. The epiglottis prevents aspiration of food and other materials into the respiratory tract. In the nasopharynx there are large masses of lymphoid tissue – the adenoids, the palatine, tubal and lingual tonsils and aggregates of lymphoid tissue which circle the pharyngeal wall (Waldeyer's ring). With antigenic stimulation, especially in childhood, they enlarge and may be the site of pathological conditions, such as lymphomas.

The Larynx, Trachea and Bronchi

The larynx is divided into the supraglottis, glottis and subglottis. The larynx acts as a vibrator via the vocal cords for speech. During normal breathing the cords are held wide open to allow air passage. With speech the folds close and air causes vibration. The intrinsic laryngeal muscles are innervated by the recurrent laryngeal branch of the vagus nerve. The epiglottis is lined by stratified squamous epithelium but in the lower half it gives way to a ciliated pseudo-stratified columnar type, characteristic of most of the larynx. The true cords are lined by stratified squamous epithelium.

The larynx is supported by a cartilaginous framework, connected by ligaments. The trachea has a series of 'C'-shaped cartilages extending into the bronchi, joined by fibroelastic membranes forming a hollow tube. Posteriorly lies the trachealis muscle. The midline cervical trachea lies anterior to the oesophagus. Subglottic tracheal lesions may cause oesophageal problems and vice versa. The isthmus of the thyroid is anterior to the second to fourth rings.

The trachea divides into left and right main bronchi. The right continues in the general direction of the trachea, the left diverges at a greater angle. Thus aspiration is commoner in the right lung, especially the middle and lower lobes. Bronchial cartilage progressively decreases with increasing distance from the trachea. At the terminal bronchiole (sixteenth division) it has disappeared. The airways continue dividing into respiratory bronchioles, alveolar ducts and finally alveoli (Figure 7.1). The terminal bronchiole is the smallest airway lined by bronchial epithelial cells. The terminal bronchiolar walls consist almost entirely of smooth muscle. The small bronchioles, i.e. terminal and those just proximal, play a larger role in determining airflow than the bronchi. This is because they have much smooth muscle, which constricts easily. As they are small, they are easily occluded, as in bronchial asthma and in chronic obstructive pulmonary disease. The respiratory bronchiole bears alveoli.

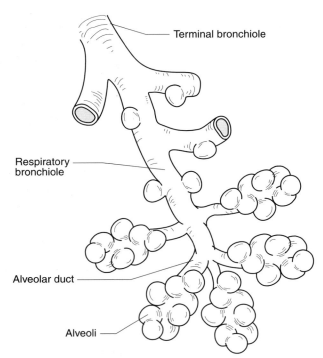

Terminal bronchiole

Respiratory bronchiole

Alveolar duct

Alveoli

FIGURE 7.1 **Model of normal respiratory acinus: each acinus is formed by branching of a terminal bronchiole into a number of respiratory bronchioles, which eventually form alveolar ducts, whose walls are lined entirely by alveoli.**

The cilia maintain the mucociliary escalator, causing upward passage of mucus and entrapped organisms or particulate matter to be expectorated. The ciliary shaft or cilium is a cytoplasmic extension from the cell surface. On transverse section the shaft shows an axial filament complex consisting of nine peripheral doublets of microtubules and two central microtubules. Radial spokes extend from central microtubules to the periphery of microtubular doublets. Each doublet has inner and outer dynein arms, essential for ciliary movement.

Just above the basement membrane are neuroendocrine cells, whose role in the adult is not known. They have clear cytoplasm and may occur as clusters, termed neuroepithelial bodies. Neuroendocrine cells contain dense core secretory granules and can secrete hormones. In the first 3 months of life, where there is relative hypoxia, they may act as chemoreceptors. These cells increase in pulmonary fibrosis and hypoxia. Neuroendocrine cell hyperplasia is also seen in association with pulmonary carcinoid tumours.

There is a surface, non-ciliated, bronchiolar secretory cell termed a Clara cell. These contain electron-dense membrane-bound inclusions and myelin bodies and produce surfactant proteins. Serous glands produce lysozyme and, if there is chronic cough, are converted to mucinous glands. The epithelium is regenerated by small pyramidal basal cells attached to the basement membrane.

The Lung

The respiratory zone of the lung begins at the respiratory bronchiole and continues into alveolar ducts and alveoli. The alveolus is cup-shaped and thin-walled. Its cells can only be identified by electron microscopy. Up to 96% of the alveolar wall is covered by type I pneumocytes. The cytoplasm is thin to facilitate gas transfer between the alveolus and the pulmonary capillary. The edges of adjacent cells are bound by tight junctions which restrict the movement of ions and water. Approximately 7% of the alveolar surface is covered by type II pneumocytes, which lie in the corners of alveolar walls. These cells form surfactant, phospholipids that lower the surface tension in the alveoli thus maintaining patency. These cells are also capable of cell division and are commonly hyperplastic following alveolar damage.

The interstitial space is the part of the septal wall which lies between the alveolar epithelial and capillary endothelial basement membrane. Normally inconspicuous, it is distended in any form of alveolar damage. It contains macrophages, myofibroblasts, mast cells and occasional collagen and elastic fibres. Any thickening of this space causes diffusion problems across the alveolar wall. The interstitial connective tissue forms a continuous sheet with that surrounding the blood vessels and bronchioles. This is important for removing fluid from alveoli to pulmonary lymphatics. Alveolar macrophages are common and may be intra-alveolar or interstitial. They are derived in the main from bone marrow precursors and are increased in cigarette smokers.

Pulmonary lymphatics are present around pulmonary blood vessels at the alveolar level and in the pleura. These drain directly into the mediastinal nodes, particularly in the upper lobes. The lymphatics can be traced to the respiratory bronchioles and continue around small bronchi and bronchioles forming a plexus outside muscle. The lungs expand and contract either by movement of the diaphragm, supplied by the phrenic nerve (C3–5), or the ribs. The diaphragm lengthens or shortens the thoracic cavity. Elevation or depression of the ribs alters the anterior/posterior diameter of the chest wall. These muscles may be affected in neuromuscular disease. The lungs lie in the pleural cavities, the parietal and visceral layers of which are lined by mesothelial cells which produce a thin film of fluid.

DISEASES OF THE UPPER RESPIRATORY TRACT

Disorders of the Nose

The Common Cold

This is a highly infectious, common disease that has economic significance. It is caused predominantly by rhinoviruses, with more than 100 antigenic types, respiratory syncytial virus (RSV), para-influenza viruses, Coxsackie A21, coronaviruses. Children may act as a reservoir in the community. Because of the large number of strains, an individual is liable to contract two to three colds a year.

Clinically there is rhinorrhoea, nasal obstruction, sneezing, pyrexia, sore throat and myalgia. Cough is due to postnasal discharge or more distal respiratory involvement by the virus. There is mucosal oedema and shedding of degenerate, columnar epithelial cells, which contain viral inclusion bodies in the first 2–3 days. Sinusitis and chest disease may complicate the common cold in susceptible patients, for example those with chronic obstructive pulmonary disease. The exudate in the sinuses becomes secondarily infected, typically by *Streptococcus pneumoniae* or *Haemophilus influenzae*. In chronic sinusitis the normal ciliated columnar epithelium is replaced by squamous epithelium, which hinders mucus clearance.

Other Upper Respiratory Tract Infections

Other upper respiratory tract infections include influenza, herpes simplex and zoster, tuberculosis, and leprosy, the last (p. 524) causing thickening of the nasal mucous membrane and perforation of the cartilage. Rhinoscleroma, caused by *Klebsiella rhinoscleromatis*, produces large deforming masses of nasal tissue. It is encountered in South America, parts of Africa, the Middle East and India.

Fungal infections, for example aspergillosis, may form fungal balls, cause sinusitis or rarely be invasive. Other fungi may affect this region, but they are more commonly seen in Asia and Africa. Rhinosporidiosis, caused by *Rhinosporidium seeberi*, is transmitted by cattle and horses and causes granulomatous nasal polyps.

Allergic Rhinitis

Allergic rhinitis can be divided into seasonal (hayfever) and perennial allergic rhinitis. Hayfever mainly affects children and adolescents, at the peak of the pollen season. The important pollen allergens come from trees, grasses and weeds, and are seen in spring, summer and early autumn, respectively. Housedust mites, furry pets, moulds or occupation (allergy to flour causing rhinitis in bakers) and rarely some foods may be allergenic. These patients have a two- to three-fold increased risk of developing perennial asthma. There is itching, watery rhinorrhoea and congestion, causing serial sneezing and 'stuffy' head. In pollen allergy, the eyes itch.

The nose suffers from allergic symptoms because of its effective filtering action for allergens. Pollen grains are 20–30 µm in size and cannot bypass the nose. There is inflammation, with CD4 T lymphocytes of the Th2 type, mast cells and eosinophils. Mast cells, stimulated by the allergen, release interleukin 3 (IL3), IL5, histamine, prostaglandins, bradykinin and platelet activating factor, which together cause many of the symptoms.

Nasal and Paranasal Polyps

These complicate allergic and perennial rhinitis. Polyps (Figure 7.2) consist of oedematous mucosa. There is respiratory epithelium with goblet cell hyperplasia and many mucous and serous glands. The basement membrane is thick and there are usually multiple eosinophils in the oedematous submucosa. There may be few eosinophils and there is chronic inflammation.

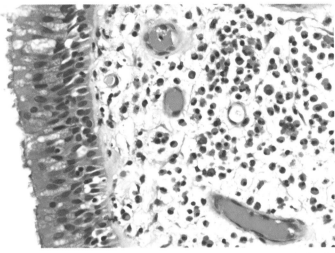

FIGURE 7.2 High-power view of a section of an allergic nasal polyp. It is lined by respiratory epithelium (left) and inflamed by masses of eosinophils and some plasma cells.

Wegener's Granulomatosis

This may be either a multisystem vasculitis or localized to one area of the respiratory tract. Over 80% of patients have nasal or paranasal involvement with 'nasal congestion'. The nasal mucosa is granular, crusted and there may be septal perforation. This disorder is discussed in more detail on p. 122.

Tumours of the Nose and Nasal Sinuses

Tumours of the nasal cavity and paranasal sinuses are rare but, because they grow into air-filled sinuses and soft tissues, they often present at an advanced stage. Sinonasal papilloma is the commonest nasal tumour, occurring most frequently in men in their sixties. The aetiology is unknown. It resembles allergic nasal polyps with a corrugated surface, although is usually unilateral. It may be exophytic or inverted, the stroma being invaginated by stratified nonkeratinizing, squamous or columnar epithelium. Mitoses are common and the greater the number the more likely the chance of recurrence. The inverted sinonasal papilloma may be accompanied or followed by carcinoma. Treatment is by total excision.

The nature of most of the remaining tumours can be deduced from knowledge of sinonasal histology. Thus there are salivary gland-like tumours, and tumours arising from bone, nerve, blood vessels or ectopic cerebral tissue. The commonest malignant nasal tumour is squamous cell carcinoma, whereas adenocarcinoma is commoner in the upper nasal cavity and sinuses especially the ethmoid, because of their presence of glands and lining respiratory epithelium. It is seen in wood and nickel workers. Carcinomas spread locally and metastasize to cervical nodes. Malignant variants of salivary gland tumours arising from minor salivary gland tissue, such as adenoid cystic carcinoma, and malignant melanoma may be seen.

Lymphomas also occur at this site. T-cell and natural killer cell tumours are commoner in Asia and South America, whereas in the West, B-cell lymphomas predominate. These are usually high grade, large cell type and cause soft tissue or osseous destruction. Epstein–Barr viral genome is seen in many of these lymphomas.

Diseases of the Larynx and Trachea

Congenital and acquired laryngeal conditions cause respiratory distress (stridor) in children. Stridor may be caused by congenital subglottic stenosis, laryngeal cysts arising from the mucous glands of the saccular appendage, laryngeal atresia and webs, viral laryngo-tracheobronchitis (croup) and acute epiglottitis often due to *Haemophilus influenzae*, type B. Diphtheria, due to *Corynebacterium diphtheriae*, may be confined to the larynx. A false membrane, composed of fibrin and neutrophils, covers the epiglottis, false and true cords, causing obstruction. Tuberculosis, sarcoidosis, leprosy and fungal infections can affect the larynx. The trachea is rarely affected by disease in adults. The commonest in children is acute laryngo-tracheobronchitis, as an extension of the laryngeal diseases mentioned above.

Laryngeal Oedema

There is no lymphatic drainage to the true vocal cord area so any oedema persists. Excess fluid in the space between the epithelium and the vocal ligaments (Reinke's space) causes vocal cord swelling (Reinke's oedema). It is commonest in smokers and there may be marked vocal cord mucosal swelling resembling a polyp.

Benign Neoplasms

Recurrent laryngeal papillomatosis is commonest in infants aged between 2 months and 5 years. It presents with hoarseness, weak cry and stridor. The disease is caused by human papilloma virus, transmitted vaginally from women with genital condylomata. The papillomas occur anywhere in the respiratory tract but the larynx, usually the true cords, is always affected. The papillomas are glistening, fleshy, irregular nodular tumours. They are covered with fronds of squamous epithelium with marked koilocytosis. Repeat chest radiographs are required to identify lung involvement. Regular follow-up is necessary. Benign connective tissue tumours, such as granular cell tumour are occasionally seen.

Malignant Tumours of the Larynx

Squamous cell carcinoma accounts for 95% of laryngeal malignancies and is classified by site as supraglottic (30%), glottic (60%) or subglottic (10%). Cigarette smoking and alcohol are the main aetiological factors; others include infection with Epstein–Barr and human papilloma viruses and coal tar products, sawdust and paints. Squamous carcinoma of the larynx is commonest on the anterior part of the true cord. It is often seen as a white plaque with a raised, well-defined margin and a variable surface ranging from furrows to ulceration. Hoarseness occurs early and supraglottic lesions can be painful. Referred pain to the ipsilateral ear, mediated by the vagus, indicates cartilaginous invasion. Stridor and dyspnoea, due to tumour bulk, occur late. Dysphagia occurs due to extension to the base of the tongue or hypopharynx. Tumour metastasizes to the cervical lymph nodes. Other rarer laryngeal tumours include adenoid cystic carcinoma, small cell carcinoma, and adenocarcinoma.

DISEASES OF THE LUNG

Pulmonary Physiology

Lung physiology is most commonly investigated by means of pulmonary function and exercise tests. In the assessment of lung function the possibility of cardiac disease, should be considered. The end result of pulmonary ventilation is adequate tissue cell oxygenation and removal of excess carbon dioxide. To achieve this the partial pressure of oxygen in the alveoli must be above that of the capillary venous blood flowing through the capillaries. It must also lower the partial pressure of carbon dioxide in the alveoli below that of the venous blood to enable excess carbon dioxide to be removed. The partial pressure of oxygen (pO_2) and carbon dioxide (pCO_2) are important measures of the adequacy of oxygenation. In arterial and mixed venous blood the pO_2 is 100 mmHg and 40 mmHg, respectively. The corresponding figures for pCO_2 are 40 mmHg (arterial) and 46 mmHg (mixed venous blood).

Lung function depends on age, size and sex, and normal values vary enormously. The forced vital capacity (total expired volume) depends on lung size, integrity of the respiratory muscles and skeleton. At the start of forced expiration, air is rapidly accelerated to a maximum flow rate at a high lung volume. As expiration progresses the speed of expulsion of air declines in a roughly linear fashion. The maximum speed is known as the peak expiratory flow rate (PEFR). This is dependent on both expiratory muscle effort and airway patency. With increasing age and airways obstruction, maximum flow rates become less dependent on effort. The more severe the airways obstruction, the less effort-dependent they become. Airway patency depends on size and the support of the surrounding elastic lung parenchyma. With expansion the lung recoils because of its elasticity. The pull of the stretched parenchyma holds airways open, especially the smaller ones. The elastic recoil also expels air from the alveoli. The PEFR is useful in assessment of severity of asthma, chronic bronchitis and emphysema.

The total amount of air expired is the forced vital capacity (FVC), which depends on lung size. Lung size is directly related to height. There is a decline in both these parameters with age. It may be affected by skeletal abnormality, weak respiratory muscles, diseases causing reduced lung volume, such as pulmonary fibrosis or large pleural effusions or most commonly severe airways obstruction as in emphysema and bronchial asthma. Forced expiratory volume in 1 second (FEV_1) is the volume of air expired during the first second of a forced maximal expiration. It is one of the most widely used lung function tests. It should be 70% or more of FVC. If the ratio of FEV_1 to FVC falls below 70% this is strong evidence of obstructive airways disease, such as asthma (reversible) or chronic obstructive pulmonary disease (irreversible). If the ratio of FEV_1 to FVC remains the same in the presence of lung disease then the inference is that both FEV and vital capacity are diminished. This happens in restrictive lung disease, such as pulmonary fibrosis, where the compliance of the lung is reduced. FEV_1 and FEV_1/FVC ratio are important markers of severity of the disease, as well as progress during treatment.

Pulmonary arterial and left atrial pressures are measured by cardiac catheterization and the blood flow through the pulmonary vessels is calculated using the Fick principle. It is also possible to determine the pulmonary vascular resistance (arterial pressure-wedge pressure). The normal pulmonary arterial pressure is 25/10 mmHg and pulmonary blood flow at rest is 4 L/min/m^2 of body surface area.

Congenital Abnormalities

Many congenital abnormalities, such as tracheal agenesis, are rare. Tracheo-oesophageal fistula, where food travels from the oesophagus into the main airways, causes choking. Lung cysts may be congenital and persist into adult life. These include bronchogenic cysts, pulmonary sequestration, congenital cystic adenomatoid malformation and congenital lobar emphysema. Acquired cysts are due to previous infection, especially staphylococcal, and also include hydatid disease, or obstruction of distal lung by a foreign body.

Pulmonary cilia dyskinesia or immotile cilia syndrome is part of Kartagener's syndrome (situs invertus, bronchiectasis, chronic rhinosinusitis and absent frontal sinuses).

Cystic Fibrosis

Key Points

- Commonest congenital lung disease, but other systems are involved.
- Inherited as autosomal recessive trait.
- The cause is a defect in the cystic fibrosis membrane conductance receptor.
- Increased viscosity of mucus leads to blockage of bronchi and ducts, with atrophy or infection.

Cystic fibrosis affects 1 in 2500 infants in the UK. It is an autosomal recessive disease, due to a defect in the gene on the long arm of chromosome 7. This gene encodes for the cystic fibrosis membrane conductance regulator (CFTR). CFTR is a cAMP-regulated, membrane protein, acting as a low conductance chloride channel across epithelium. This causes reduced chloride permeability across epithelial membranes, altering mucus composition, making it thicker and therefore able to cause obstruction. There are over 250 genetic mutations in cystic fibrosis, some giving different clinical presentations. The commonest is delta F508, which removes a phenylalanine residue at position 508 of the CFTR protein.

Cystic fibrosis is a multisystem disease, but the lung is often worst affected. It involves bowel (meconium ileus or steatorrhoea) and liver (biliary cirrhosis), causes male infertility (blockage of the seminal vesicles but the patient produces normal sperm), recurrent pancreatitis (pancreatic duct obstruction) and nasal polyps (part of chronic sinusitis). There is excessive sweat chloride, sodium and potassium, leading to the diagnostic sweat test.

Bronchial mucus is poorly hydrated and pulmonary mucociliary is transport impaired due to increased mucus viscosity and abnormal sulphated mucins. In any organ stasis causes infection. Cystic fibrosis causes recurrent pneumonia with organisms such as *Pseudomonas aeruginosa*, *Staphylococcus aureus* and *Aspergillus*. These infections weaken the bronchi and the negative intrathoracic pressure pulls them outwards, causing bronchiectasis (Figure 7.3). This is defined as permanent bronchial dilatation and bronchi crowd together and are filled with pus. There is acute or chronic bronchial inflammation and purulent bronchiolitis, progressing to obliteration. Pneumothorax is common, secondary to emphysematous blebs.

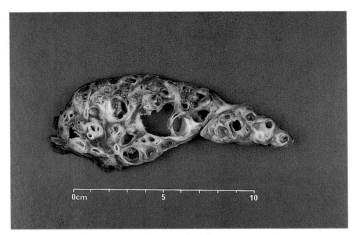

FIGURE 7.3 Bronchiectasis. A slice of left lung showing markedly dilated bronchi, scarring and loss of lung parenchyma.

α_1-Antitrypsin Deficiency

α_1-Antitrypsin (AAT) is a major serum protease inhibitor. It is a glycoprotein, produced in hepatocytes and macrophages. Deficiency results from mutations in a gene located on chromosome 14q 31–32.3. Approximately 75 alleles have been identified at the AAT locus. The phenotype (Pi type) is determined by isoelectric examination of serum. The commonest British phenotype is PiM, but low serum AAT levels are seen in PiZ and PiS. The condition is an autosomally recessive condition seen in 1/3000 Caucasians.

Hyaline Membrane Disease (Respiratory Distress Syndrome)

This disorder affects preterm babies weighing less than 1500 g who develop cyanosis, chest wall retraction and grunting respiration within an hour of birth. Chest radiographs show a ground glass appearance. Immature lungs lack surfactant, causing terminal airway collapse. The lungs are heavy at autopsy. The earliest change is necrosis of epithelium in distal bronchi and bronchioles. Hyaline membranes (composed of protein-rich exudate) block terminal bronchioles and developing alveolar ducts, as well as lining immature alveoli.

If the patient survives ventilation, bronchopulmonary dysplasia (BPD) develops. There is bronchiolar and bronchial damage with obliterative bronchiolitis. Hyaline membranes continue to form and involve peripheral alveoli. Interstitial fibrosis develops and alveoli are lined by prominent type II cells. The lung is firm and nodular with focal emphysema. The vessels are thick walled with intimal fibrosis.

The underlying cause of BPD is epithelial/endothelial barrier damage. There is continued interstitial fluid and protein leakage, causing hyaline membranes and stimulating fibrosis. High ventilatory oxygen concentrations probably play an important part. The preterm infant is susceptible to relatively normal inspired oxygen concentrations.

Bronchial Asthma

> **Key Points**
>
> - Asthma presents with bronchospasm, which can be life-threatening. Immune mechanisms are important.
> - Asthma is associated with many environmental factors, including pollens, animal fur, chemicals and diet.
> - Asthma is increasing in prevalence.
> - The important cells in asthma are mast cells, eosinophils and lymphocytes.
> - Histamine, leukotrienes and other cytokines cause smooth muscle contraction, vasopermeability and oedema of the bronchiolar wall.

Asthma is the main reversible cause of airflow limitation. Patients have wheezing, chest tightness, shortness of breath, often worse at night, and cough. Cough may be prominent, causing a misdiagnosis of chronic bronchitis. There is a decrease in FEV_1 and PEFR, the latter showing variability.

Asthma occurs in 12–15% of children, and the incidence increased by 50% between the mid-1970s and mid-1980s in industrialized countries. The prevalences of eczema and hayfever similarly rose, suggesting an increase in allergy.

Aetiology

Atopy is an established risk factor. One gene governing bronchial hyperresponsiveness and regulating serum IgE levels is located near a major locus on chromosome 5q. The cytokine genes which regulate IgE, mast cell, basophil and eosinophil functions, cells common in asthma, i.e. IL3, 4, 5, 9, 13 and granulocyte macrophage-colony stimulating factor (GM-CSF), are on chromosome 5. No single gene accounts for the major part of the expression of the disease. This phenotypic variability is probably in keeping with the aetiological heterogeneity and environmental influences. Exposure to allergen in the first 2–3 years appears important, providing the stimulus for airways sensitization.

Environmental determinants include sensitizing chemicals, air pollution by allergens (e.g. soya bean) or indoor allergens (e.g. tobacco smoke, viral infections and house dust mite). Over 200 materials can cause occupational asthma. Diet may be important, either directly or perhaps as a surrogate for other markers. High salt diets and those containing much 'junk' food are linked with an increased prevalence of asthma while those high in oily fish appear protective. Breastfeeding protects babies against the disease. Infections such as measles are protective, especially if occurring in the first year. The keeping of pets may be important, since animal dander is an aero-allergen.

Asthma is exacerbated by atmospheric pollution, high concentrations of sulphur dioxide, nitrogen dioxide, ozone, cigarette smoke and dust, cold air and exercise. Similarly drugs, such as aspirin or other non-steroidals, may provoke attacks.

Pathology and Pathophysiology

In death from status asthmaticus, the lungs are hyperexpanded, due to mucus plugging. Bronchial and bronchiolar walls are infiltrated by eosinophils, neutrophils, plasma cells and lymphocytes. These inflammatory cells cause hyperaemia, mucosal and submucosal oedema. Eosinophils are not seen in normal mucosa. The surface epithelium is focally sloughed in areas. In the surviving epithelium there is goblet cell hyperplasia, especially in the peripheral airways. The basement membrane may be thickened by deposition of collagen. There is prominent bronchiolar smooth muscle, causing contraction and luminal narrowing (Figure 7.4). Biopsies from non-fatal cases show a similar cellular infiltrate, with or without basement membrane thickening.

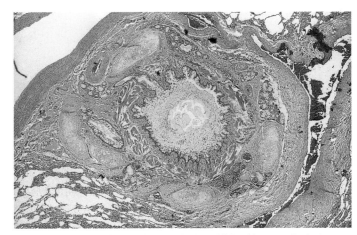

FIGURE 7.4 Asthma. Microscopic view of a bronchiole with mucus in the lumen, submucosal oedema and inflammation, and prominent smooth muscle.

Charcot–Leyden crystals, derived from eosinophils, may be seen in bronchial lumina whereas if epithelium is shed, it forms casts called Curschmann spirals.

The physiological and clinical features in asthma are the result of interaction between the resident and infiltrating inflammatory cells and the airway epithelium. This results in a release of chemical mediators from the cells. The lymphocytes are of Th2 progeny and secrete cytokines including IL4, IL5, IL6, tumour necrosis factor (TNF)α, platelet-derived growth factor (PDGF) and GM-CSF. Interleukin 4 and IL6 are needed for the recruitment of mucosal mast cells and IL5 and GM-CSF for maturation and priming of the eosinophils. Mast cell activation releases histamine causing bronchoconstriction, leukotrienes and prostaglandins. In addition these cells increase microvascular permeability and initiate neutrophil and eosinophil recruitment. Mast cells cause smooth muscle contraction, vasopermeability and oedema. Their sulphapeptide leukotrienes initiate fluid and mucus secretion. Mast cells synthesize cytokines, including IL3, IL4, IL5, IL6 and TNFα.

Eosinophils are attracted to endothelial cells, initially attaching to intercellular adhesion molecule-1 (ICAM-1) and vascular cell adhesion molecule-1 (VCAM-1), then migrating out of the vessel. They release toxic granule proteins, such as eosinophil cationic protein (ECP) and neutrophil basic protein (NBP), oxygen free radicals, leukotrienes, platelet activating factor (PAF), cytokines and growth factors. Toxic granule proteins cause shedding of bronchial epithelium. Airway epithelial cells, fibroblasts and endothelial cells produce cytokines, including IL6, IL8, GM-CSF, TNFα, PDGF and IG-1. This production is in response to cytokines released within the airways.

Complications

Pneumothorax is caused by overdistended lungs and popping of pleural blebs. Mucoimpaction may show contamination with *Aspergillus* (Figure 7.5). This fungus may itself provoke asthma. Bronchiectasis due to persistent mucus plugging is an occasional complication.

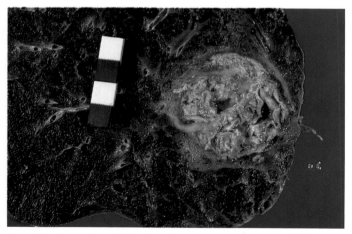

FIGURE 7.5 Aspergilloma. This slice of lung shows a large pale ball of fungus (*Aspergillus*) mixed with mucus in a markedly dilated bronchus (see p. 179).

THE EFFECTS OF CIGARETTE SMOKING ON THE BODY AND CHRONIC OBSTRUCTIVE PULMONARY DISEASE

Key Points

- Cigarette smoke contains carcinogens and addictive agents, among many injurious factors.
- Smoking causes many diseases, including chronic obstructive pulmonary disease, coronary atheroma and many cancers.
- Passive smoking results in fetal damage, increased childhood infections and disease in adults.
- Chronic obstructive pulmonary disease consists of chronic bronchitis, small airways disease and pulmonary emphysema.
- COPD produces fixed airway obstruction, with decreased FEV_1 and PEFR.

Constituents of Cigarette Smoke

Cigarette smoke yields more than 4000 constituents. These include carbon monoxide, hydrogen cyanide, aldehydes, cadmium (linked to emphysema), ammonia, nicotine and benz(a)anthracene and benzopyrene (both potent carcinogens). These are suspended in water droplets with resinous cores, which are absorbed onto bronchial walls and propelled on the mucociliary escalator, back to the mouth; 98% of these particles are removed by cilia within 24 hours. Smaller particles enter alveoli and if undissolved, are ingested by macrophages and removed to lymphatics.

Nicotine is elaborated by the tobacco root and makes cigarettes addictive. The lungs absorb 85% and it causes increases in heart rate, blood pressure and cardiac output. Passive smoking increases the risk of lung cancer and ischaemic heart disease and is linked to an increased incidence of asthma and chest infections in children. The diseases caused or associated with cigarette smoking are given in Table 7.1.

Chronic Obstructive Pulmonary Disease

Key Points

- Chronic obstructive pulmonary disease consists of chronic bronchitis, small airways disease and pulmonary emphysema.
- It produces irreversible airway obstruction.
- In chronic bronchitis the submucosal glands are hyperplastic, causing mucus hypersecretion.
- The basis of hypoxic pulmonary hypertension is the muscularization of pulmonary arteries.
- Death is from bronchopneumonia, respiratory or cardiac failure or other cigarette-induced disease, such as myocardial infarction or lung cancer.

TABLE 7.1 Diseases associated with cigarette smoke (the effects of cigarette smoke are many and varied, with few organs unaffected)

Target	Disease	Examples	Effects
Arteries	Atherosclerosis	Coronary artery occlusion	Myocardial ischaemia, infarction
		Carotid arteries	Risk of cerebrovascular accident
		Aorta and other arteries	Hypertension, peripheral ischaemia
Lung	Chronic obstructive pulmonary disease	Chronic bronchitis and emphysema	Breathlessness, irreversible airway obstruction, cyanosis
	Carcinoma	Squamous and other carcinomas	Local airway obstruction, haemoptysis, systemic spread, cachexia
	Asthma		
	Lung infections		
Bladder	Transitional cell carcinoma		Haematuria
Pancreas	Adenocarcinoma		Biliary obstruction
Cervix uteri	Squamous carcinoma	Cofactor synergizing with human papillomavirus infection	Bleeding per vagina
Colon	Adenoma and adenocarcinoma	Cofactor with other factors such as diet, inherited genetic susceptibility	Per rectum bleeding, faecal occult blood

Chronic obstructive pulmonary disease (COPD) encompasses three pathologic entities, which are considered separately pathologically, but often coexist: chronic bronchitis, pulmonary emphysema and small airways disease.

Epidemiology

In the UK, 6% of male and 3% of female deaths are caused by COPD. The reason for the male predominance is unknown. The most important aetiologic factor in COPD is tobacco smoking; others include occupation, especially dust-associated such as coal mining, and AAT deficiency. The wide variation in susceptibility of smokers to the development of COPD is at least partly genetic.

Clinical Features

Chronic bronchitis was defined functionally by the Medical Research Council as 'chronic or recurrent increase in the volume of bronchial secretions, sufficient to cause expectoration on most days for a minimum of three months of the year, for not less than two successive years, which cannot be attributed to other cardiac or pulmonary disease.' The presence of chronic bronchitis (very common in smokers) is not a good marker of functional impairment. The symptoms have insidious onset, with a morning smoker's cough and gradually worsening exertional dyspnoea, especially in damp weather. There are increasing numbers of chest infections with *H. influenzae* and *S. pneumoniae*. The chest radiograph shows hyperinflation with an enlarged heart and prominent hila if there is cor pulmonale, due to the prominent pulmonary arteries. There are upper, and sometimes lower, lobe emphysematous bullae. There is fixed airways obstruction with a decrease in FEV_1 and PEFR. These measure airflow limitation and reflect loss of elastic recoil and/or narrowing of the airways. Goblet cells in smokers extend to the terminal bronchioles. In chronic bronchitis there is an increased mass of serous and mucous glands (Figure 7.6). Most mucus is produced by the submucosal glands, but hypersecretion does not probably contribute to the pathologic basis of the fixed airway obstruction in COPD (see p. 168).

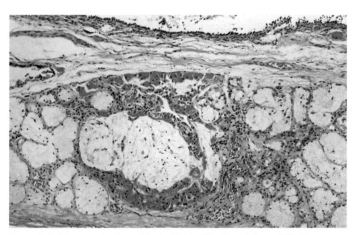

FIGURE 7.6 Microscopic view of bronchial wall in chronic bronchitis. There are prominent mucous glands in the submucosa.

Pulmonary Emphysema

This is defined as a condition of the lung characterized by a permanent increase beyond normal size of the air spaces distal to the terminal bronchiole, either from dilatation or destruction of their walls. A simpler definition is permanent dilatation, distal to the terminal bronchiole. It excludes pulmonary overinflation, as in bronchial asthma or post-pneumonectomy. Emphysema can be categorized as:

● centriacinar (centrilobular)
● panacinar (panlobular)

- bullous
- paraseptal
- scar.

The classification depends on an understanding of the functional unit of the lung (the respiratory acinus) (see Figure 7.1). Thus centriacinar emphysema is characterized by an increase in size of the respiratory bronchioles, which are dilated and often have black pigment (carbon) in their walls (Figure 7.7). The adjacent alveoli may also show dilatation. Panacinar emphysema (Figure 7.8) usually shows an upper lobe distribution and is characterized by persistent enlargement and fusion of air spaces involving the entire acinus. If there is lower lobe panacinar emphysema, one should consider if the patient has AAT deficiency.

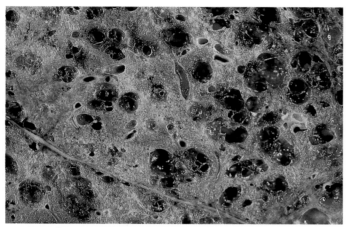

FIGURE 7.7 Centriacinar emphysema. This slice of lung shows expanded air spaces around respiratory bronchioles.

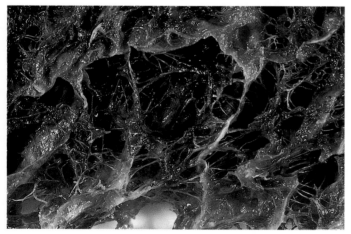

FIGURE 7.8 Panacinar emphysema. This slice of upper lobe shows more diffuse enlargement of air spaces than seen in Figure 7.7.

Bullous emphysema occurs usually either at anterior margins or the apices of the upper lobes and shows air spaces with few strands of alveolar tissue. A bulla is defined as an emphysematous space with a diameter of more than 1 cm. Bullae and blebs, which are less than 2 mm in diameter, may

rupture causing a pneumothorax and lung collapse. This may precipitate respiratory failure. Blebs are commoner in young, tall men with some 'Marfanoid' features, suggesting in this group there is an underlying collagen disease. At post mortem emphysematous lungs are overexpanded and fill the chest. Computed tomography provides the diagnosis in life. Surgeons excise apical bullous emphysema to remove useless tissue and allow the more preserved lower lobes to provide better respiratory function. Centriacinar, panacinar and bullous emphysema often coexist and cause diagnostic problems as to the predominant type of emphysema. Paraseptal and scar emphysema may be associated with other primary diseases, for example tuberculosis (scar emphysema), and are localized and seldom cause a clinical problem.

Emphysema is basically an 'apparent' dilatation of airspaces but is, in fact, due to destruction of alveolar walls (see Special Study Topic 7.1). The destruction has two major effects:

- Loss of pulmonary surface area for gas exchange (leading to hypoxia).
- Loss of elastic support for small airways. This is the means by which airways collapse and narrowing occurs (and thus destruction).

The patient becomes a respiratory cripple and may develop cor pulmonale. This is a consequence of hypoxia and is defined by the World Health Organization as 'hypertrophy of the right ventricle resulting from diseases affecting the function and/or structure of the lungs, except when the pulmonary alterations are the result of diseases that primarily affect the left side of the heart, as in congenital disease'. The most accurate way of determining right ventricular hypertrophy at autopsy is to weigh the free wall of the right ventricle. The upper limit of normal is 65 g. Right ventricular hypertrophy is associated with both panacinar and centriacinar emphysema but a smaller percentage of lung tissue needs to be involved by centriacinar than panacinar emphysema to produce right ventricular hypertrophy. Usually the type, rather than the severity of emphysema, is associated with the development of right ventricular failure. In centriacinar emphysema the percentage of lung tissue functionally destroyed is greater than in the panacinar variety. In centriacinar emphysema, the functional air space around the abnormal respiratory bronchiole is hypoxic. This gives a larger total area of hypoxic tissue than if an entire upper lobe is destroyed by panacinar emphysema.

Causation of Right Ventricular Hypertrophy in Emphysema

In the normal adult there is no muscle in pulmonary arteries less than 100 μm in diameter. In chronic hypoxia there is growth of muscle from more proximal arteries into arterioles, which are then termed 'muscularized'. Intimal longitudinal muscle grows in muscular pulmonary arteries and pulmonary arterioles and in time is replaced by intimal fibrosis. The increase in pulmonary vascular resistance causes pulmonary arterial hypertension.

Small Airways Disease

This refers to abnormality of terminal and small bronchioles. There may be an asthmatic component to COPD with smooth muscle contraction, subepithelial fibrosis and chronic inflammation, causing luminal narrowing and airflow obstruction. The lumen may be further occluded by mucus and necrotic cells. Goblet cell and sometimes squamous cell metaplasia impede the mucociliary escalator flow.

Cause of Death in COPD

Death in COPD is from bronchopneumonia, congestive cardiac failure or respiratory failure.

7.1 SPECIAL STUDY TOPIC

EMPHYSEMA IN CHRONIC OBSTRUCTIVE PULMONARY DISEASE

Emphysema, together with chronic bronchitis and small airways disease, make up the clinical entity chronic obstructive pulmonary disease (COPD), which tends to be progressive, is irreversible, and is characterized by obstruction to air flow resulting in hypoxia, breathlessness and eventually respiratory failure. Often overshadowed by lung cancer in public awareness, it is a major health problem and affects about 8/1000 worldwide, being among the top 10 causes of mortality and causing even more morbidity. Cigarette smoking is strongly implicated; thus COPD is a growing problem in developing countries where smoking is actively promoted and the market is increasing each year. Emphysema, defined as a loss of lung parenchyma without significant scarring, is perhaps the more significant component of COPD with serious clinical sequelae.

Aetiology and Pathogenesis of Emphysema

The most important known cause of emphysema is cigarette smoking. However, not every smoker develops emphysema and not all patients with emphysema have smoked. The aetiology is therefore more complex; other modifying factors must be important. A clue comes from patients with genetically determined deficiency of AAT, who may develop both emphysema and cirrhosis of the liver. As AAT deficiency causes an imbalance of proteases favouring tissue destruction, the theory is that these patients are more susceptible to the effects of proteases released from inflammatory cells in the lung causing tissue destruction. While this seems likely to be true for this particular disease it has been less than convincingly demonstrated that this is generally applicable. For instance, the emphysema in cases of AAT deficiency tends to affect the whole acinus (panacinar), in keeping with a circulating overall reduction in antiprotease protection. By contrast, most cases of cigarette-smoking-associated emphysema have predominantly focal damage at the entrance to the acinus (centriacinar) in keeping with local damage perhaps as a result of deposition of reactive particulate components of smoke. So we can conclude that emphysema is heterogeneous, both in aetiology and pattern, but there are several common principles which can be elucidated and are currently being investigated further. There is now a developing literature on genetic susceptibility in this area.

Genetic Susceptibility

In about 2% of cases of COPD AAT deficiency may be important. AAT opposes the effects of neutrophil proteases. The normal M allele is the most common (>95%). The S allele (3%) is associated with mildly reduced plasma levels of AAT. However, the Z allele (1%) is associated with low levels: homozygosity for Z (protease inhibitor phenotype PiZZ) has less than 10% normal levels of AAT in plasma. Not all PiZZ individuals develop emphysema and smoking certainly increases the likelihood, in keeping with the thesis that susceptibility to emphysema is multifactorial. This gave rise to the protease/antiprotease theory and led to a number of abortive attempts at treatment based on faith rather than evidence. Similarly, but less strikingly, other enzymes involved in metabolism of oxidant components of smoke have been shown to be polymorphic. The polymorphisms may affect the inducibility of the gene, the amount of product protein produced or its activity. A large number of studies have provided inconclusive evidence on the roles of glutathione-S-transferases, microsomal epoxide hydrolases and a host of other enzymes. Thus, although there is some support for an oxidant/antioxidant balance, the attempts to exploit this therapeutically have also failed to impress. This does not mean that genetic susceptibility is irrelevant, rather it emphasizes the complex and multifactorial nature of the disease.

Inflammation

In COPD there is chronic inflammation in small airways, comprising neutrophils, resident and incoming macrophages and CD8+ T lymphocytes. This recurrent, low level damage causes tissue remodelling and ultimately disruption of alveolar wall to airway attachments that are crucial for maintaining airway patency. Loss of these attachments leads to collapse of airways on expiration, which obstructs airflow.

Remodelling of Extracellular Matrix

In a number of human and animal settings emphysema is associated with activation of tissue metalloproteinases (MMPs). MMP1 degrades perlecan and collagens and can inactivate AAT. MMP9 and 12 expression is altered in emphysema. These MMPs can also liberate and activate latent transforming growth factor β and other cytokines. Of late it has been appreciated in areas as diverse as bone repair and cardiology that remodelling is influenced by mechanical force. It comes as no surprise that the lung is particularly influenced by mechanical forces and that the interpretation of any *in vitro* studies must be tempered by this awareness.

Lessons from Transgenic Studies

The use of transgenic mice alongside other animal models has led to a plethora of possible candidates for the tissue damage seen in emphysema. Surfactants, integrins, extracellular matrix, MMPs and cytokines have all

been implicated. The take home message is that the aetiology and pathogenesis of emphysema is complex! There is no single cause but rather a matrix of susceptibility factors, both genetic and environmental that conspire in some cases to cause disease.

Conclusion

Emphysema as part of COPD excites less enthusiasm and concern than perhaps it should. This is in part because it is difficult to study. Several very strongly held, and opposing, views on its cause have been tried, tested and found wanting. Each has contributed to our understanding of the disease but highlighted how heterogeneous and complex it is. But from the extensive information now emerging new ideas for treatment are being suggested.

Further Reading

Al-Jamal R, Wallace WAH, Harrison DJ. Gene therapy for chronic obstructive pulmonary disease: twilight or triumph? *Expert Opin Biol Ther* 2005; **5**: 333–346.

ACUTE AND CHRONIC INTERSTITIAL LUNG FIBROSIS

This group includes a number of fibrosing conditions of lung of varying aetiology all characterized functionally by a restrictive physiological abnormality. The term interstitial is used but in practice there is evidence of both intra-alveolar and interstitial fibrosis at some stage of the disease. In bronchiolitis obliterans-organizing pneumonia (BOOP), the process is predominantly in alveolar and bronchiolar lumina. Sarcoidosis is included in this group of conditions.

Adult Respiratory Distress Syndrome

Adult respiratory distress syndrome (ARDS) is an extreme form of acute lung injury associated with a variety of pulmonary and extrapulmonary insults (Table 7.2).

TABLE 7.2 Clinical scenarios associated with acute respiratory distress syndrome

Respiratory	Non-respiratory
Infection (viral, bacterial)	Sepsis
Aspiration	Trauma (with hypotension)
Toxin inhalation	Burns
Oxygen therapy	Pancreatitis
	Ingested toxins (e.g. Paraquat)

Key Points

- Adult respiratory distress syndrome presents with severe dyspnoea, hypoxaemia and diffuse pulmonary infiltrates.
- It is mediated by polymorphs and complicated by fibrosis.
- Pathology shows hyaline membranes, and fibrin thrombi, progressing to intra-alveolar and interstitial fibrosis.
- Adult respiratory distress syndrome is characterized by uncontrolled activation of inflammatory mediators especially TNF, IL1, IL6 and IL8.

Adult respiratory distress syndrome has multiple causes but the basic pathology is identical, irrespective of aetiology. In up to 40% of cases no predisposing cause is found. It represents early interstitial lung disease. The term has many synonyms, the best being diffuse alveolar damage (DAD). It may occur as part of multiorgan failure. Early in the disease there is disseminated intravascular coagulation in the lung. This may also affect the central nervous system, heart, gastrointestinal tract and kidneys.

Clinically the patient develops severe dyspnoea, marked hypoxaemia with cyanosis and tachypnoea, and is refractory to oxygen. There is decreased lung compliance with diffuse bilateral pulmonary infiltrates. There is a latent period varying from several hours to days following the insult, during which the clinical features are those of the underlying illness.

The early changes have been little studied in humans, for obvious reasons. These vary depending on which side of the basement membrane the insult occurs. The initial changes probably affect type I pneumocytes, which separate from the basement membrane. There is also type II pneumocyte damage, affecting surfactant production, and focal endothelial damage. There is interstitial oedema and fibroblast ingrowth to repair the gap left by the damaged type I cells. With loss of type I cells, fibrin leaks through epithelial cell junctions. The mixture of fibrin, dead cells, and plasma proteins makes up hyaline membranes (Figure 7.9). This is the characteristic pathology of ARDS of any cause. The pathogenesis of ARDS is summarized diagrammatically in Figure 7.10.

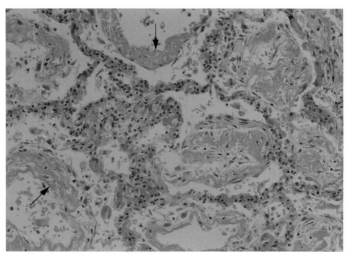

FIGURE 7.9 Lung section from autopsy on a patient who developed adult respiratory distress syndrome following peritonitis. Neutrophil polymorphs are packed in the alveolar capillaries and fibrin is present in alveoli, in places forming hyaline membranes (arrows).

This condition is associated with a high mortality. At post mortem the lungs are blue, heavy, haemorrhagic and oedematous, each weighing over 1000 g (normal weight 3–400 g each). After 10–14 days they become solid, fleshy and reddish/grey, due to early fibrosis. Early alveolar wall congestion progresses to give rise to fibrin thrombi in arteries and capillaries (disseminated intravascular coagulation) and an increase in megakaryocytes in the pulmonary capillaries releasing platelets. As early as 48 hours, loose myxoid interstitial and sometimes intra-alveolar fibrosis begins.

Complications

The major complications in survivors are as follows. Pulmonary fibrosis is the most common residual problem, as myofibroblasts, which are active in lung remodelling, migrate from the interstitium through gaps in the epithelial basement membrane. The damage may progress to diffuse

fibrosis and cystic change, but fibrosis is not inevitable and the lung may sometimes recover. Pulmonary hypertension, due to hypoxia, and pneumonia are also significant complicating diseases.

Fibrosing Alveolitis (Interstitial Pulmonary Fibrosis, Cryptogenic Pulmonary Fibrosis)

Key Points

- Fibrosing alveolitis is a lung fibrosis of unknown cause.
- Typically there is restrictive defect in lung function.
- It may result in respiratory failure or cor pulmonale.

There are many causes of pulmonary fibrosis. These include sarcoidosis, Langerhans' cell histiocytosis and collagen diseases, such as rheumatoid disease, systemic lupus erythematosus and systemic sclerosis and asbestosis. Drugs, such as methotrexate used for cancer or amiodarone for treating cardiac disease, are also implicated and there is an increased incidence among metal or wood dust workers. In many cases, however, no cause is found, as seen in the term 'cryptogenic' pulmonary fibrosis. Fibrosing alveolitis is classified into:

- Acute interstitial pneumonia.
- Usual interstitial pneumonia (cryptogenic fibrosing alveolitis, CFA). The term CFA is a clinical one and is not used by pathologists.
- Desquamative interstitial pneumonia (DIP)//respiratory bronchiolitis.
- Non-specific interstitial pneumonia (NSIP).
- Chronic interstitial pneumonia.
- Giant cell interstitial pneumonia.

Acute interstitial pneumonia may not be a discrete entity. The picture is that of organizing ARDS with no predisposing cause. SARS gives a similar histological picture but in cases before the Asian and Canadian outbreaks, no causative virus was found. There is a prodromal upper respiratory tract viral illness, followed by increasing dyspnoea and non-productive cough.

Usual interstitial pneumonia is commonest in male smokers in the fifth decade. It has an insidious onset of exertional dyspnoea because of the large pulmonary functional reserve and possible relative inactivity in this age group. Clinically there is a dry, non-productive cough and lower lobe end-inspiratory crackles (Velcro crackles). With progression there is finger clubbing and central cyanosis and death usually results within 5 years of diagnosis from infection, respiratory failure or cor pulmonale. In addition, there is an increased incidence of lung cancer. Lung function tests are typically restrictive but may show a mixed restrictive and obstructive picture, due to associated emphysema. Computed tomography reveals a lower lobe with fine, ground-glass appearance, progressing to honeycombing (Figure 7.11). On early CT scans the disease is typically subpleural but at post mortem involves all lobes.

Airway insults
e.g. infection, aspiration, smoke, hyperoxia

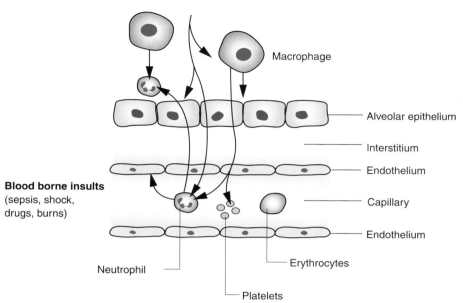

FIGURE 7.10 Pathogenesis of adult respiratory distress syndrome. Initial injury is to the capillary endothelium or the alveolar epithelium. The endothelial damage is often initiated by endotoxin and is sustained by interactions between neutrophils, macrophages, cytokines, oxygen radicals, complement and arachidonate metabolites. Fluid and proteins leak from the capillary into the interstitium and alveoli.

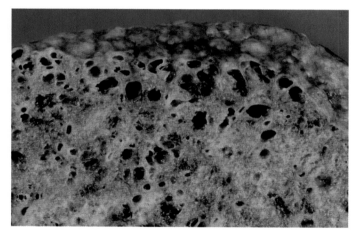

FIGURE 7.11 Honeycomb lung. This can be the end result of a number of fibrosing lung diseases, including cryptogenic fibrosing alveolitis.

The acute phase of cryptogenic fibrosing alveolitis may resemble the exudative phase of ARDS but is rarely seen. In some cases, even at post mortem, there may be hyaline membranes indicating active disease. The fibrosis is unevenly distributed in the affected lobe(s), unlike non-specific interstitial pneumonia. In the proliferative phase there is intra-alveolar but predominantly interstitial fibrosis, centred round alveoli, ducts and respiratory bronchioles. A key feature in active disease is the presence of fibroblastic foci. These are areas of myxoid fibrosis, which are becoming incorporated into the alveolar wall. There is cuboidalization of the epithelium, and squamous metaplasia, mucinous or ciliated metaplasia.

Smooth muscle proliferation is due to myofibroblast proliferation and differentiation. There is variable interstitial inflammation with lymphocytes, plasma cells, macrophages and some neutrophils. Cases with no fibroblastic foci and a well-defined chronic inflammatory reaction have the best prognosis. In the late stages there is honeycomb lung with cystic change and metaplasia of the lining epithelium. The arteries show medial hypertrophy and pulmonary arterioles are muscularized and the lumina of arteries and veins are obliterated by intimal fibrosis as a reaction to the surrounding fibrosis and pulmonary hypertension.

Desquamative Interstitial Pneumonia (DIP)

The alveoli are filled with macrophages, with little fibrosis and it is steroid-reversible. It is rare and presents with dyspnoea. It is part of a spectrum of disease with respiratory bronchiolitis. Both are related to cigarette smoking. A DIP-picture is caused by asbestos and other inorganic particles. Patients with DIP/respiratory bronchiolitis present with cough, dyspnoea, bi-basal end-inspiratory crepitations, interstitial radiological infiltrates and a restrictive or mixed restrictive/obstructive pattern. There is prominent proliferation of brown pigmented macrophages in respiratory bronchioles and alveoli. The pigment is due to the products of cigarette smoke.

Non-specific Interstitial Pneumonia (NSIP)

In this disorder fibrosis is less severe and more even than in usual interstitial pneumonia. The importance of recognizing this pattern on biopsy is that it has a much better prognosis.

Sarcoidosis

Sarcoidosis is a multisystem granulomatous disorder, affecting people in the 20–40-year age group. The aetiology is unknown. In Europe the incidence ranges from 3 to 500 cases per 100 000 population. There are geographic and racial differences in that it is commoner in the African American population.

A quarter of patients have dry cough, dyspnoea and exercise intolerance and another quarter present with eye, skin or nasal complaints. A third have fever, fatigue, malaise and weight loss. Only in 15% of patients is the disease progressive and 40% have few symptoms. Hilar lymphadenopathy is common. There is decreased diffusion capacity due to interstitial fibrosis. Depending on the degree of lung damage, there may be loss of lung volume. The inflammatory process extends through the lymphatics to hilar and mediastinal lymph nodes and terminates with diffuse pulmonary fibrosis and cavity formation. (See also Case History 4.1, p. 62).

Pathogenesis

Bronchoalveolar lavage shows increased T lymphocytes. The helper:suppressor T cell ratio in active sarcoid is 4–10 times greater than normal while in inactive lesions suppressor T cells predominate. The elevated helper:suppressor T cell ratio suggests an immunoregulatory imbalance but BAL cell profiles cannot predict prognosis or steroid response. The granulomas produce angiotensin-converting enzyme (ACE), with elevated serum levels. This may be a marker of body granuloma burden and is sensitive in predicting relapse or remission.

T lymphocytes from active sarcoid release monocyte chemotactic and inhibition factors. The factor switching on the T cells is unknown. Though the disease resembles tuberculosis, *Mycobacteria* do not seem to be the cause. Inhaled antigens, such as pine pollen, talc and peanut dust have been incriminated. Genetic factors may be involved, as there are familial clusters.

Pathology

The earliest events are a lymphocytic alveolitis with granulomas (Figure 7.12). These follow the lymphatics to the lymph nodes. The lymph nodes and lung are involved in 80% of cases. Other organs involved in decreasing order of frequency are liver, spleen, heart, skin, central nervous system, kidney, eyes and parotid glands, thyroid, intestine, stomach and pituitary. The granulomas and lymphocytic alveolitis may progress to pulmonary fibrosis and honeycombing, more marked in the upper lobes. There may be bronchiectasis and cavity formation, sometimes with *Aspergillus*. Histology is characterized by non-caseating granulomas, which are interstitial and follow the lymphatics. Non-specific intracellular inclusions, such as asteroid bodies, are seen. Sarcoid may affect the pleura and vessels. The Kveim test, an intradermal injection of sarcoid tissue, is now rarely used not least because of the risk of transmission of other infections.

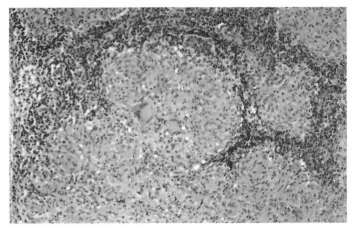

FIGURE 7.12 Sarcoidosis. Microscopic view of non-caseating granulomatous inflammation, including giant cells.

Bronchiolitis

The term bronchiolitis describes various inflammatory diseases of the distal bronchioles. Patients have dyspnoea, cough, variable amounts of sputum, rales or rhonchi. The chest radiograph shows hyperinflation with interstitial or alveolar infiltrates. The main causes are:

- inhalation injury,
- infection, e.g. RSV, *Mycoplasma pneumoniae*
- drug or chemical-induced reactions
- connective tissue diseases
- organ transplantation
- idiopathic.

Bronchiolitis may occur as part of other diseases, for example asthma and COPD. Acute bronchiolitis is common in children after viral infections, with acute inflammation filling the bronchiolar lumina and extending, with fibrosis, into the adjacent peribronchiolar tissue. Bronchiolitis is classified histologically into:

- acute bronchiolitis
- small airways disease (constrictive bronchiolitis)
- respiratory bronchiolitis
- mineral dust airways disease
- follicular bronchiolitis
- constrictive bronchiolitis (obliterative bronchiolitis)
- cryptogenic organizing pneumonia (COP or BOOP).

These histological pictures have varying aetiologies. Constrictive bronchiolitis occurs most commonly with rheumatoid disease. There may be bronchiolar inflammation, peribronchiolar fibrosis and obliterative fibrosis of the bronchiolar lumen. In the early stages there is intraluminal, mucosal, submucosal and peribronchiolar inflammation in membranous and respiratory bronchioles. The inflammatory infiltrate has variable numbers of polymorphs, lymphocytes and plasma cells.

OCCUPATIONAL LUNG DISEASE

Key Points

- Occupational lung disease must be considered in any patient with respiratory problems.
- Occupational lung disease follows exposure to fumes, inorganic or organic dusts.
- Coal dust pneumoconiosis, silicosis and asbestosis are decreasing in the West due to legal controls. There is widespread use of asbestos in India and the Far East.
- Organic dusts, such as fungi, can cause asthma in the workplace.

Occupational lung disease occurs in diverse forms and is due to fumes, vapours, gases dusts, or immunologic processes.

Coal Worker's Pneumoconiosis

Coals, rich in carbon, are complex minerals and their composition varies from mine to mine. Inorganic material may be present in coals, including muscovite and kaolin, as well as trace elements such as arsenic, titanium and beryllium. Miners constructing communicating shafts may work on hard siliceous rocks and develop silicosis rather than coal worker's pneumoconiosis (CWP). The incidence and progression of CWP relates to the cumulative exposure of dust inspired, as well as the coal rank, i.e. the amount of volatile matter within the coal. The higher-ranked coals, containing the least amount of volatile matter, have a higher incidence and severity of CWP. The assessment of pneumoconiosis is on the prevalence and size of the radiological opacities in a system devised by the International Labour Organization. The condition is divided into several forms.

Simple CWP is a radiological or pathological diagnosis with no associated symptoms or signs. The earliest change is the collection of dust-laden macrophages around respiratory bronchioles and adjacent alveoli. In time, multiple bilateral, stellate black (macular) lesions not exceeding 1 cm are found especially in the upper two-thirds of the lungs, with associated focal (centrilobular) emphysema. Macules are small foci of fibrosis. The peripheral lymph nodes contain whorled, pigmented nodules. Complicated CWP gives no symptoms or signs at an early stage but when extensive and associated with bullous emphysema, the affected person has breathlessness, cough and exertional dyspnoea. This progresses to cor pulmonale. The lesions of progressive massive fibrosis are larger than 1 cm and occur on a background of severe simple CWP. They are commoner in the upper lobes. They are soft, black, well-delineated, may reach several centimetres and can destroy a lobe or lobes. There are varying degrees of cavitation due to ischaemic necrosis. On histological examination dust is seen, free and within macrophages and admixed with collagen.

Kaplan's syndrome is an eponymous term denoting pneumoconiosis in coal miners with rheumatoid disease. Chest radiographs show large, round, peripheral shadows, not restricted to the upper lobes, as in progressive massive fibrosis. Pulmonary lesions can precede joint manifestations. The lesions are round to oval, firm nodules, may be discrete or confluent and vary from several millimetres to several centimetres. These nodules can show cavitation and calcification. They represent a combination of rheumatoid nodules and dust-related fibrosis. The central zone has necrotic collagen, coal dust, the latter often lying in rings. The periphery has palisading fibroblasts. Care should be taken to exclude tuberculosis, which is associated with histiocytes and giant cells and is a complication of PMF.

Asbestos Exposure and Asbestosis

Key Points

- Asbestos is a group of fibrous silicates.
- Exposure is associated with ship building and the construction and demolition industries.
- Asbestos causes lung cancer and mesothelioma of pleura, peritoneum and pericardium.
- Asbestosis denotes pulmonary fibrosis due to asbestos.
- Pleural plaques indicate asbestos exposure *not* necessarily asbestosis.

Asbestos refers to a group of naturally occurring fibrous silicate minerals that are still mined in Canada, Australia, South Africa and the former Soviet Union. There are two major groups of fibres, serpentine and amphibole which vary in their crystalline structure. The serpentine group consists of chrysotile (white asbestos), accounting for 90% of world production. The amphiboles, which include crocidolite (blue) and amosite (brown) are the more carcinogenic.

Asbestos bodies, in most cases amphiboles, have a central fibrous core coated with iron, which gives a typical golden brown, beaded, dumb-bell appearance (Figure 7.13). Chrysotile fibres have a higher effective fibre diameter than amphiboles and impact on bifurcations of larger, proximal airways. Amphiboles are short, straight fibres, usually less than $0.5\,\mu m$ in diameter, and can penetrate deep into the lung and through the visceral pleura. The longer, thinner fibres are most hazardous and show the greatest carcinogenic effects. Industrial exposure is seen in shipbuilding, construction, especially as asbestos is removed during demolition, increasingly with men who worked in the building and electrical trades, and in car mechanics who worked with brake linings. Patients may be exposed due to living close to an asbestos factory or because a close relative has carried the mineral home from work.

Asbestos is associated with many pleuropulmonary reactions: pleural plaques (denoting exposure) asbestosis (interstitial pulmonary fibrosis caused by asbestos), diffuse

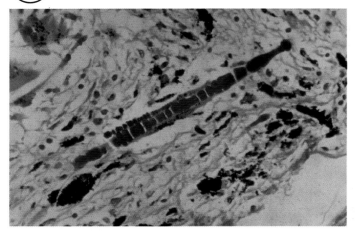

FIGURE 7.13 Asbestos body in a high-power view of a section of scarred lung tissue. It appears golden brown and beaded as it is coated with iron.

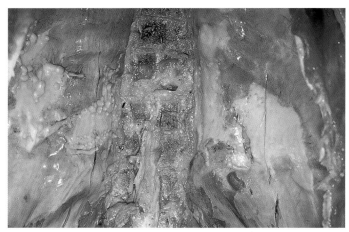

FIGURE 7.14 Pale yellowish-white fibrous plaques on the posterior parietal pleural surface at autopsy on a patient who had a history of occupational exposure to asbestos.

pleural fibrosis and asbestos-induced pleural effusions. Asbestos causes lung cancer and malignant pleural and peritoneal mesothelioma.

Asbestosis

Asbestosis occurs after prolonged, substantial exposure. The latency from the first exposure to the development of symptoms is in excess of 20 years. Asbestosis prevalence is associated with age, fibre type, smoking and cumulative exposure. Asbestos plaques are seen on the diaphragmatic and parietal pleura, lying parallel to the ribs. They vary in size and may calcify. Clinically asbestosis is associated with a non-productive cough, basal crackles, dyspnoea and, in advanced stages, finger clubbing and cor pulmonale.

The earliest changes are fibrosis in and around respiratory bronchiolar walls. This extends distally causing obliteration of the acinus. The traction of the fibrosis causes bronchial and bronchiolar dilatation, i.e. honeycomb lung. Asbestosis resembles UIP pathologically but asbestos bodies are identified in lung smears or sections. There is visceral and parietal pleural fibrosis and pleural plaques (Figure 7.14). The lungs are contracted and show honeycomb change, more marked in the lower and subpleural zones.

Lung cancer and asbestos exposure are related. This has previously been thought to be due to the fibrosis. Asbestos is carcinogenic and small pulmonary burdens can be associated with lung cancer. Cigarette smoking and asbestos exposure have a multiplicative effect in causing lung cancer. Mesothelioma is discussed on p. 187.

Silicosis

Silicosis is defined as a fibrotic disease of the lungs caused by inhalation of dust, containing crystalline silicon dioxide. Its development depends on particle size, mineral form and individual susceptibility. Most rocks contain silica, either in its free form (silicon dioxide), or combined as various silicates. Silica exists in crystalline and amorphous forms, the latter including flint and opal. The commonest form of crystalline silica is quartz, seen in many rock types. Sandstone contains almost 100% quartz, slate and shale up to 40%. Silica exposure occurs in quarrying, stone cutting, mining and tunnelling, as well as foundry work, due to crystoballite, containing silica.

The clinical presentation depends on the length and intensity of exposure. Long-term exposure to dust with little quartz causes slowly progressive nodular changes. Higher concentrations cause progressive nodularity, often with massive upper zone fibrosis (progressive massive fibrosis).

Complications of silicosis include pulmonary tuberculosis, due to the toxic effect of silica on macrophages, the main defence against the organism, and other opportunistic infections, such as tuberculosis and aspergillosis, complicate cavitating progressive massive fibrosis. Pneumothorax is related to bullous emphysema. Silicosis is associated with collagen diseases: the aetiological connection may be the antinuclear antibodies in silicosis.

Pathology and Pathogenesis

In chronic silicosis there are firm, greyish/black, sometimes calcified, well circumscribed nodules, commonest in the upper zones. These vary from several millimetres to large massive lesions (progressive massive fibrosis), occupying a lobe or extend into several upper and middle lobes. The centres may cavitate, containing greyish/black fluid. This is due to ischaemic necrosis or tuberculosis. Hilar nodes are enlarged with calcified nodules.

Histologically the silicotic nodule has concentric layers of hyaline fibrous tissue with a peripheral zone of dust-laden macrophages and chronic inflammation. There may be a necrotic centre. Interaction between silica and macrophages damages lysosomal membranes, releasing cytokines, increasing macrophage production and release. Macrophage death causes release of the silica, which is then re-phagocytosed.

Hypersensitivity Pneumonitis (Extrinsic Allergic Alveolitis, EAA)

This disease, of which the classic form is farmer's lung, shows a diffuse interstitial pulmonary infiltrate involving small airways. It is caused by inhalation of different antigens (Table 7.3). The majority of these are small enough to enter alveoli but some deposit on larger airways and become solublized. Chemicals are absorbed with antigen or antigenic determinants. The disease is acute or chronic. Acute EAA does not progress to chronic disease, without continuous long-term, low level exposure. In acute attacks, 4–8 hours after exposure to the causative allergen, there is cough, dyspnoea, chest tightness and fever. Symptoms subside in 12–16 hours, without repeated antigen exposure. Bilateral fine nodularity is seen radiologically.

TABLE 7.3 Some factors associated with extrinsic allergic alveolitis

Humidifier	Bacterial antigens associated with humid conditions
Farmer's lung	Dust from hay, thermophilic *Actinomycetes*
Pigeon fancier's lung Woodworkers Mushroom pickers Unknown	Feather antigens, excreta

In chronic disease there is dyspnoea, chronic cough and weight loss, progressing to respiratory failure with clubbing. There are coarse reticular and nodular upper and midzone infiltrates, terminating in honeycomb lung. The fibrosis usually involves the upper lobes.

Immunopathogenesis

Bronchoalveolar lavage (BAL) shows a T-cell lymphocytosis, up to 70%. The CD4: CD8 ratio may be normal or low. The T lymphocytes are responsive to a specific antigen. A relative BAL lymphocytosis is seen in asymptomatic farmers and pigeon breeders. Thus the T-cell response does not fully explain the causation of this disease. Patients with active disease show a defect in antigen-specific, T-lymphocyte suppressor function. This may allow inspired allergen to provoke T-lymphocyte-dependent inflammation. Mast cells are increased in EAA.

Pathology

The lungs are rarely seen in the acute phase but are yellow and indurated. The lower lobe is most affected. The yellow appearance is due to bronchiolar obstruction, with an excess of foamy macrophages. In the chronic phase there is interstitial fibrosis in the upper lobes, with superimposed cystic change.

There is an interstitial infiltrate with alveolar walls thickened predominantly by lymphoplasmacytic cells, scanty neutrophils, mast cells and eosinophils. Intra-alveolar foamy macrophages and loose-knit, ill-defined interstitial,

non-caseating, granulomas are seen in 70% of cases. The granuloma distribution is different from sarcoidosis, which follows the lymphatics. With progression, interstitial fibrosis develops.

LUNG INFECTIONS

Key Points

- Infection is common in the lungs, because they are open to the air and receive organisms from the blood.
- Most pulmonary infection is spread by aerosols and thus incidence is increased in overcrowded conditions.
- Common predisposing causes for pneumonia are obstruction, aspiration, cigarette smoking and immunosuppression.
- Complications of pneumonia are lung abscess, empyema, non-resolution and pulmonary fibrosis.

Pneumonia is pulmonary infection, caused by viruses, bacteria, fungi or parasites. A predisposing factor, such as undeclared lung cancer, with obstruction behind it, cystic fibrosis, immunosuppression, aspiration, etc., should always be sought.

Lung infections are classified based on anatomy or aetiology. Pneumonias may be localized, affecting a lobe (lobar pneumonia) or diffuse, affecting lung lobules, bronchi and bronchioles (bronchopneumonia). A causative organism should be sought, though this may be difficult in viral infection. Molecular probes are becoming highly sensitive for the detection of microorganisms. They detect DNA and RNA sequences unique to a particular organism. The method has the advantage of detecting small numbers of organisms, undetected by other means. However, the clinical significance of small numbers of organisms has still to be clarified.

Bacterial Pneumonia

Bacterial infections cause lobar pneumonia, bronchopneumonia or both.

Lobar Pneumonia

Smoking, chronic bronchitis, alcoholism and overcrowding predispose to classic lobar pneumonia (typically caused by *S. pneumoniae*). There is abrupt onset with high fever, tachypnoea, dry cough and severe pleuritic chest pain, progressing to respiratory distress. Rusty, thick tenacious sputum is produced and the typical signs of consolidation are present. Pneumonia due to organisms such as *H. influenzae* or *Legionella* has a similar clinical picture. These classic signs and symptoms change with early antibiotic treatment. There are four distinct pathological phases:

- Spreading inflammatory oedema – rarely seen and resembles pulmonary oedema.

- So-called 'red hepatization' – when the affected lobe is firm and brick-red, resembling liver (Figure 7.15) and small bronchi are plugged with fibrin. Alveoli are filled with red blood corpuscles and fibrin but there are few polymorphs. The alveolar capillaries are congested.
- In grey hepatization – the lung is firm, grey/yellow and there is overlying fibrinous pleurisy. Alveoli are filled with fibrin, many polymorphs and a few red blood corpuscles. The pulmonary arterioles may become thrombosed.
- Resolution – macrophages remove the exudate from the alveoli, the normal architecture is restored and the lung is re-inflated.

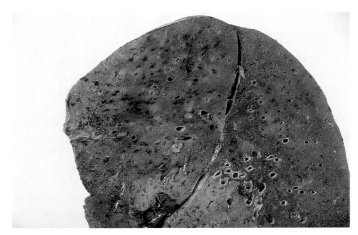

FIGURE 7.16 Bronchopneumonia. There is patchy consolidation (paler areas) of this lung. This case was due to aspiration of gastric contents (not shown).

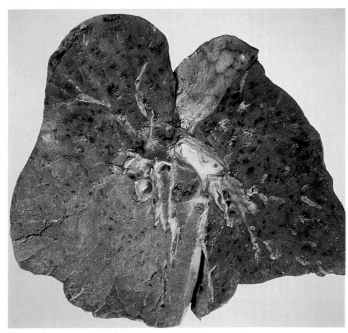

FIGURE 7.15 Lobar pneumonia affecting the whole of the lower lung on the left of the picture. This is solid and dull red (red hepatization) due to inflammatory exudates filling alveoli and small bronchi.

Bronchopneumonia

Bronchopneumonia typically occurs in infancy, old age, in debilitated individuals in whom there is retention of pulmonary secretion and with aspiration of gastric contents or a foreign body and diminished coughing (Figure 7.16). There is often a history of a pre-existing viral infection, chronic bronchitis, bronchiectasis or cystic fibrosis. Bronchopneumonia typically involves the lower lobes. The infection is centred around bronchioles and spreads into the adjacent alveolar spaces. There is more patchy consolidation than in lobar pneumonia. Lung abscesses may develop and infection may spread to the adjacent pleura or pericardium. At autopsy, the lungs are bulky and dark with blood-stained, purulent fluid filling bronchi and much of the parenchyma. Bronchial and bronchiolar walls are infiltrated by polymorphs and mononuclear cells, with shedding of the epithelium. Alveolar and bronchiolar lumina are filled with debris, pus cells and oedema. If the pneumonia is treated, a subsequent radiograph may detect an underlying cause, such as a carcinoma which may have caused bronchial obstruction. A recurrent pneumonia should *always* trigger a search for an underlying cause.

Other Bacteria

Haemophilus influenzae is a commensal in the respiratory tract and is seen especially in the yellow/green sputum of patients with COPD. Pneumonia may be lobar or bronchial. Gram-negative pneumonia is an important cause of septicaemia and hospital-based death. It occurs in patients in intensive care units or in those on broad-spectrum antibiotics, immunosuppressives or steroids. The causative organisms may be multiple and include *Pseudomonas aeruginosa*, *Proteus* and *Escherichia coli*. Diagnosis may be difficult and the presenting feature may be septicaemic shock with fever, lymphocytosis and mucopurulent sputum. Gram-negative bacilli in the sputum are present in any hospitalized patient and are insufficient for a diagnosis of this type of septicaemia.

Two specific Gram-negative organisms should be mentioned. *Klebsiella pneumoniae* usually occurs in the smoking, alcoholic male but may occur in malignancy and diabetes. It presents with rigors, fever and purulent sputum. The patient is *in extremis* with frank haemoptysis. There is lobar or lobular consolidation, proceeding to abscess formation. The disease is usually seen in the right upper lobe or in an apical segment of the lower lobe, suggesting previous inhalation.

Pseudomonas pneumoniae is important in cystic fibrosis and patients with burns, tracheostomies or on ventilators. There are multiple indurated haemorrhagic foci which resemble infarcts or yellow, irregular areas of consolidation, progressing to abscess formation.

Legionnaires' Disease

This is caused by *Legionella pneumophila*. There are three types of infection:

- Outbreaks in previously fit individuals, exposed to contaminated shower or cooling systems.

- Sporadic cases, where the source of infection is unknown. It occurs in middle-aged and elderly people, often smokers.
- Immunocompromised patients.

The organism grows in water and is spread by aerosols. Males are more commonly affected. Symptoms vary but characteristically there is headache, myalgia and rigors and half of patients have nausea, vomiting, diarrhoea and abdominal pain. There may be mental confusion in severely ill patients. Respiratory symptoms include tachypnoea and cough, initially dry then purulent. Multilobular shadowing is seen in radiographs. There is confluent bronchopneumonia and less commonly a lobar pattern. Diagnosis is by demonstration of the organism by antibody staining.

Complications of Pneumonia

While in optimal circumstances pneumonia may resolve, frequently this is not the case. Lung abscess is a local cavity, usually with a fluid level. The commonest cause is aspiration, inhalation of a foreign body or obstruction by a bronchial carcinoma. Abscesses are commoner with organisms, such as *K. pneumoniae*, *Streptococcus pyogenes* or septic infarcts. There is foul-smelling sputum, because of an overgrowth of the cavity by anaerobes.

Direct extension of the infection from the lung to the pleural cavity results in empyema, a collection of pus. Non-resolution of pneumonia may follow incorrect treatment, commonly due to mycobacteria, actinomyces or fungi, or in pneumonia complicating tumour, thromboembolism or collagen diseases. Pulmonary fibrosis is usually intra-alveolar.

Pulmonary Tuberculosis

> **Key Points**
>
> - The causative organism is *Mycobacterium tuberculosis*.
> - Incidence is rising once again.
> - It has two forms: primary and secondary.
> - Spread is to draining lymph nodes and by blood.

The general features of tuberculosis are discussed in Chapter 19. This disease apparently conquered in the West, is now increasing in incidence. The declining rate was largely due to better living standards with a smaller contribution from chemotherapy. The increase is due to human immunodeficiency virus (HIV) infection, immunosuppression and multiple drug resistance, especially in the poorer developing countries. In the West, immigrants from the southeast Asian subcontinent and the West Indies are more susceptible to the disease.

Primary Tuberculosis

Infection with *M. tuberculosis* causes a caseous granulomatous focal lesion, called a Ghon focus, situated subpleurally. The organisms then travel to the regional hilar nodes, causing granulomatous caseation. The Ghon focus (primary lung lesion) and the involved regional nodes are termed the primary complex. This is usually clinically silent, apart from calcification on a chest radiograph. In children under 2 years there may be bronchial or vascular erosion, resulting in tuberculous bronchopneumonia or miliary tuberculosis.

Secondary Pulmonary Tuberculosis

This is probably due to re-infection, not reactivation of a dormant primary lesion. The second dose of *M. tuberculosis* causes a hypersensitivity reaction with tissue necrosis. Histologically, there are lymphocytes, histiocytes, plasma cells and Langhans'-type giant cells with central caseation. This lesion, usually in the upper lobe, heals by fibrosis and calcification if there is a high degree of immunity. The predilection for upper lobe involvement is probably due to its better ventilation.

Cavitation occurs at the apex of the upper lobe (Figure 7.17). There may be significant haemoptysis due to erosion of vessels. Some cases present as hilar or mediastinal lymphadenopathy, when an extrinsic tuberculoma impinges on the trachea or bronchus. This may erode a bronchus, oxygen aiding growth of the organism, causing dissemination and tuberculous bronchopneumonia. Alternatively miliary tuberculosis, due to rupture of a tubercle into a vein, may develop. The name miliary is because of the similarity with millet seeds. Miliary spread enables the disease to establish itself in organs such as bone, meninges and kidney. There may be a pleural effusion.

Typically there is central caseation, a lymphoplasmacytic reaction with surrounding epithelioid (histiocytic) cells and Langhans' cells, due to fusion of histiocytes.

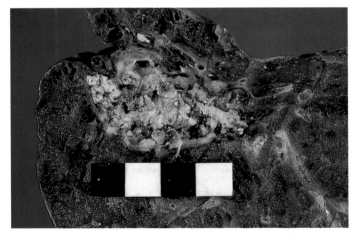

FIGURE 7.17 Secondary pulmonary tuberculosis. There is caseation, fibrosis and developing cavitation toward the apex of the upper lobe.

Clinical Features

Primary tuberculosis may be asymptomatic but there can be a vague illness with cough and wheeze and erythema nodosum. Lymphadenopathy compresses bronchi, causing segmental or lobar collapse. If chronic this causes bronchiectasis, usually in the middle lobe (Brock's syndrome).

In adult post-primary pulmonary tuberculosis there is tiredness, anorexia, weight loss, cough, pleural effusion and fever but drenching night sweats are now uncommon. The chest radiograph shows patchy or nodular upper lobe shadowing as well as fibrosis with/without cavitation. Miliary tuberculosis presents in a non-specific manner with weight loss, fever and few physical signs. The chest radiograph may show normal findings, as tubercles are only 1–2 mm in diameter. A Mantoux skin test is usually positive, but may be occasionally negative in severe disease. Bone marrow culture may be helpful.

Atypical Mycobacterial Infection

This is difficult to distinguish from TB. Mycobacteria, other than those causing tuberculosis, are increasingly recognized as a cause of chronic lung disease. The causative organisms include *M. kansasii*, *M. avium-intracellulare* and *M. fortuitum*. These organisms are commoner in patients with HIV, silicosis, and in the immunocompromised. There are four main pulmonary patterns:

- solitary nodules
- chronic bronchitis or bronchiectasis
- tuberculous-like and diffuse infiltrates, seen especially in HIV
- pleural involvement, but this is rare.

There are granulomas with varying degrees of necrosis. Bilateral diffuse interstitial infiltration is seen in the *M. avium-intracellulare* group.

Viral Infections

Key Points

- All viruses are cytopathic, stripping epithelium and enabling secondary invaders to cause bronchopneumonia.
- Influenza causes pandemics because of its ability to undergo antigenic drift, enabling new strains to evolve.
- RSV, measles and adenovirus cause morbidity and mortality in children, HIV in adults and children.
- Animal-to-human transmission is becoming more important with new threats identified such as severe acute respiratory syndrome (SARS) and avian influenza.

The histological diagnosis of viral infection is only possible if there are specific intracytoplasmic or intranuclear inclusion bodies.

Influenza

This is caused by an RNA virus that belongs to the orthomyxovirus family, with three main types A–C. The structural proteins are haemagglutinin, major protein and neuraminidase. Haemagglutinin is recognized by neutralizing antibody. Influenza A virus can undergo antigenic drift, because of changes in both the haemagglutinin and neuraminidase antigens. Strains evolve that are different from the original pandemic virus. The virus is cytopathic to respiratory epithelium, leaving a bare basement membrane on which staphylococci and other organisms grow. The virus impairs chemotaxis in polymorphs and macrophages.

The disease is seen every year and in the temperate climates, usually during winter months. There is headache, non-productive cough, myalgia and a high temperature. Viral spread is by droplets and spread is increased by close contact or crowding. The disease is only usually fatal in its acute stage if there is underlying cardiopulmonary disease. Death is usually due to staphylococcal pneumonia.

The acute changes vary from a patchy fibrinous intra-alveolar exudate and hyaline membranes with interstitial oedema to severe alveolar haemorrhage and necrosis of bronchiolar mucosa. Repair of the alveolar wall occurs with type II cell proliferation and there are mild chronic interstitial cell infiltrates.

Respiratory Syncytial Virus Infection

This is commoner in young children due to the close proximity of the upper and lower respiratory tracts. Epidemics in temperate climates are in winter and early spring. Transmission is by droplets, via the nose or eyes. There is fever, cough and rhinorrhoea. It is commoner in premature infants or those with pre-existing cardiopulmonary disease. The virus replicates in epithelial cytoplasm and lymphoid tissue. The epithelial cells die and form mucus plugs, causing partial or complete airway obstruction. There is an associated lymphoplasmacytic and neutrophilic infiltrate in bronchiolar walls. Typical multinucleated giant cells suggest a giant cell pneumonia. These cells contain intracytoplasmic, acidophilic inclusions. Respiratory syncytial virus pneumonia complicates measles and influenza.

Measles

This is a serious disease in malnourished children in developing countries. It is spread by aerosol. The virus replicates in respiratory lymphoid tissue, causing rhinorrhoea and cough. The respiratory epithelium sloughs, leaving a bare basement membrane. Multinucleated cells with intranuclear inclusions are present, especially in alveoli. There is a peribronchiolar lymphoplasmacytic infiltrate. Secondary bacterial pneumonia often supervenes.

Adenovirus

These are DNA viruses, causing severe bronchiolitis. Infection is a complication of immunosuppression. The lungs have small, dark collapsed foci. There is bronchial ulceration. Shedding of bronchial and bronchiolar epithelium, containing some nuclei with eosinophilic inclusions and a clear halo, are seen. These coalesce and stain basophilically, causing smudge cells.

Cytomegalovirus Infection

This is an important complication of solid organ transplantation and HIV infection. It can cross the placenta and cause perinatal disease. In adults there is fever, non-productive cough, dyspnoea and hypoxia. The characteristic intranuclear, acidophilic inclusions surrounded by a clear zone are seen in bronchiolar and alveolar epithelium. There is an associated lymphoplasmacytic infiltrate.

Other viruses causing pulmonary damage include parainfluenza, chickenpox (varicella), herpes simplex, rubella and hantavirus.

Atypical Pneumonias

Mycoplasma pneumoniae is an important cause of community-acquired pneumonia transmitted by droplets. A quarter of infections are asymptomatic, and the clinical illness varies from a mild upper respiratory tract infection to pneumonia with uni- or multilobular consolidation. The lungs are heavy, dark red with subpleural haemorrhages.

Chlamydia spp. are Gram-negative bacteria. *C. pneumoniae* is a common cause of pneumonia. The infection may present as a pharyngitis, with pneumonia occurring several weeks later. The pneumonia is mild, except in the elderly, with fever, cough and crackles. The pathology is ill-described as there have been few deaths or biopsies. Diagnosis is made serologically or by specific monoclonal antibody. *C. psittaci* causes psittacosis/ornithosis, which is highly infectious, transmitted by aerosol or by direct handling of infected bird tissues. Budgerigars, pigeons and many species of wild birds carry the organism. It causes cough, sputum, chest pain, dyspnoea, haemoptysis and fever and lower lobe consolidation. The bronchial and bronchiolar epithelium show desquamation, necrosis and lymphocytic inflammation. Alveolar cells show intracytoplasmic inclusions. Diagnosis is made by an immunofluorescence ELISA test or by serology. *C. trachomatis* causes oculogenital infections and is a rare cause of neonatal pneumonia.

Fungal Infections

Some of the fungi causing lung disease are purely saprophytic and grow along pre-existing cavities or necrotic lung tissue. Others, such as blastomycosis and coccidiomycosis, are seen in well-defined geographic zones, where the fungal spores are found in the soil. They cause primary invasive infections in previously healthy people, in the absence of predisposing factors. Fungi cause a variety of effects from tissue necrosis, as in coccidiomycosis and histoplasmosis, to allergic-type reactions, such as asthma due to absorption and sensitization to fungal products in *Aspergillus* infection.

Aspergillosis

Aspergillus is widespread, being found in soil, decaying organic matter, such as manure and hay. Spores are disseminated by air currents. Infection is most likely in the immunosuppressed. Allergic manifestations include asthma, eosinophilic pneumonia, mucoid impaction of bronchi, allergic bronchopulmonary aspergillosis and bronchocentric granulomatosis. Cystic fibrosis patients develop hypersensitivity to *Aspergillus*. The main forms of aspergillosis are:

● Aspergilloma or fungal ball colonizes a pre-existing cavity, such as old sarcoid, tuberculosis or bronchiectasis (see Figure 7.5). Cavities are commoner in the upper lobes. They cause haemoptysis and a radiograph shows a round opacity, surrounded by a radiolucent crescent of air. The ball is necrotic, brownish/yellow and the surrounding lung is fibrotic.
● Invasive aspergillosis is confined to immunosuppressed patients. The affected lung resembles an infarct, is dark red, haemorrhagic and shows coagulative necrosis with fungal hyphae. Fungal involvement of arteries produces infarction.
● Granulomatous pulmonary aspergillosis resembles tuberculosis.
● Tracheobronchial aspergillosis is seen in immunosuppressed patients. A necrotic membrane lines the trachea and main bronchi. If it separates, bronchial obstruction occurs.

Cryptococcosis

This is caused by *Cryptococcus neoformans*, found in bird excreta contaminating soil worldwide. The disease is often asymptomatic even with marked radiologic changes which include nodular infiltrates, pleural effusions and lobar consolidation. Patients have fever, weight loss, dyspnoea and night sweats. Sporadic cases with no predisposing condition occur, but it is seen in the immunocompromised.

The disease may resemble tuberculosis and form a primary cryptococcal complex in any lobe. There are foci of caseation surrounded by fibrosis with hilar lymph node involvement. Localized granulomatous lesions (cryptococcomas or toruliomas) are solitary, round, subpleural shadows, several centimetres in diameter which may undergo central necrosis and cavitation. The disease may also disseminate to give diffuse pneumonia or a miliary picture. Silver stains show budding yeasts.

Pneumocystis *jirovecii (carinii)* Pneumonia

Reactivation of latent infection is probably the cause of the disease in immunosuppressed patients (p. 515). *Pneumocystis jirovecii (carinii)* causes diffuse disease with consolidation. The lungs are bulky with firm yellow/pink foci. There is an interstitial plasmalymphocytic infiltrate with characteristic foamy intra-alveolar eosinophilic material. Methenamine silver or monoclonal antibodies demonstrate the organism.

MISCELLANEOUS LUNG DISEASES

Bronchiectasis

Key Points

- There is abnormal and irreversible dilatation of bronchi.
- It follows bronchiolitis and pneumonia.
- It is a complication of cystic fibrosis, tuberculosis.
- It becomes chronically infected and causes abscesses, for example in brain.

Bronchiectasis is defined as an abnormal and irreversible dilatation of bronchi (see Figure 7.3). It may affect one lung segment or be widely distributed. Bronchiectasis is the result of episodes of infection, usually with some degree of lung collapse. The bronchial walls are weakened and lack support and are expanded by the force of inspiration. Bronchiolitis and bronchopneumonia in childhood, cystic fibrosis and chronic pulmonary tuberculosis are common precursors. An obstructing lung cancer can also cause bronchiectasis in the distal segment.

The dilated bronchi become crowded together with loss of the intervening lung parenchyma. Although they are initially lined by respiratory epithelium, squamous metaplasia often follows and eventually the cavities become chronically infected. The patient has a chronic cough with foul-smelling breath and sputum. Bacteraemia may lead to the formation of systemic abscesses, classically in the brain. Amyloidosis may supervene.

The Lung in Systemic Disease

Systemic diseases may affect the lungs. The commonest are the connective tissue disorders, which can affect the lungs in diverse ways. They may produce interstitial disease and more commonly a CFA picture, BOOP, lymphocytic interstitial pneumonia, rheumatoid nodules, alveolar haemorrhage, bronchiectasis and pulmonary hypertension. The commonest collagen diseases affecting the lung are rheumatoid disease (p. 357), systemic lupus erythematosus and scleroderma. In rheumatoid disease pulmonary involvement may precede the joint manifestations. There may be pleural effusions, interstitial fibrosis and rheumatoid nodules, which may cavitate and cause haemorrhage.

Systemic lupus erythematosus causes ARDS, pulmonary haemorrhage and pleural effusions as the main manifestations. Scleroderma most commonly causes interstitial pulmonary fibrosis but 30% of patients have pulmonary hypertension and the Crest syndrome (calcinosis, Raynaud's phenomenon, oesophageal involvement, sclerodactyly and telangiectasia). Pulmonary hypertension is caused by medial hypertrophy of pulmonary arteries and concentric intimal thickening with myxoid connective tissue. Sjögren's syndrome is an autoimmune disorder characterized by keratoconjunctivitis, sicca syndrome and xerostomia. It affects women in the fourth and sixth decades of life. There is xerotrachea (dessication of the bronchial tree) and lymphocytic infiltration, which extends to the bronchial tree. It may progress to malignant lymphoma. Patients have cough, dyspnoea and recurrent pneumonitis. The lung may be affected by amyloidosis which may be primary or myeloma-associated or secondary (inflammation or malignancy associated).

Pulmonary Vascular Disease

The normal pulmonary vasculature is a low pressure system. Any prolonged rise in pulmonary arterial or venous pressure produces morphologic vascular changes. A rise in either pulmonary venous or arterial pressure causes an increase in pulmonary capillary pressure, forcing fluid into alveoli-pulmonary oedema. Pulmonary arteries are divided into three groups. Elastic arteries are greater than $500\,\mu m$ in diameter and have multiple elastic laminae and smooth muscle. Muscular arteries are between $80\,\mu m$ and $500\,\mu m$ in diameter, with internal and external elastic laminae, between which is a thin media, reflecting the low pressure system. Pulmonary arterioles, less than $80\,\mu m$ in diameter, lose their media with decreasing calibre and have a single elastic lamina. Pulmonary veins contain muscle, collagen and elastic fibres, the latter forming an internal elastic lamina. The alveolar capillaries have a single layer of endothelium resting on a continuous basal lamina. They lie in the alveolar walls.

Pulmonary Embolism

Key Points

- These are usually derived from deep venous thrombosis of calf and ilio-femoral veins.
- They may cause sudden death, pulmonary infarction or be asymptomatic.
- If recurrent it may cause pulmonary hypertension.

Pulmonary embolism accounts for 10% of hospital deaths. Thromboembolism (p. 106) follows venous stasis, vessel injury and coagulation changes in the deep calf veins, the ilio-femoral and pelvic veins. Less commonly emboli derive from intravascular catheters, right atrial thrombosis due to atrial fibrillation and right ventricular thrombus following myocardial infarction. It is much more common in sedentary people and has recently been described in individuals spending many hours in front of computer screens (e-emboli).

Pulmonary thromboembolism is frequently silent. Very large emboli may present with shock, due to an acute increase in right ventricular and pulmonary arterial pressure and are often fatal; coiled thromboemboli lie in the pulmonary trunk and main pulmonary arteries. These are the end event, a search of the pulmonary arteries histologically will show many old or organizing emboli.

Large emboli may result in lung infarcts: these are wedge-shaped haemorrhagic areas with a pleural base and apex pointing toward the embolus (Figure 7.18). The

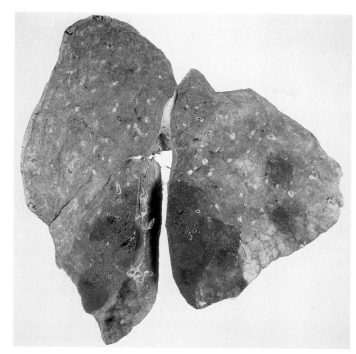

FIGURE 7.18 Pulmonary infarction. The dark haemorrhagic areas towards the periphery of the lung in the lower part of the field are infarcted.

lesion heals by fibrosis and rarely may become infected. Other symptoms are dyspnoea, substernal or central chest pain and haemoptysis. Unexplained dyspnoea should raise the clinical suspicion of pulmonary embolism. Ventilation: perfusion scans and ECGs are most useful diagnostically. Duplex ultrasound, using Doppler flow, is helpful in diagnosing deep venous thrombosis.

Recurrent pulmonary thromboembolism typically affects young women who present insidiously with dyspnoea, syncope, chest pain and pulmonary hypertension. There are eccentric recanalization channels in the pulmonary arteries, the rest of the lumen being replaced by intimal fibrosis. The media shows hypertrophy.

Pulmonary Oedema

This is a life-threatening emergency. The patient is acutely breathless, wheezing, anxious and sweaty, produces frothy, blood-tinged sputum and is tachypnoeic with peripheral shutdown. The paO_2 falls. The chest radiograph shows diffuse haziness, secondary to intra-alveolar fluid and Kerley B lines, due to interstitial oedema.

The lung is well suited to the development of oedema as it lacks solid tissue support. The organ consists predominantly of alveolar walls, suspended in air with only a thin tissue barrier separating capillaries from alveoli. Fluid is kept inside the pulmonary capillaries by a combination of factors including low haemodynamic pressure, plasma colloid osmotic pressure, active reabsorption of excessive alveolar fluid and the efficiency of pulmonary lymphatics. Pulmonary oedema can be due to haemodynamic (hydrostatic) causes and increased vascular permeability. There are other types: due to high altitude, neurogenic causes and uraemia.

Haemodynamic Pulmonary Oedema

Haemodynamic pulmonary oedema is usually caused by increases in capillary transmural pressure, usually due to congestive cardiac failure. An increased plasma volume has a similar effect. Initially there is interstitial oedema, the septa are widened and the lymphatics dilated. Fluid leaks through the alveolar wall but lies in the corners of the alveoli. Because the thin parts of the alveolar capillary wall are intact at this stage, there is little disturbance to gas exchange. If the fluid continues to increase, the oedema covers the entire alveolar surface, giving a low paO_2. This causes diminished diffusion through the thickened alveolar wall.

The commonest cause of haemodynamic pulmonary oedema is increased pulmonary venous pressure typically due to left ventricular failure (p. 134) secondary to systemic hypertension, ischaemic or valvular heart disease. With raised left atrial pressure the pulmonary capillaries are distended and red blood corpuscles leak into the alveoli. They are ingested by macrophages, causing pulmonary haemosiderosis. The small pulmonary arteries show medial hypertrophy, and pulmonary veins form a media between internal and external elastic laminae, i.e. arterialization.

High-altitude, Neurogenic and Uraemic Pulmonary Oedema

High-altitude pulmonary oedema, whose mechanism is unknown, develops on rapid ascent to altitudes above 3000 m. Pulmonary hypertension secondary to hypoxia occurs, increasing the hydrostatic pressure and there may also be a component of permeability oedema, caused by mechanical damage to the alveoli. Neurogenic pulmonary oedema is associated with a rapid rise in intracranial pressure. Uraemic pulmonary oedema shows a bat's wing pattern on chest radiograph leaving the peripheral lung translucent, and flooding the perihilar alveoli. This is a type of permeability oedema since the oedema fluid contains high concentrations of plasma proteins. It is probably caused by toxic byproducts of renal failure.

Drug-induced Lung Disease

There may be a direct pulmonary toxic effect related to dose. Toxicity can be enhanced by factors such as age, radiotherapy and oxygen. The main drugs causing pulmonary damage are cytotoxics, especially busulphan used in chronic myeloid leukaemia. This produces atypical epithelial cells with large hyperchromatic nuclei, suggesting malignancy, and progresses to interstitial fibrosis. Other drugs can produce pulmonary oedema, haemorrhage, pulmonary hypertension and systemic lupus erythematosus.

Pulmonary Haemorrhage

Pulmonary haemorrhage syndromes are a heterogeneous group of diseases characterized by haemoptysis, pulmonary infiltrates and anaemia. Pathologically there is a haemorrhagic alveolitis. It may occur secondary to venous hypertension and vasculitides. Antibasement membrane antibody formation on alveolar septa and immune complex deposition in systemic vasculitis are important causes.

Antibasement membrane antibody disease (Goodpasture's syndrome, p. 387) consists of pulmonary haemorrhage and proliferative glomerulonephritis. There may be massive pulmonary haemorrhage and little renal disease or vice versa. There is an alveolar capillaritis with fibrin thrombi and alveolar haemorrhage resembling ARDS. Diagnosis is by detection of antibody to anticollagen-α3 (IV).

Idiopathic pulmonary haemosiderosis is rare, affecting mainly males. There is progressive alveolar replacement by haemosiderin-laden macrophages, interstitial and intraalveolar fibrosis. The diagnosis is one of exclusion.

Pulmonary vasculitis

Rarely the lung may be a major focus of damage in vasculitis. Wegener's granulomatosis is a necrotizing granulomatous vasculitis that also affects kidneys and upper respiratory tract (p. 122). Churg–Strauss syndrome is usually characterized by a raised eosinophil count.

LUNG TUMOURS

Key Points

- Lung tumour is one the major cancers.
- It is mainly smoking related.
- Small cell, squamous and adenocarcinoma are the main forms.
- Secondary tumours commonly affect the lung,

The WHO produced a revised lung and pleural tumour classification in 2004. The main tumour variants are given in Table 7.4.

Tumours in the lung may be primary or secondary, benign or malignant. Because the lung receives the entire cardiac output, tumour metastases are common. Lung tumours are classified anatomically as central, that is arising from the main bronchi or peripheral, from the lung parenchyma. This is important as the site determines the signs and symptoms. All central lung tumours present with similar symptoms, i.e., cough, recurrent chest infections and haemoptysis, due to ulceration of the surface of the tumour. They often cause collapse of a lobe or lung, while recurrent infection may lead to bronchiectasis. Peripheral lung tumours are often detected as a chance radiological finding, known as 'a solitary pulmonary nodule'. As a rough guide 40% of solitary nodules are malignant and 60% are benign. The benign lesions may well be inflammatory or non-neoplastic rather than benign tumours. For any individual patient these figures do not help with diagnosis. By convention a nodule is between 4 cm and 6 cm in diameter; a larger lesion is termed a mass often suggesting malignancy. Radiologically benign lesions tend to have a smooth circumscribed periphery, malignant ones are larger with irregular margins. If a nodule has been radiologically stable in size for 2 years and the patient is below 35 years, it is malignant in only 1–5% of cases. Positron emission tomog-

TABLE 7.4 Histological classification of lung tumours

Epithelial origin	
Benign primary	e.g. Squamous papilloma
Malignant primary	Squamous carcinoma
	Adenocarcinoma – papillary, acinar, solid, bronchioloalveolar subtypes
	Small cell undifferentiated
	Large cell undifferentiated
	Mixed types combining several of the above
	Neuroendocrine (carcinoid) with varying malignant potential
Metastatic	For example carcinoma from kidney, colon
Mesenchymal origin	
Benign primary	Inflammatory pseudotumour (inflammatory myofibroblastic tumour)
	Mesenchymoma
Malignant primary	Primary sarcomas from blood vessels, muscle, etc. (all are rare)
Metastatic	Osteosarcoma
Other	Lymphoma

raphy (PET) scans are now increasingly used to try and differentiate benign from malignant disease but they are not 100% accurate. The usual treatment for remaining solitary nodules of unknown aetiology is resection.

Benign and Peculiar Lung Tumours

It is unnecessary for any medical student to memorize every benign lung tumour. If one remembers the normal bronchial wall components, i.e. epithelium, connective tissue, muscle, cartilage, fat, nerves, neuroendocrine cells, and that the mucous and serous glands of the bronchial wall act as a minor salivary gland, the nature of the majority of benign tumours can be predicted. Two important benign neoplasms, one low-grade malignant tumour, and one debatably neoplastic lesion are considered here.

Mesenchymoma

These lesions were originally called bronchial hamartomas but because they grow in adulthood and have an abnormal karyotype, characteristically an exchange of material between 6p21 and 14q24, they are now regarded as neoplasms. Twice as common in smokers, they are usually peripheral and range from 1 cm to 4 cm in diameter. The cut surface is grey or yellow if fat is prominent. They consist of cartilage, bone, fat, loose myxoid tissue and islands of ciliated or columnar epithelium.

Papilloma of the Bronchus

Papillomas may be solitary or multiple. They are rare and present in middle age as a central tumour, consisting of squamous epithelium, and growing exophytically into the bronchial lumen. A third show carcinoma *in situ* or invasive carcinoma and those without these changes require close follow-up.

Carcinoid Tumours

Carcinoid tumours are low-grade malignant neuroendocrine tumours similar to those seen, for example in the gut. They are divided into typical (TC) and atypical (AC) forms. The latter is smoking-related. The division is based on the mitotic rate, TC having fewer than 2 mitoses per $2\,mm^2$, but no necrosis, AC having 2–10 mitoses per $2\,mm^2$ and/or foci of necrosis. TC have a good prognosis if surgically excised.

Langerhans' Cell Histiocytosis

The lung may be involved in this tumour-like disorder characterized by proliferation of Langerhans' cells; the cause is unknown but there is strong association with cigarette smoking. In adults there is often interstitial lung disease. Women, typically in their third and fourth decades, are affected three times as often as men. They present with dyspnoea, cough, chest pain and wheezing and radiologically there are reticulonodular infiltrates. Pulmonary function tests may be normal or have a restrictive or obstructive pattern.

Early in the disease there are nodules up to 1 cm in diameter but these may progress to honeycomb change and associated pulmonary emphysema. There is an interstitial proliferation of Langerhans' cells; these show nuclear grooving and stain with CD1a and S100. Ultrastructurally the Langerhans' cell shows cytoplasmic laminar, racket-shaped bodies (Birbeck granules).

Carcinoma of Lung

Clinical Presentation

Central tumours cause obstructive symptoms, including cough, haemoptysis, wheezing, dyspnoea and stridor. Pancoast tumours (superior sulcus tumours) are localized neoplasms arising posteriorly at the apex of the upper lobe near the brachial plexus. They infiltrate the C8, T1 and T2 nerve roots, causing pain, temperature changes and muscle atrophy in the shoulder and arm innervated by these nerve roots. Horner's syndrome, consisting of unilateral enophthalmos, ptosis and miosis, is caused by involvement of the sympathetic chain and stellate ganglion. Superior vena caval obstruction causes oedema and plethora of the face, as well as dilated neck and upper torso veins. Hoarseness due to recurrent laryngeal nerve entrapment is seen particularly in left upper lobe tumours, because the left recurrent laryngeal nerve loops around the aortic arch. Tumour can involve the phrenic nerve, paralysing a hemi-diaphragm. The oesophagus may be infiltrated, causing dysphagia and if the pleura is involved, an effusion occurs.

Metastases are common in small cell lung carcinoma (SCLC), with 20% metastatic at presentation. Squamous cell carcinoma tends to remain intrathoracic whereas adeno- and large cell carcinoma metastasize to regional nodes, liver, adrenals, central nervous system and bone. Small cell carcinoma, because of its ability to produce hormones can present with paraneoplastic or neuromuscular syndromes (see below). All lung tumours show histological heterogeneity. If there is a common stem cell, it is not surprising there are mixtures of squamous and adeno or SCLC. Major heterogeneity is only found in 5% of cases.

Small Cell Lung Carcinoma

This is a rapidly growing and metastasizing tumour which may present with secondaries without any visible primary tumour. It presents as a hilar mass with extension into lymph nodes (Figure 7.19). The tumour is soft, white and shows extensive necrosis. In advanced cases the bronchial lumen is obstructed by extrinsic compression. In classic SCLC there are sheets of small, hyperchromatic nuclei with nuclear moulding and little cytoplasm (Figure 7.20). There is a high mitotic rate, apoptosis and necrosis. This

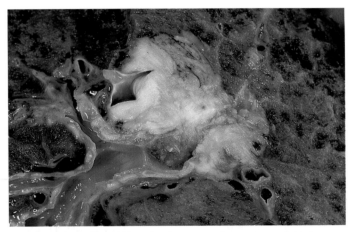

FIGURE 7.19 Slice of lung hilum showing an invasive carcinoma (white) originating in the wall of a bronchus. This is a small cell carcinoma, but one could not tell that without microscopy.

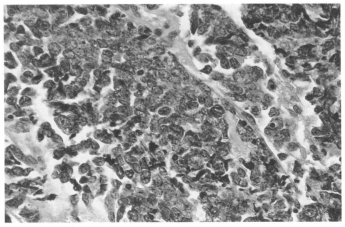

FIGURE 7.20 Small cell carcinoma of lung. Microscopic view showing sheets of small, hyperchromatic nuclei with nuclear moulding.

tumour stains positively with NCAM (neural cell adhesion molecule, CD56), synaptophysin, chromogranin and thyroid transcription factor 1 (TTF-1). The term combined SCLC implies a tumour with this pattern combined with an adenocarcinoma, squamous or large cell carcinoma component. Small cell carcinoma may also be primary in the upper respiratory tract, oesophagus and cervix. Lymphovascular invasion occurs early and distant metastases are common. These are seen in bone marrow, liver, kidney, adrenals, cerebrum, cerebellum, meninges, regional and cervical lymph nodes. This tumour is extremely responsive to chemotherapy, at least initially, and this is the main modality of treatment. After chemotherapy, recurrent tumour may be predominantly squamous or adenocarcinoma. SCLC has many neuroendocrine features.

Squamous Cell Carcinoma

These are more often central, in main or segmental bronchi than peripheral and present earlier than other types of carcinoma because of obstructive symptoms. They may show an endobronchial growth or infiltrate between, or destroy, the cartilaginous rings to invade surrounding tissue. The tumour is solid, greyish/white and may show cavitation (Figure 7.21). There is often related bronchiectasis and obstructive pneumonitis. Adjacent to the tumour there may be carcinoma *in situ* as well as chronic bronchitic changes. The tumour shows varying degrees of differentiation; tumour giant cells imply a poor prognosis.

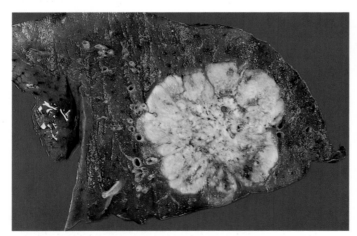

FIGURE 7.21 A large squamous cell carcinoma of lung. Such tumours generally metastasize later than small cell carcinomas and are thus more often amenable to surgery.

Adenocarcinoma

This type of lung cancer is increasing, especially in smoking females. Most adenocarcinomas are peripheral, well-circumscribed masses. If they involve the pleura it becomes fibrosed and puckered. Central adenocarcinomas arise from bronchial mucous glands and have a male predominance. There is no significant survival difference between the two variants. Adenocarcinomas vary in size and may occupy an entire lobe. They sometimes contain carbon pigment and may show marked scarring (Figure 7.22). The term 'scar carcinoma' is no longer used, since most authors regard the stroma as a desmoplastic response rather than indicating origin in a pulmonary scar. Adenocarcinomas may be multiple and this may create confusion with metastases. Pleural seeding is common and it may mimic a mesothelioma.

Histologically there are different growth patterns with tubular, papillary, acinar and signet ring variants. The cells are large and polygonal and tend to be discohesive with a high nuclear/cytoplasmic ratio. Spindle cell and giant cell foci may be identified. The tumour spreads aerogenously and may show a bronchioloalveolar pattern. This should not be called bronchioloalveolar carcinoma. Adenocarcinoma rapidly invades lymphatics, blood vessels, the pleura and spreads to distal sites.

The traditional difficulty in distinguishing a lung primary from secondary adenocarcinoma, for example of stomach or pancreas, is simplified by the frequent expression of thyroid transcription factor by primary adenocarcinoma of lung.

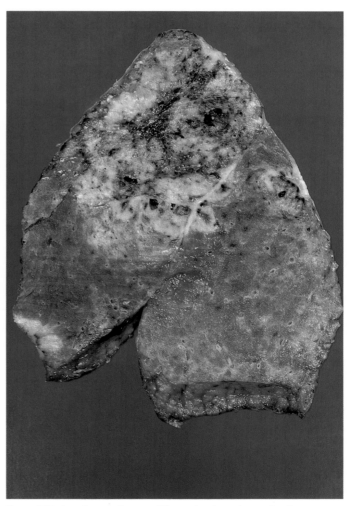

FIGURE 7.22 An adenocarcinoma with associated scarring and carbon pigmentation occupies most of the upper lobe of this lung and extends into the fissure and lower lobe.

Bronchioloalveolar Carcinoma (Alveolar Carcinoma)

This term refers to a variant of adenocarcinoma in which the tumour cells spread along the alveolar walls without invading the underlying stroma. Tumour does not usually infiltrate the pleura. There are two main histological subtypes. Mucinous tumours have a glistening appearance and are composed of tall columnar mucinous or goblet cells. These cells produce much mucin and patients may produce copious sputum. Non-mucinous tumours consist of Clara or type II cells which are cuboidal with eosinophilic, ciliated cytoplasm and prominent nuclei. Discrete satellite nodules are seen in either type. This variant tends to have a good prognosis, especially if detected early and surgically removed.

Large Cell Carcinoma

Large cell carcinoma is a diagnosis of exclusion, in a tumour in which no acinar or squamous differentiation, or mucin production is seen. It consists of sheets and nests of large cells with prominent vesicular nuclei and nucleoli (Figure 7.23). The cell borders are easily visualized. Necrosis and haemorrhage are frequent and there may be acute and/or chronic inflammation. They form large necrotic masses, which frequently invade the overlying pleura and grow into adjacent structures.

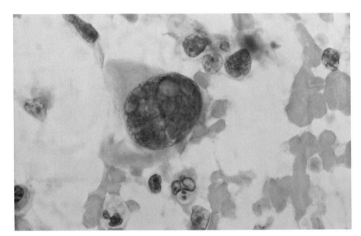

FIGURE 7.23 Cytological preparation from a large cell carcinoma of lung showing an enormous malignant cell (compare size with adjacent red blood cells) with prominent vesicular nucleus and nucleoli. Papanicolaou.

Paraneoplastic Syndromes

This term identifies symptoms and signs secondary to cancer, occurring at a site distant from the tumour or its metastases. They are caused by the production of products such as polypeptide hormones, hormone-like peptides, antibodies, immune complexes, etc. by the tumour. Cushing's syndrome, the commonest, is due to ectopic adrenocorticotropic hormone (ACTH) production, usually seen in SCLC. Non-metastatic hypercalcaemia is commonest in squamous cell carcinoma. The squamous carcinoma cells secrete parathyroid hormone-related peptide (PTH-rP) which shows a limited sequence homology with parathyroid hormone.

The syndrome of inappropriate antidiuretic hormone secretion (SIADH) is seen mainly with SCLC. In half the cases there is ectopic vasopressin secretion from the tumour. In the remainder there is abnormal release of this peptide from the posterior pituitary because of altered or defective chemoreceptor control. Gynaecomastia develops because of increased levels of βhCG (human chorionic gonadotrophin). Neurological syndromes associated with carcinomas are discussed on p. 320.

Epidemiology and Aetiology

The lung is the commonest site of cancer worldwide and is in first place in all areas of Europe and North America. In the European Union, lung cancer accounts for 21% of all cancer deaths in men and the corresponding figures for women are 14%. This latter figure is increasing and worldwide lung cancer is the fifth most frequent cancer in women.

The major contribution of cigarette smoking to lung cancer has been known since four retrospective studies showing the relationship were published in the 1950s, each showing a consistent statistically significant association. The relative risk increases in a stepwise fashion with the increased number of cigarettes smoked. This association is strongest for squamous and small cell lung cancer. The age at which the subject begins to smoke is also critical. Other types of tobacco inhalation, ranging from pipes and cigars in the West, to bidis in Asia, also correlate with a significant risk for lung cancer. Passive smoking, too, is associated with an increased risk of lung cancer, for example in non-smoking women married to smokers; it is now estimated that this causes about 2000 deaths per year in the USA.

Only 10–15% of smokers who consume 20 or more cigarettes a day will develop lung cancer implying that host factors may be important in altering the risk/predisposition to the development of this disease. There is mounting evidence that some of the genetic changes predisposing to lung cancer are inherited in a mendelian character. First-degree relatives of lung cancer relatives have a 2.4-fold increased risk of lung cancer or other non-smoking-related cancers. More tangible evidence of linkage between heredity and lung cancer has been shown in relatives of patients with retinoblastoma, with a 15-fold risk, and in some families with the Li–Fraumeni syndrome who inherit one mutated copy of the p53 tumour suppressor gene. Both the retinoblastoma and the p53 gene are mutated or inactivated in most small cell and non-small lung cancers.

To determine the role of occupation is complex since employees may be exposed to more than one potentially carcinogenic substance. The proportion of lung cancer attributable to occupational exposure has been estimated at 10–15%. Tobacco smoke acts as a strong confounder in the association. A prime example of industrially-induced cancer is asbestos-related disease. Cigarette smoke and asbestos have a multiplicative effect in increasing the incidence of lung cancer.

Arsenic and its compounds, chromates, nickel, beryllium and cadmium, all cause an excess of lung cancer deaths.

A 48-year-old steelworker presented with a history of weight loss, persistent cough and occasional flecks of blood in his sputum. His elder brother died 3 years ago from lung cancer. On examination his fingers were heavily nicotine-stained and there was a loss of the nailbed angle and increased fluctuation at the nail bed, a feature known as finger clubbing. There was dullness to percussion at the right lung base. The liver was palpable three finger breadths below the costal margin. A chest radiograph showed shadowing in the right base of lung and ultrasound showed multiple echogenic areas within the liver.

Blood biochemistry revealed deranged liver function tests, particularly an elevated alkaline phosphatase, indicating obstruction of biliary drainage. Sputum was sent for cytological examination but this showed only inflammatory cells. Microbiological culture grew *Haemophilus influenzae*, sensitive to broad-spectrum antibiotics.

However bronchoscopy showed obstruction of the right lower lobe bronchus with bleeding. Brushings for cytology showed only inflammatory cells but a biopsy showed squamous carcinoma undermining the bronchial mucosa. Further imaging showed widespread metastases in hilar and mediastinal lymph nodes. The patient's condition deteriorated rapidly and he died within 3 weeks of presentation.

This case illustrates a number of key points about lung cancer:

- smoking is its main cause
- it has often metastasized by the time of clinical presentation (most common with small cell carcinoma, but sometimes, as here, also with non small cell carcinoma) commonly to lymph nodes and liver
- negative cytology (or biopsy) does not exclude carcinoma.

Hydrocarbons, derived from coal or petroleum and polycyclic aromatic hydrocarbons, such as dibenzanthracene and benzo (a) pyrene are known carcinogens and an increased lung cancer risk is seen in coke oven workers, gas house workers and aluminium workers, exposed to pitch volatiles (tar). The increased risk of lung cancer in radiation was first shown in the Schneeberg mines due to radon gas, a decay product of naturally occurring uranium.

An increased incidence of lung cancer complicates cryptogenic fibrosing alveolitis and other significant causes of pulmonary fibrosis.

Other Lung Tumours

Pulmonary lymphomas are similar to non-Hodgkin's lymphomas elsewhere, most being B cell in origin. Primary pulmonary sarcomas are also rare. The lung is frequently the site of secondary carcinomas and sarcomas, especially osteogenic and high-grade soft tissue sarcoma. Because of advances in chemotherapy it may be beneficial to treat these patients with localized resection.

PLEURA

Key Points

- Effusions and pleurisy are common having many causes.
- Pneumothorax may follow rupture of bullae or penetrating injury.
- Mesothelioma is commonest tumour, and is due to asbestos exposure in most cases.

The pleural cavity is formed by the parietal and visceral pleura. The former covers the inner surface of the thoracic cage, mediastinum and diaphragm and the latter covers the lung surfaces. Both layers consist of a single layer of mesothelial cells, basement membrane and layers of collagen and elastic tissue. Mesothelial cells vary in shape from flat, cuboidal or columnar and ultrastructurally have long bushy microvilli.

Pleural Effusion

This is a common problem and is detected clinically when approximately 0.5 L is present. It appears first in the costophrenic angle. The effusion is categorized as a transudate or exudate. Normal pleural fluid has a protein concentration of 0.4 g/dL. A transudate has a protein concentration less than 30 g/L and is usually due to haemodynamic disorders, such as cardiac failure or severe hypoalbuminaemia. Exudates are due to inflammatory or neoplastic processes, where vascular permeability is increased and have a protein content greater than 30 g/L. The causes of pleural effusions are given in Table 7.5.

Empyema is a collection of pus in the pleural cavity, usually secondary to an underlying pneumonia, sometimes due to a stab wound to the chest or rarely post-thoracic surgery. Haemothorax, a collection of blood, follows thoracic trauma or rupture of a thoracic aortic aneurysm. Chylothorax, is a collection of opalescent lymph, usually due to obstruction of the thoracic duct, typically by tumour.

Pneumothorax

The accumulation of air in the pleural space is commonly caused by rupture of an emphysematous bulla, but may also follow penetrating chest wall injuries. Air leaks into the pleural space, causing collapse of the underlying lung. Occasionally a valve-like mechanism allows accumulation of air and build-up of pressure with compression of the mediastinal structures and contralateral lung. This is called as a tension pneumothorax.

TABLE 7.5 Causes of pleural effusion

General cause	Specific cause	Effect
Trauma	Direct trauma	Haemothorax
	Fractured ribs	Haemothorax
	Bleeding dyscrasia, for example warfarin therapy	Haemothorax
Neoplasia	Extension of primary lung carcinoma	Exudative, may also be bloody
	Primary malignant mesothelioma	Exudative, may also be bloody
	Metastatic carcinoma, for example from breast or ovarian primary	Exudative
Inflammation and infection	Pneumonia	Exudative
	Pulmonary embolus	Exudative
	Pleurisy (infection)	Suppurative
	Systemic lupus erythematosus	Exudative, may also be bloody
Organ failure	Cardiac, renal or liver failure	Hydrothorax, transudate
Lymphatic obstruction	Caused by tumour	Chylous (lymph)

Pleural Plaques

Pleural plaques are well circumscribed discs of acellular hyaline collagen seen mostly on the parietal and diaphragmatic pleura and occasionally on the visceral surface. Typically they are located in the posterolateral aspects of the lower part of the thorax and the upper part of the dome of the diaphragm. In the chest they lie parallel to the ribs (see Figure 7.14). They may calcify and appear in the chest radiograph. Their importance is that they are evidence of asbestos exposure but otherwise have no intrinsic clinical importance.

Pleural Tumours

Malignant Mesothelioma

The disease may present in the pleura, peritoneum or rarely the pericardium. It is due largely to exposure to asbestos, especially crocidolite (blue asbestos) and amosite. In the Cappadocia region of Turkey, where erionite, a non-asbestos zeolite fibre, is present in the soil, mesothelioma and asbestos-related disease are endemic. The incidence in Great Britain is rising and is expected to peak in the year 2020. This gives a lag period from exposure to development of disease of 40+ years. The age-adjusted incidence in the USA is shown in Figure 7.24. Pleural mesothelioma is rare before the age of 40 and shows a male predominance. Women exposed to the asbestos dust on their husband's clothes are at risk. There is dyspnoea, pleural effusion, chest pain, weight loss, cough and fever. Most patients are dead within a year.

Malignant mesothelioma is usually unilateral, starting as small nodules over the visceral pleura and extending to cover the entire lung (Figure 7.25). As the pleural cavity is obliterated, it is impossible to define the origin of the tumour. The tumour encases the pericardium, myocardium, mediastinum, aorta, oesophagus and other great vessels. These tumours are divided into epithelioid, sarcomatoid and mixed. The epithelioid have tubulo-papillary foci,

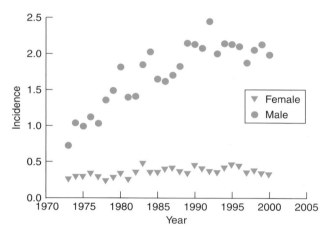

FIGURE 7.24 Age-adjusted mesothelioma incidents in USA (cases per 100 000) by gender. Source: Weill H, Hughes JM, Churg AM. Changing trends in US mesothelioma incidence. *Occup Environ Med* 2004; **61**: 438–441.

consisting of cuboidal cells with fibrous tissue cores. There may be complex acini and microcystic foci. Tumour grows into underlying lung, along the septae. Sarcomatoid mesothelioma consists of malignant fibroblast-like cells among collagen. Mixed mesothelioma shows both patterns. The diagnosis of mesothelioma and its differentiation from reactive mesothelium and from metastatic adenocarcinoma is difficult. Mucin stains are negative in mesothelioma and a panel of immunostains is helpful. Peritoneal mesothelioma is less common than pleural and is often associated with frank asbestosis. There is vague abdominal discomfort and distension with decreased appetite and constipation.

Localized Fibrous Tumour

This is rare, often asymptomatic but some patients have cough, dyspnoea, finger clubbing and hypoglycaemia. The tumours are round or oblong and may be attached to the pleura by a pedicle. They are greyish/white, nodular or lobulated, and usually cured by surgical excision.

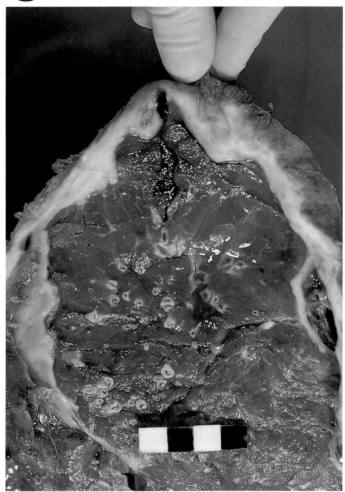

FIGURE 7.25 Malignant mesothelioma encasing most of the lobe shown in this field.

SUMMARY

The lung is unique in forming an interface with the heart, and thus diseases of one system impact on the other. In addition, as the organ of respiration and being open to the atmosphere, it is susceptible to infection, the causes of occupational lung disease, as well as inhaled allergens and cigarette smoke. Diseases of the respiratory tract are of great importance to all doctors, since asthma, COPD, lung infections and lung cancer will form the bulk of many general practioner's workload. In many developing countries, diseases such as tuberculosis, are a major health problem. With the advent of readily available air travel, such infections are easily transported to this country, causing disease in susceptible individuals. The pleural cavity may give rise to a unique tumour, mesothelioma, an asbestos-related tumour that is due to peak in incidence in the UK by 2020.

FURTHER READING

Cagle PT, Allen T, Barrios R, *et al. Color Atlas and Text of Pulmonary Pathology*. Philadelphia: Lippincott Williams and Wilkins, 2004.

Corrin B, Nicholson AG. *Pathology of the Lungs*. 2nd edn. Edinburgh: Churchill Livingstone, 2005.

Travis WD, Brambilla E, Muller-Hermelink HK, Harris CC. *World Health Organization Classification of Tumours. Pathology and Genetics of Tumours of the Lung, Pleura, Thymus and Heart*. Lyon: IARC Press, 2004.

Tomashetski JF, Cagle PT, Farver CF, Fraire AE (eds). *Dail and Hammars' Pulmonary Pathology*. Berlin: Springer Verlag, 2008.

THE LYMPHORETICULAR SYSTEM AND BONE MARROW

Robert Jackson, Frederick Lee and Paul Van der Valk

8

INTRODUCTION

The lymphoreticular system is involved in the defence of the body against microorganisms and foreign substances – i.e. the immune response. The system consists of two discrete organs, the thymus and spleen, together with an extensive network of lymph nodes which is distributed throughout the body. In addition, there is diffuse lymphoid tissue, which is closely associated with mucosal surfaces, most prominently in the gut (p. 243), and also in the upper respiratory tract in Waldeyer's ring – the tonsils and adenoids. Lymphoid cells are also well represented within the bone marrow. This is, of course, the site of haemopoiesis – the process by which mature blood cells are produced.

In this chapter, diseases of lymph nodes, spleen and thymus will be described. While the pathology of the bone marrow will be discussed and brief mention will be made of haematological disease, no attempt has been made to provide any comprehensive account of all 'blood diseases' which properly fall into the subject of haematology. Hence, readers are referred to standard textbooks on this topic.

DISEASES OF LYMPH NODES

Key Points

- Lymph nodes are the frontier posts of the lymphatic system.
- Enlargement is usually due to an inflammatory process.
- Sometimes, the underlying cause (tuberculosis, toxoplasmosis, HIV) can be deduced from the nature of the cellular response.
- Lymph nodes are commonly involved in malignancy, both primary (lymphomas) and secondary (carcinoma, melanoma).

Under normal conditions lymph nodes are small bean-shaped structures, which even in their major peripheral locations (e.g. cervical, axillary or inguinal) are seldom palpable. Their primary function is to entrap – and if needs be – to mount an immune response to foreign agents or unwanted materials which have gained access to the tissue spaces. The structure of a lymph node and its basic functions are illustrated diagrammatically in Figure 8.1.

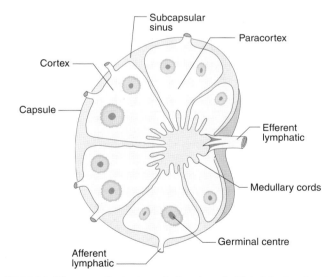

FIGURE 8.1 Diagrammatic structure of a lymph node. Material enters the sinus network of the lymph node via the afferent lymphatics. The phagocytic cells which line the sinuses entrap the antigenic material and deliver it to antigen-presenting cells within the B- and T-cell areas. A B-cell reaction results in germinal centre formation within the cortex, which leads to the production of plasma cells and memory cells which re-circulate. T-cell reactions occur mainly within the deep paracortical areas.

Lymph node enlargement is an important clinical finding. The main causes are listed in Table 8.1, where they are classified under the patterns of the histological appearances

TABLE 8.1 Important causes of lymphadenopathy

Reactive states
Acute lymphadenitis
  Pyogenic infections
Follicular hyperplasia
  Non-specific reaction
  HIV infection
  Rheumatoid arthritis, SLE and other connective tissue
    diseases
Paracortical reactions
  Drug hypersensitivity, e.g. anticonvulsants
  Viruses, e.g. Epstein–Barr virus, cytomegalovirus
Histiocytic reactions
  Foreign material, e.g. anthracosis, silicone
  Dermatopathic lymphadenopathy
Granulomatous reactions
  Infection, e.g. tuberculosis, toxoplasmosis, fungi
  Unknown, e.g. sarcoidosis, Crohn's disease,
    reaction to tumours
Neoplastic
Metastatic tumours
  Carcinoma, melanoma
Primary tumours
  Hodgkin lymphoma
  Non-Hodgkin lymphoma

seen. In most cases lymphadenopathy is a reaction to inflammatory disturbances taking place in the tissue spaces, even though in some cases the nature of the provoking agent cannot be identified. Only in a minority of cases is nodal enlargement caused by a neoplastic process, but this must always be borne in mind, especially if lymphadenopathy is persistent and unexplained.

Reactive Lymphadenopathy

Lymph nodes are commonly enlarged due to transient acute inflammation taking place during pyogenic infections involving the tissue spaces (acute lymphadenitis). Lymphadenopathy may also arise as a consequence of chronic inflammation. While it is convenient to classify these reactions according to the predominant reactive element (see Table 8.1), mixed patterns are commonly seen.

Acute Lymphadenitis

This is an acute inflammatory reaction to organisms or toxins which have gained entry to lymphatics from tissue spaces. It may be preceded by inflammation of the lymphatics themselves (lymphangitis), and the initial reaction takes place within the sinuses. In some cases suppuration follows. This type of lesion is seen in cervical lymph nodes draining acute streptococcal tonsillitis. Historically, bubonic plague is more dramatic: a bubo is an acutely inflamed lymph node following entry of the plague bacillus through a flea bite in the lower limb.

Follicular Hyperplasia

Germinal centre formation within the cortical B-cell population is an expression of antigenic exposure, and not surprisingly becomes exaggerated in reactive states (Figure 8.2). It is not specific, and can be seen in relation to many inflammatory conditions. It is especially pronounced in some infections, most notably HIV, cytomegalovirus (CMV) and toxoplasmosis, and autoimmune disorders such as rheumatoid arthritis.

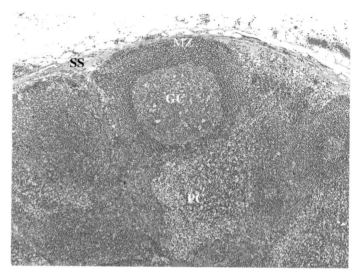

FIGURE 8.2 A lymph node displaying follicular hyperplasia. GC = germinal centre; MZ = mantle zone; SS = subcapsular sinus; PC = paracortex.

Paracortical Hyperplasia

This reactive process takes place in the deeper parts of the lymph node cortex (T-cell zones) and is recognized by the presence of numerous large transformed lymphocytes (immunoblasts). This change is usually seen in viral infections, most notably infectious mononucleosis, and drug reactions, especially anticonvulsants. The degree of lymphoid proliferation is so florid in these latter conditions that the unwary pathologist can mistake the histological features for malignant lymphoma.

Histiocytic Reactions

Sinus histiocytosis – a proliferation of histiocytes in the sinuses – is a common reaction most often seen in nodes draining malignant tumours. Reactions with increased histiocytes within the nodal parenchyma are usually related to foreign material or cellular debris. Accumulation of anthracotic carbon pigment is prominent within the mediastinal and hilar nodes of older city dwellers due to soot inhalation. Other materials which produce these reactions include silicone used in artificial finger joints and in breast implants. In dermatopathic lymphadenitis, lymph nodes draining skin disorders – especially lichenoid conditions and mycosis fungoides (p. 505) – may be considerably enlarged due to a paracortical proliferation of Langerhans cells and histiocytes containing melanin pigment.

Granulomatous Reactions

Granulomas are seen in lymph nodes in many circumstances (Table 8.2), and infections, especially tuberculosis (TB), are one of the most important causes. The granulomas in TB, unlike those in sarcoidosis, commonly show central necrosis. Necrotizing granulomas are also a typical feature of cat-scratch disease and lymphogranuloma venereum. Sarcoid-like granulomas can occur in reactive nodes draining carcinomas and lymphomas (especially Hodgkin lymphoma) and in mesenteric nodes in Crohn's disease.

TABLE 8.2 Causes of granulomatous lymphadenopathy

Infectious causes
    Tuberculosis
    Cat scratch disease
    Yersiniosis
    Spirochaetal disease
    Fungal infection, e.g. histoplasmosis
    Leishmaniasis
    Schistosomiasis
Idiopathic
    Sarcoidosis
    Crohn's disease
    Primary biliary cirrhosis
Reactive
    Foreign material, e.g. silicone from prosthesis
    Draining tumour/carcinoma/Hodgkin lymphoma/non-Hodgkin lymphoma
    Drug reactions

Miscellaneous Lymph Node Lesions

Kikuchi's disease is a self-limiting disease characterized by painful cervical lymphadenopathy mainly in young females. Langerhans' cell histiocytosis (pp. 183 and 352) may affect lymph nodes. The hyaline vascular variant of Castleman's disease is another idiopathic condition that gives rise to a mediastinal mass composed of abnormal lymphoid tissue with prominent follicular structures containing a central blood vessel. Another form exists in which there is massive infiltration by numerous plasma cells, often associated with fever, anaemia, weight loss and other systemic symptoms.

Malignant Lymphomas

This term describes primary tumours of the lymphoreticular system, almost all of which arise from lymphocytes. They vary greatly in their behaviour, and while most prove fatal if untreated, considerable advances have been made in their management. Most lymphomas arise in lymph nodes, but 30–40% develop in extranodal sites such as the stomach, though almost any organ may be primarily involved. They usually produce lymph node enlargement which may be localized or generalized, with widespread involvement of the lymphoreticular system at presentation. This latter tendency is a reflection of the normal recirculating behaviour of lymphocytes. Ironically, more aggressive lymphomas may remain localized, at least for a time, and tend to spread to adjacent nodes, rather like carcinomas.

Classification of Lymphomas

It is customary to distinguish between Hodgkin lymphoma and non-Hodgkin lymphomas. Although this is to some extent a historical and rather arbitrary distinction, it remains of major importance in determining therapy and prognosis. In view of the complexity of lymphoma diagnosis, there have been many classifications over the years. With the advent of modern investigative techniques, the accuracy and reproducibility of classification is now high. The World Health Organization (WHO) classification published in 2001 is now accepted throughout the world (Table 8.3). It combines haematoxylin and eosin (H&E) morphology, immunophenotyping, genetic information and clinical features to define specific disease entities with a particular clinical course and prognosis. As the number of therapeutic options increases and specific treatments become linked to defined entities, accurate classification and a standardized nomenclature become increasingly important.

Hodgkin Lymphoma

Key Points

- These tumours are characterized by the presence of Reed–Sternberg cells, with an appropriate cellular background.
- Patients present with lymphadenopathy, often painless.
- Systemic symptoms are common.
- The extent of the tumour (clinical stage) correlates with the prognosis.
- Epstein–Barr virus (EBV) is aetiologically important.

First described in 1832, Hodgkin's disease was subsequently defined pathologically by the presence of distinctive large tumour cells known as Reed–Sternberg cells. Approximately 25% of cases of malignant lymphoma fall into this category. While it was always suspected that Hodgkin's disease was a lymphoma, proof that the Hodgkin cells were in fact unusual germinal centre-derived B cells has come to light only in recent years – hence the use of the term 'Hodgkin lymphoma' rather than 'Hodgkin's disease' in the 2001 WHO classification.

TABLE 8.3 The World Health Organization classification of lymphomas (2001) – simplified

B-cell neoplasms
Precursor B cell neoplasm
Precursor B-lymphoblastic leukaemia/lymphoma

Mature B-cell neoplasms
Chronic lymphocytic leukaemia/small lymphocytic lymphoma
Lymphoplasmacytic lymphoma
Hairy cell leukaemia
Plasma cell myeloma
Extranodal marginal zone B-cell lymphoma
Follicular lymphoma
Mantle cell lymphoma
Diffuse large B-cell lymphoma
Burkitt lymphoma
Post-transplant lymphoproliferative disorder

T-cell neoplasms
Precursor T-cell neoplasms
T-lymphoblastic lymphoma/leukaemia

Mature T-cell neoplasms
T-cell prolymphocytic leukaemia
Adult T-cell leukaemia/lymphoma
Mycosis fungoides
Sézary syndrome
Peripheral T-cell lymphoma
Enteropathy-type T-cell lymphoma
Angioimmunoblastic T-cell lymphoma
Anaplastic large-cell lymphoma
Primary cutaneous CD30-positive T-cell lymphoma
Extranodal NK/T-cell lymphoma, nasal type

Hodgkin lymphoma
Nodular lymphocyte predominant HL
Classical HL
   Nodular sclerosis
   Mixed cellularity
   Lymphocyte-rich
   Lymphocyte-depleted

Clinical Features

Hodgkin lymphoma (HL) has a bimodal incidence with peaks in early adult life and in late middle age (4 in 100 000 of the population per annum). Cases in childhood are sometimes seen, especially in developing countries. Clinically, HL usually presents with enlargement of peripheral lymph nodes, the diagnosis then being made by lymph node biopsy. Extranodal involvement is extremely rare and is usually due to direct extension from a nodal mass. Patients with large mediastinal masses may present with superior vena caval obstruction. There may be systemic symptoms, most notably an intermittent low-grade fever, sweating, weight loss and pruritus. The disease may be complicated by concurrent infection due to immunological impairment. The extent of involvement by HL is defined by the Ann Arbor

staging system (Table 8.4), and is highly relevant for planning treatment. The tumour spreads early from one nodal group to another, while liver and bone marrow involvement are late events.

TABLE 8.4 The Ann Arbor staging system for Hodgkin lymphoma

Stage*	Description of lymphoma
I	Disease is confined to one lymph node group or involvement of a single extranodal site (I_E)
II	Disease confined to several lymph node groups on the same side of the diaphragm**
III	Disease is present in lymph node groups on both sides of the diaphragm with minimal involvement of an adjacent extranodal site (III_E)
IV	Diffuse involvement of one or more extranodal tissues, e.g. bone marrow or liver

*Each stage is subdivided according to whether there are systemic symptoms (B) or none (A).
**Spleen is regarded as a lymph node for staging purposes.

Macroscopic Pathology

The affected lymph nodes are usually discrete and rubbery, but may be matted together. They have a grey-pink cut surface, often with areas of necrosis. There may be dense bands of fibrous tissue around and within the node (see Figure 8.8.

Histological Appearances

The two main histological features of HL are first, the presence of a small population of large neoplastic cells, the Hodgkin/Reed–Sternberg cell, and second a large population of non-neoplastic inflammatory cells. Two distinct forms of HL are now recognized: classical Hodgkin lymphoma and nodular lymphocyte-predominant Hodgkin lymphoma. These appear to be separate tumours biologically, and their distinction is important clinically.

Classical Hodgkin Lymphoma (CHL)

CHL accounts for 94% of all HL, and is characterized by the presence of typical Reed–Sternberg cells and their mononuclear variants collectively termed Hodgkin/Reed–Sternberg cells (HRS cells). As cells similar to HRS cells can sometimes be seen in other conditions, it is important that there is also a mixed inflammatory background consisting of small lymphocytes, histiocytes, plasma cells, eosinophils and neutrophils (Figure 8.3) The Reed–Sternberg cells each have a single bilobed nucleus (so that they may appear binucleate in sections), with a large eosinophilic nucleolus (Figure 8.4); the cytoplasm is abundant. Mononuclear and pleomorphic variants are common. The HRS cells have a particular phenotype

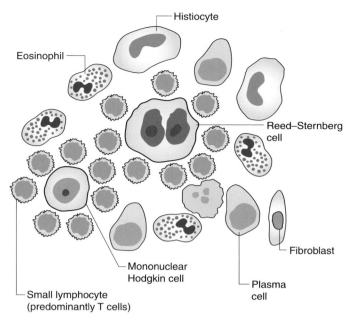

FIGURE 8.3 Schematic diagram of the cellular composition of classical Hodgkin lymphoma. The Reed–Sternberg and mononuclear Hodgkin cells are the neoplastic component and may account for only 5% of the total cellularity. The Hodgkin/Reed–Sternberg (HRS) cells secrete cytokines (e.g. interleukins, tumour necrosis factor) which invoke the inflammatory cellular reaction. Cytokine production is also likely to account for the fever and sweats experienced by some patients.

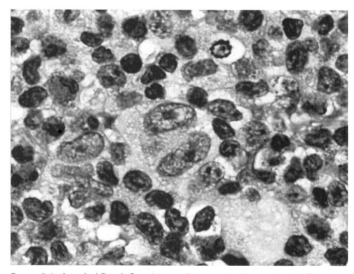

FIGURE 8.4 A typical Reed–Sternberg cell surrounded by a mixed infiltrate of small lymphocytes, a single histiocyte and eosinophils.

that can easily be established by immunocytochemistry on paraffin sections. They are positive for CD30 and CD15, and negative for the standard B- and T-cell antigens (see Figure 8.10, p. 197). Surprisingly they are also negative for CD45, the common leucocyte antigen that is expressed on all lymphocytes. While the pathologist is usually fairly certain of the diagnosis based on the H&E morphology, it is good practice to perform immunophenotyping to support this impression. If the immunocytochemical profile does not fit, an alternative diagnosis should be considered, as there are many mimics of HL.

Classical HL can be divided into four major subtypes based on variations in their histological features:

- Nodular sclerosis (NS): this is the most common subtype, and represents 70% of all CHL. The tumour consists of mixed cellular nodules surrounded by thick bands of collagen. The Reed–Sternberg cells show cytoplasmic vacuolation (lacunar cells). Typically, NS HL occurs in young adult females, and mediastinal involvement is common (see Case History 1).
- Mixed cellularity (MC): representing 20% of all CHL, this variant is characterized by a mixed cell population often including granulomas, but lacks the fibrosis seen in NS. This subtype is more common in the elderly and HIV-positive patients, and is more frequently associated with EBV.
- Lymphocyte-rich CHL (LRCHL): a variant in which the stromal response consists almost exclusively of small lymphocytes. It occurs predominantly in males and usually presents in low stage. Immunocytochemistry is required to distinguish it accurately from NLPHL.
- Lymphocyte-depleted (LD): the HRS cells predominate and are highly pleomorphic. Reactive lymphocytes are markedly reduced in number. Many tumours which were formerly included in this group have now been reclassified as high-grade non-Hodgkin lymphoma following detailed immunophenotyping. The LD subtype tends to occur in later life and presents in high stage.

Prognosis

In the past, the MC and LD variants have been regarded as having a poorer prognosis. Many of the prognostic differences formerly seen between the subcategories have been eradicated by modern chemotherapy. If CHL is untreated, death generally occurs in 6 to 24 months, but with treatment there is an 85% cure rate. The elderly generally have a poorer outcome.

Nodular Lymphocyte-predominant Hodgkin Lymphoma (NLPHL)

In this form – which typically arises in young adult males and represents 6% of all HL cases – the tumour cells differ from classic Reed–Sternberg cells. They have folded, multilobated nuclei, less-prominent nucleoli, and less-abundant cytoplasm: they are known as 'popcorn cells'. These cells express B-cell markers (e.g. CD 20) and, unlike CHL, are capable of producing immunoglobulin and are usually negative for CD30 and CD15. In general, this variant has a very good prognosis. In 5% or so of cases, it evolves into a high-grade B-cell lymphoma.

Aetiology

There is now little doubt that EBV plays a major role in the causation of CHL (see Special Study Topic 8.1), but not of NLPHL.

EPSTEIN–BARR VIRUS AND LYMPHOMA

In addition to being the causative agent of infectious mononucleosis (IM) and being linked to the development of nasopharyngeal carcinoma, the Epstein–Barr virus (EBV) is also closely associated with a variety of lymphoid neoplasms (see Table 8.5). Evidence of latent infection can be detected in 90% of normal adults. In the developed world, exposure tends to occur during adolescence, and this can give rise to the acute syndrome of IM, though in the majority of patients the acute episode is asymptomatic. The virus resides in memory B cells, and low levels of infected cells can be detected in blood and excised lymph nodes of normal individuals.

TABLE 8.5 Lymphomas associated with EBV

Burkitt lymphoma
Classical Hodgkin lymphoma
Immunosuppression-related lymphomas
Post-transplant lymphoproliferative disorder
Primary immunodeficiency disorders
HIV-related
Drug-related (methotrexate, cytotoxics)
Lymphomatoid granulomatosis
Extranodal natural killer cell lymphoma/nasal type
Angioimmunoblastic T-cell lymphoma
EBV-positive diffuse large B-cell lymphomas (DLBCL)

Biology

EBV is a human herpes-type virus containing a genome of double-stranded DNA, 172 kilobases in length encoding approximately 100 genes. The virus is capable of infecting many different types of human cells, but it preferentially infects B lymphocytes via its capacity to bind to the B-cell surface protein CD21. Entry into cells other than lymphocytes is likely to be related to different types of receptors.

There are two consequences of infection – lytic and latent. In lytic infection (as occurs in acute IM), the virus enters epithelial cells and replicates, with the release of many virions which in turn infect neighbouring cells, including B lymphocytes. Many viral proteins are expressed on the cell surface and are recognized by host cytotoxic T cells, and this brings about destruction of the infected cell. In latent infection, the normally linear DNA of the EBV genome forms a circular structure (an episome) by fusion of terminal repeat segments at either end of the viral genome. In contrast to lytic infection, only a small number of viral genes are expressed by the host cell, and this allows it to avoid recognition by cytotoxic T cells and so escape destruction. Each newly infected cell contains a viral episome of unique size due to variations in the length of terminal repetitive sequences. Viral replication occurs as the cell itself divides, each daughter cell containing an identical copy of the viral genome. Analysis of viral DNA by PCR or Southern blotting can provide evidence as to the clonality of the viral genome. There are three different expression patterns of the latent genes in immortalized B cells, and these patterns can be seen in the various EBV-elated lymphomas (Table 8.6).

In cell culture experiments, B lymphocytes infected by EBV continue to grow – they are immortalized. This is a reversible phenomenon, unlike true neoplastic transformation. All the latent gene products are important for cell immortalization. For example, latent membrane protein 1 (LMP1) has been found to activate antiapoptotic genes in cell lines, and also to induce permanent activation of various signal transduction pathways resulting in up-regulation of Nuclear Factor kappa B (NFκB).

Detection of EBV

EBV can be detected in paraffin-embedded tissue sections using either immunocytochemistry (ICC) or *in-situ* hybridization (ISH) (Figures 8.5–8.7). Southern blotting and PCR methods performed on fresh tissue are also available and are useful in determining clonality of the viral genome.

TABLE 8.6 Gene expression profile in three different patterns of viral latency: EBERs (Epstein–Barr encoded small RNAs are present within all patterns of latency)

Latency pattern	EBERs	EBNA1	EBNA2	EBNA3 A,B,C	EBNALP	LMP1	LMP2
Type 1	+	+	–	–	–	–	+
Type 2	+	+	–	–	–	+	+
Type 3	+	+	+	+	+	+	+

EBNA 1, 2, 3A, 3B, 3C, LP = Epstein–Barr nuclear antigen; LMP = latent membrane protein. A type 1 pattern is seen in Burkitt lymphoma; type 2 in classical Hodgkin lymphoma; and type 3 in post-transplant lymphoproliferative disorder.

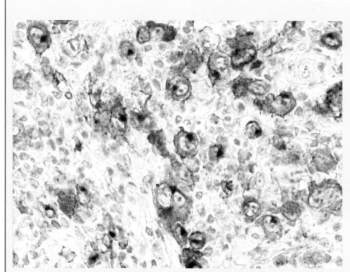

FIGURE 8.5 Immunocytochemistry for EBV latent membrane protein 1 (LMP1) in CHL. Numerous HRS cells are positive.

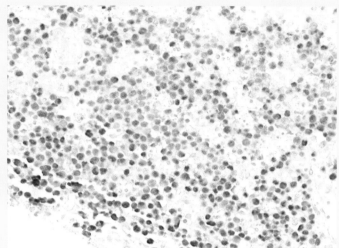

FIGURE 8.7 *In-situ* hybridization for EBV EBER in a case of Burkitt lymphoma. The nucleus of every tumour cell is positive.

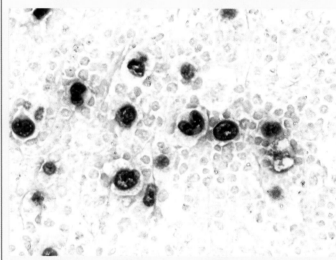

FIGURE 8.6 *In-situ* hybridization using an oligonucleotide probe to EBV-encoded RNA (EBER) in a case of CHL. The nuclei of Reed–Sternberg and mononuclear Hodgkin cells contain large amounts of EBERs. The surrounding reactive T cells are negative.

Subtypes of Lymphoma Associated with EBV

Burkitt Lymphoma

Virus-like particles were detected in cell cultures of endemic Burkitt lymphoma (BL) in 1964. EBV genomes of identical clonality are found in all tumour cells, in keeping with infection prior to the monoclonal expansion of the lymphoid population (Figure 8.7). The occurrence of BL in particular geographic areas is related to coexistent endemic falciparum malaria, which results in a decreased T-cell immunity that allows growth of the infected cells. Although EBV is present in all tumour cells in endemic BL, it is the occurrence of a chromosomal translocation involving the C-MYC locus on chromosome 8 that is the most important event in malignant transformation. It is possible that the EBV-induced immortalization of B lymphocytes increases the likelihood of this genetic event occurring.

The incidence of EBV positivity in sporadic BL in western countries is much lower (30%). Cases related to immunosuppression as a consequence of HIV or immunosuppressive drugs are often positive.

Classical Hodgkin Lymphoma

EBV can be detected in the Reed–Sternberg and mononuclear Hodgkin cells in 30–40% of cases, especially in those with the mixed cellularity variant and in the elderly (see Figures 8.5 and 8.6). There is a three-fold increase in the incidence of EBV-positive HL in those with a history of IM. The median interval between IM and the development of HL is 4–5 years, although the increased risk remains for 20 years. There appears to be no increase in EBV-negative HL after IM. In absolute terms, only 1 patient in 1000 with a history of IM will develop HL, which implies that there are likely to be other important factors required for lymphomagenesis.

Post-transplant Lymphoproliferative Disorder (PTLD)

Perhaps the best evidence for a role for EBV in lymphoma pathogenesis is the development of lymphoproliferative disorders in patients who are receiving immunosuppressive therapy following allogeneic organ transplantation. The vast majority of PTLD cases are positive for EBV. The incidence varies depending on the organ transplanted (1% in renal and 8% in lung transplantation), presumably reflecting the different levels of immunosuppression required for each system. In the normal individual, latently infected cells

SPECIAL STUDY TOPIC CONTINUED . . .

remain in the bone marrow and tonsillar area, and further proliferation of virally infected cells is prevented by an NK and cytotoxic T-cell response. When this immunosurveillance is decreased as a result of immunosuppressive therapy, EBV induces cell proliferation. Initially this may be a polyclonal reactive proliferation of plasma cells, but as further genetic events occur, evolution to a monoclonal proliferation takes place, for example diffuse large B-cell lymphoma. The majority of lymphomas are of B lineage, but 10–14% are derived from T cells. In some cases a reduction of immunosuppression can bring about a sustained remission, though this may not be possible in many cases because of the risk of rejection of the transplanted organ. In these cases chemotherapy will be required.

EBV-driven Lymphomas (not transplant-related)

Immunosuppression for other causes may be complicated by EBV-driven diffuse large B-cell, Burkitt or Hodgkin lymphoma. These include primary immune disorders, such as Wiskott–Aldrich syndrome and common variable immunodeficiency. The incidence of NHL, often extranodal, is increased approximately 100-fold in HIV infection. Immunosuppressive drugs such as methotrexate (which is used to treat severe psoriasis and autoimmune diseases) may give rise to lymphoma, 50% of which are positive for EBV. Regression is seen in 60% of cases if methotrexate can be withdrawn. Some EBV-driven lymphomas occur in patients who are not apparently immunosuppressed. The best example of this category is the extranodal natural killer/T-cell lymphoma of nasal type which causes massive destruction of the tissues of the face, maxilla and skull. This is most prevalent in Asia, Central and South America, and almost 100% of cases are associated with the presence of EBV. Up to 5% of all diffuse large B-cell lymphomas (DLBCLs) occurring in previously well patients are EBV-positive. It is possible that these patients have some specific defect in immune surveillance that has not yet been identified.

Conclusion

There is a clear association between the development of various types of lymphoma and EBV infection. EBV can cause immortalization of cells, but other factors are required to cause neoplastic transformation. The importance of detecting EBV in human lymphomas is that it may highlight a potentially reversible cause of immunosuppression. Immunosuppression reduction, where possible, can result in regression in a significant proportion of cases. New therapies directed at improving deficient T-cell immunity in EBV-driven lymphomas are being developed. Autologous in-vitro-activated and even allogeneic cytotoxic T lymphocytes directed specifically towards EBV antigens expressed by the tumour cells have already been used in the management of post-transplant lymphoproliferative disorder. Immunization against EBV, though not available at the present time, may have a role in lymphoma prevention in the future.

Further Reading

Niedobitek G, Meru N, Delecluse HJ. Epstein–Barr virus infection and human malignancies. *Int J Exp Pathol* 2001; **82**: 149–170.

Hjalgrim H, Askling J, Rostgaard K, Hamilton-Dutoit S, *et al*. Characteristics of Hodgkin's lymphoma after infectious mononucleosis. *N Engl J Med* 2003; **349**: 1324–1332.

Papadopolous EB, Ladanyi M, Emanuel D, *et al*. Infusions of donor lymphocytes to treat Epstein–Barr virus associated lymphoproliferative disorders after allogeneic marrow transplantation. *N Engl J Med* 1994; **330**: 1185–1191.

Jaffe ES, Harris NL, Stein H, Vardiman JW. *World Health Organization Classification of Tumours. Pathology and Genetics of Tumours of the Haemopoeitic and Lymphoid Tissues*. IARC Press: Lyon, 2001.

CASE HISTORY 8.1

CLASSICAL HODGKIN LYMPHOMA

A 19-year-old man presented to his general practitioner with an enlarged lymph node in his neck. The GP initially suspected a reactive condition because the boy recently had a tooth abscess on the same side. He decided to watch and wait. A month later, the patient returned and it was clear that the node had increased in size. The young man was now also suffering from night sweats and had experienced some weight loss. An urgent appointment was made for the neck lump clinic in the local hospital. An excision biopsy was performed (Figure 8.8).

Histological examination revealed a nodular infiltrate divided by thick collagenous bands (Figure 8.9). The nodules were composed of large numbers of small lymphocytes, histiocytes, neutrophil polymorphs, eosinophils and plasma cells. There was also a moderate number of mononuclear Hodgkin and classic Reed–Sternberg cells present. On immunocytochemical analysis, the large cells were positive for CD30 (Figure 8.10) and CD15, but negative for CD45, B- and T-cell lineage markers. The pathological features were characteristic of classical Hodgkin lymphoma – nodular sclerosis subtype.

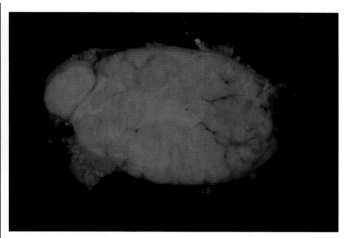

FIGURE 8.8 Photograph of the cut surface of the excised lymph node (3 cm maximum) which has a nodular architecture with fibrotic bands between the nodules.

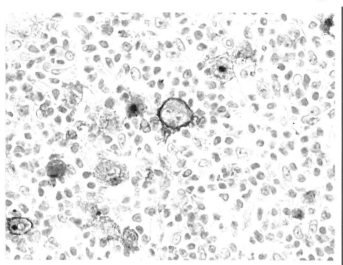

FIGURE 8.10 Immunohistochemistry for CD30. Several HRS cells display membrane and perinuclear dot positivity for CD30.

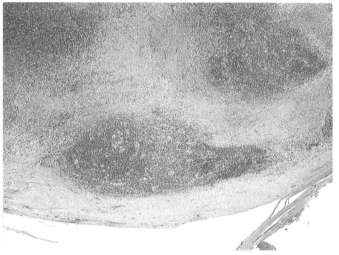

FIGURE 8.9 Low-power view of the nodal histology. Thick bands of collagen divided the node into cellular nodules. There is also a thickened capsule.

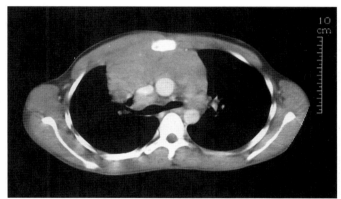

FIGURE 8.11 Computed tomography scan of the thorax, showing a large mediastinal mass.

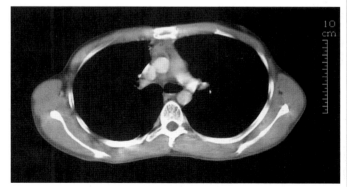

FIGURE 8.12 Computed tomography scan of the thorax after treatment; the mass is no longer apparent.

The patient was referred to the haematologist who arranged for staging to be carried out. Computed tomography (CT) scanning revealed a large mediastinal mass (Figure 8.11), in addition to abdominal and para-aortic lymphadenopathy. A bone marrow trephine biopsy was negative. The Ann Arbor stage was 3B. The man was informed that Hodgkin lymphoma is a malignant condition, which will progress if left untreated, but that with chemotherapy and radiotherapy a cure can be achieved in 85% of patients. The patient underwent six cycles of chemotherapy over a 6-month period, during which the patient experienced hair loss and mild nausea. He also required intravenous antibiotics for an episode of sepsis related to a transient neutropenia. A repeat CT scan at the end of therapy showed complete resolution of the mediastinal mass (Figure 8.12). The patient remains in complete remission at 5 years after therapy, and is now regarded as cured.

Non-Hodgkin Lymphoma

> **Key Points**
> - These are a heterogeneous group of tumours, with a complex classification.
> - There is a wide range of clinical behaviours between subtypes.
> - Low-grade tumours are often widely disseminated at presentation and grow slowly, but are seldom cured.
> - High-grade tumours are often localized and grow rapidly, but may be cured by chemotherapy.
> - In Western countries B-cell lymphomas predominate.

These tumours show great diversity in their behaviour and morphology. The accurate diagnosis and WHO classification of NHL is essential in planning rational treatment and requires a combination of histological, immunocytochemical, and molecular genetic techniques. The incidence in Britain is approximately 16 per 100 000 per annum.

Diagnosis of NHL

H&E Morphology

Distinguishing between a reactive lymphoid infiltrate and a lymphoma can sometimes be difficult, as individual neoplastic lymphocytes – unlike the situation in carcinoma – often look identical to their normal counterparts. However, the distribution of the neoplastic lymphocytes and the low-power architecture of the excised lymph node give important clues to the diagnosis; hence the importance of a relatively large biopsy.

Immunophenotyping

Different categories of normal lymphocytes express various surface antigens which can be detected either by flow cytometry in liquid cell suspensions or by immunocytochemistry on paraffin blocks of formalin-fixed tissue. Many lymphomas have a characteristic pattern of antigen expression, and therefore a panel of antibodies is applied to lymph node biopsies in routine diagnostic practice (see Table 8.7).

Detection of Clonality

Reactive lymphoid infiltrates are derived from many different clones, all directed against different antigens. The cells in a lymphoma are genetically identical and represent the progeny of a single cell (monoclonal). In a B-lymphocytic proliferation, the demonstration that the cells produce only one of the two types of immunoglobulin light chain (κ or λ), either by immunocytochemistry or by in-situ hybridization, effectively establishes the presence of monoclonality and thus of neoplasia. Monoclonality can also be determined by detecting clonal rearrangements of immunoglobulin and T-cell receptor genes in B- and T-cell lymphomas, respectively.

Cytogenetics

Many lymphomas are associated with a specific reciprocal chromosomal translocation, and detection of these either by classical cytogenetics or by molecular techniques (fluorescence in-situ hybridization and PCR) may be very helpful in establishing a diagnosis (Table 8.7). In some instances the protein product of the translocation may be detected by immunocytochemistry.

TABLE 8.7 Immunocytochemical profile and cytogenetic abnormalities of the most common B-cell lymphomas

Tumour	CD20	CD5	CD10	CD23	CyclinD1	Cytogenetics
Small lymphocytic lymphoma/CLL	+	+	–	+	–	13q14 del, trisomy 12, 17p13 del, 11q22–23 del, 6q-
Follicular lymphoma	+	–	+	+	–	t(14;18)(q32;q21)
Mantle cell lymphoma	+	+	–	–	+	t(11;14)(q13;q32)
Marginal zone lymphoma	+	–	–	–	–	Trisomy 3, t(11;18)(q21;q21)
Diffuse large B-cell lymphoma	+	–	–/+	–/+	–	t(14;18) in 15%, 3q27 abnormalities, complex
Burkitt lymphoma	+	–	+	–	–	t(8;14),t(8;22),t(2;8)

Antibody numbers are preceded by 'CD', which stands for 'cluster of differentiation'.
CD20 is expressed by most B cells.
CD5 is a T-cell marker, but is expressed by B cells in SLL and MCL.
CD10 is a marker of germinal centre cells.
CD23 is expressed by follicular dendritic cells and a population of normal mantle zone lymphocytes.
Cyclin D1 is a cell cycle regulatory protein which is not detectable in normal lymphocytes. Its expression by lymphoma cells is almost always diagnostic of MCL.
+ = positive in most cases, –/+ = usually negative but positive in a minority of cases.

A combination of these techniques demonstrates that in Western Europe and North America most NHLs are of B-cell derivation. T-cell tumours are uncommon, except in specific locations such as the skin and small bowel. In oriental countries, T-cell tumours are much more prevalent. The relative frequencies of lymphoma types in Great Britain are shown diagramatically in Figure 8.13.

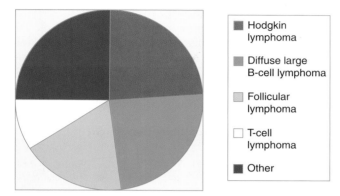

- ■ Hodgkin lymphoma
- ■ Diffuse large B-cell lymphoma
- ■ Follicular lymphoma
- □ T-cell lymphoma
- ■ Other

FIGURE 8.13 Relative frequency of lymphoma types in Great Britain.

Within each NHL subtype the degree of aggressiveness varies, and the outcome depends upon factors such as age at diagnosis, the presence of systemic symptoms, the stage of the disease, the origin of the disease (nodal versus extranodal) and the general condition of the patient (performance status). NHL can be staged in much the same way as HL. As a generalization, low-grade lymphomas are slowly progressive but incurable, while high-grade tumours advance rapidly but are susceptible to aggressive chemotherapy.

The aetiology of NHL is largely unknown, although a number of viruses are closely associated with some categories, for example EBV and Burkitt lymphoma (see SST), human herpes virus 8 (HHV8) and primary body cavity lymphoma in HIV patients, hepatitis virus C and primary splenic lymphomas and human lymphotropic virus 1(HTLV1) and T-cell lymphoma/leukaemia in adults. *Helicobacter pylori* has an aetiological role in primary gastric B-cell lymphomas. The incidence of lymphoma in autoimmune conditions is higher than normal.

B-cell Lymphomas

These are tumours of B cells at various stages of differentiation, which largely correspond to the stages of normal B-cell maturation. The major forms of B-cell lymphoma include the following.

Follicular Lymphoma (FL)

These are tumours derived from germinal centre (follicle centre) cells, and they at least partially retain a follicular architecture. FL usually arises within lymph nodes, and at presentation is often found to be disseminated with involvement of multiple nodes, spleen and bone marrow. The cells are a mixture of small cleaved centrocytes and larger centroblasts, with the number of the latter determining the grade. Lower-grade tumours are indolent but seldom curable and will transform into a more aggressive form, diffuse large cell lymphoma, in 25% of cases (see Case History 8.2). A proportion of grade 3 tumours is potentially curable by chemotherapy. The follicle centre cells in FL express the antiapoptotic protein bcl2 as a result of the t(14;18) translocation, and this promotes cell proliferation (Figure 8.14).

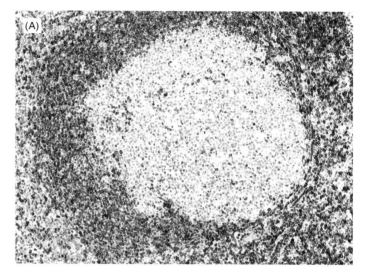

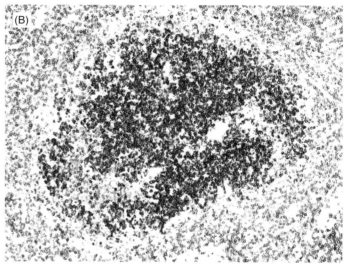

FIGURE 8.14 Immunostaining for bcl2. (A) Reactive follicle: the germinal centre (GC) cells are negative. A small number of intrafollicular T-cells are positive. (B) In contrast, the GC cells in the neoplastic follicle in follicular lymphoma are strongly positive. Overexpression is a consequence of the t(14;18) translocation where the promoters on the IgH gene on chromosome 14 cause transcription of the bcl2 gene on chromosome 18 and is a useful tool to distinguish between reactive and malignant follicular lesions.

FOLLICULAR LYMPHOMA

A 61-year-old woman presented to the ENT department with a 3-month history of a swelling on the left side of her neck. She also complained of weight loss of 4 kg. A clinical examination revealed multiple enlarged lymph nodes on the left side of her neck. A fine-needle aspirate of the node was performed at the clinic by the consultant cytologist, and this showed a pattern highly suspicious of a low grade non-Hodgkin lymphoma (NHL). A formal excision biopsy of the lymph node was performed under general anaesthesia 4 days later. This revealed the typical features of a grade 1 follicular lymphoma (Figure 8.15A, B). Immunophenotyping carried out by immunocytochemistry on the paraffin-embedded material supported this diagnosis (see Table 8.8).

TABLE 8.8 Immunocytochemistry results

Antibody	CD3	CD5	CD10	CD20	CD23	bcl2	CyclinD1
Case 1	–	–	+	+	–	+	–

The patient was referred to the local haematologist who specialized in haemato-oncology. A staging computed tomography (CT) scan revealed bilateral cervical and axillary lymphadenopathy in addition to a 12-cm para-aortic nodal mass near the pancreas. Extensive paratrabecular lymphomatous infiltration was noted on bone marrow trephine biopsy (Figure 8.16). The patient was informed of her diagnosis and that the disease was involving multiple sites including the bone marrow (Ann Arbor

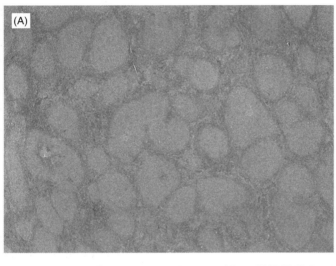

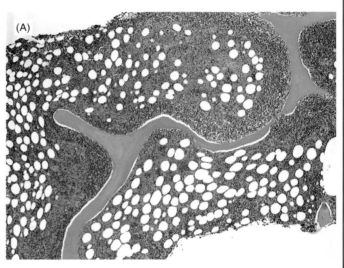

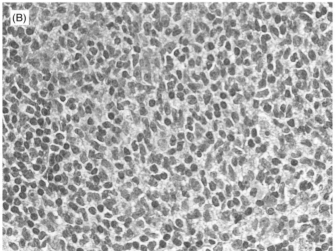

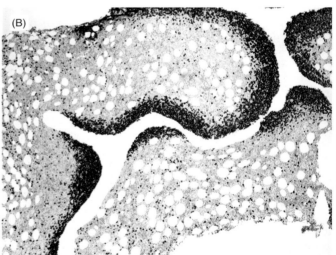

FIGURE 8.15 (A) Low-power view of the lymph node biopsy: the node is replaced by numerous follicular structures. At high power (B), there is a mixture of germinal centre-type cells comprising large cells (centroblasts) and smaller cells with a cleaved nucleus (centrocytes). Tingible body macrophages are absent. This pattern is characteristic of follicular lymphoma. The number of large cells is less than 5 per high-power field and therefore the lesion is regarded as grade 1.

FIGURE 8.16 The bone marrow is extensively involved by follicular lymphoma. (A) This low-power H&E view shows a band of small lymphoid cells involving the area immediately adjacent to the bony trabecula (paratrabecular). (B) A parallel section is stained for CD20 (a B-lymphocyte marker) by immunocytochemistry, thus confirming the B-cell nature of the infiltrate.

Stage 4B). It was explained that whilst it was unlikely that this low-grade lymphoma could be cured, much could be done to alleviate the symptoms and bring about a temporary remission.

The patient was treated with a chemotherapeutic regimen, and this resulted in disappearance of the cervical and axillary nodes. Cervical lymphadenopathy recurred after a further 3 years, and a further course of

chemotherapy was required. Two years later, the patient developed a rapidly growing para-aortic abdominal mass which involved the porta hepatis and caused obstructive jaundice that was complicated by ascending cholangitis and septicaemia. It was suspected that high-grade transformation had occurred. The patient died as a consequence of the septicaemia at 66 months after the initial presentation.

Small Lymphocytic Lymphoma/Chronic Lymphocytic Leukaemia

This disorder of the elderly frequently arises in the bone marrow, and most commonly presents with a raised peripheral small lymphocyte count, i.e. that is, chronic lymphocytic leukaemia. The spleen, liver and lymph nodes are usually enlarged, and bone marrow failure eventually occurs late in the disease. In 5% of cases the patient presents with lymphadenopathy only, with no leukaemic component. This is a low-grade tumour, but it may be accompanied by immunological impairment and autoimmune disease, and occasionally is complicated by high-grade transformation (Richter syndrome). Cytogenetic abnormalities provide useful prognostic information; for example, 17p13 deletion is associated with a more aggressive disease. The median survival is 7 years.

Mantle Cell Lymphoma

As the name suggests, this tumour is thought to arise from cells of the mantle zone of the follicle. Often a nodal tumour, it may also arise in the gastrointestinal tract, but quickly becomes disseminated so that most patients present with Stage III or IV disease (see Case History 8.3). Hepatosplenomegaly and marrow involvement are common. The tumour is characterized by a translocation t(11;14) (q13;q32) which leads to overexpression of the *cyclinD1* gene, which in turn leads to cell progression from G_1 to S phase in the cell cycle. Despite an apparent 'low-grade' appearance this lymphoma has, despite therapy, a poor median survival of only 3 years.

MANTLE CELL LYMPHOMA

A 69-year-old man presented to the accident and emergency department with a 2-day history of bleeding per rectum. He also admitted to a 2-month history of general malaise and some weight loss. On examination, he was found to have cervical lymphadenopathy. A full blood count revealed an iron-deficiency anaemia (Hb 9.6 g/dL)

in addition to a mild lymphocytosis. The initial clinical impression was of colonic carcinoma with metastatic spread. A flexible sigmoidoscopy revealed multiple focally ulcerating polyps in the colon. An endoscopic biopsy was performed. The histology, immunophenotype and FISH result were diagnostic of mantle cell lymphoma (Figure 8.17A, B; Figure 8.18; also see Table 8.9).

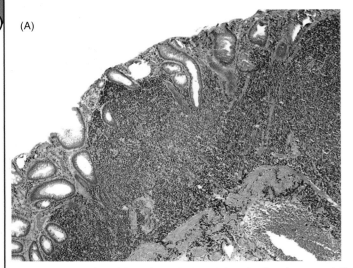

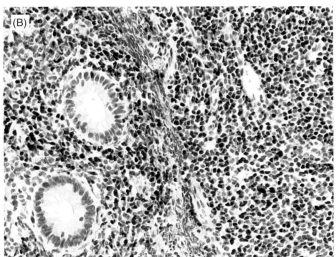

FIGURE 8.17 (A) H&E staining of colonic biopsy. There is a lymphomatous infiltrate within the mucosa and submucosa which is composed of a diffuse infiltrate of lymphoid cells resembling centrocytes. (B) Immunocytochemistry for *cyclinD1*. There is nuclear expression of *cyclinD1* in the neoplastic lymphoid population (not normally seen in other types of lymphoma).

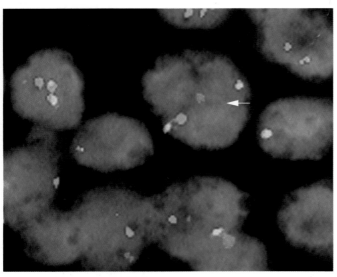

FIGURE 8.18 Fluorescence *in-situ* hybridization (FISH) for the t(11;14) translocation is performed on a 1 μm paraffin section from the biopsy. Red and green signals indicate the 11 and 14 chromosomes, respectively. In a cell containing a t(11;14) reciprocal translocation (arrowed), one red and one green signal (corresponding to the normal chromosomes) and two fusion signals (where the red and green probes are brought together by the translocation giving rise to emission of yellow light) are seen.

TABLE 8.9 Immunocytochemical profile of the lymphoma: the coexpression of CD5 by the CD20-positive B cells and nuclear positivity for cyclinD1 is characteristic of MCL

Antibody	CD3	CD5	CD10	CD20	CD23	Bcl2	CyclinD1
Case 2	–	+	–	+	–	+	+

Staging CT scan revealed lymphadenopathy in the cervical, axillary, intrathoracic, abdominal para-aortic and iliac regions. There was also bilateral tonsillar enlargement. A bone marrow trephine biopsy showed diffuse infiltration by lymphoma.

This patient therefore had presented with stage 4B mantle cell lymphoma. Extranodal involvement is not unusual in this lymphoma and the pattern of colonic involvement with multiple polyps is well described, so-called 'lymphomatous polyposis'. Despite the small cell size, this is an aggressive lymphoma. As expected, the patient responded only transiently to chemotherapy and died from the disease 9 months after the first presentation.

Extranodal Marginal Zone Lymphoma

Most extranodal lymphomas (e.g. in the stomach and thyroid) are in this category. They usually develop against a background of reactive lymphoid proliferations due either to infections (e.g. *Helicobacter pylori*; p. 243) or to autoimmune disease (e.g. Hashimoto's thyroiditis). Most patients present with localized disease and experience an indolent course and prolonged disease-free intervals. Interestingly, regression of early gastric lymphomas occurs in a significant number of cases following the eradication of *H. pylori* by antibiotics. Transformation to high-grade tumours may occur. Similar tumours can arise within lymph nodes.

Diffuse Large B-cell Lymphoma

This is the most common type of non-Hodgkin lymphomas in Western countries. These tumours arise in nodal and extranodal sites usually *de novo*, but sometimes they evolve from low-grade lymphomas. They tend to present with expansive and invasive lesions, which initially remain localized, but rapidly spread to adjacent lymph nodes and become widely disseminated (Figure 8.19). Approximately 50% are curable with appropriate chemotherapy. Much work is being directed at identifying at presentation those tumours that will not be cured by standard chemotherapy. BCL2 expression is regarded as a poor prognostic factor. Recently, the expression pattern of approximately 12 000 genes was examined using gene array technology. As a result, two patterns – a germinal centre and an activated B-cell pattern – were identified, the former being more often

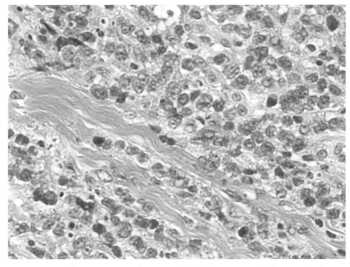

FIGURE 8.19 Diffuse large B-cell lymphoma. The lymph node is completely replaced by a diffuse infiltrate of large lymphoid blast cells.

associated with a good outcome. In the future, it is likely that further molecular research will identify factors that will determine choice of therapy in individual cases.

Burkitt Lymphoma

This highly aggressive B-cell tumour is found mainly – but not exclusively – in tropical parts of the globe. This endemic form mainly affects young children and has a distinctive extranodal pattern of growth involving in particular the jaws in males and the ovaries in females. Patients are at risk of developing central nervous system involvement. The characteristically rapid growth of the tumour is reflected in the high mitotic rate and the 100% labelling of the tumour cells with the proliferation marker Ki-67 (which labels those cells in cell cycle, but not those in G_0). There is a high apoptotic rate, and the numerous macrophages ingesting apoptotic debris account for the typical 'starry sky' histological appearance (Figure 8.20).

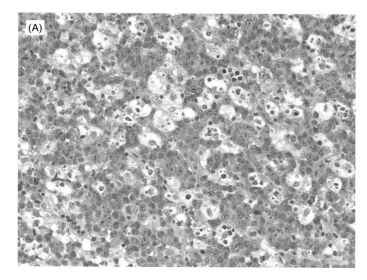

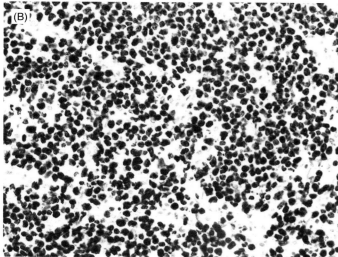

FIGURE 8.20 Burkitt lymphoma. (A) Diffuse infiltrate of small blast cells in addition to numerous macrophages with abundant pale cytoplasm phagocytosing cellular debris. (B) Almost 100% of tumour cells display nuclear positivity for the proliferation marker Ki67.

Epstein–Barr virus has an important role in the development of Burkitt lymphoma, and its genome is found in the cells in most endemic cases. Both endemic and sporadic variants are characterized by a translocation involving chromosome 8 which causes deregulation of the C-MYC gene, resulting in cell proliferation. Intensive chemotherapeutic

regimens have led to a cure rate of 60–90% depending on stage in this highly aggressive lymphoma.

These tumours and their characteristic immunoprofile and chromosomal rearrangements are summarized in Table 8.7.

T-cell Lymphomas

These account for 10–14% of all lymphomas in Western countries. In general, they are difficult to treat and carry a poor prognosis. Some present with lymphadenopathy, but they may be leukaemic at early stages and not infrequently arise in extranodal sites such as skin and bowel. Adults are most often affected.

In the past, T-cell lymphomas have been difficult to classify, and many are now included under the general category of peripheral T-cell lymphoma, unspecified. Most of these are nodal tumours showing as a rule a pleomorphic cellular picture due to varying admixtures of small lymphoid elements and transformed cells (immunoblasts) with a correspondingly unpredictable, but usually poor, prognosis.

Some T-cell tumours, however, present as distinctive clinicopathological entities.

T-cell Prolymphocytic Lymphoma

This usually presents with a high peripheral T-lymphocyte count, hepatosplenomegaly and skin infiltration. It is much more aggressive than B-CLL; the median survival is less than 1 year.

Mycosis Fungoides (MF)

This tumour presents as a skin rash (p. 505), initially with patches and plaques and later with nodules. Histologically there is infiltration of dermis and epidermis by CD4+ T cells. It can be difficult to diagnosis in its early stages as it can resemble dermatitis. MF tends to be indolent in its behaviour, at least initially. A minority of patients develop high-grade transformation and die as a consequence.

Sézary Syndrome

Possibly a variant of MF, this is characterized by erythroderma, lymphadenopathy and circulating neoplastic lymphocytes with an atypical 'cerebriform' nucleus. It is aggressive, and has a poor survival rate.

Angioimmunoblastic T-cell Lymphoma

Adults in later life are usually affected by this tumour which causes widespread lymphadenopathy, hepatosplenomegaly and striking systemic symptoms such as fever, weight loss, haemolytic anaemia and skin rashes. Hypergammaglobulinaemia may be a feature. The outlook is poor despite treatment.

Adult T-cell Leukaemia/Lymphoma

This is found mainly in the Far East, and is associated with viral infection (HTLV1). It varies in behaviour, but is generally aggressive. Usually it presents with lymphadenopathy, hepatosplenomegaly, leukaemic changes and skin rashes. There may be lytic bone lesions and associated hypercalcaemia.

Enteropathy-type T-cell Lymphoma

This is a tumour of the small bowel arising from intraepithelial T lymphocytes which, as a rule, is associated with coeliac disease. It is often highly aggressive, and usually presents with bowel obstruction or perforation (Figure 8.21). The majority of patients presenting with this tumour have no antecedent history of coeliac disease, but are found to have evidence of subclinical disease during investigations for their lymphoma.

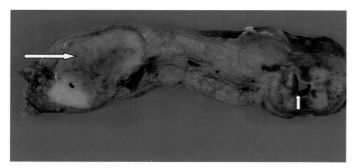

FIGURE 8.21 Cross-section of small bowel and mesentery in enteropathy-type T-cell lymphoma complicating coeliac disease. The patient presented with small bowel obstruction and malabsorption. Note the markedly narrowed bowel lumen (short arrow) and the involved lymph node within the mesentery (long arrow).

Anaplastic Large-cell Lymphoma

This lymphoma is composed of large pleomorphic cells which express the lymphocyte activation marker CD30. These tumours may show a translocation t(2;5)(p23;35) with expression of the chimaeric protein derived from the *ALK* gene (a tyrosine kinase receptor). The 5-year survival of treated ALK-positive tumours is 80%, in contrast to only 40% in ALK-negative cases. A primary cutaneous variant, negative for t(2;5) occurs, and has a very good prognosis.

Metastatic Tumours

It cannot be overemphasized that tumours found in lymph nodes are more often metastatic than primary (Figure 8.22). Almost all carcinomas tend to spread initially by the lymphatic system, and some non-epithelial tumours such as melanoma and, much less commonly, sarcomas can behave in a similar way. Lymph node enlargement is therefore a feature commonly associated with these tumours, and may indeed be the first indication of their presence; a carcinoma of the stomach may be diagnosed after the appearance of an enlarged supraclavicular lymph node (Troissier's sign). It needs to be stressed that lymphadenopathy does not equate with metastatic disease and may be reactive in nature. It is therefore important to examine these nodes histologically or cytologically for confirmation. If the nearest regional node, the sentinel node, is clear of tumour, this is a good sign.

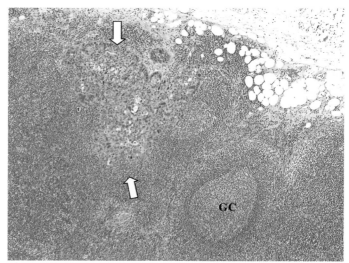

FIGURE 8.22 A deposit of metastatic adenocarcinoma is present in the subcapsular sinus of this lymph node (between arrows). GC = germinal centre.

DISEASES OF THE THYMUS

Key Points

- The thymus is responsible for T-lymphocyte development.
- Enlargement is often asymptomatic, but can cause superior vena cava obstruction.
- Thymic hyperplasia is often associated with autoimmune diseases, especially myasthenia gravis.
- Thymoma is an epithelial tumour, which may be locally aggressive.
- Lymphoma and germ cell tumours may involve the thymus.

The thymus lies in the superior anterior mediastinum, overlying the pericardium. It is basically an epithelial structure, the cortical part being derived from ectoderm and the medulla from the endoderm of the third and fourth branchial pouches. Within the microenvironment of the cortex, T-lymphocyte precursors of bone marrow origin undergo antigen-independent proliferation and development. This process is maximal in childhood, the thymus enlarging from infancy until puberty, and then gradually decreasing throughout adult life. Failure of development of the epithelial component results in severe immunodeficiency (Di George syndrome).

Thymic Enlargement

Thymic enlargement is an uncommon clinical finding and may be found only on routine chest X-radiography. Occasionally, a rapidly enlarging thymus may compress the superior vena cava and threaten life. The main causes of thymic enlargement are listed in Table 8.10.

TABLE 8.10 Major causes of thymic enlargement

Follicular hyperplasia, associated with:
  Myasthenia gravis
  Systemic lupus erythematosus
  Rheumatoid arthritis
Tumours:
  Thymoma
  Thymic carcinoma
  Lymphoma (Hodgkin lymphoma, T-lymphoblastic, mediastinal large B cell)
  Germ cell tumours (seminoma, teratoma)

Non-neoplastic thymic enlargement is usually due to the presence of lymphoid follicles with germinal centres within the medulla – a phenomenon related in most instances to autoimmune diseases and especially to myasthenia gravis (p. 371). Removal of the thymus often results in remission of the disease.

Thymic Tumours

Thymoma is a primary epithelial tumour of the thymus which behaves like a low-grade carcinoma, invading surrounding structures but seldom metastasizing (less than 10% of cases). The lesion consists of epithelial cells often interspersed with so many thymic lymphocytes that it can be misdiagnosed as a lymphoma. While often found incidentally, thymoma may be associated with myasthenia gravis, pure red cell aplasia, hypogammaglobulinaemia and autoimmune diseases such as polymyositis. Several forms of lymphoma may affect the thymus, most notably classical Hodgkin lymphoma and mediastinal large B-cell lymphoma, both typically in young women. T-lymphoblastic leukaemia which usually occurs in childhood may present with a large anterior mediastinal mass. Germ cell tumours, similar to those found in the gonads, can arise at this site.

DISEASES OF THE SPLEEN

Key Points

- The spleen removes effete blood cells and foreign material from the blood.
- Moderate splenomegaly in the Western world is often due to portal hypertension or blood diseases.
- Massive splenomegaly in the Western world is usually due to haemopoietic neoplasia, and in the tropics to infections (e.g. malaria, leishmaniasis).
- Hypersplenism results in pancytopenia.
- Removal of the spleen results in susceptibility to disseminated pneumococcal infection.

In normal adult life the spleen weighs 120–160 g, and is the only lymphatic tissue specialized to filter the blood. This function is intimately related to its structure, and particularly to its vascular arrangements (Figure 8.23). The spleen removes foreign materials, microorganisms and time-expired and otherwise abnormal red blood cells. It can also remove inclusion bodies (e.g. residual DNA, denatured haemoglobin) from red cells. The spleen has important immunological functions, and has a major role in counteracting blood infection, largely by producing IgM. Enlargement of the spleen and a reduction in its size or its surgical removal may have important clinical effects.

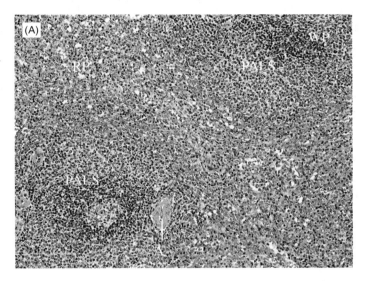

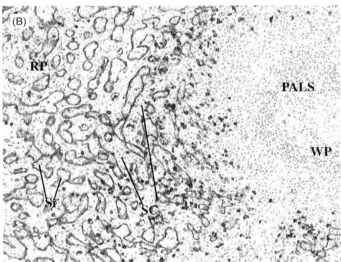

FIGURE 8.23 Microanatomy and function of the spleen. (A) High-power view of the spleen (this field is 2 mm in diameter). (B) Immunocytochemical staining of spleen for CD8, highlighting the CD8+ splenic sinusoidal lining cells. The spleen contains white pulp (WP) which consists of periarteriolar lymphoid sheaths (PALS) comprising both T and B lymphocytes, and the red pulp (RP) which acts as a filter for the blood. Blood leaves the arterioles, enters sinusoids (Si), flows through fenestrae in the sinusoidal lining cells, percolates through the cellular splenic cords (SC) containing macrophages and fibroblasts, and eventually reaches the efferent capillaries. Effete and damaged red cells are removed from the circulation within the splenic cords.

Splenic Enlargement

Splenic enlargement has many causes, the most important of which are summarized in Table 8.11. Worldwide, protozoal infections (e.g. malaria) represent the most important cause of massive splenomegaly. In the Western world, this is usually due to myeloproliferative disorders (Figure 8.24) and chronic lymphocytic leukaemia, though other rarer causes such as Gaucher's disease (p. 215) may also be responsible. Moderate

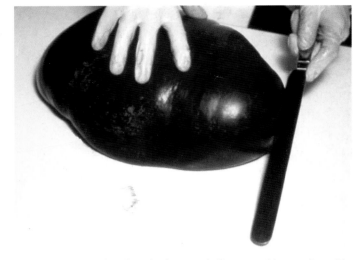

FIGURE 8.24 Massively enlarged spleen surgically removed from patient with chronic idiopathic myelofibrosis.

enlargement occurs in chronic bacterial and viral infections, portal hypertension, the haemolytic anaemias and some lymphomas. Most lymphomatous involvement of the spleen is secondary, though true primary lymphomas do occur, for example splenic marginal zone lymphoma (Figure 8.25). Metastatic carcinoma or melanoma rarely involve the spleen.

TABLE 8.11 Causes of splenomegaly

Hereditary causes	
Storage disease	Gaucher's disease
	Niemann–Pick disease
Haemolytic anaemia	Sickle cell disease
	Congenital spherocytosis
	Thalassaemia
Infective causes	
Protozoal	Malaria
	Leishmaniasis
	Schistosomiasis
Bacterial	Tuberculosis
	Secondary syphilis
	Bacterial endocarditis
	Brucellosis
Viral	Infectious mononucleosis
Fungal	Histoplasmosis
Tumour	
Lymphoma	Chronic lymphocytic leukaemia
	Lymphoplasmacytic lymphoma
	Splenic marginal zone lymphoma
	Classical Hodgkin lymphoma
Myeloproliferative disorders	Chronic myeloid leukaemia
	Idiopathic myelofibrosis
	Polycythaemia vera
Metastatic tumours	Carcinoma (rarely metastasizes to spleen)
Non-neoplastic haematological conditions	
	Haemolytic anaemia
	Autoimmune idiopathic thrombocytopenia
Vascular	
Portal hypertension	Cirrhosis
	Portal vein thrombosis
	Budd–Chiari syndrome
Autoimmune	Systemic lupus erythematosus
	Felty's syndrome
Miscellaneous	Sarcoidosis
	Amyloidosis
	Idiopathic splenomegaly

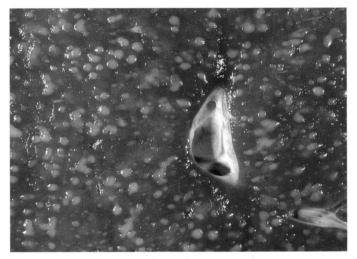

FIGURE 8.25 Cut surface of spleen showing expansion of periarteriolar lymphoid sheaths by splenic marginal zone lymphoma.

Clinical Effects

Usually, the first indication of splenomegaly is that the spleen becomes palpable on examination. When enlargement is substantial there may be abdominal discomfort and even pain, although this is usually due to infarction which often occurs in a spleen enlarged for any cause. More importantly, when a spleen exceeds approximately 1 kg, there is increased sequestration and premature destruction of the formed elements of the blood (hypersplenism), resulting in pancytopenia and compensatory marrow hyperplasia. Splenic rupture – either spontaneously or with minimal trauma – is a serious complication occurring particularly in infectious mononucleosis.

Hyposplenism

Hyposplenism occurs most often as a result of splenectomy. Congenital absence may be associated with cardiac anomalies such as dextrocardia. Atrophy of the spleen is seen in coeliac disease as part of generalized immunodeficiency, and in sickle cell disease due to progressive microvascular occlusion. Splenic hypofunction is usually evident from examination of the peripheral blood in which there is an accumulation of abnormal red cells and inclusions (e.g. Howell–Jolly bodies) which are usually removed by the spleen. Splenectomy – both in childhood and adult life – predisposes to severe infections, especially with pneumococci.

DISEASES OF THE BONE MARROW

From approximately 7 months of foetal life, the bone marrow is entirely responsible for haemopoeisis. Diseases involving the marrow result in two basic effects for the patient:

- a deficiency of one or more of the cell lines producing anaemia, agranulocytosis or thrombocytopenia, causing fatigue, increased susceptibility to infection and a bleeding tendency, respectively
- an overproduction of cells as a result of neoplastic transformation of a stem cell causing an increase in circulating cells (i.e. leukaemia).

Frequently both effects coexist. Much can be learned regarding marrow function by close examination of a peripheral blood film. However, a full assessment requires aspiration and trephine biopsy of bone marrow from the iliac crest.

Normal Haemopoiesis

Normal haemopoiesis (Figure 8.26) is the process by which pluripotent stem cells develop into all the different lineages while at the same time maintaining their numbers by self-renewal so that production can go on throughout the life of the individual. In normal individuals, the marrow is composed of a mixture of fatty and haemopoeitic components, the ratio of which varies with age. An infant's marrow is almost 100% haemopoeitic, while in the elderly this value is closer to 30% (Figure 8.27).

Disorders of Red Blood Cells

This group of disorders comprises the anaemias (reduced haemoglobin), polycythaemia (increased haemoglobin) and a group of miscellaneous conditions resulting in the occurrence of red cell inclusions. The normal blood smear

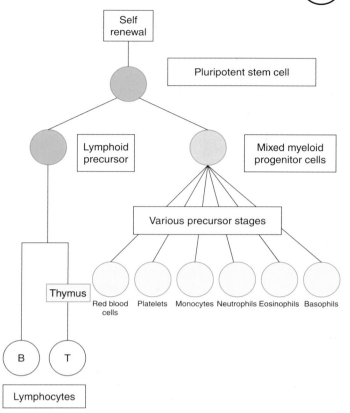

FIGURE 8.26 Simplified diagram of normal haemopoiesis. The pluripotent stem cell in the marrow gives rise to a number of progenitor cells that in turn proliferate and differentiate to produce all the cellular constituents of blood, including lymphoid cells. This process is controlled by various growth factors, produced by a range of cells including lymphocytes and endothelial cells, the secretion of which is partially dependent on environmental factors; for example hypoxia induces erythropoietin secretion, resulting in increased red cell production. The marrow stroma provides the appropriate environment for stem cells to grow and proliferate. The stem cell, which is capable of producing approximately 10^6 mature blood cells, is also capable of self renewal.

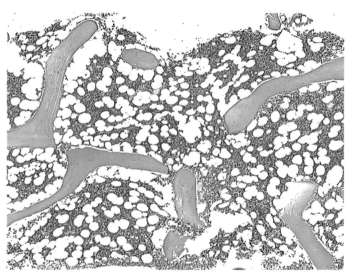

FIGURE 8.27 Trephine biopsy of ileum from a normal adult. The cellular haemopoietic red marrow accounts for 40–50% of the marrow space. The remainder consists of fat cells.

contains biconcave erythrocytes of uniform size and shape measuring 7 μm in diameter (Figure 8.28). The normal haemoglobin (Hb) concentration is 13.5–17.5 g/dL for males, and 11.5–15.5 g/dL for females.

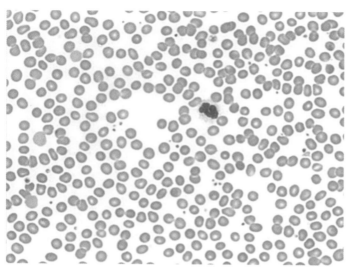

FIGURE 8.28 The normal blood film. Contrast this with the abnormal smears on the following pages.

The Anaemias

Key Points

- Anaemia is defined by a haemoglobin concentration below the normal range.
- Anaemia may be caused by insufficient production of red cells or excess loss or destruction.
- The causes of anaemia correlate with the appearances of peripheral blood and bone marrow.

A shortage of red blood cells (RBCs) may occur due to insufficient production, or to excessive destruction or loss. The clinical symptoms and signs will depend on the severity of the anaemia and on the speed at which it has developed. Low oxygen tension in the tissues will usually manifest itself by fatigue, dizziness, palpitations and, when severe, by angina or cardiac failure. In long-standing anaemia, compensatory erythropoiesis – driven by erythropoietin produced in response to hypoxia – will cause replacement of fatty marrow by haemopoietic marrow and may even cause thinning of the bone cortex. The major forms of anaemia are listed in Table 8.12. Investigation requires estimation of total Hb concentration and microscopic examination of a

TABLE 8.12 An aetiological classification of anaemia

1. Blood loss	Acute or chronic	
2. Increased erythrocyte destruction (haemolytic)	(a) Intrinsic red blood cell (RBC) defect	*Congenital* Thalassaemia, RBC enzyme deficiencies Abnormal haemoglobins, e.g. sickle cell disease RBC membrane defects, e.g. hereditary spherocytosis
	(b) Factors extrinsic to RBC	*Acquired* Paroxysmal nocturnal haemaglobinaemia Autoimmune haemolytic anaemia Haemolytic disease of the newborn Drugs/chemicals Microangiopathic haemolytic anaemia Hypersplenism Mechanical factors
	(c) Combined	G6PD deficiency Red cell instability caused by exposure to oxidizing agents
3. Inadequate RBC production	(a) Deficiency states (b) Anaemia of chronic disease	Iron, vitamin B$_{12}$, folate, protein Connective tissue disorders Renal failure Liver failure
	(c) Primary bone marrow failure	Aplastic anaemia Selective red cell aplasia
	(d) Bone marrow infiltration	Carcinoma, lymphoma, myeloma Leukaemias
	(e) Myelodysplastic conditions	e.g. Sideroblastic anaemia
	(f) Storage diseases	Gaucher's disease

TABLE 8.13 Red blood cell indices in the common anaemias

	Iron deficiency	B₁₂/folate deficiency	Anaemia of chronic disease	Hereditary spherocytosis	Thalassaemia
Cell size	↓	↑	N or ↓	↓	↓
Hypochromasia	+ +	0	0 or +	0	+ + +
Poikilocytosis	+ +	+ + +	+	0	+ + +
Hb (g/dL)	↓	↓	↓	↓	↓
MCV	↓	↑	N or ↓	↓	↓
MCH	↓	N or ↑	N	N	↓
MCHC	↓	N	N	↑	↓

Hb = haemoglobin concentration; MCV = mean corpuscular volume; MCH = mean corpuscular haemoglobin; MCHC = mean corpuscular haemoglobin concentration.
↑ = increase; ↓ = decrease; N = normal; + = present; + + = prominent; + + + = very prominent.

blood film which may reveal reduction in staining intensity (hypchromasia), change in size (anisocytosis) and changes in shape (poikilocytosis) of the RBCs. Red cell parameters can be determined accurately by modern automated equipment providing essential information in determining aetiology of the anaemias (Table 8.13). Subtle variations in these indices can occur prior to a drop in the blood haemoglobin concentration facilitating early diagnosis.

Iron-deficiency Anaemia

Key Points

Iron-deficiency anaemia is:
- a hypochromic microcytic anaemia
- most often caused by prolonged blood loss
- common in women of reproductive age
- may be the first sign of an occult gastrointestinal carcinoma
- hookworm infestation is a common cause in much of the world.

This condition is one of the most common forms of anaemia, and results from chronic blood loss or insufficient iron uptake. In women of reproductive age, menstrual blood loss is the usual explanation. It may also result from chronic gastrointestinal tract bleeding, for example from a chronic peptic ulcer or an occult caecal or gastric carcinoma. In some parts of the world helminthic infections (e.g. hookworm infestation) are important. Iron deficiency may result from a diet which is low in iron, or from malabsorption, for example in coeliac disease. Achlorhydria also aggravates poor iron uptake.

In iron-deficiency anaemia, the bone marrow shows erythroid hyperplasia and there is a loss of stainable iron stores. Haemoglobin synthesis is impaired and red cell precursors are incompletely haemoglobinized. As a consequence, the erythrocytes in the peripheral blood are small and pale (Figure 8.29). Iron deficiency is the prototype of a hypochromic/microcytic anaemia (low mean corpuscular volume [MCV], low mean corpuscular haemoglobin [MCH]). In addition, blood chemistry data will reveal low serum iron, low ferritin level, and undersaturation of transferrin, i.e. an increased iron-binding capacity.

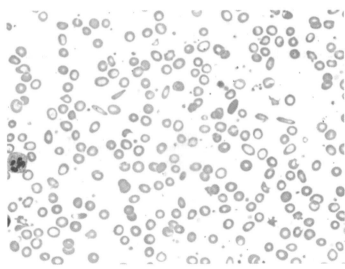

FIGURE 8.29 Blood film in iron-deficiency anaemia. Note the hypochromic and microcytic red blood cells and pencil-shaped poikilocytes.

Anaemia of Chronic Disease

This condition is related to iron deficiency as it is caused by the inability of the body to mobilize iron from the macrophages where most of it is stored. It occurs as a complication of chronic infection, rheumatoid arthritis or malignancy. The anaemia persists as long as the underlying condition is present. Unlike iron deficiency, the bone marrow shows no or only mild erythroid hyperplasia and there is sufficient stainable iron. There is a low serum iron level, but reduced iron binding capacity and normal or raised ferritin.

Disorders of Lymphocytes

Lymphopenia

Lymphopenia, a reduction in peripheral lymphocyte numbers, is normal in the elderly. It may occur in immunodeficiency disease such as HIV infection in which the number of CD4+ cells is low. Lymphopenia can also occur in autoimmune diseases such as SLE, in some acute infections, and following treatment with steroids and cytotoxic drugs.

Lymphocytosis

A lymphocytosis, increased peripheral lymphocytes, is normal in the first year of life. In older children and adults, reactive lymphocytosis is usually caused by viral infections. Infectious mononucleosis causes a striking lymphocytosis with numerous very atypical forms which can raise the possibility of malignancy. The other main cause of lymphocytosis in adults is lymphomatous disorders such as chronic lymphocytic leukaemia and mantle cell lymphoma (see Case History 3).

Neoplastic Conditions of the Bone Marrow

> **Key Points**
>
> Primary:
> - leukaemia
> - myeloproliferative disorders
> - myelodysplasia
> - some lymphomas
> - plasma cell myeloma.
>
> Secondary:
> - metastatic malignancy
> - lymphomas.

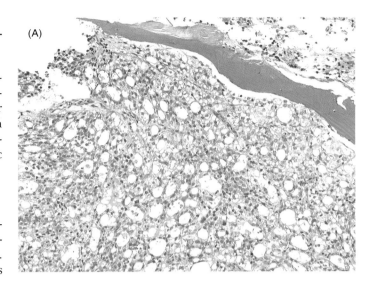

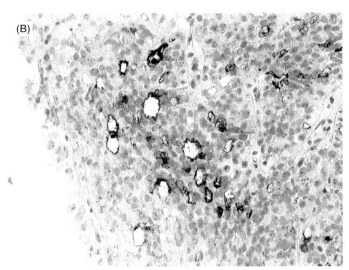

FIGURE 8.34 Bone marrow trephine biopsy in metastatic prostatic carcinoma. (A) Haematoxylin and eosin staining; (B) immunocytochemistry for prostate-specific antigen is positive, confirming an origin from the prostate.

Metastatic malignancy involving the bone marrow most commonly complicates carcinomas arising in lung, breast, thyroid, kidney and prostate (Figure 8.34). Malignant melanoma is another well-recognized cause. Marrow replacement gives rise to a leucoerythroblastic blood film (Figure 8.35), which may also be seen in storage diseases (Figure 8.36) and myelofibrosis. Low-grade lymphomas commonly involve the marrow (see Case Histories 2 and 3) and some primarily arise there.

Primary malignancies of the bone marrow are clonal stem cell disorders producing varying degrees of proliferation and differentiation. The acute leukaemias are tumours showing proliferation, but little if any differentiation. These tumours consist of primitive blast cells with a high proliferative rate as no cells leave the pool of dividing cells to differentiate. They are thus fast-growing and clinically aggressive. Those processes – characterized by proliferation and differentiation – are known as 'myeloproliferative disorders'. Both the bone marrow and peripheral blood are highly cellular, but all stages of differentiation are seen. Differentiation draws cells out of the dividing pool – hence the apparent proliferation rate is lower and the clinical course is more protracted. In the myelodysplastic syndromes there is proliferation and differentiation, but the latter is abnormal. The high rate of proliferation causes increased marrow cellularity, but the abnormal differentiation results in destruction of defective cells and so peripheral blood counts are low. Multiple myeloma – a tumour composed of mature plasma cells – typically arises in the bone marrow.

The Leukaemias

Leukaemia is defined as a tumour with an increased number of white cells in the peripheral blood. In a small proportion

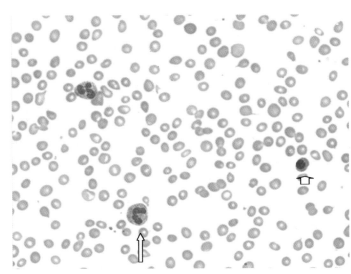

FIGURE 8.35 Leucoerythroblastic blood film: a nucleated red blood cell precursor (short arrow) and an immature granulocyte (long arrow) are present. Immature precursors are not normally seen in the peripheral blood but, when present, indicate replacement of the normal marrow and consequent extramedullary haemopoiesis. Tear-drop poikilocytes are also a feature.

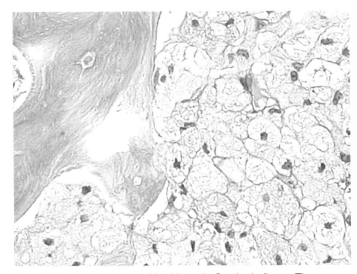

FIGURE 8.36 Bone marrow trephine biopsy in Gaucher's disease. The marrow is replaced by macrophages filled with glucocerebroside.

of cases the white cell count may not be raised, and this is the so-called 'aleukaemic leukaemia'. The acute leukaemias comprise acute myeloid leukaemia and acute lymphoblastic leukaemia, the latter now being classified with the lymphoproliferative disorders as it is derived from primitive precursor B or T lymphocytes (see Table 8.3 on p. 192). The chronic leukaemias include chronic myelogenous leukaemia, which is classified with the myeloproliferative disorders, and chronic lymphocytic leukaemia with the lymphoproliferative disorders (p. 192).

The Acute Leukaemias

Key Points

- Marrow is replaced by blast cells which spill into peripheral blood.
- The clinical effects are due largely to marrow replacement and marrow failure.
- The tumours are aggressive, but often susceptible to chemotherapy.
- Cytogenetic abnormalities have a prognostic importance.

Clinically, all acute leukaemias are similar in that their effects are due to bone marrow failure. The proliferating malignant cells crowd out the normal haemopoietic elements, leading to anaemia, infections and bleeding. The onset is often abrupt with fever, malaise and sometimes bone pain. Rarely, acute leukaemia involves tissues other than the bone marrow such as the skin and gingiva. Occasionally, infiltrating myeloid leukaemia cells produce a tumour mass (myeloid sarcoma) in soft tissue or beneath the periosteum. This usually occurs when leukaemia is manifest, but it may precede the onset of overt disease by months.

Diagnosis and classification involve an assessment of cell morphology by microscopy, cytochemistry, immunophenotyping performed by flow cytometry, and increasingly on genotyping. Without treatment, patients with acute leukaemia would die within weeks or months. Chemotherapy has greatly improved the outlook, especially in the lymphoblastic leukaemias of childhood. The acute myeloid leukaemias have a much poorer prognosis, and although most patients achieve complete remission, a significant proportion relapse and eventually die of the disease.

Acute Myeloid Leukaemia (AML)

AML is defined as a clonal expansion of myeloid blasts in bone marrow, blood or other tissue (Figure 8.37). The incidence among the UK population is 3 per 100 000, and the median age of onset is 60 years. Risk factors for AML include ionizing radiation, viruses, chemicals (e.g. benzene) and cytotoxic chemotherapy. Traditionally, AML has been classified morphologically by a system devised by French, American and British haematologists (FAB classification). The discovery of a number of genetic abnormalities that predict clinical behaviour better than morphology alone led to the modified classification produced by the WHO in 2001 (Table 8.14). The presence of a t(8;21)(q22;q22) or an inversion 16 is associated with an improved outcome. The t(15;17) defines a variety of AML (acute promyelocytic leukaemia) which has a high risk of association with DIC. Though the latter may be fatal, early recognition and treatment with the differentiating agent trans-retinoic acid, can control this complication. Those cases arising on a background of a myelodysplastic or myeloproliferative disorder

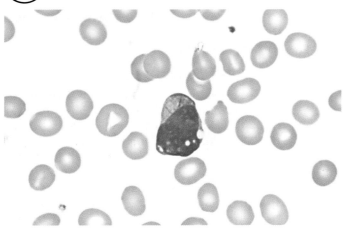

FIGURE 8.37 Blood film in acute myeloid leukaemia. A single blast cell containing an Auer rod (cytoplasmic crystalline structure specific for myeloid differentiation) is depicted.

TABLE 8.14 WHO classification of acute myeloid leukaemia (simplified version)

a) AML with recurrent cytogenetic abnormalities
t(8;21)(q22;q22)
inversion(16)(p13q22)
t (15;17), acute promyelocytic leukaemia
11q23 abnormalities
b) AML with multilineage dysplasia
c) AML/myelodysplastic syndrome – therapy-related
d) AML not otherwise categorized*
e.g. AML minimally differentiated
AML without maturation
Acute myelomonocytic leukaemia
Acute monoblastic leukaemia
Acute erythroid leukaemia
Acute megakaryoblastic leukaemia
Acute panmyelosis with myelofibrosis
Myeloid sarcoma

*Category 'd' is based on the FAB morphological classification and includes those cases not fitting into the other three categories.

tend to occur in older patients, and have a poorer prognosis. A significant proportion of long-term cancer survivors develop AML as a consequence of cytotoxic chemotherapy. The remaining cases are subdivided according to their morphology based on the FAB classification.

The diagnosis of AML requires the demonstration of more than 20% myeloid blasts in the blood or marrow. Differentiation from acute lymphoblastic leukaemia can be difficult on morphology alone, and immunophenotyping by flow cytometry is often required. The detailed laboratory techniques used in subclassifying these tumours is beyond the scope of this textbook.

Acute Lymphoblastic Leukaemia (ALL)

ALL is a clonal proliferation of lymphoid precursor B or T cells which usually results in an acute leukaemia, though sometimes it can produce lymph node or mediastinal enlargement in the absence of circulating blasts. The latter presentation is termed 'lymphoblastic lymphoma', though for management purposes this is regarded as being equivalent to ALL. In the UK the incidence is 4 per 100 000, and each year this results in approximately 450 new cases. ALL usually affects children, the median age of onset being between 4 and 7 years. The aetiology of the condition is largely unknown, though both genetic and environmental factors are felt to play a role.

ALL broadly falls into two main groups: those of B-cell and T-cell type. Diagnosis requires detailed immunophenotyping to establish whether the neoplastic cells are of B or T lineage, and to differentiate them from myeloid leukaemia. Immunoreactivity for the enzyme terminal deoxynucleotidyl transferase (TdT), distinguishes lymphoblasts from mature lymphocytes (Figure 8.38).

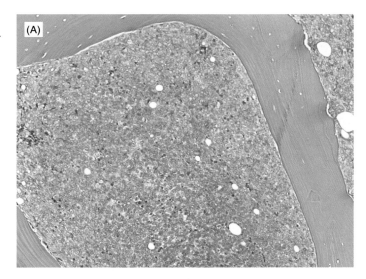

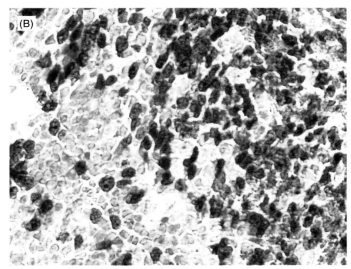

FIGURE 8.38 Trephine biopsy of bone marrow in acute lymphoblastic leukaemia. (A) The marrow cellularity is almost 100% and is replaced by an infiltrate of small blast cells. (B) Nuclear positivity for terminal deoxynucleotidyl transferase (TdT) is identified in the majority of cells by immunocytochemistry.

B-cell acute lymphoblastic leukaemia (B-ALL), representing 85% of cases, is predominantly a disorder of childhood but also affects adults. Patients present with symptoms and signs of marrow replacement (anaemia, infection, haemorrhage), bone pain, lymphadenopathy and splenomegaly. There is a tendency to involve other tissues, especially the central nervous system, with signs of raised intracranial pressure and cranial nerve palsies (especially VI and VII). Central nervous system involvement is a poor prognostic sign as treatment is difficult. The testes are also frequently involved. Cure can be achieved in 80% of children, and this represents one of the greatest achievements in cancer therapy during the past 30 years. Good prognostic factors for children are age between 4 and 10 years, a low leucocyte count at presentation, and hyperdiploid chromosomes or a t(12;21)(p13;q22). Adverse factors include age <1 year, and the t(9;22) and t(4;11) translocations. The survival rate for adults is less good.

Some 15% of ALL in children is due to T-lymphoblastic leukaemia/lymphoma, which tends to affect adolescent males and may present with a mass in the anterior mediastinum. Here, the tumour cells mimic the normal development of T lymphoblasts by migrating from the bone marrow to the thymus. Although initially associated with a poorer prognosis than B-ALL, modern therapies are producing a substantial cure rate in children.

Chronic Myeloproliferative Disorders

Key Points

- Clonal haemopoeitic stem cell disorders with effective haemopoeisis.
- Excess production of mature cells usually producing high peripheral counts.
- The clinical presentation varies depending on the predominant differentiated component.
- There can be overlap in clinical and laboratory features between the different subtypes.
- They may be complicated by gout.
- There is a risk of progression to acute leukaemia or myelofibrosis.

The chronic myeloproliferative disorders are clonal haemopoeitic stem cell disorders characterized by the proliferation of one or more of the myeloid lineages (granulocytic, erythroid or megakaryocytic) associated with relatively normal and effective maturation. This results in a raised peripheral white cell, red cell and/or platelet count. Although only one lineage may appear to be primarily involved (e.g. red cells in polycythaemia vera), all lineages are found to be abnormal on further investigation. This derangement at stem cell level is proven by the demonstration of chromosomal abnormalities in all lineages in one given disorder.

The aetiology is largely unknown, though association with exposure to benzene, ionizing radiation and genetic factors is recorded. The overall incidence is 6–9 per 100 000 population.

There are four main categories.

Chronic Myelogenous Leukaemia (CML)

CML results from a genetic abnormality at the level of the pluripotent stem cell. Its typical chromosomal abnormality – the Philadelphia chromosome (Ph) – can be found in all haemopoietic cells including the lymphoid series.

The disease occurs at any age, but usually in patients during their fifth and sixth decades of life. It has an incidence of 1.5 per 100 000 population.

The symptoms are mostly non-specific with fatigue, anorexia, weight loss and hepatomegaly. On occasion, abdominal swelling due to splenomegaly, often massive, is the presenting feature. Splenic infarction may lead to sudden abdominal pain. In approximately 30% of cases, the patient is asymptomatic and the diagnosis is made from a routine full blood count. This reveals anaemia and a markedly raised white cell count (often $>10 \times 10^9$/dL) composed mainly of myeloid cells of varying maturation (Figure 8.39). The bone marrow is hypercellular with a predominance of the granulocytic series, though there is often also an increase in

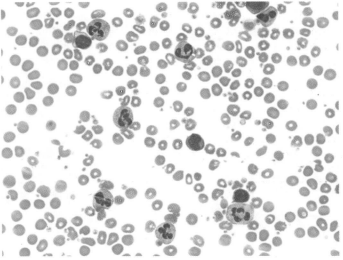

FIGURE 8.39 Blood film from patient with chronic myelogenous leukaemia (CML). There is a marked increase in the number of granulocytes compared to the normal blood film (see Figure 8.28).

megakaryocytes and erythroid precursors. Genetic studies reveal the translocation t(9;22)(q34;q11) in 95% of cases (Figure 8.40). The course of the disease is indolent for some years (chronic phase), but almost inevitably it evolves into an 'accelerated' phase, which becomes refractory to therapy. Blast crisis and evolution to acute leukaemia, either myeloid or lymphoblastic, may follow. The median survival is 3–4 years, with death occurring from acute transformation or from infection or haemorrhage. Chemotherapy is useful for controlling symptoms in the chronic phase, but does not affect overall survival. Bone marrow transplantation also has a role. Recently, a signal transduction inhibitor specifically targeting the pathways activated by bcr-abl has been developed (imatinib), and this is proving beneficial in clinical trials (Figure 8.40), notably as it also seems to be effective for gastrointestinal stromal tumours (p. 243).

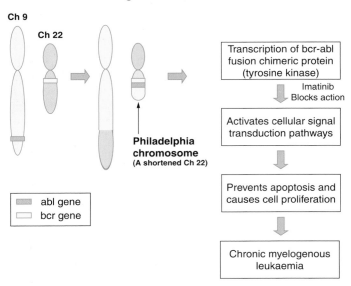

FIGURE 8.40 Cytogenetic abnormality in chronic myelogenous leukaemia (CML). This diagram depicts the classical t(9;22)(q34;q11) translocation associated with CML. This was the first cytogenetic abnormality ever detected in a human malignancy. There is a reciprocal translocation between the long arms of Ch 9 and Ch 22 bringing together the abl and bcr genes in the derivative Ch 22 (the Philadelphia chromosome).

Polycythaemia Vera

This condition is characterized by an increased red cell production and a lesser degree of proliferation of the myeloid and megakaryocytic lineages. It is more common among males, and the mean age of diagnosis is 60 years. The incidence is 0.8 per 100 000 population. The clinical symptoms are caused by the increase in red cell mass resulting in headache, tiredness, a plethoric complexion and itching, especially after hot baths. There is increased blood viscosity and a tendency to thrombosis leading to strokes, myocardial infarction and deep vein thrombosis. Sometimes, as the platelets produced are dysfunctional, there may be haemorrhage, especially from the gastrointestinal tract. The increased cell turnover may lead to gout. Splenomegaly is common.

The diagnosis is established by identifying both a raised haemoglobin concentration (>18.5 g/dL in men, >16.5 g/dL in women) and an increased red cell mass. Oxygen saturation is usually normal, and erythropoietin levels low, allowing distinction from secondary polycythaemia. Both the white cell and platelet counts are usually raised. The bone marrow is hypercellular due to proliferation of mainly erythroid and megakaryocyte series. The clinical course is usually prolonged, though regular venesection is required.

Death may result from vascular complications. In 15% of cases, myelofibrosis supervenes; another 5% evolve into acute myeloid leukaemia, particularly in those who have received chemotherapy.

Chronic Idiopathic Myelofibrosis

This is a clonal proliferation of mainly megakaryocytes and granulocytes associated with extensive fibrosis of the marrow which often prevents acquisition of an aspirate sample (a dry tap). This fibrosis is probably caused by the release of growth factors (e.g. platelet-derived growth factor) from the neoplastic megakaryocytes. The bones eventually become sclerotic. Haemopoiesis is displaced and there is extramedullary haemopoiesis primarily in the spleen, liver, lymph nodes and sometimes other organs. The peripheral blood shows a leucoerythroblastic reaction (see Figure 8.35). Splenomegaly may be massive, resulting in hypersplenism (see Figure 8.24). The incidence is less than 1 per 100 000 population per annum. Patients may present with vague symptoms of fatigue, night sweats and weight loss. Many are asymptomatic at diagnosis and come to light due to the detection of splenomegaly or abnormalities found on a routine blood film. The prognosis is poor (median survival 3–5 years), with many patients dying from infection, haemorrhage or bone marrow failure; acute myeloid leukaemia may supervene in 10%.

Essential Thrombocythaemia

In this condition, the megakaryocytic lineage is mainly involved resulting in sustained elevation of platelet counts, usually in excess of 600×10^9/L. Between 20% and 50% of patients present with either a thrombotic event or haemorrhage, the remainder being detected by a routine blood test. Otherwise, the disease is indolent, but may progress to myelofibrosis, and rarely to acute leukaemia.

The Myelodysplastic Syndromes (MDS)

This group of conditions is characterized by a clonal stem cell disorder causing bone marrow proliferation with abnormal differentiation resulting in ineffectual haemopoiesis in the face of a hypercellular marrow. Myelodysplasias present mainly in the elderly, with symptoms attributable to pancytopenia. As these conditions have a tendency to evolve into AML, they were formerly known as 'preleukaemias'. Myelodysplasia may be primary or occur secondary to previous chemotherapy or HIV infection. There are a number of subtypes with varying risks of leukaemic transformation.

Plasma Cell Myeloma

Key Points

- Monoclonal proliferation of plasma cells within bone marrow.
- Multifocal osteolytic bony lesions.
- Hypercalcaemia.
- Signs and symptoms of marrow replacement.

- Excess production of monoclonal immunoglobulin (M-protein in serum, Bence–Jones protein in urine).
- May be complicated by AL amyloidosis.
- Many patients present with acute renal failure.

Plasma cell myeloma is a malignant tumour arising in the bone marrow, and is composed entirely of monoclonal plasma cells. It is one of the most common haematological malignancies, and affects adults with an incidence of 10 per 100 000 of the population per annum. The median age of diagnosis is 68 years. Chemicals, viruses and ionizing radiation have been reported as aetiological factors, though none is identified in the majority of cases. Myeloma affects the patient by several mechanisms. First, by the direct effects of the tumour eroding bones – especially those of the vertebral column, ribs and skull; this results in pain, pathological fractures and vertebral collapse. Second, by causing replacement of the marrow resulting in pancytopenia with consequent immunosuppression, thrombocytopenia and anaemia. The third mechanism is related to the secretory product of the neoplastic plasma cells. Neoplastic plasma cells – like their normal counterparts – are capable of producing immunoglobulin, and almost all cases are associated with a serum or urine monoclonal gammaglobulin, the M-component. A monoclonal immunoglobulin light chain (Bence–Jones protein) is detected in the urine in 75% of cases. When the level of the latter is high, precipitation may occur in the renal tubules, resulting in acute renal failure. In some situations the protein may be deposited in the tissues as AL amyloid. Hyperviscosity syndromes may also occur.

The diagnosis is usually suspected from the clinical and radiological features, and is confirmed by bone marrow biopsy and serum electrophoresis. The diagnostic criteria are listed in Table 8.15. The bone marrow may show an interstitial infiltrate or confluent sheets of plasma cells, which display varying degrees of atypia. The monoclonal plasma cells are capable of producing only one light chain – a feature which can be exploited in determining monoclonality (Figure 8.41). Monosomy 13 occurs in 15–40% of cases.

TABLE 8.15 WHO diagnostic criteria for plasma cell myeloma

Diagnosis requires a minimum of 1 major and 1 minor criterion or 3 minor criteria in a patient with progressive symptomatic disease
Major criteria: Marrow plasmacytosis greater than 30%
Plasmacytoma on biopsy
M-component
Serum: IgG >3.5 g/dL; IgA >2 g/dL
Urine: 1 g/24 h of Bence–Jones protein
Minor criteria: Marrow plasmacytosis (10–30%)
M component present but less than above
Lytic bone lesions
Reduced normal immunoglobulins (<50% normal), IgG <600 mg/dL; IgA <100 mg/dL; IgM <50 mg/dL

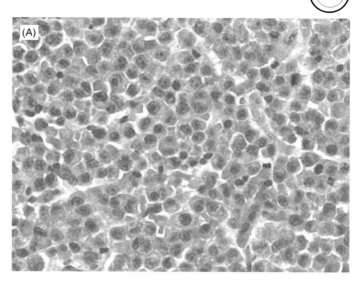

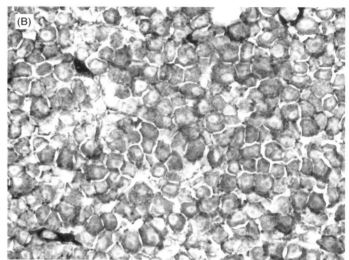

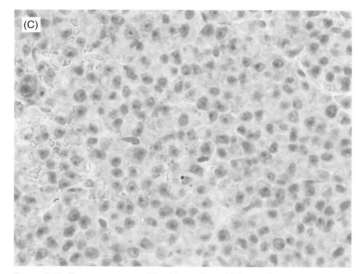

FIGURE 8.41 Bone marrow trephine biopsy in multiple myeloma. (A) Haematoxylin and eosin staining shows confluent sheets of atypical plasma cells. (B) The neoplastic plasma cells stain only for kappa light chain using immunocytochemistry and are therefore monoclonal. (C) The same population of cells is negative for lambda light chain.

Despite treatment the prognosis of plasma cell myeloma is poor, with a median survival of 3 years. A small proportion of patients may survive for 10 years.

Some patients presenting with a low level of serum paraprotein are found to have less than 10% monoclonal plasma cells in the bone marrow. These patients display none of the clinical features of myeloma and lack bony lesions. This condition is called *monoclonal gammopathy of undetermined significance* (MGUS) and has a high prevalence (3%) after the age of 70 years. The majority of patients require no treatment, though plasma cell myeloma or amyloidosis will develop in 25% of cases.

Solitary plasmacytoma is a tumour occurring in bone or upper respiratory tract, and is composed of monoclonal plasma cells identical to those of plasma cell myeloma. As these lesions are localized, radiotherapy can induce a cure in a significant proportion of cases. Plasma cell myeloma will occur in 50% of patients within 10 years of initial presentation.

SUMMARY

- Conditions involving the lymphoreticular system and bone marrow are common and present in a wide variety of ways.
- Diseases involving lymph nodes usually present with lymphadenopathy and include reactive conditions such as tuberculosis and sarcoidosis in addition to neoplastic disorders such as metastatic carcinoma or lymphoma.
- Lymphoma is a malignant tumour derived from lymphocytes which may affect lymph nodes or extranodal sites.
- The bone marrow may be affected by congenital, infective, autoimmune and neoplastic disorders resulting in varying degrees of bone marrow failure. Anaemia, thrombocytopenia and decreased white cell count are the consequences of bone marrow failure and lead to fatigue, haemorrhage and increased susceptibility to infection.

- Leukaemia is a malignant condition characterized by an increase in white cells in the peripheral circulation as a result of a clonal proliferation of bone marrow stem cells.
- There are many different types of leukaemia and lymphoma with different clinical presentations and prognoses. Their accurate diagnosis is complex and requires correlation of morphologic, immunophenotypic, cytogenetic and clinical data.
- Many lymphomas and leukaemias are curable with modern therapy.

ACKNOWLEDGEMENTS

We wish to acknowledge the contribution of Professor CJLM Meijer, VU University Medical Center, Amsterdam, for input to the first draft of this chapter. We thank Drs Mike Leach, Noelle O'Rourke, Grant McQuaker and Andy Clarke for assistance with the figures and case histories.

FURTHER READING

Bain BJ, Clark DM, Lampert IA, Wilkins BS. *Bone Marrow Pathology*, 3rd edn. Oxford: Blackwell Science, 2001.

Hoffbrand AV, Moss PAH, Pettit JE. *Essential Haematology*, 5th edn. Oxford: Blackwell Science, 2006.

Jaffe ES, Harris NL, Stein H, Vardiman JW. World Health Organization Classification of Tumours. *Pathology and Genetics of Tumours of the Haemopoeitic and Lymphoid tissues*. Lyon: IARC Press, 2001.

Knowles DM (ed), *Neoplastic Haematopathology*. Lippincott, 2nd edn. Baltimore: Williams & Wilkins, 2001.

Stansfeld AG, d'Ardenne AJ. *Lymph Node Biopsy Interpretation*, 2nd edn. Edinburgh: Churchill Livingstone, 1992.

Weiss LM (ed). *Pathology of Lymph Nodes. Contemporary Issues in Surgical Pathology*, Volume 21. Edinburgh: Churchill Livingstone, 1996.

Wilkins BS, Wright DH. *Illustrated Pathology of the Spleen*. Cambridge: Cambridge University Press, 2000.

David A Levison, D Gordon McDonald and Francis A Carey

THE ORAL CAVITY, SALIVARY GLANDS AND OROPHARYNX

The Oral Cavity

The mouth is subject to the same types of lesions as other sites in the body, but these often show distinct features peculiar to the mouth. In addition, there are a number of specific lesions related to the teeth and their supporting tissues. Dental caries and non-specific chronic inflammation of the soft tissues related to the teeth, probably the most common diseases of humankind, are caused principally by oral bacteria. A highly complex bacterial flora is found in saliva, adherent to epithelium and in deposits on tooth surfaces. The dental plaque on teeth consists of many types of bacteria in an organic matrix of salivary and bacterial origin. This may calcify to form dental calculus.

The Teeth

Teeth consist of three specialized calcified tissues (Figure 9.1). The dentine is a thick layer of calcified collagenous tissues surrounding the soft tissues of the pulp. The enamel, which forms the hard outer layer of the crown is acellular, consisting largely of calcium apatite crystals in a delicate organic matrix. The cementum overlies the root dentine. At the apex of each root is one or more foramina through which vessels and nerves enter the pulp.

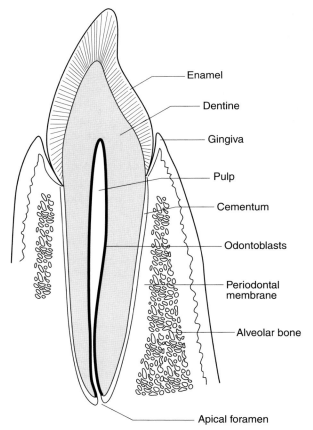

FIGURE 9.1 **The tooth and its supporting tissues.**

(Labels: Enamel, Dentine, Gingiva, Pulp, Cementum, Odontoblasts, Periodontal membrane, Alveolar bone, Apical foramen)

Dental Caries

> ### Key Points
>
> - Dental caries is a bacterial disease, related to adherent dental plaque.
> - Plaque forms in stagnation areas in fissures and between teeth.
> - Acid demineralization of enamel leads to cavitation.
> - Bacteria invade dentine and cause pulpitis (toothache).

Dental caries is the progressive destruction, by bacteria and their products, of the calcified tissues of the teeth exposed to the oral environment. Caries itself, and consequent inflammation of the tooth pulp, are the commonest causes of tooth loss up to middle age. Caries can involve any tooth surface, but usually starts in two principal areas of the tooth: the fissures on the occlusal or biting surfaces of posterior teeth and the areas between teeth (proximal caries). Both of these are areas of relative stagnation in which bacterial plaque is likely to accumulate. The bacteria within the plaque produce various organic acids, the resulting pH depending on factors such as the thickness of the plaque and the concentration of dietary sugars. The initial attack on enamel is by the acid, which produces decalcification. At first this is a painless process, but, as the lesion extends through the enamel, the dentine and pulp are involved and the individual starts to get a toothache. Bacteria do not enter the enamel until decalcification has so weakened the structure that it breaks down to form a cavity. Bacteria initially penetrate the dentinal tubules, but then cause softening and distortion of the dentine by a combination of decalcification and proteolytic breakdown of the collagen matrix. The carious dentine becomes yellow by absorption of pigment from bacterial metabolic products and from the mouth. The process then extends through the dentine towards the dental pulp. Caries may also start at the neck of the tooth often by involving the cementum and then the dentine, or, if cementum is deficient, by directly attacking the dentine. This form of caries is more common in older patients in whom recession of the gingiva is common. In the early stages of enamel caries, the damage is reversible, but thereafter caries of enamel and dentine is progressive except in unusual circumstances where the area becomes self-cleaning and the lesions may be arrested.

Pulpitis

The dental pulp is a vascular connective tissue confined within the pulp chamber and root canals in the dentine. Pulpitis is the most common and clinically significant lesion of the pulp. It occurs most often due to the extension of the carious process into dentine and then to the pulp. Physical injury, such as heat and chemical irritation from filling materials, may also give rise to pulpitis, which may be acute or chronic. Because the changes are occurring within the rigid confines of the pulp chamber, there is increase in pressure due to inflammatory exudate. Consequently acute pulpitis is very painful. The pain of pulpitis is poorly localized and patients frequently cannot indicate the tooth involved. If the inflammation spreads to the apical periodontal ligament the patient can localize the tooth involved and it becomes tender to percussion. If the insult to the pulp is less severe, chronic pulpitis may result. The pulp may undergo necrosis following acute or chronic pulpitis. Clinically, a non-vital tooth lacks lustre and may be discoloured by the leaching of products of the necrotic pulp into the dentine. In children, a large carious cavity penetrating quickly to the pulp may result in a large opening into the pulp chamber, leading to open pulpitis from which exudate can drain. Granulation tissue may extend as a pulp polyp into the carious cavity.

Periodontal Disease

> ### Key Points
>
> - Periodontal disease is caused by bacterial plaque.
> - There is chronic inflammation with net tissue loss.
> - Inflammation and tissue loss involve complex immunologically mediated processes.
> - Destruction of periodontal ligament causes tooth loss.

Periodontal disease involves the gingiva (gums), the periodontal ligament and the related bone. Acute inflammation of the gingiva can arise from various physical, chemical and infective causes. Acute necrotizing ulcerative gingivitis (Vincent's infection) is a distinct condition in which there is necrosis of the interdental papillae with variable spread to other parts of the gingiva. There is overgrowth of two commensal organisms, *Fusobacterium fusiforme* and *Borrelia vincentii*, but the exact relationship of these to the disease is not clear. A similar, but more destructive type of gingivitis is seen in acquired immune deficiency syndrome (AIDS).

Chronic periodontitis (Figure 9.2) is very common, increasing in frequency and severity with age. It is the most common cause of tooth loss in older individuals. A number of local and systemic factors are involved, but of these the most important is the bacterial plaque around the neck of the tooth. For clinical convenience the lesions are divided into chronic gingivitis where the disease is confined to the gingiva, and chronic periodontitis where the process involves the deeper tissues, causing recession of the gingiva. Many mechanisms of tissue destruction have been described involving polymorphonuclear leucocytes, macrophages and both humoral and cell-mediated immune mechanisms. It is probable that all of these are operating in different situations. The later stages of the disease involve osteoclastic resorption of the alveolar bone supporting the teeth. Deepening of the gingival sulcus occurs with the formation of periodontal pockets. Infrequently there is an acute exacerbation of infection in such pockets and a periodontal abscess can arise.

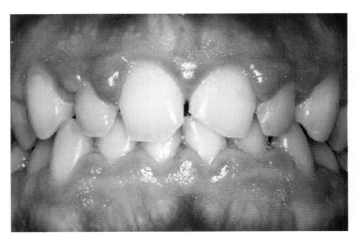

FIGURE 9.2 Chronic periodontitis, with redness and swelling of the attached gingiva.

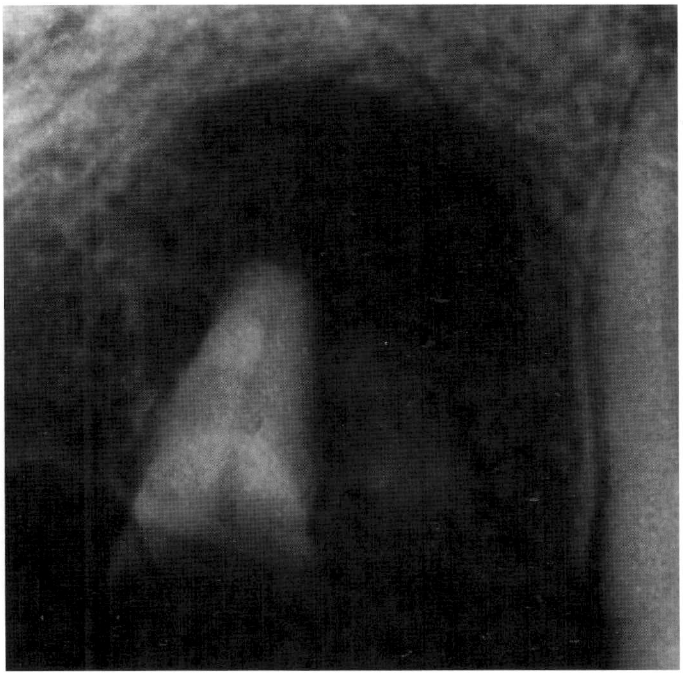

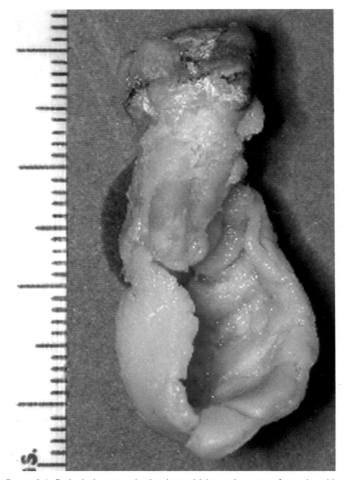

FIGURE 9.3 Periapical radiolucency, indicating resorption of bone and replacement by either inflammatory soft tissue or a cyst.

Periapical Pathology

Key Points

- Periapical pathology usually results from pulpitis.
- Periapical granuloma results in a periapical radiolucency.
- A periapical cyst develops from a periapical granuloma.

The periapical tissues are the site of a variety of lesions related to the root apices of teeth. The most frequent of these arise from spread of infection from pulpitis, through the apical foramina of the tooth, to reach the periodontal ligament. This can result in an acute periapical abscess, a very painful condition which may be accompanied by cervical lymphadenopathy and generalized fever and malaise. Pus tracks through the adjacent bone and, after the periosteum is breached, a soft tissue abscess – a gumboil – develops and later discharges. More frequently, following low-grade pulpitis, a periapical granuloma develops. This consists of a mass of granulation tissue heavily infiltrated with chronic inflammatory cells. There is resorption of surrounding bone, seen radiographically as a periapical radiolucency (Figure 9.3). Acute exacerbation may result in a secondary acute periapical abscess and conversely, a periapical granuloma can develop after an acute periapical abscess has pointed and drained. Remnants of the odontogenic epithelium in the periapical tissue can be stimulated to grow within a periapical granuloma and these give rise to the most common cysts of the jaws, a periapical cyst, also known as a radicular cyst or a dental cyst (Figure 9.4).

FIGURE 9.4 Periapical cyst, projecting into which are the roots of a molar with a large amalgam restoration.

Epithelial-lined Cysts of the Jaws

> **Key Points**
> - Most jaw cysts are derived from odontogenic epithelium.
> - Jaw cysts may be inflammatory or developmental.
> - The odontogenic keratocyst is prone to recurrence.

Several types of epithelial-lined cysts occur in the jaws. The most frequent are derived from the dental epithelial tissues. These odontogenic cysts are subdivided into inflammatory and developmental cysts and categorized by their position in relation to the teeth. The commonest is the periapical cyst described above, which is an inflammatory cyst developing from a periapical granuloma. If the affected tooth is extracted, the cyst may remain as a residual cyst. The most frequent developmental odontogenic cyst is the dentigerous cyst which develops around the crown of a tooth which has failed to erupt. Closely related is the eruption cyst which presents as a bluish fluctuant swelling overlying the crown of an erupting tooth.

The odontogenic cysts described above are lined by non-keratinized stratified squamous epithelium which may include a few mucus-secreting cells. These cysts are usually symptomless unless infected and can grow to several centimetres with considerable bone destruction. They must be differentiated from the odontogenic keratocyst which has a distinctive keratinized stratified squamous epithelial lining (Figure 9.5). Its relationship to the teeth is variable and it occurs anywhere in the jaws, the most common site being in the mandibular molar area, often extending up into the vertical ramus of the mandible. The importance of this cyst lies in the frequency with which it recurs after attempted surgical removal, because of the friable nature of the lining and the presence of the related small daughter cysts.

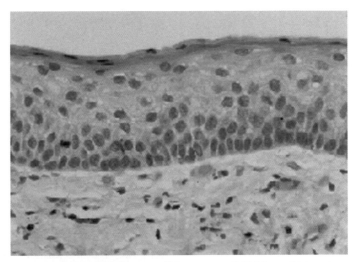

FIGURE 9.5 Odontogenic keratocyst lining: a one-cell thick layer of intensely eosinophilic parakeratin on the surface of otherwise unremarkable benign stratified squamous epithelium.

Cysts derived from non-odontogenic epithelium are less frequent. The nasopalatine cyst arises in the midline of the anterior hard palate. The nasolabial cyst is very uncommon and presents as a soft tissue swelling at the ala of the nose.

Other Tooth-related Pathology

Tooth development begins at about 3 months of intrauterine life and extends over about 20 years until the completion of root formation of the third molars. During this period many developmental abnormalities can occur in the number of teeth, in the form and colour, in the structure of individual tooth elements and the times of eruption and shedding of teeth. These abnormalities result from various factors, both genetic and environmental. An example of iatrogenic disease is the permanent staining of the calcified dental tissues caused by administration of some tetracyclines during tooth development.

Odontogenic tumours are rare lesions, of widely differing pathology, derived from the dental soft and hard tissues. Some of these lesions are neoplasms, but several are hamartomas. The most important is the ameloblastoma which is an epithelial neoplasm of distinct appearance. Ameloblastomas are most frequent in the molar region of the mandible and are locally aggressive, often producing extensive bone destruction (Figure 9.6). The most frequent odontogenic tumours are odontomes. These are hamartomatous lesions containing enamel and dentine. A complex odontome consists of a disorganized mass of dental tissues, whereas a compound odontome consists of numerous small teeth.

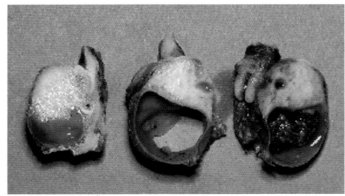

FIGURE 9.6 Ameloblastoma: slices from this example show a partially cystic tumour with a solid tumour nodule within the cyst wall.

Oral Mucosa

The oral mucosa is subjected to numerous physical insults. It is exposed to vast numbers of microorganisms and to food and other material introduced into the mouth. Oral epithelium has a high rate of cell turnover. In almost all lesions of oral mucosa, physical trauma and infection have a role and this may be superimposed on a previously normal or abnormal mucosa. It is not surprising that these circumstances produce complex changes in diseases which are not yet fully documented or understood.

Developmental Abnormalities of Oral Epithelium

Apart from Fordyce's disease – the presence of pale yellowish sebaceous glands in the lining mucosa, especially the cheeks – developmental abnormalities of oral mucosa are rare.

Oral Candidiasis (Candidosis)

Candida spp. are part of the oral flora in about half the population. *Candida albicans* is the most frequent of these. Opportunistic infection by *C. albicans* occurs in a number of situations. Thrush is an acute condition found most often in young children or debilitated adults and is characterized by detachable white fungal plaques on the epithelium. Erythematous candidosis is found under upper dentures and is an inflammatory reaction to fungi which are found mainly in the interstices of the fitting surface of the denture. Candidal hyphae may also be found in adherent hyperkeratotic lesions as chronic hyperplastic candidiasis (candidal leucoplakia). Persistent oral candidal infections are a common problem in patients with AIDS. Angular cheilitis is described as a *Candida*-associated lesion, but is often associated with other contributory causes.

ORAL FUNGAL INFECTION

A 70-year-old woman complained of discomfort at the angles of her mouth and a sore tongue. Clinically, angular cheilitis was present (Figure 9.7). The tongue was atrophic with loss of the normal pattern of papillae (Figure 9.8). The patient had full dentures which she had worn for several years. The wear on the teeth had resulted in the lower jaw closing beyond the normal position and there was a tendency for saliva to leak out onto the skin at the angles of the mouth. Examination of the palate revealed a red, inflamed area corresponding to the outline of the upper denture (Figure 9.9).

Microbiological examination revealed heavy growth of *C. albicans* in cultures of swabs from the angle of the mouth and from the fitting surface of the upper denture. In addition, haematological investigation revealed microcytic anaemia with a haemoglobin level of 95 g/L.

Investigations were conducted for iron deficiency anaemia. No obvious source of blood loss was found. In particular, possible blood loss from neoplasms was excluded. It was felt that the cause of the iron deficiency was related to poor diet in an elderly person living alone and with limited finances. The iron deficiency responded to oral administration of iron. The fungal infestation was treated with appropriate antifungal drugs. New dentures were designed to increase the vertical dimension, in other words to open the mouth slightly and prevent the leakage of saliva. The patient was also counselled about

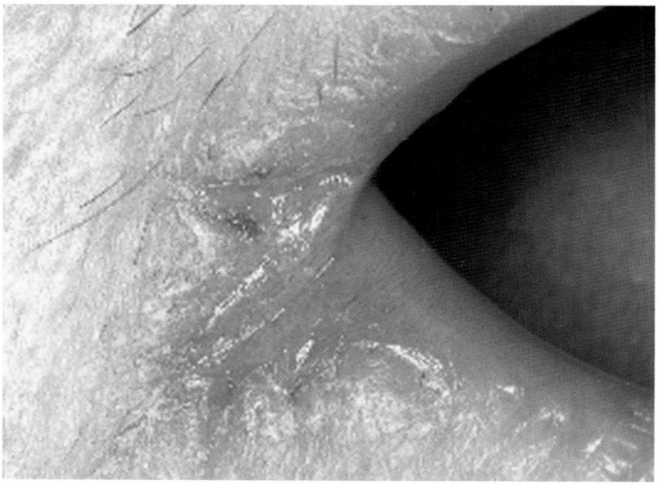

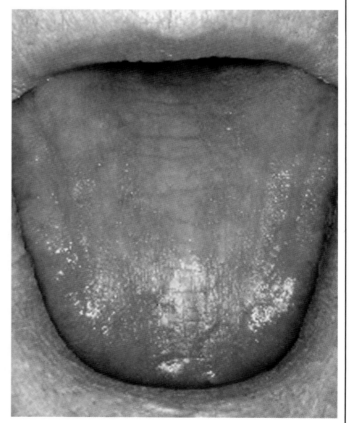

FIGURE 9.8 Atrophic tongue: the rough filiform papillae of the dorsum of the tongue are replaced by flat mucosa; causes include chronic candidal infection, acute candidal infection after antibiotic treatment and various vitamin/mineral deficiencies.

FIGURE 9.7 Angular cheilitis: inflammation and fissuring at the labial commissure is often a marker of chronic candidal infection.

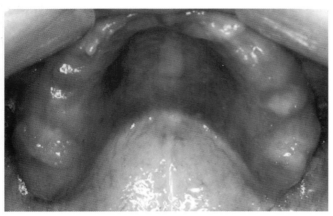

FIGURE 9.9 Chronic erythematous candidosis: the pattern of inflammation on the hard palate mirroring the outline of the upper denture strongly suggests candidal infection.

denture hygiene to keep the denture free from fungal colonization. The clinical situation resolved satisfactorily. Lessons to be learned from this case are:

- oral lesions often have a multifactorial aetiology
- both local and systemic factors need to be considered
- treatment of only some of the involved factors is unlikely to resolve the whole clinical situation.

Viral Infections

The most frequent viral infection of oral epithelium is caused by herpes simplex virus types I and II. Acute herpetic gingivostomatitis is characterized by extensive painful ulceration and occasionally generalized upset. Secondary or recurrent herpetic lesions are more common, especially at mucocutaneous junctions round the lips and nose, where the initially vesicular phase is followed by ulceration and crusting.

Recurrent Oral Ulceration (Aphthous Ulceration)

Recurrent painful fibrin-covered ulcers, either singly or in crops, are a common and troublesome problem said to occur in about 20% of the population. The aetiology is not fully determined, but some cases may be associated with vitamin B group deficiencies, iron deficiency or various food allergies.

Dermatoses

A number of diseases can involve the skin and mucosae. The skin manifestations of these are discussed in Chapter 18. The oral mucosal features are similar, but frequently not so clear cut, making diagnosis more difficult. Lichen planus (Figure 9.10) is the most frequent of the dermatoses which affect the mouth. Other examples include pemphigus, mucous membrane pemphigoid, erythema multiforme and lupus erythematosus.

Premalignant (Potentially Malignant) Lesions

Key Points

- Leucoplakia, white patch, has a low risk of malignancy.
- Erythroplakia, red patch, has a high risk of malignancy.
- The more severe the dysplasia microscopically, the greater risk of malignancy.
- High-risk sites for malignant change are floor of mouth, and ventral and lateral tongue.

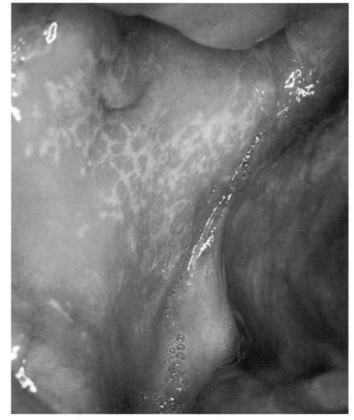

FIGURE 9.10 Lichen planus: a lacy network of white striae on the buccal mucosa is usually symmetrical; other lesions of lichen planus include atrophy, erosions and white plaques (the last often on the tongue).

Leucoplakia and erythroplakia are potentially malignant lesions. Leucoplakia (Figure 9.11) is a clinical descriptive term for a white patch which cannot be attributed to any specific disease and erythroplakia is the analogous term for the less frequent red patches. These are not pathological entities and cover a variety of histological changes. Leucoplakia is due to keratinization of a normally unkeratinized site or hyperkeratosis of a site where keratin is normally present. Smoking and frictional irritation are common aetiological factors, but many cases are of unknown aetiology, or idiopathic. Histologically the epithelium may show acanthosis or atrophy and a variable inflammatory infiltrate is present. A small proportion of leucoplakias and many erythroplakias show dysplasia. The more severe the dysplasia in an individual case, the greater is the likelihood of progression to carcinoma. On the floor of the mouth and the ventral surface and lateral margins of the tongue, leucoplakia is more prone to become malignant, particularly in elderly people. Leucoplakia arising on an atrophic epithelium or showing as areas of white upon an erythematous background, non-homogeneous leucoplakia, is also more likely to proceed to carcinoma.

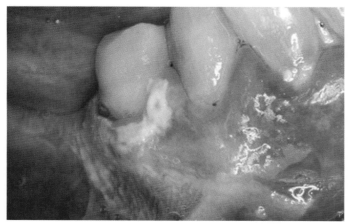

FIGURE 9.11 Leucoplakia: irregular white patch on the gum due to keratin production by the gingival squamous epithelium.

Pigmentation

The most frequent pigmentation of oral mucosa is exogenous pigmentation due to an amalgam tattoo. Melanocytes are more numerous in oral epithelium than in skin, but less often produce melanin. Melanin pigmentation, especially of the gingiva, roughly parallels skin pigmentation, being more common in coloured races. Reactive or secondary melanosis is seen in smokers, following chronic dermatoses and in Addison's disease. Unexplained pigmentation in the mouth should always be regarded with suspicion as malignant melanoma can occur, particularly in the palate, and has a bad prognosis.

Soft Tissue Swellings

Fibrous overgrowths of the oral mucosa are a common response to chronic irritation. An epulis is a localized swelling on the gingiva. The common type is a reaction to chronic irritation, for example from dental calculus (calcified plaque) or the rough margin of a carious cavity or filling. It consists of a mass of cellular fibrous tissue frequently

with metaplastic bone formation. Pyogenic granulomas are a mass of granulation tissue resulting from irritation at any intraoral site, but most often on gingiva as a vascular epulis or in pregnancy, as a pregnancy epulis. Giant cell epulis is a distinct lesion consisting of numerous multinucleated giant cells in a vascular stroma. The giant cell epulis is a superficial lesion with minimal bone involvement, but intraosseous lesions, such as central giant cell granuloma or osteitis fibrosa cystica in hyperparathyroidism may mimic a giant cell epulis if they extend to involve the gingival soft tissues.

Tumours of the Oral Mucosa

Key Points
- Oral cancer is increasing incidence.
- Oral cancer has a poor prognosis if not treated early.
- Small oral cancers are mainly red.
- Floor of mouth is a high risk site for small, symptomless cancers.
- Larger cancers commonly involve tongue.
- Lymphatic spread is associated with poor prognosis.

Squamous cell papillomas can occur at any intraoral site. They are caused by human papilloma virus and their incidence is increasing. Squamous cell carcinoma accounts for more than 90% of oral malignancies. Despite the fact that early recognition should be possible, many oral cancers have a poor prognosis because the tumours are not recognized and treated when small. Distinction should be made between lip cancer and intraoral cancer. Cancer of lower lip presents as a non-healing ulcer or a small lump (Figure 9.12). Sunlight is the most frequent aetiological agent. Such tumours grow slowly and are slow to metastasize to lymph nodes.

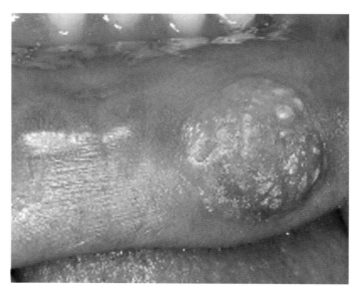

FIGURE 9.12 Lip cancer: squamous cell carcinoma presenting as a raised berry-like tumour on the mucosal aspect of the lower lip.

Intraoral carcinomas generally have a poorer prognosis the further posteriorly in the mouth they arise. Although some appear to develop from recognized premalignant lesions, over three-quarters of carcinomas in developed countries arise in clinically normal mucosa. The earliest lesions are red rather than white and are symptomless. They most often originate in the floor of the mouth (Figure 9.13) or soft palate area. Larger tumours most often involve the lateral margins of the tongue (Figure 9.14). The initial spread of oral cancer is local spread to adjacent tissues. This is followed by spread to local lymph nodes, which is associated with a significantly poorer prognosis. Haematogenous spread is a late complication.

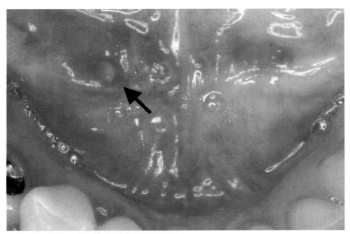

FIGURE 9.13 'Early' cancer of floor of mouth: squamous cell carcinoma presenting as a small non-healing ulcer in the floor of mouth; this is a 'high-risk area' for development of oral cancer particularly in smokers who drink alcoholic spirits.

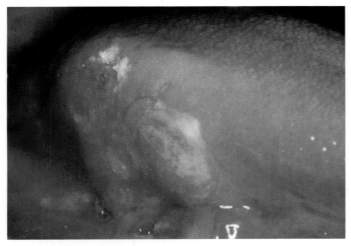

FIGURE 9.14 Advanced cancer of tongue: squamous cell carcinoma typically presents as an indurated plaque-like mass in the ventral and lateral aspects of the tongue.

Successful treatment of squamous cell carcinoma of the mouth is dependent on early diagnosis. It is important that lesions of the oral mucosa which do not relate to obvious causes, or which fail to respond to the removal of obvious causes, undergo biopsy. The incidence of intraoral cancer is rising in Europe, probably due to increased smoking and alcohol consumption.

The Salivary Glands

Key Points

- Mumps is a common viral infection of major salivary glands.
- Mucocoeles arise from trauma causing mucus leakage.
- Chronic sialadenitis involves endogenous infection secondary to duct obstruction.
- Sjögren's syndrome is an autoimmune exocrinopathy.

There are three pairs of major salivary glands –parotid, submandibular and sublingual – and numerous intraoral minor salivary glands. The most common lesion of minor salivary glands is the mucocoele (Figure 9.15). The common site is the lower lip. The lesion is due to leakage of mucus from a damaged duct which is surrounded by granulation tissue. A ranula is a larger variant occurring in the floor of the mouth involving sublingual ducts.

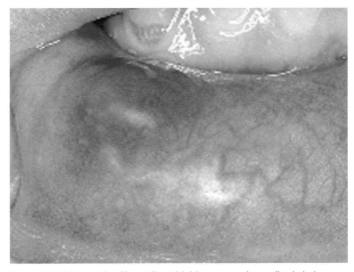

FIGURE 9.15 Mucocoele of lower lip: a bluish-grey cyst immediately below the labial mucosa caused by damage to a minor salivary gland duct and liberation of salivary juice into the loose connective tissues of the lip; traumatic injury to the lip by the teeth after a fall is typical.

Inflammatory Lesions

Mumps is the commonest acute inflammatory lesion of the salivary glands. This viral infection has an incubation period of 3 weeks and infected individuals secrete the virus in their saliva for about a week before the main symptom of painful salivary gland swelling is evident and for just over a week thereafter. Both parotid glands are usually involved and sometimes also the submandibular glands. The salivary enlargement usually subsides without permanent damage to the glands. Mumps may be accompanied by orchitis or pancreatitis. Mumps virus is also a relatively frequent cause of aseptic meningitis.

Suppurative parotitis is an uncommon infection caused by pyogenic cocci and can occur as a postoperative complication in dehydrated patients. It may also occur in elderly debilitated patients, sometimes as a sequel to septicaemia. Chronic sialadenitis arises as an endogenous infection related to obstruction and can occur in either the parotid or submandibular glands. In the latter it is often associated with salivary calculi. Sialadenitis leads to atrophy with marked acinar loss and interstitial fibrosis.

Sjögren's Syndrome

Sjögren's syndrome is an autoimmune condition in which there is a generalized exocrinopathy. The salivary glands and the lacrimal glands are the most obviously involved. It is the second most common non-organ-specific autoimmune disease. Patients complain of dryness of the mouth (xerostomia) and eyes (xerophthalmia). The dry eyes and mouth may occur in isolation (sicca syndrome or primary Sjögren's syndrome) or as secondary Sjögren's syndrome associated with another non-organ-specific autoimmune condition, most frequently rheumatoid arthritis. Biopsy of lower labial minor salivary glands, which show focal lymphocytic infiltration, is used as a diagnostic tool. In major glands, particularly the parotids, there is acinar loss and extensive infiltration of lymphocytes. This may give obvious parotid swelling. In longstanding cases there is a risk of malignant lymphoma developing in the parotid.

Tumours of Salivary Gland Epithelium

Key points

- Epithelial salivary gland neoplasms are a complex group, mostly benign.
- 80% of salivary gland tumours involve the parotid gland.
- Pleomorphic adenomas account for over 70% of tumours.
- There is a higher relative incidence of carcinomas in minor glands.

These tumours are uncommon and comprise approximately 2% of all tumours in man. Approximately 80% occur in the parotid gland, 10% each in the submandibular and minor salivary glands. The classification of salivary gland tumours is complex and not entirely satisfactory. About 17 benign tumour types and 22 malignant types have been identified. About 85% of tumours are benign. A higher relative frequency of malignant variants is found in minor salivary glands

By far the most frequent salivary gland neoplasm is the pleomorphic adenoma. This shows very varied patterns of differentiation with combinations of glandular epithelium and myoepithelium (Figure 9.16). The tumours are variably

encapsulated and if they are inappropriately treated, particularly in the parotid, residual tumour can give rise to multiple recurrences from which the patient may never be cured. A further complication is the possibility of adenocarcinoma arising in about 10% of pleomorphic adenomas over time.

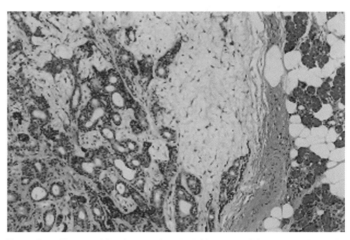

FIGURE 9.16 Pleomorphic adenoma (on the left) separated from normal parotid tissue (on the right) by a thin capsule of collagenous tissue. Pleomorphic adenoma is a benign epithelial neoplasm of 'mixed patterns', here represented as fused glands (left) and spindle-celled cartilage-like tissue (centre).

The most frequent of the malignant neoplasms are the adenoid cystic carcinoma and the mucoepidermoid carcinoma which together account for about 10% of salivary neoplasms. Adenoid cystic carcinomas often show a distinctive cribiform (sieve-like) growth pattern. They have a particular tendency for local spread and are difficult to eradicate surgically. Mucoepidermoid carcinomas show a variable mixture of squamous epithelium and glandular epithelium. They are tumours of variable behaviour showing local invasion and sometimes spread to local lymph nodes.

The Oropharynx

Infections of the Oropharynx

Sore throat and tonsillitis are caused by infection. *Streptococcus pyogenes* is a common cause of sore throat in children whereas infection by various viruses is more common in adults. The streptococcal infection can precede rheumatic fever or glomerulonephritis. Infectious mononucleosis, glandular fever, is caused by Epstein–Barr virus and is a cause of lymphadenopathy. It can lead to a particularly troublesome sore throat in adolescents and young adults.

Diphtheria, caused by *Corynebacterium diphtheriae*, is an acute inflammation which most frequently affects the fauces, soft palate and tonsils. It was previously a serious killer disease, but immunization programmes are largely responsible for the present low incidence of diphtheria in many parts of the world.

Tumours of the Oropharynx

The most important tumours of the oropharynx are carcinomas and lymphomas. Squamous cell carcinoma is the most frequent and has similarities to oral cancer being associated with smoking. A poorly differentiated nasopharyngeal carcinoma which has an association with Epstein–Barr virus can occur in the oropharynx. It is uncommon in white people, but has a much higher incidence in individuals of southern Chinese origin. Various types of lymphoma, usually non-Hodgkin's lymphoma, occur in the oropharynx.

THE OESOPHAGUS

Normal Structure and Function

Averaging some 25 cm in length, the oesophagus is a muscular tube with a well-defined origin at the cricoid cartilage. Its function is a simple one, namely the conduction of food from the pharynx to the stomach. This simplicity is reflected in its structure. The mucosal lining is of stratified squamous epithelium, while the underlying submucosa includes numbers of mucinous glands which lubricate the lining. The muscle coat is prominent, being for the most part arranged, as in the rest of the gut, in inner circular and outer longitudinal coats. Striated (voluntary) muscle fibres are present proximally, contributing to the upper oesophageal sphincter, thus allowing voluntary initiation of swallowing. The so-called lower oesophageal sphincter is in reality the smooth muscle of the wall acting under autonomic control to prevent reflux of gastric contents. There is no clearly defined anatomical lower sphincter. Partly for this reason the lower end of the oesophagus is much less well defined than the upper.

Because of its simplicity of function, the oesophagus produces a relatively limited range of symptoms in disease. The retrosternal burning pain of heartburn is a common effect of reflux of gastroduodenal contents into the oesophagus. Dysphagia (difficulty in swallowing) is an important and sometimes sinister symptom (see Neoplasia, p. 233). Oesophageal disease is also an important cause of haematemesis (vomiting of blood).

Congenital Abnormalities, Disorders of Motility and Vascular Abnormality

Key Points

- Atresia, with and without tracheo-oesophageal fistula, occurs in neonates.
- Achalasia is a motor disorder of the lower oesophageal sphincter.
- Hiatus hernia is strongly associated with acid reflux.
- Oesophageal varices are an important cause of upper gastrointestinal haemorrhage in portal hypertension.

Atresia

The oesophagus and trachea both derive from the embryonic foregut. Congenital abnormalities of the oesophagus and trachea are commonly related. Duplication cysts, lined either by squamous or respiratory epithelium, are recognized. More importantly, oesophageal atresia is a cause of neonatal dysphagia resulting from failure of canalization (lumenal development) of the oesophagus. It is commonly associated with tracheo-oesophageal fistula and a high risk of neonatal aspiration pneumonia (Figure 9.17).

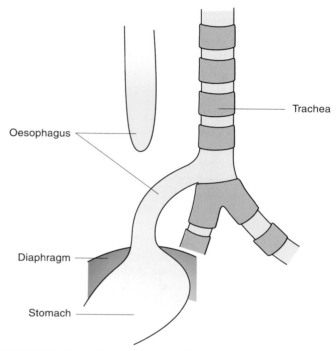

FIGURE 9.17 In the most common variant of oesophageal atresia the upper oesophagus is a blind-ended tube, while the lower part is in communication with the trachea.

Achalasia

Achalasia is a Greek term meaning 'failure to relax'; this is a good description of this disorder, which is characterized by poor relaxation of the functional lower oesophageal sphincter. The disease is of unknown cause, and may present at any stage in life, usually with dysphagia and regurgitation of undigested food material. Aspiration pneumonia is a significant problem. Microscopically, the disease is characterized by a reduction in the numbers of neurones in the muscular (myenteric) plexus of the lower oesophagus. In advanced disease, the proximal oesophagus may show dilatation, inflammation and ulceration. There is also a slightly increased risk of carcinoma. Other diseases leading to loss of lower oesophageal motility include systemic sclerosis (muscle fibrosis and atrophy) and South American trypanosomiasis (Chagas' disease, where there is direct parasitic infection of the myenteric neurones).

Hiatus Hernia

This is an acquired abnormality defined by abnormal location of the oesophagogastric junction and (part of) the gastric cardia above the diaphragm. Formerly thought to be due to congenital shortening of the oesophagus, it is now considered to be due to a combination of diaphragmatic weakening and increased intra-abdominal pressure. It is therefore associated with the Western diet, and particularly with obesity. In a less common abnormality (para-oesophageal or 'rolling' hiatus hernia), part of the stomach protrudes into the mediastinum alongside the oesophagus (Figure 9.18).

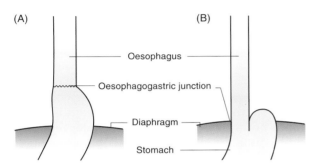

FIGURE 9.18 Hiatus hernia. (A) In a sliding hiatus hernia the proximal stomach is 'pulled' into the mediastinum. (B) In the 'rolling' variant, part of the fundus of the stomach protrudes through an abnormally large diaphragmatic orifice.

The major clinical effect of hiatus hernia is loss of the lower oesophageal sphincter mechanism, leading to reflux oesophagitis.

Diverticula

Abnormal outpouchings of the oesophageal wall can occur either by pulsion (increased intraoesophageal pressure, as may occur in achalasia) or by traction ('pulling' from an external neoplasm or inflammatory focus). Diverticula can regurgitate food and/or become distended, leading to dysphagia.

Varices

The venous drainage of the oesophagus is through a network of veins lying in the adventitial soft tissue. At the lower end, some blood drains from this plexus into the portal venous system. In portal venous hypertension (most commonly seen in association with liver cirrhosis), back-pressure in this system can lead to massive dilatation of submucosal veins (oesophageal varices) (Figure 9.19). The superficial position of the varices renders them particularly prone to rupture, often with catastrophic haemorrhage.

Inflammatory Disease

Inflammation of the oesophagus, manifested endoscopically by the cardinal signs of congestion and redness of the

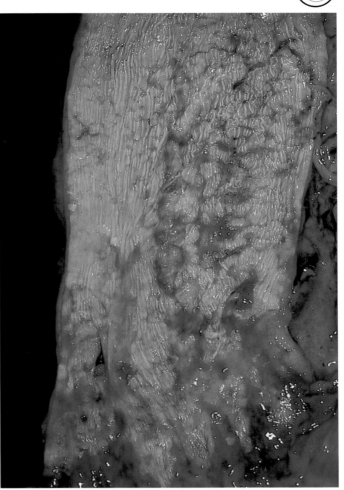

FIGURE 9.19 Oesophageal varices. Markedly dilated lower oesophageal veins in a patient dying from the effects of cirrhosis.

mucosa, is usually caused by the chemical irritation of refluxed gastroduodenal contents (reflux oesophagitis). A limited number of infectious agents (*Candida*, herpes simplex virus) may be a direct cause of oesophagitis. The oesophagus may be involved in Crohn's disease and in systemic sclerosis. Oesophageal obstruction (tumour, achalasia) leads to a secondary proximal oesophagitis.

Reflux Oesophagitis

The oesophageal squamous epithelium is not well equipped to deal with the injurious effects of gastric fluid (a potent mix of acid, pepsin and smaller quantities of bile acids and trypsin). The main natural defence mechanism is the functional integrity of the lower oesophageal sphincter. This may be compromised by increased intra-abdominal pressure (obesity, pregnancy), and by intrinsic relaxation or incompetence of the muscle sphincter (alcohol, tobacco, hiatus hernia). Other mechanisms such as acid clearance time are likely to be important in determining the severity of the disease. The issue is further complicated in that some patients with severe tissue manifestations of disease (e.g. ulceration) have no history of heartburn, while markedly symptomatic patients with proven reflux may show no histo-logical evidence of inflammation.

Reflux causes cell damage to the superficial squamous epithelium. The cell loss causes compensatory basal cell hyperplasia, and this – together with some inflammatory cell exudation – constitutes the histological picture of reflux oesophagitis. More severe disease leads to complications such as oesophageal peptic ulceration and, in long-standing disease, oesophageal fibrous stricture, the latter occurring on a background of chronic ulceration. Barrett's oesophagus is a further important consequence of gastro-oesophageal reflux (see below).

Infective Causes of Oesophagitis

The oesophagus is relatively resistant to infection, and most cases of infective oesophagitis occur in immunocompromised individuals. *Candida albicans* is a relatively common fungal cause of erosive inflammation in this situation. Viruses such as herpes simplex and cytomegalovirus may infect the oesophagus.

Barrett's Oesophagus

Key Points

- Barrett's oesophagus is an acquired glandular metaplasia of the oesophagus.
- It is caused by reflux of gastroduodenal contents.
- There is a risk of progression to adenocarcinoma.

Some individuals with long-standing reflux disease develop this condition, which is characterized by a metaplastic change in the oesophageal epithelium from stratified squamous to columnar (glandular) type (Figure 9.20). This change, which is also known simply as columnar lined oesophagus (CLO), appears to have increased in frequency

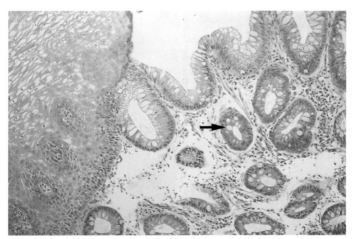

FIGURE 9.20 Biopsy of the squamocolumnar junction in an endoscopically obvious case of Barrett's oesophagus. There is glandular epithelium in addition to the normal squamous mucosa. Intestinal metaplasia is indicated by the presence of goblet cells (arrow).

over the past 30 years. The main importance of Barrett's oesophagus is that it is undoubtedly associated with an increased risk of progression to adenocarcinoma. Microscopically, the columnar epithelium can show a range of appearances, with three basic patterns being recognized:

- junctional (resembling gastric cardia)
- gastric fundic (including acid- and pepsin-secreting cells)
- intestinal (with small intestinal-type goblet cells).

Clinical follow-up has shown that it is the intestinal type that is most often associated with malignancy. Dysplastic changes can sometimes be recognized in biopsy specimens as an intermediate stage between metaplastic epithelium and invasive malignancy.

Clinicopathological Problems in Barrett's Oesophagus

When first described (by Norman Barrett, a thoracic surgeon at St Thomas Hospital, London during the early 1950s), columnar epithelium in the apparent oesophagus was thought to reflect a congenitally short oesophagus with 'pulling up' of the stomach into the thorax. It is now clear that this is not the case. There are two major related practical problems in the identification and management of this disorder in clinical practice.

Definition of the Normal Lower Limit of Squamous Epithelium

It is usually considered that the squamocolumnar junction in normal individuals is synonymous with the gastro-oesophageal junction, although some authorities state that the distal 1–2 cm of the normal oesophagus is lined by columnar epithelium of junctional type. A major source of confusion is identification of the gastro-oesophageal junction in practice. Endoscopists rely on the funnel-like appearance at the transition from the tubular oesophagus to the more capacious stomach, and also on the appearance of the beginnings of gastric mucosal folds. Because these landmarks are rather fluid in life, published studies on Barrett's oesophagus have often allowed an upward margin of error of 1–5 cm before columnar epithelium on biopsy was considered abnormal. It is therefore not surprising that the reported prevalence of the condition at endoscopy has varied widely. More recently, some workers have attempted to bypass the anatomical problems by redefining Barrett's oesophagus as the presence of metaplastic intestinal epithelium in the region of the squamocolumnar junction, reasoning that it is the presence of intestinal metaplasia which defines those who are at high risk of progression to malignancy.

Clinical Follow-up in Barrett's Oesophagus

Patients identified as having Barrett's oesophagus are at increased risk of developing adenocarcinoma. The risk for the individual case is, however, small. Follow-up of all patients with Barrett's oesophagus (by endoscopy and multiple biopsy) has not been demonstrated to be a cost-effective measure. Often, follow-up is reserved for those patients with long segment disease, intestinal metaplasia, and particularly those with dysplasia. High-grade dysplasia caries a very high risk of progression to invasive malignancy, and may be an indicator for prophylactic oesophagectomy.

Oesophageal Neoplasms

Benign neoplasms

Benign tumours of the oesophagus are uncommon. The epithelium occasionally gives rise to squamous cell papillomas, but the most frequently occurring type is of mesenchymal origin – the leiomyoma (benign smooth muscle tumour).

Malignant Neoplasms

Key Points

- Squamous cell carcinoma is related to diet and smoking, and shows a marked geographical variation.
- Adenocarcinoma is increasing in incidence, and occurs mostly in Barrett's oesophagus.
- Both types of carcinoma have a poor prognosis.

Almost all malignancies of the oesophagus are of epithelial origin (Figure 9.21A). The clinical presentation is usually with dysphagia that often rapidly progresses to inability to swallow fluids. Of the two major histological types, squamous cell carcinoma (Figure 9.21B) arises in the oesophageal squamous lining, while adenocarcinoma is mostly associated with Barrett's oesophagus (Figure 9.21C) and is now the more common type in the Western world.

Squamous carcinoma of the oesophagus shows a wide geographical variation in incidence, with particularly prominent epidemiological hotspots being sites around the Caspian Sea and in parts of China. Rare cases have a defined genetic component, being associated with a characteristic palmar and plantar hyperkeratosis (tylosis). Other cases may occur following the ingestion of corrosives, or as a result of long-standing mucosal irritation in achalasia. Macroscopically, squamous carcinomas present as irregular ulcerated, exophytic masses that partly or almost totally occlude the lumen. At the time of presentation, they have usually invaded through the oesophageal muscularis and, in the absence of a serosal covering, they commonly have infiltrated surrounding structures and may have spread to mediastinal or supraclavicular lymph nodes. The clinical prognosis is very poor.

Adenocarcinomas generally arise in Barrett's oesophagus. This is a disease of Western society, being associated with obesity and oesophageal reflux. These tumours have shown a remarkable rise in incidence during the past 20–30 years (paralleled by the rising prevalence of Barrett's oesophagus). The reasons for this changing epidemiology are, as yet, unclear. Macroscopically, they are similar to squamous carcinomas, but the surrounding mucosa often

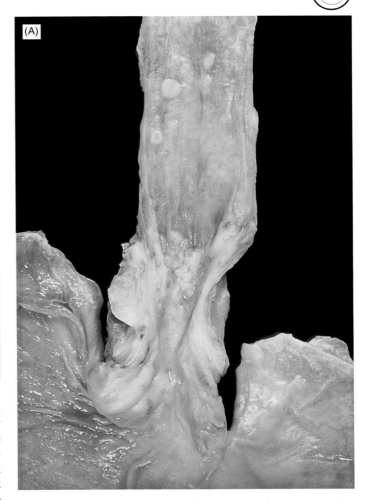

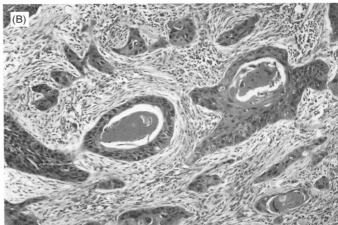

FIGURE 9.21 (A) Macroscopic view of an ulcerated, stenosing carcinoma of the lower oesophagus. (B) Squamous cell carcinoma with islands of neoplastic cells showing central keratin formation.

has the velvety pink appearance of Barrett's metaplasia, in distinction to the normal silvery grey squamous mucosa. Again, the lesion is commonly of advanced stage at presentation but, arising as it does in the lower oesophagus, the spread is more commonly to nodes along the greater and

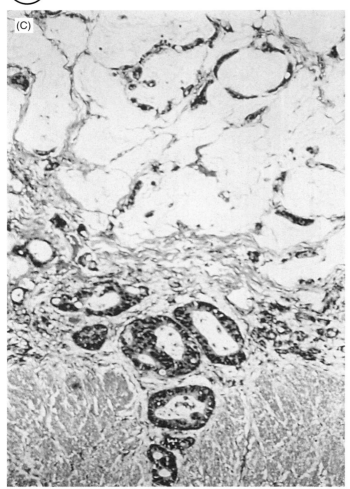

FIGURE 9.21 (C) Adenocarcinoma showing obvious gland formation.

the antrum, extends from the incisura to the pylorus, where there is a well-defined muscular sphincter. Mucosal crypts are shorter and less densely packed in the antrum. Parietal cells are still present, but chief cells are rare in this region. Gastrin-secreting G cells are identified in pyloric crypts. Small numbers of neuroendocrine cells may be seen throughout the stomach. The microscopic features of a gastric gland are summarized in Figure 9.22.

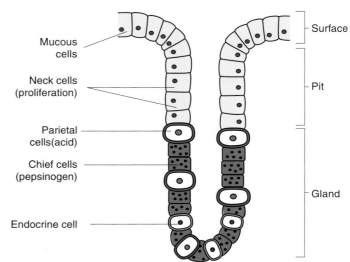

FIGURE 9.22 Schematic representation of the microscopic structure of a gastric gland. The relative proportion of different cell types varies across the stomach. In the cardia, mucous cells predominate. The body ('fundic') glands contain the great bulk of secretory parietal and chief cells. In the antrum, gastrin-producing endocrine cells are prominent.

lesser curves of the stomach and to the liver. The prognosis, again, is dismal.

THE STOMACH

Normal Structure and Function

The stomach is a roughly J-shaped dilatation of the gut, functioning as a reservoir of ingested food and controlling the release of manageable quantities into the duodenum, which has a much smaller capacity. The process of digestion is also begun in the stomach with the secretion of acid and pepsinogen. The so-called intrinsic factor required for vitamin B_{12} absorption is also produced by the gastric epithelium. Both macroscopically and histologically the stomach is divided into three regions. The cardia is an ill-defined region lying just below the oesophagogastric junction. The mucosal crypts are relatively simple and contain mainly mucin-secreting cells. The body or fundic mucosa occupies most of the gastric lining extending distally to the incisura angularis. It is in this region that large numbers of acid-secreting parietal (or oxyntic) cells and pepsinogen-producing chief cells are located. The third major region,

Congenital Abnormalities

Congenital defects of the stomach are uncommon. Cysts and duplications may occur. In diaphragmatic hernia there is a failure of development of part of one dome of the diaphragm with herniation of all or part of the stomach, usually together with intestine, into the thoracic cavity. The main presenting problem is respiratory embarrassment.

In congenital pyloric stenosis there is hypertrophy of the circular muscle at the pyloric sphincter, leading to gastric outflow obstruction that presents clinically with projectile vomiting. This condition is about five times more common in males than in females.

Inflammatory Disorders

Key Points

- Acute gastritis is associated with alcohol and drug injury.
- Chronic gastritis may be due to bacterial infection, chemical injury or autoimmunity.

Gastritis, in its many forms, is a source of considerable confusion to the student, clinician and pathologist. Gastritis may be classified histologically, endoscopically, by topographic distribution in the stomach, or by aetiology. The terminologies used do not always correspond. Thus, the endoscopic appearance of 'gastritis' is very poorly correlated with the biopsy appearances. The histological changes and topographical distribution of abnormality have been found to be the best markers of aetiology, and thus form the basis of a rational approach to classification and, ultimately, clinical treatment.

In the past the causes of acute gastritis have been relatively well understood, but it is only during the past 10–20 years that the aetiology and pathogenesis of most cases of chronic gastritis have become clear.

Acute Gastritis

Acute inflammation of the gastric mucosa has long been associated with chemical injury, particularly by alcohol and non-steroidal anti-inflammatory drugs (NSAIDs). More recently, another form of acute gastritis occurring in the early stages of *Helicobacter pylori* infection has been described. Acute gastritis may be subclinical, or may present with abdominal pain, vomiting and/or haemorrhage. Macroscopically, the mucosa is oedematous and congested and may show superficial mucosal erosion (the site of blood loss). Histologically, there is capillary congestion and leakage of blood cells into the lamina propria. In erosive gastritis the superficial epithelium is lost. This picture of haemorrhagic, erosive gastritis is typical of chemical injury. *H. pylori* acute gastritis is characterized by a more prominent neutrophil response. Occasionally other more virulent organisms (particularly streptococci) may cause a severe, usually fatal, purulent gastritis.

Chronic Gastritis

The discovery, usually attributed to the Australians Warren and Marshall in 1983, of *H. pylori* has radically changed our concepts of chronic gastritis. In the past it was recognized that a small subset of patients with chronic gastritis were suffering from an autoimmune attack on the gastric mucosa, but the majority of instances were put down to vague dietary or endogenous (acid, bile) agents. It is now clear that three major types exist – *H. pylori*-induced, autoimmune and chemical (reactive) – with a few exceptional cases having unusual causes and often characteristic histological features.

Helicobacter-associated Chronic Gastritis

Helicobacter pylori is a spiral bacterium which has become remarkably well adapted to life at the interface between the surface epithelium of the stomach and the covering layer of secreted mucus. The organism causes direct epithelial cell injury, and also excites a vigorous immune response – two mechanisms of development of a chronic inflammatory reaction. Histologically, the mucosa shows a mixed inflammatory cell response with neutrophil infiltration of the

epithelium and a lymphocyte and plasma cell infiltrate in the stroma (this mixed pattern is often referred to as 'active chronic gastritis') (Figure 9.23). Severe, long-standing epithelial injury may lead to glandular atrophy. The epithelium may also show an adaptive response termed 'intestinal metaplasia' in which a partial or almost complete change in epithelial cell differentiation towards small intestinal type occurs. This benefits the host insofar as the intestinal mucosa is resistant to *H. pylori* infection.

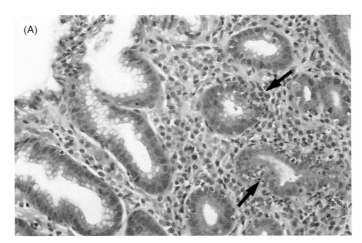

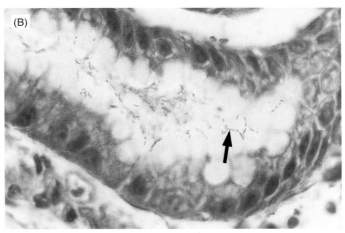

FIGURE 9.23 (A) Active chronic gastritis. Chronic inflammatory cell infiltration of the lamina propria with neutrophil movement into crypts (arrows). (B) *Helicobacter pylori* organisms in the surface mucus are better seen (arrow) in a Giemsa stain.

Two topographic patterns of *H. pylori* infection are recognized, although the distinction may not be clear in an individual patient. Many patients have a predominantly antral active chronic gastritis. These are the individuals who are most at risk of developing duodenal ulceration. Somewhat less commonly infection and inflammation involve both body and antrum ('pangastritis'). This disease pattern is associated with gastric ulcer and adenocarcinoma.

Autoimmune Chronic Gastritis

The association has long been recognized between vitamin B_{12} deficiency, macrocytic anaemia and a form of chronic gastritis. This syndrome – which is referred to clinically as pernicious anaemia – is associated with circulating anti-bodies to gastric parietal cells and is a good example of organ-specific autoimmunity. Histologically, there is chronic gastritis (not usually showing neutrophil 'activity') involving mainly the body of the stomach. In long-standing cases, mucosal atrophy is prominent and there is commonly extensive intestinal metaplasia. The associated anaemia is explained by gastric parietal cell loss with consequent deficiency of intrinsic factor and inadequate vitamin B_{12} absorption in the terminal ileum.

Chemical (Reactive) Gastritis

This pattern of mucosal response is often termed 'bile reflux gastritis'. Indeed, reflux of bile and alkaline small intestinal material is a common cause of gastric epithelial cell injury in patients with gastroduodenal motility disturbances which may be an isolated (primary) phenomenon, or may follow surgery to the pyloric region. Similar patterns of mucosal change may be seen following other chemical injuries, particularly long-term NSAID ingestion, and the term chemical gastritis is therefore preferred. Histologically, there is marked hyperplasia in the proliferative compartment of the gastric pits (the neck cells) with oedema of the mucosa (Figure 9.24). A cellular inflammatory infiltrate is often remarkably absent or scant. *H. pylori* are not usually seen.

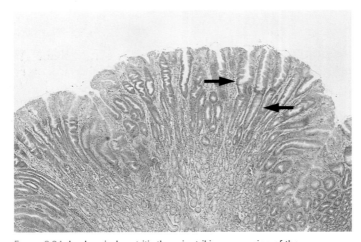

FIGURE 9.24 In chemical gastritis there is striking expansion of the proliferative 'neck' cell compartment of the pits (arrows).

Epidemiology, Pathogenesis and Diagnosis of H. pylori Infection

Helicobacter pylori is a microaerophilic, motile, spiral bacterium which is Gram-negative by conventional bacteriological analysis. These organisms can be identified in, and cultured from, the stomachs of healthy individuals. In Western society, infection is more prevalent among older age groups, whilst in developing countries infection is very commonly acquired in childhood and is almost universal by

middle age. Once infected, a few individuals can eliminate the organism, but the great majority develop a persisting chronic gastritis. *H. pylori* is transmitted from person to person, but the exact route (oral–oral, faecal–oral) is not clear. Infection is associated with low socio-economic status and crowded living conditions.

Gastric mucosal colonization by *H. pylori* and the consequent superficial active chronic gastritis is not necessarily (or even commonly) associated with clinical disease. In the absence of ulceration there is a very poor correlation between infection and dyspeptic symptoms. Infection is, however, associated with varying degrees of certainty, with a number of important conditions ranging from peptic ulceration to atrophic gastritis, adenocarcinoma and lymphoma (Figure 9.25). There is also an epidemiological link with extraintestinal disease such as abnormally short stature and ischaemic heart disease, although the link in these instances is unlikely to be causal. The ability of *H. pylori* to cause disease is dependent (as in many chronic infectious diseases) both on bacterial virulence factors and on variations in host response. Studies of mutant organisms have shown that bacterial motility and urease activity are essential for survival. The organism also produces adhesion factors, including a haemagglutinin which binds to sugar moieties on the gastric epithelial cell membrane. Virulent strains have also been shown to produce a number of tissue injuring factors, including Gram-negative lipopolysaccharide and the highly antigenic CagA and VacA proteins as well as a number of heat shock proteins. The host cell response (polymorph leucocytes and lymphoplasmacytic) is characterized by high levels of proinflammatory cytokines including interleukins IL-1, IL-8 and tumour necrosis factor α (TNFα). Cytokine production is thought to be important in the increased gastrin secretion seen in *H. pylori* gastritis. Other physiological changes have been identified, including an increased gastrin response to infused gastrin-releasing peptide (GRP). These changes are most

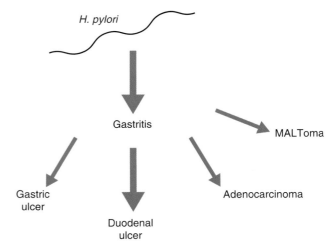

FIGURE 9.25 *Helicobacter pylori* disease associations. The size of the arrow is a rough indication of the clinical magnitude of the association. MALToma = mucosal associated lymphoid tumours.

marked in patients with duodenal ulceration. Some individuals show a tendency to low gastric acid output, and these tend to develop a severe pangastritis, gastric ulceration and possibly adenocarcinoma.

Diagnosis of *H. pylori* infection is not simple. Direct culture is difficult and is not routinely used, although it can provide useful information on antibiotic sensitivity. Minimally invasive tests include the urease breath test (measuring radio-labelled carbon released from ingested urea) and serology. The latter is useful in epidermiological studies, but suffers from the fact that circulating antibodies can be detected after elimination of infection. Endoscopy offers the most reliable diagnosis. Mucosal biopsies can be directly tested for urease activity when placed on gel-covered slides. Histological examination of specially stained sections is still the 'gold standard', and also allows assessment of inflammation, atrophy, intestinal metaplasia and dysplasia.

Special Forms of Gastritis

A few uncommon, but well recognized, patterns of gastritis are worth noting. Granulomatous gastritis may be seen in the context of sarcoidosis and Crohn's disease. While both of these diagnoses must be considered when granulomatous inflammation is identified in a gastric biopsy, a significant number of patients in this circumstance show no evidence of disease elsewhere. The cause of this isolated granulomatous gastritis is unclear.

In lymphocytic gastritis there is an increase in numbers of lymphocytes *within* the gastric mucosal epithelium. This pattern is similar to that seen in coeliac disease (see p. 245). Some cases are indeed associated with coeliac disease and some with *H. pylori* infection but, in many, the cause is unclear.

Eosinophilic gastritis is characterized by a dense infiltrate of eosinophil leucocytes in the wall of the stomach. A hypersensitivity response to ingested antigen is strongly suspected, but a specific source is not always identified.

Peptic Ulceration

Key Points

- Ulcers are caused by loss of balance between mucosal defence and acid attack.
- Acute ulcers are seen in chemical injury and severe stress (shock).
- Chronic ulcers are strongly associated with *Helicobacter* gastritis.
- Complications include haemorrhage, perforation, stenosis.

Peptic ulceration is defined by the fact that it occurs only in mucosal surfaces exposed to the potentially injurious effect of gastric acid and pepsin. It is seen (in decreasing order of frequency) in the duodenum, stomach, distal oesophagus and, following surgery, in relation to gastroenterostomy stomas. Although acid–pepsin attack is a prerequisite for disease ('no acid, no ulcer' is a hallowed catchphrase), the precise pathogenesis involves consideration of a number of factors, including mucosal defence mechanisms, prostaglandin metabolism, mucosal blood flow and, crucially, the effect of *H. pylori* infection. The relative importance of the different mechanisms is well illustrated by comparing gastric and duodenal peptic ulcers (see below and Table 9.1). Peptic ulcers are usually considered in separate acute and chronic categories.

Acute Peptic Ulcers

Mucosal erosion (loss of continuity of the epithelial lining) is a common feature of acute gastritis. If the defect is severe enough to penetrate the muscularis mucosae to involve the submucosa, this becomes – by definition – an ulcer. Acute ulcers can be distinguished morphologically from chronic by the lack of fibrosis in the former. The importance of distinguishing between erosions and acute ulcers is that ulcers are

TABLE 9.1 Comparison of important features of chronic gastric and duodenal ulcers

Parameter	Ulcer type	
	Gastric	**Duodenal**
Causal factor	• 'Undermined mucosal defences'	• 'Increased acid attack with weakened defences'
Epidemiology	• Risk increases with age (50+ years)	• Occurs at younger age than GU (35+ years) • More common than GU (3:1) • Associated with blood group O
Gastric acid output	• Low → normal	• Normal → high
H. pylori infection	• Commonly involves antrum and body ('pangastritis')	• Yes (90+%) • Commonly confined to antrum • Organisms may be seen in foci of duodenal gastric metaplasia

There are at least four mechanisms for the production of diarrhoea and steatorrhoea in Zollinger–Ellison syndrome:

- Extensive gastrin causes increased gastric acid and fluid production.
- Low pH in the small intestine causes mucosal damage.
- Bile salts are precipitated in an acid environment resulting in a failure of micelle production and fat emulsification.

- Pancreatic enzymes are denatured by acid, leading to functional pancreatic insufficiency.

Further Reading

Kingham JGC, Levison DA, Fairclough PD. Diarrhoea and reversible enteropathy in Zollinger–Ellison syndrome. *Lancet* 1981; **11**: 610–612.

---

from the surface epithelium. The importance of this mechanism in GU occurring in the intact stomach is less well established.

Apart from mucus, gastric surface epithelial cells also secrete bicarbonate – which is also a major factor in maintaining the pH gradient between the mucosa and the gastric contents. The epithelial cells themselves form a significant barrier to acid. The apical cell membranes of these cells and the tight intercellular junctions combine to effect this role. This function can be disrupted by the direct cytotoxic effect of *H. pylori*, or by the indirect damage caused by the inflammatory response to this organism. Mucosal blood flow is an important fallback mechanism for clearing up any hydrogen ions that may have escaped through the mucus/epithelial barrier. Loss of this mechanism is likely to be an important contributor to acute ulcers in shock, but there is some evidence that mucosal blood flow is also decreased in some patients with chronic peptic ulcers. Prostaglandins appear to have a protective effect against mucosal epithelial cell damage. Interference in this pathway is the probable mechanism of ulceration in NSAID patients.

A number of endogenous peptide/protein factors are important in maintaining epithelial cell integrity and, indeed, in effecting repair in areas of damage. Growth factors such as epidermal growth factor (EGF) and transforming growth factor-α (TGFα) are important in this regard, as are the trefoil peptides – a family of mucin-associated molecules which have important effects in maintaining a protective mucous layer and in stimulating motility of epithelial cells across areas of ulceration. The importance of trefoil peptides is emphasized by their close association with regeneration and repair of ulcers at a number of sites in the gastrointestinal tract (e.g. Barrett's oesophagus, peptic ulcer and in inflammatory bowel disease).

Gastric Neoplasms and Polyps

Polyps and Benign Tumours in the Stomach

A number of conditions give rise to mucosal elevations in the stomach, all of which are described macroscopically (and endoscopically) as 'polyps'. Many such lesions are non-neoplastic. Polyps of hyperplastic and inflammatory type occur on a background of gastritis and are of little clinical significance. Not uncommonly, multiple mucosal polyps are seen in the body and cardia of the stomach which, histologically, are seen to be due to marked dilatation of the fundic glands (fundic cyst polyps). The pathogenesis of these is unclear, but it is interesting that they are more common in patients with familial adenomatous polyposis (FAP) of the colon. True benign neoplastic epithelial polyps are unusual. These adenomas are morphologically very similar to the much more common colorectal adenomas. Their recognition is very important as they have a very high risk of progression to invasive malignancy (adenocarcinoma).

Malignant Neoplasms

> **Key Points**
>
> - Gastric carcinoma shows marked geographic variation in incidence.
> - Its incidence is decreasing in Western populations.
> - The intestinal subtype is associated with chronic gastritis and *H. pylori* infection.
> - The diffuse type is not related to gastritis.

Adenocarcinoma

Carcinoma of the stomach is a disease notable for its variable geographical incidence. The highest incidence is seen in the Far East, notably Japan. From the pathologist's viewpoint, the disease is interesting in that the two major histological subtypes (intestinal and diffuse; see below) have quite different epidemiological and genetic profiles. Migrant studies have shown that the geographical variation in incidence of gastric cancer is largely due to environmental influences, and the consumption of smoked foods rich in nitrates has been implicated. Fresh fruit and vegetables appear to have a protective effect, possibly mediated by antioxidants such as ascorbic acid. An improved diet has been proposed as a major contributory factor in explaining the declining overall incidence of gastric cancer in Western society over the past few decades.

Morphology

Gastric carcinomas can be classified by their site of origin (e.g. antral, fundic, cardiac). The topographical site of the tumour is of no prognostic significance, but is of considerable importance in tumour epidemiology. The recent overall decline in the incidence of gastric carcinoma appears to involve mainly tumours of the distal stomach, while cancers of the cardiac mucosa have actually increased in incidence. These cardiac tumours appear to share the epidemiological associations of carcinomas arising in Barrett's oesophagus.

Gastric carcinomas can be classified macroscopically as either polypoid, exophytic, ulcerative or infiltrative (Figure 9.29). These categories again are of little independent clinical significance, but the diffusely infiltrative lesions give rise to a rigid immobile ('leather bottle') stomach known as linitis plastica. This can give a characteristic appearance radiologically on barium meal examination.

Microscopic examination has yielded a number of classifications. The most useful is the Lauren system, which defines two major subgroups (Figure 9.30). Intestinal carcinomas are gland-forming neoplasms which, as the term would suggest, resemble carcinomas of the large and small intestines (and indeed oesophageal adenocarcinoma). Diffuse carcinomas are characterized by non-cohesive, mucin-containing 'signet ring' cells that infiltrate widely through the wall of the stomach, often being associated with the macroscopic pattern of linitis plastica. This classification is of clinical use since, for tumours of equivalent stage, the prognosis is worse in diffuse cancers. These two categories are also different in epidemiology and pathogenesis. Intestinal cancers tend to occur in older individuals and have declined in incidence in recent years. Diffuse adenocarcinomas now make up about 50% of gastric cancers, and tend to occur in a younger age group.

Aetiology and pathogenesis

Intestinal adenocarcinomas frequently develop on a background of chronic gastritis with atrophy. As in oesophageal

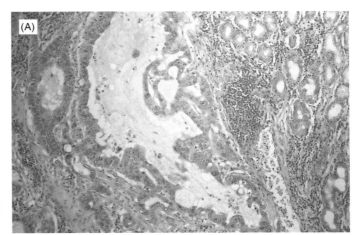

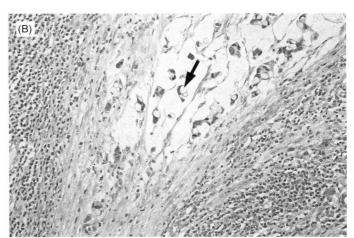

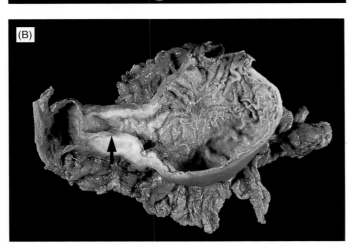

FIGURE 9.29 (A) Large ulcerated gastric carcinoma. (B) Infiltrative carcinoma showing marked thickening of the wall in the region of the antrum and pylorus (arrow).

FIGURE 9.30 (A) Intestinal-type gastric adenocarcinoma with well-formed glands. (B) Diffuse carcinoma made up of dissociated mucin-producing, signet-ring cells (arrow).

adenocarcinomas, there is an association with intestinal metaplasia, and a preinvasive state of dysplasia can be recognized. Chronic gastritis of all types shows an association with carcinoma but, in view of its frequency, there has recently been a considerable focus of attention on the role of *H. pylori* as a potential carcinogenic agent.

H. pylori is not directly mutagenic, but infection is associated in some patients with decreased acid production. This hypochlorhydria allows the proliferation of other organisms, some of which are capable of generating mutagenic compounds from dietary nitrates. DNA damage from reactive oxygen species (generated directly by *H. pylori* and also by inflammatory neutrophils and macrophages) is an important factor, and also highlights the previously mentioned protective effect of antioxidants in the diet (see p. 240). Increased epithelial cell proliferation, resulting from the cytotoxic effects of *H. pylori* and possibly also from cytokine stimulation, is important in providing the fertile ground of DNA synthesis in which mutagenic agents can operate.

Diffuse carcinomas are not associated with chronic gastritis and do not have a clearly defined precursor dysplastic lesion. At the molecular genetic level, there are also some differences between the tumour types, confirming the epidemiological differences. Intestinal cancers are characterized by up-regulation of growth factor receptors such as Her 2, while diffuse neoplasms show down-regulation or mutation of the E-cadherin gene coding for an important epithelial cell adhesion molecule.

Prognostic Factors in Gastric Cancer

As mentioned above, the outcome in adenocarcinoma of the stomach depends to some extent on the tumour type (intestinal or diffuse). A number of other prognostic indicators have been studied but, as in most human malignancies, tumour stage is of prime importance. Most patients in

---

 ## 9.1 SPECIAL STUDY TOPIC

GASTRIC LYMPHOMA: A DISEASE OF MUCOSA-ASSOCIATED LYMPHOID TISSUE

The gastrointestinal tract is the most common primary site of mucosa-associated lymphoid tissue (MALT) lymphoma (also known as marginal zone lymphoma). Within the gut, the majority of such tumours arise in the stomach. Clinical presentation of gastric lymphoma is variable. Low-grade lesions present with non-specific symptoms such as dyspepsia. Higher-grade tumours may present with anorexia and weight loss, and are easily confused clinically with gastric carcinoma. Macroscopically, MALT lymphomas are often poorly defined, but higher grade examples present as solid ulcerated tumour masses. Microscopically and immunophenotypically, these tumours are mostly low-grade B-cell lymphomas of marginal zone origin. They are made up of small- to medium-sized lymphocytes which may show some plasma cell differentiation. They often infiltrate around reactive follicles. The most characteristic histological feature is tumour cell infiltration of the epithelium of gastric glands (the lymphoepithelial lesion; Figure 9.31). Regional lymph nodes may be involved by tumour. Unlike other low-grade B-cell lymphomas, it is unusual to have systemic disease (distant lymph node or bone marrow involvement) at presentation. High-grade MALT lymphomas are made up of larger blast-like cells. Many high-grade tumours show residual elements of lower-grade neoplasm, and it is thought that some arise by progression from these pre-existing neoplasms.

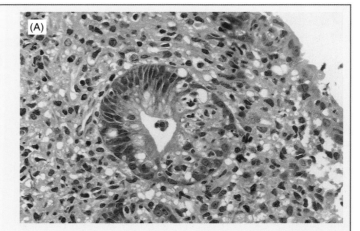

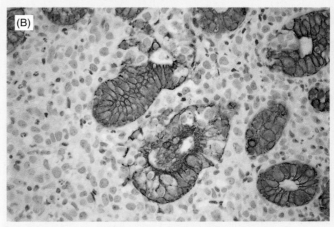

FIGURE 9.31 Gastric B-cell lymphoma of MALT origin (marginal zone lymphoma). (A) The characteristic lymphoepithelial lesion shows atypical lymphoid cells invading a gastric gland. The extent of this process is emphasized in (B), where the glands are highlighted by an immunohistochemical demonstration of cytokeratin.

Western society present at an advanced stage of disease, when the malignant cells have invaded through the stomach wall and spread to local and regional lymph nodes and/or the liver. In Japan where, because of a high incidence, there is a screening programme for gastric carcinoma, survival following resection of 'early' gastric cancer (defined as carcinoma invading no deeper than the submucosa of the stomach) is much better than in North America or Europe.

Other Gastric Neoplasms

Neuroendocrine (carcinoid) tumours of the stomach are rare and, although malignant, have a better prognosis than adenocarcinoma. Gastric malignant lymphomas are a source of considerable biological and clinical interest. These neoplasms are almost invariably of B-cell lineage. They are the best and most common example of lymphoma arising in the mucosa-associated lymphoid tissue (MALT). As with adenocarcinoma, there is a strong epidemiological link with *H. pylori* colonization. These organisms are antigenic and provoke a chronic inflammatory cell reaction in the mucosa. This is the background upon which clonal populations of cells may arise and progress to a clinical lymphoid neoplasm. Prognosis depends on the grade and stage of the tumour. The link to *H. pylori* is emphasized by regression of histologically proven neoplasms following antibiotic therapy, which is now the initial treatment for most such tumours.

Gastrointestinal Stromal Tumours (GIST)

It is an interesting paradox that, while most of the tissue of the gastrointestinal tract is mesenchymal in origin, the great majority of neoplasms are epithelial. Nevertheless, connective tissue tumours are an important clinical problem. They are seen throughout the gut, but are most common in the stomach. It was formerly thought that these were of smooth muscle origin and they were labelled as leiomyomas or leiomyosarcomas to indicate likely benign or malignant clinical course. In fact, with the exception of the oesophagus, most mesenchymal tumours show no evidence of muscle differentiation and are usually referred to as gastrointestinal stromal tumours (GIST). In fact, the cells in GIST resemble the pacemaker cells of the gut – the interstitial cells of Cajal.

These tumours can present with ulceration and bleeding, as an obstruction, or as abdominal masses. On gross examination of resected specimens, these tumours are usually well demarcated from surrounding tissues (Figure 9.32). Microscopically, they are usually made up of spindle-shaped cells

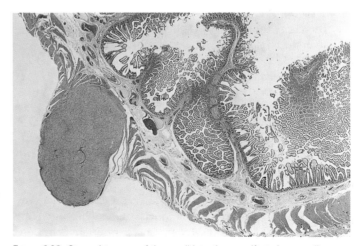

FIGURE 9.32 Stromal tumour of the small intestine manifested as a well-demarcated nodule in the muscularis.

and there may be evident necrosis. Some tumours behave in an entirely benign fashion while others can progress rapidly to metastatic disease. It can be difficult to predict prognosis in an individual patient, but tumour size and the frequency of mitotic figures are important (thus, for example, tumours of more than 10 cm or showing more than 10 mitoses per high power microscopic field are at very high risk of malignant behaviour).

It has been shown that most GIST show a mutation of the c-*kit* oncogene, and overexpress the gene product CD 117 on the cell membrane. Detection of this is a useful diagnostic test for the neoplasm. It is also of great therapeutic importance, as the tyrosine kinase-inhibiting drug imatinib acts directly to inhibit the effect of the oncogene mutation. This drug is remarkably effective in controlling inoperable and metastatic GIST, and is an excellent example of how understanding tumour biology can lead to development of specific, effective non-toxic therapy.

THE INTESTINES

Normal Structure and Function

Small Intestine

The small intestine is the main site of enzymatic digestion and absorption of nutrients. In the duodenum, the gastric contents are mixed with bile and pancreatic secretions and the main process of digestion begins. Absorption then proceeds in the jejunum and ileum. The mucosa of the small intestine provides a vast area for absorption through its villous structure. The villi themselves are covered by specialized absorptive cells (enterocytes) which have microvilli on their luminal surfaces, further increasing the surface area. Enterocytes produce hydrolytic enzymes such as disaccharidases and peptidases.

Other cells present in the small intestinal mucosa include:

- Epithelial stem cells in the intestinal crypts. These can divide and differentiate into all other epithelial cell types.
- Endocrine cells: these produce a variety of hormones such as enteroglucagon, cholecystokinin, gastrin, motilin, secretin, vasoactive intestinal polypeptide (VIP), and serotonin (5-hydroxytryptamine; 5-HT).
- Paneth cells: these are present at the bases of the crypts, and contain prominent large lysozyme-rich granules. Their secretions modulate the intestinal flora.
- The mucin-producing cells of Brunner's glands: these submucosal glands are mainly present in the duodenum, and produce mucus and epidermal growth factor (EGF). They are, therefore, considered to have a role in mucosal repair.
- The cells in the lamina propria, namely lymphocytes, plasma cells, eosinophils and mast cells. These occupy the space between the crypts and prominent lymphatics and blood capillaries. The lymphoid cells belong to the MALT. In some parts of the intestine the lymphoid

cells are aggregated; this is particularly prominent in the terminal ileum, where they form Peyer's patches.

Large Intestine

This is composed of the caecum, ascending colon, transverse colon, descending colon, sigmoid colon and rectum. Its functions include:

- storage and elimination of food residues
- maintenance of fluid and electrolyte balance
- the large intestine is the main site for the bacterial degradation of complex carbohydrates and other nutrients.

The mucosa of the large bowel differs from that of the small in the following important respects:

- it is flat with no villi
- it contains straight crypts lined by absorptive and mucus-producing goblet cells
- the endocrine cells and Paneth cells are less numerous, the latter normally being found only on the right side of the colon and in very small numbers
- the lamina propria is less prominent and contains very few lymphatics; thus, malignancy confined to the mucosa has a very limited metastatic potential.

It is important to know the blood supply of the intestines, as this determines the site and pattern of ischaemic damage, and is also followed by lymphatics, thereby determining the routes of spread of carcinoma. The superior mesenteric artery supplies the entire small intestine apart from the first half of the duodenum. This artery also supplies the right side of the colon and most of the transverse colon. In the small intestine, the terminal branches of the superior mesenteric artery are end arteries, there being few anastomoses between them. In the large bowel there is a degree of distal and proximal anastomosis between all of the supplying vessels. The inferior mesenteric artery supplies the distal transverse, descending, sigmoid colon and upper part of rectum. The middle and inferior rectal arteries, branches of the internal iliac and internal pudendal arteries, supply the remainder of the rectum. The venous drainage of the bowel, apart from the anal canal, is via the portal system to the liver. This is the reason why primary gastrointestinal malignancies frequently develop hepatic metastases.

The sympathetic nervous supply to the gut originates in the coeliac and mesenteric plexuses. Parasympathetic ganglia lie within the gut wall, where, together with other neurones, they form the submucosal (Meissner's) plexus and the muscular (Auerbach's) plexus. Parasympathetic stimulation increases muscular contraction, blood supply and secretory activity, while sympathetic activity has the opposite effect. There are also sensory receptors in the mucosa and bowel wall which respond to changes in volume and composition of bowel contents; by releasing neurotransmitters such as VIP, cholecystokinin and somatostatin, these receptors produce motor and secretory responses.

Congenital Disorders

Atresia

Failure of development or canalization of part of the gut is most often described in the duodenum and the anorectal area. Duodenal atresia is strongly associated with trisomy 21 (Down syndrome).

Malrotation

Failure of the caecum to descend into the right iliac fossa can lead to positioning of the entire large bowel to the left side of the abdominal cavity.

Diverticula and Duplications

Congenital diverticula of the upper small intestine may be a source of abnormal bacterial overgrowth, with consequent malabsorption (see p. 246). Meckel's diverticulum is a well-recognized vestigial remnant of the embryological vitellointestinal duct, and is found attached to the wall of the distal ileum. It may become inflamed and mimic acute appendicitis. Occasionally, heterotopic gastric and/or pancreatic epithelium may be present in the diverticulum, leading to local ileal peptic ulceration.

Hirschsprung's Disease

This condition is characterized by a lack of normal ganglion cells in the myenteric plexus of part of the bowel. It is due to the failure of migration of primitive neuroblasts into the developing gut. The distal large bowel is usually affected, but the abnormality may extend to involve the entire colon and even part of the small intestine. Diagnosis can be made on biopsies by demonstrating a lack of ganglia and the associated unchecked proliferation of parasympathetic acetylcholinesterase-producing nerves in the mucosa.

Malabsorption

Malabsorption can be due to a range of mechanisms:

- inadequate digestion: due to pancreatic insufficiency; hepatobiliary disease; post-gastrectomy
- intestinal damage: causes include coeliac disease; tropical sprue; post-infective malabsorption; Crohn's disease; parasitic disease; drugs; radiation enteritis; Whipple's disease; lymphoma; immunodeficiency; amyloidosis; and intestinal resection
- altered intestinal flora (bacterial overgrowth): jejunal diverticulosis; blind loops
- biochemical abnormality; causes include abetalipoproteinaemia; disaccharidase deficiency; specific amino acid malabsorption (e.g. Hartnup disease); and bile acid deficiencies
- lymphatic obstruction: intestinal lymphangiectasia (congenital or acquired)
- inadequate absorptive surface: intestinal resection or bypass
- endocrine disturbances: carcinoid syndrome; Verner–Morrison syndrome (vipoma, due to a VIP-producing tumour); diabetes mellitus; hypothyroidism
- circulatory disturbance: mesenteric vascular insufficiency.

Coeliac Disease

> **Key Points**
>
> - Coeliac disease results from an abnormal immune response to wheat gliadin.
> - Epithelial cell damage leads to small intestinal villous atrophy.
> - Coeliac disease is associated with dermatitis herpetiformis and intestinal lymphoma.

Coeliac disease is the most common intestinal cause of malabsorption in the Western world. It affects about 1 in 2000 individuals in the UK, but 1 in 300 in the west of Ireland. The condition usually presents in infancy or early childhood, but may only become manifest in adult life. It is due to a genetically determined, abnormal cell-mediated immune response to gliadin, a derivative of the wheat protein gluten (hence its alternative name gluten-sensitive enteropathy). There is a strong familial tendency and an association with HLA-B8. The skin disease dermatitis herpetiformis is also associated with HLA-B8, and most patients with this skin disease appear also to have coeliac disease.

The diagnosis is usually suspected in a child who fails to thrive, and suspicion is heightened if the stools are bulky and pale due to malabsorption of fat. Serological testing usually reveals the presence of antibodies to gliadin, and endomysium including tissue transglutaminase. However, the diagnosis can only be firmly established on a mucosal biopsy of distal duodenum or jejunum that reveals the typical picture of villous atrophy and crypt hyperplasia (Figure 9.33). These features are associated with increased numbers of plasma cells and lymphocytes in the lamina propria and increased numbers of intraepithelial cytotoxic T lymphocytes. Absolute confirmation of the diagnosis depends on return of these features to normal on re-biopsy after several weeks on a gluten-free diet.

Villous atrophy is due to damage to the surface enterocytes brought about by the immune reaction to gliadin. This results in a marked increase in cell death among the enterocytes, which is compensated for by an increased production of enterocytes in the crypts – hence crypt hyperplasia.

The immediate effects of coeliac disease are impaired nutrition and development due to malabsorption of fats, proteins, carbohydrates and vitamins. Long-term effects are an increased risk of T-cell lymphoma of the small intestine (enteropathy-type T-cell lymphoma). There also appears to be an increased incidence of certain other tumours, for example small intestinal and oesophageal carcinoma. Splenic atrophy – the cause of which is uncertain – is also commonly observed.

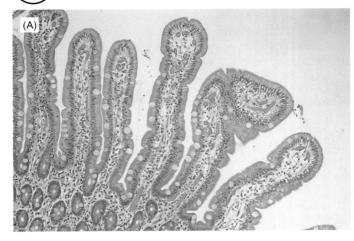

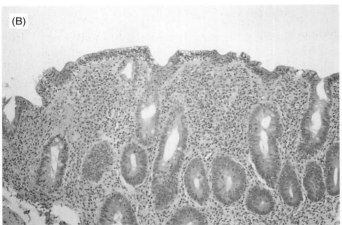

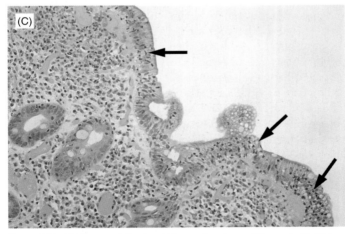

Figure 9.33 (A) A normal duodenal biopsy, showing well-formed villi. (B) In this case of coeliac disease the villous architecture is lost ('subtotal villous atrophy'). (C) There is an increased complement of intraepithelial lymphocytes (arrows).

Tropical Sprue

Identical, but usually less severe, changes to those found in coeliac disease are seen in tropical sprue. This is a form of malabsorption found in the tropics and subtropics, but not in Africa. It usually presents with diarrhoea, weight loss and a macrocytic anaemia due to folate or vitamin B_{12} deficiency. It is not due to gluten sensitivity, but may be relieved by broad-spectrum antibiotics, or may resolve spontaneously when the patient leaves the tropics. Its aetiology is uncertain, but abnormal bacterial colonization of the upper small intestine is the likely cause.

Giardiasis

Ingestion of water containing the encysted form of *Giardia lamblia* is the cause of giardiasis, which may give rise to mild malabsorption. Diagnosis is made by small intestinal biopsy which reveals the trophozoite phase of the parasite close to, or attached to, surface mucosa.

Altered Intestinal Flora

This occurs in bowel stasis as in diverticula or blind loops following operative bypass procedures. Abnormal overgrowth of organisms may compete for nutrients such as vitamin B_{12}, interfere with the action of bile salts, or inactivate mucosal enzymes.

Whipple's Disease

This is a rare multisystem disease caused by infection by bacteria (*Tropheryma whippelii*, a Gram-positive actinomycete). The disease may present with symptoms due to the infection of lymph nodes, joints, heart valves, lung or the central nervous system, but the most common presentation is with malabsorption. The disease responds to broad-spectrum antibiotics.

Bacterial Infections

Bacterial infection of the intestinal tract is a major cause of disease and death throughout the world. Often, infection is acquired through drinking contaminated water.

Cholera

This is due to infection with *Vibrio cholerae*, which produces a powerful exotoxin causing enterocytes to secrete abundant fluid and sodium ions. Massive watery diarrhoea may result, with devastating fluid loss and a rapidly fatal outcome. The toxin binds to epithelial cells, causing increased adenylate cyclase activity which results in high cyclic AMP levels in the intestinal mucosa. Histological changes in the mucosa are minimal.

Salmonella

Infection by *Salmonella typhi* or *Salmonella paratyphi* causes typhoid and the milder paratyphoid fever. These diseases are seen only rarely in Western countries, due largely to the availability of clean drinking water supplies. However, food poisoning by less virulent salmonellae is becoming increasingly common in the United Kingdom. Symptoms usually relate to the upper intestinal tract with colicky periumbilical pain, vomiting and watery diarrhoea, but sometimes they relate to the large intestine with frequent bloody stools and tenderness over the sigmoid colon.

WHIPPLE'S DISEASE

The patient, a 45-year-old male, presented with non-specific symptoms of feeling unwell, vague joint pains, and significant weight loss. A physical examination revealed the presence of generalized moderate lymphadenopathy, but no other abnormalities. The results of basic laboratory tests were all within normal ranges. A lymph node biopsy showed no evidence of malignancy, but a reactive picture characterized by the presence of large numbers of macrophages with prominent eosinophilic cytoplasm (Figure 9.34). A periodic acid–Schiff (PAS) stain, which stains for mucin, carbohydrate and certain organisms, was positive on these macrophages. On the basis of these appearances and the clinical findings, a diagnosis of Whipple's disease (a rare infection due to *Tropheryma whippelii*) was suggested. As lymph node appearances are not specific in this disease, it was decided to seek confirmation of the diagnosis by performing a duodenal biopsy. This showed slight shortening and swelling of the villi, prominent dilated mucosal lymphatics, and an increased inflammatory infiltrate in the lamina propria including large numbers of swollen pink macrophages (Figures 9.35 and 9.36), confirming the diagnosis of Whipple's disease. The patient was immediately placed on the broad-spectrum antibiotic tetracycline, and within a few weeks his symptoms had disappeared, he felt much better, and he had begun to put on weight. A follow-up duodenal biopsy performed 6 months after the commencement of the course of tetracycline therapy revealed a nearly normal small bowel mucosa (Figure 9.37).

The patient was then lost to follow-up for over a year, after which time he represented with unmistakable signs of dementia. A reappraisal of the management of the case by the physician raised the possibility that the dementia might also be due to Whipple's disease, as tetracycline does not cross the blood–brain barrier. The patient was immediately started on a prolonged course

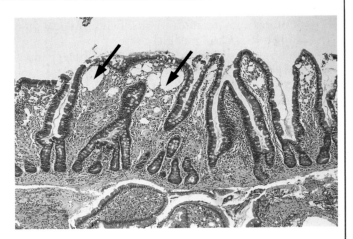

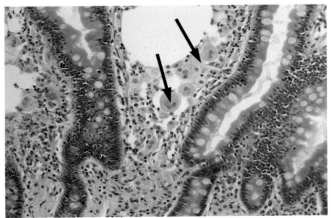

FIGURES 9.35 (TOP) AND 9.36 Low-power and higher-power views of duodenal biopsy, showing features described in the text. Arrows indicate dilated lymphatics in Figure 9.35, and macrophages in Figure 9.36.

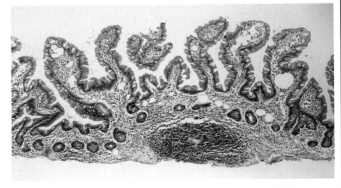

FIGURE 9.37 Duodenal biopsy following broad-spectrum antibiotic therapy. Note the normal villus architecture, no dilated lymphatics, and normal inflammatory cell component in the lamina propria.

of trimethoprim, and within a few weeks the clinical signs of dementia had all but disappeared.

Lessons to be learned from this case are:

- Whipple's disease, due to an unusual bacterium capable of intracellular survival, is a relatively rare systemic infection usually affecting middle-aged men.

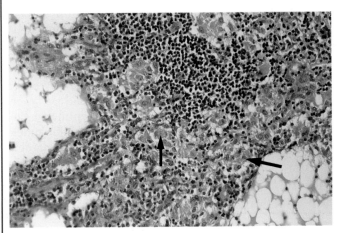

FIGURE 9.34 Haematoxylin and eosin staining of lymph node, showing fat and large numbers of pink swollen macrophages (arrows).

- Symptoms may relate to joints, lymph nodes, skin, brain, or the gastrointestinal tract.
- The diagnostic gold standard is small bowel (duodenal) biopsy.
- The condition can be fatal if not treated, but readily responds to broad-spectrum antibiotics. An antibiotic which crosses the blood–brain barrier should be used.
- Whipple's disease is a rare, but curable, cause of malabsorption.

Sigmoidoscopy in the latter case reveals changes which are very similar, both macroscopically and microscopically, to those of ulcerative colitis (see below).

Bacillary Dysentery

This is an acute infection of the large bowel causing painful diarrhoea with blood and mucus in the stools. *Shigella flexneri* and *Shigella dysenteriae* can produce mucosal appearances very similar to those of ulcerative colitis, though the more common *Shigella sonnei* produces less severe pathology.

Campylobacter *Colitis*

Campylobacter jejuni and *Campylobacter coli* are relatively frequent causes of severe gastroenteritis and colitis. Histological changes in rectal and colonic biopsies are non-specific and similar to those seen in other forms of infective colitis.

Escherichia coli *Diarrhoea*

E. coli is associated with a variety of diarrhoeal illnesses. Most are due to toxin formation. Some bacterial serogroups, particularly 0157:H7 are important causes of food-borne epidemics associated in some individuals with development of the haemolytic–uraemic syndrome and a mortality of approximately 10%.

Neonatal Diarrhoea

Specific enteropathogenic serotypes of *Escherichia coli* cause a significant proportion of diarrhoeal illness seen in neonates and infants. The resulting diarrhoea may be so severe that it leads to dehydration and death.

Staphylococcal Enterocolitis

This infection is relatively rare, but is a real threat among hospitalized patients receiving broad-spectrum antibiotics. These drugs alter the normal bowel flora such that infection with *Staphylococcus aureus* can then occur. This may result in severe diarrhoea accompanied by shock and dehydration, and can be life-threatening. The symptoms are caused by a powerful endotoxin released by the organisms. Occasionally, the disease is relatively mild and may respond to treatment, but more often it is severe and can be fatal. The small intestine is predominantly involved with ulceration.

Tuberculosis

This usually affects the terminal ileum. The primary infection – usually caused by drinking milk infected by bovine tuberculosis – is now rarely seen in the UK following the pasteurization of milk supplies. The condition results in a trivial lesion in the ileal mucosa associated with enlarged, caseating mesenteric nodes. Secondary tuberculosis is the result of swallowing infected sputum in the presence of severe pulmonary tuberculosis. This results in deep transverse ileal ulcers which heal by scarring, and cause strictures. Sometimes the disease can involve the ileocaecal valve and cause a picture which is macroscopically indistinguishable from that of Crohn's disease. Antibiotic therapy is the treatment of choice for intra-abdominal tuberculosis, but surgery is often required for complications, or to obtain tissue for diagnosis. Complications include obstruction by adhesions, perforation of ulcers (rare) and malabsorption due to extensive mucosal damage or lymphatic obstruction.

Actinomycosis

This usually presents as an inflammatory mass in the region of the appendix and caecum. The organism, *Actinomyces israelii* – a Gram-positive filamentous bacterium normally present in the mouth – may escape acid digestion in the stomach and infect the bowel. The disease is characterized by the formation of sinuses linking the bowel lumen to the skin surface, and fistulae. Yellowish (sulphur) granules composed of colonies of the organism are often visible to the naked eye in the watery pus.

Antibiotic-associated Colitis

This is due to overgrowth of *Clostridium difficile* in the colon following suppression of the normal bowel flora by broad-spectrum antibiotics. The disease can be mild or severe. Histologically, there is superficial loss of epithelial cells which become embedded in an exudate containing mucin, polymorphs, and abundant fibrin, forming a pseudomembrane on the surface – hence the term 'pseudomembranous colitis' (Figure 9.38).

Viral Infections

Most UK cases of acute gastroenteritis are due to viral infections. It is often not possible to confirm the diagnosis by laboratory means because of the relative insensitivity of

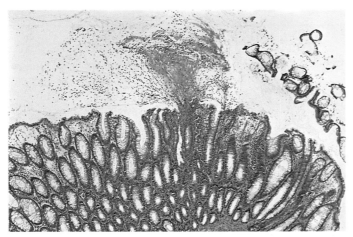

FIGURE 9.38 Pseudomembranous colitis. The colonic mucosal surface shows an erupting fibrinous 'pseudomembrane'.

available tests, and the fact that only tiny doses of viruses may cause illness. The main causative agents are parvoviruses and 'small round structured' viruses. These infect the small intestine, damage enterocytes, and cause mild villous atrophy and crypt hyperplasia and inflammation of the lamina propria.

The large bowel is occasionally infected by cytomegalovirus, which can cause an acute haemorrhagic colitis. It may occur *de novo* or complicate ulcerative colitis. The virus can be recognized due to the large intranuclear inclusions it produces in mucosal cells, both epithelial and endothelial.

Some cases of AIDS (especially in Africa) show severe malabsorption and nutritional disturbances. Sometimes, the symptoms appear to be directly due to the effects of the HIV virus, though often a superimposed opportunistic intestinal infection can be identified such as those due to coccidial protozoa (cryptosporidiosis) or *Mycobacterium avium intracellulare*.

Fungal and Chlamydial Diseases
(see also Chapter 19)

Fungal infections of the alimentary tract are rare, but are being seen increasingly in immunocompromised patients. In such instances, normally non-pathogenic phycomycetes are often found. Lymphogranuloma venereum is a venereal infection caused by specific serotypes of *Chlamydia trachomatis*. It is usually seen in females, and may cause rectal strictures due to spread to the rectum via lymphatics. The histological picture is characterized by granulomas and non-specific chronic inflammation.

Parasitic Infection (see also Chapter 19)

Giardiasis has been mentioned previously in relation to malabsorption and cryptosporidiosis in relation to AIDS. Other important protozoal parasitic diseases of the intestine are amoebiasis and schistosomiasis.

Amoebiasis affects the large intestine, and is the result of infection by the protozoan *Entamoeba histolytica*. It is more prevalent in the tropics than in temperate climates. Infection is by the faecal–oral route. Ingested as cysts, the organism is passed unharmed through the stomach, eventually reaching the large intestine where the cyst wall is dissolved, liberating active amoebae. These invade the mucosa by means of release of a cytolytic enzyme. They cause characteristic undermining 'flask-shaped' ulcers (recognizable in sections), or they may cause a more diffuse colitis. Organisms can be recognized in faeces or in the tissues, and often contain ingested red blood cells.

Large intestinal schistosomiasis is usually due to *Schistosoma mansoni* or *S. japonicum*, but is sometimes seen with *S. haematobium*. For an account of the lifecycle of the parasites, see Chapter 19. The pathological changes in schistosomiasis are the result of the inflammatory response to the presence of eggs embedded in the wall of the intestine. Left-sided lesions are almost always due to *S. mansoni*, whereas right-sided colonic and appendiceal lesions may be caused by *S. haematobium*.

Idiopathic Chronic Inflammatory Bowel Disease

There are two main idiopathic inflammatory bowel diseases, namely Crohn's disease and ulcerative colitis. Their main features are summarized and contrasted in Table 9.2. It is very important to remember that before a diagnosis of idiopathic inflammatory bowel disease is made, infective causes of inflammation must be excluded.

Crohn's Disease

Crohn's disease is more common in women than men, and usually presents in the 20- to 60-year-old age group. It most often affects the terminal ileum, but may also involve the large bowel either alone or together with the small bowel. Less often, the disease may affect other parts of the intestine from the mouth to the anus, and may also give rise to discontinuous skin lesions. The macroscopic appearances of the bowel vary according to the stage of the disease. The initial lesion is mucosal swelling due to submucosal oedema. This obscures the normal transverse folds of the mucosa. In this setting small superficial (aphthous) ulcers develop. In turn these deepen, giving rise to fissures. In the established, more chronic, form of the disease the mucosa shows a distinct cobblestone pattern due to the oedematous swollen mucosa being divided into segments by deep fissuring ulcers. The bowel wall at this stage is thickened due to a combination of oedema, inflammation and fibrosis which may lead to stricture formation. Regional lymph nodes are usually enlarged. Characteristic of bowel involvement by Crohn's disease is the fact that these areas of abnormality are separated by macroscopically normal segments. These discrete, diseased areas of bowel are referred to as 'skip lesions'. Thickened segments

TABLE 9.2 Comparison of the main features of Crohn's disease and ulcerative colitis

Feature	Crohn's disease	Ulcerative colitis
Characteristics	Chronic, relapsing, inflammatory condition of unknown aetiology	Chronic, relapsing, inflammatory condition of unknown aetiology
Presentation	Abdominal pain or obstruction	Bloody diarrhoea
Sites	Anywhere in the GI tract. Commonest in distal ileum, then colon	Confined to large bowel. May be localized to rectum or, in continuity, with any length of the colon
Inflammation	Transmural, patchy, often partly granulomatous	Mucosal, diffuse, non-granulomatous
Complications	<ul><li>Malabsorption</li><li>Fistula formation</li><li>Anal lesions</li><li>Malignancy (slight ↑ incidence of adenocarcinoma)</li><li>Amyloidosis</li><li>Perforation</li></ul>	<ul><li>Blood loss</li><li>Electrolyte disturbances</li><li>Toxic dilation</li><li>Malignancy (↑ incidence of adenocarcinoma in extensive colitis)</li><li>Extracolonic complications: (a) skin: pigmentation, erythema nodosum (b) liver: sclerosing cholangitis (c) eye: iritis, uveitis (d) joints: ankylosing spondylitis, arthritis</li></ul>

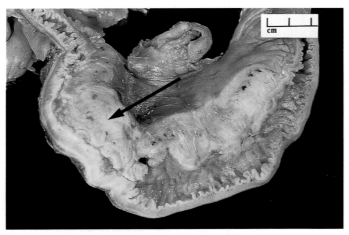

FIGURE 9.39 In this case of Crohn's disease, a segment (arrow) in which the wall is thickened by inflammation and fibrosis obstructs the small intestine.

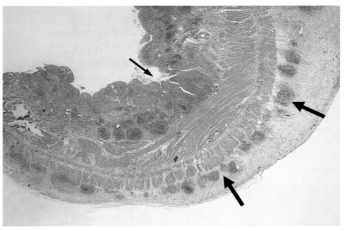

FIGURE 9.40 Low-power histology of Crohn's disease. Fissures (small arrow) disrupt the mucosa, and lymphoid chronic inflammation extends through the wall to the subserosal fat (large arrows).

of bowel wall can lead to narrowing of the lumen with partial obstruction (Figure 9.39).

Histologically, Crohn's disease is characterized by inflammation of all layers of the bowel (transmural inflammation; Figure 9.40). The submucosa is usually oedematous, and the ulcers extend from the mucosa deep into the bowel wall, forming fissures. Fibrous scarring becomes prominent with time. The full-thickness inflammation is characterized by focal aggregates of lymphocytes and, in many cases, non-caseating granulomas (Figure 9.41).

Local complications of Crohn's disease include inflammatory adhesions to other loops of the bowel, the parietal peritoneum or bladder. Deep fissuring ulcers may extend through the full thickness of the bowel wall into an adjacent viscus and cause a fistula. If a track is formed between the bowel and the skin surface, this is referred to as a 'sinus'. Sinuses are particularly common in the perianal region. Other complications include intestinal obstruction due to stricture formation or fibrous adhesions, perforation of the bowel by a deep fissuring ulcer leading to an intra-abdominal abscess, perianal fistulae, fissures and abscesses, a small increased risk of carcinoma of the bowel after many years, and occasionally heavy bleeding from ulcers. Crohn's disease usually follows a relapsing and remitting pattern, but because the scarring of the bowel wall and adhesions are permanent the likelihood of obstructive symptoms increases with time. Crohn's disease is also characterized by systemic complications (see Table 9.2).

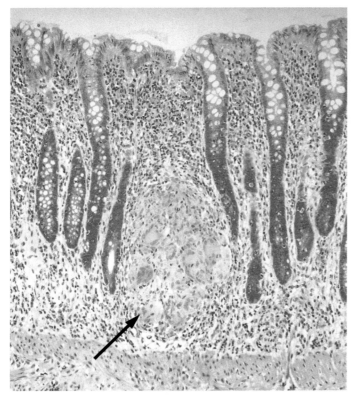

FIGURE 9.41 Inflammatory infiltration of the lamina propria and a granuloma (arrow) in a colonic biopsy from a patient with Crohn's disease.

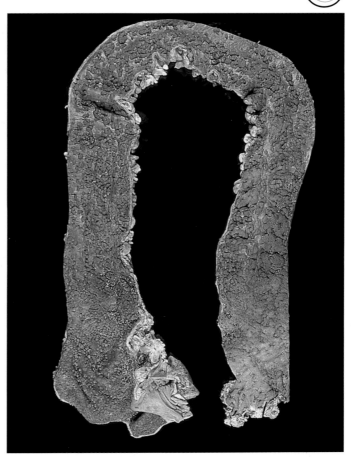

FIGURE 9.42 Specimen from a total colectomy performed for refractory ulcerative colitis. The mucosa is diffusely red and inflamed. Many inflammatory pseudopolyps are present.

Ulcerative Colitis

Ulcerative colitis contrasts with Crohn's disease in a number of important respects (see Table 9.2). Patients with active ulcerative colitis typically develop diarrhoea in which faecal matter is mixed with blood, mucus and pus. The disease begins in the rectum; if confined to the rectum it is referred to as proctitis. It may extend proximally in continuity throughout part or the whole of the large bowel (Figure 9.42). The term 'extensive colitis' is usually applied to disease affecting the colon right back at least to the hepatic flexure.

As with Crohn's disease, the appearances vary depending on the activity of the disease process. In active or early disease the mucosa appears to be congested and friable, and shows areas of shallow ulceration which eventually become confluent. The ulceration is typically superficial, extending no deeper than the submucosa. Histology at this stage shows marked congestion and oedema of the mucosa, a diffuse increase in chronic inflammatory cells in the lamina propria, cryptitis (neutrophil polymorphs infiltrating between epithelial cells of the crypts), and crypt abscesses (collections of neutrophil polymorphs in distended crypts) and a reduction in number of mucus cells in the glands (Figure 9.43). Such inflamed mucosa is often seen adjacent to an area of ulceration. The submucosa and deeper layers of the bowel wall are generally not inflamed.

In quiescent or treated colitis, the bowel mucosa usually appears macroscopically slightly reddened, granular and thinned, but is not ulcerated. Histology shows mild chronic inflammation of the lamina propria, but usually no cryptitis nor crypt abscesses. Glands may appear shortened or distorted but usually in inactive disease mucous cell numbers are not reduced, in contrast to the appearances in active disease.

Relatively infrequently the disease may present or relapse in a fulminant form in which the colon shows extensive confluent mucosal ulceration. This is associated with oedema and inflammation extending into the muscle layer. The damaged bowel wall progressively dilates, leading to the situation known as acute toxic megacolon. This can be life-threatening due to rapid loss of fluid, blood and electrolytes, or to perforation.

Local complications of ulcerative colitis include blood and fluid loss that may be severe, toxic dilatation and perforation; dysplasia and carcinoma may develop in long-standing extensive disease. Systemic complications of ulcerative colitis include erythema nodosum, pyoderma gangrenosum, iritis, arthritis, ankylosing spondylitis and chronic liver disease – particularly sclerosing cholangitis.

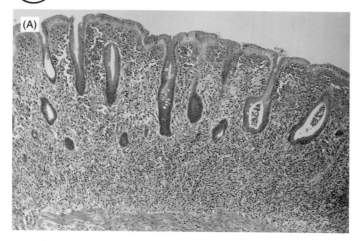

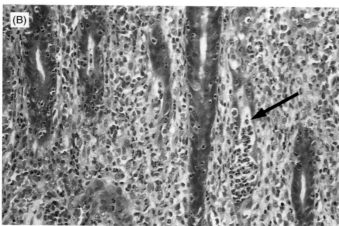

FIGURE 9.43 (A) Diffuse mucosal inflammation and crypt shortening in ulcerative colitis. (B) A higher-power view of a crypt abscess (arrow).

The natural history of ulcerative colitis is very variable, with small numbers of patients requiring early surgery, and small numbers having persistent active disease despite medical treatment, but most patients being generally reasonably controlled by medical treatment though suffering occasional relapses. Long-standing extensive colitis, i.e. colitis present for over 10 years and extending from the rectum to at least the hepatic flexure, is associated with a significantly increased risk of the development of rectal or colonic carcinoma. The development of carcinoma in ulcerative colitis is believed usually to be preceded by a non-invasive phase in which mucosal epithelial cells show varying degrees of dysplasia. It is suggested that patients who have had extensive colitis for over 10 years should undergo regular colonoscopy with biopsy in order to try to diagnose preinvasive neoplastic lesions. Repeated biopsies showing high-grade dysplasia even without invasion are regarded as an indication for colectomy.

The aetiologies of both ulcerative colitis and Crohn's disease are unknown. Both show a familial tendency and a number of candidate genes are under investigation. Mutations in CARD15 (NOD2) appear to account for 10–15% of patients with Crohn's disease. The clinical and pathological differences between the two conditions suggest that they probably have different aetiologies, although cases of overlapping

clinical and pathological findings are not rare. The granulomatous nature of Crohn's disease has led to extensive investigations for a bacterial causative agent, particularly a mycobacterium, but so far no convincing candidate has been identified. Smoking appears to predispose to Crohn's disease. With ulcerative colitis, possible aetiological factors include stress, infective and immunological causes. It is suggested that some sort of infection may trigger an inappropriate autoimmune response which leads to destruction of the colonic mucosa. Steroids and anti-inflammatory agents are usually effective in ulcerative colitis, suggesting that an immune activation may be important. Smoking appears to protect against ulcerative colitis.

Vascular Disease of the Intestines

Intestinal ischaemia may result from sudden occlusion of vessels. This may be by thrombosis on an atheromatous plaque, or by an embolus lodging in a mesenteric vessel. Ischaemic injury may also occur in the presence of patent vessels if the blood supply is inadequate to maintain gut nutrition, for example in hypotensive shock or non-occlusive arterial narrowing. Venous thrombosis is a rarer cause of ischaemia, but may occur in hypercoagulable states or, locally, in an impacted hernia (Figure 9.44). Systemic vasculitis is a further cause of ischaemia.

From a pathogenetic viewpoint, ischaemia can be considered as acute or chronic in type.

Acute Ischaemia

A sudden critical decrease in blood supply to the intestines threatens the viability of the bowel and the life of the

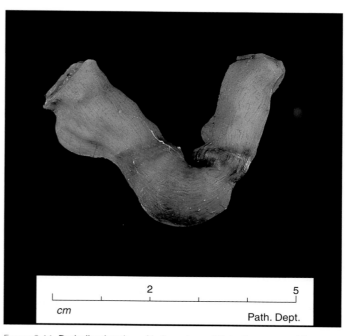

FIGURE 9.44 Dark discoloration of ischaemic small intestine removed from an inguinal hernia.

patient. The most common cause is arterial thrombo-embolus, followed by *in-situ* thrombus formation and non-occlusive vascular disease. Cellular injury is caused by anoxia and also often by reperfusion injury, in a manner analogous to that seen in the myocardium (see Chapter 6). The clinical features and severity of injury depend on the depth of intestinal damage. If infarction is confined to the mucosa, then complete regeneration is possible. Submucosal extension (mural infarction) can lead to fibrous stricture. Transmural infarction (gangrene) will lead to perforation if not surgically resected. Even before perforation, septicaemia may ensue as a result of unimpeded bacterial invasion.

Chronic Ischaemia

This condition is almost always seen in association with widespread atherosclerosis. Classically, it presents as 'mesenteric angina' – that is, post-prandial abdominal pain due to an inability to increase blood supply in response to the increased physiological demands of the digestive and absorptive process. These individuals are at extremely high risk of superimposed acute ischaemia, and frequently have areas of fibrous stricture due to previous mural infarcts. Diagnostic difficulty can arise in the investigation of patients with bloody diarrhoea in that microscopic features of ischaemia on biopsy can be confused with inflammatory bowel disease, pseudomembranous colitis or solitary rectal ulcer.

Necrotizing Enterocolitis

This is a condition, mainly seen in infants, in which there is intestinal gangrene caused partly by ischaemia and partly by overwhelming bacterial infection. Vasculitis is characteristic and inflammatory changes are seen in thrombosed blood vessels.

Vascular Malformations

A number of conditions are characterized by an abnormal proliferation of mature blood vessels in the wall of the bowel. Classification of these is complex. Some are congenital, while others appear to develop in adult life. Angiodysplasia is one such lesion, presenting in later life as colonic bleeding from abnormal submucosal vessels, often in the right side of the colon.

Acquired Disorders of Gut Motility

Diverticular Disease

Non-congenital intestinal diverticula are abnormal outpouchings of mucosa, often extending through the bowel wall to reach mesenteric or subserosal fat (Figure 9.45). The presence of such diverticula (diverticular disease) is common in the colon, and particularly in the sigmoid. Diverticula occur near the taenia coli at the points of penetration of blood vessels. There is marked muscular hypertrophy, and the mucosa can be thrown up into a complex pattern of

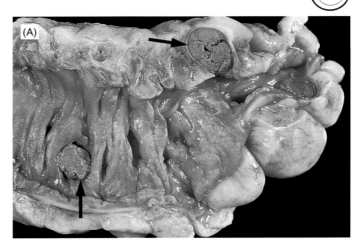

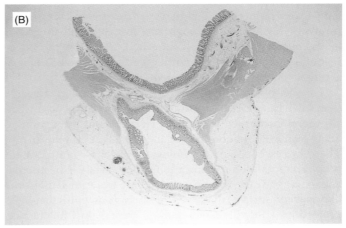

FIGURE 9.45 **(A)** Sigmoid colon resected for diverticular disease. Multiple mucosal outpouchings are visible, some with impacted hard faeces (faecoliths; arrows). **(B)** A full-mount histological preparation showing a mucosal diverticulum extending through the muscle wall of the colon.

folds. Diverticular disease is a condition of older individuals, and is associated with increased intraluminal pressure probably as a result of a low-fibre diet. Patients complain of colicky lower abdominal pain. Complicated disease occurs when diverticula become ulcerated, often due to an impacted faecolith. Bacterial infection can ensue, leading to a localized abscess or, worse, disseminated peritonitis with septicaemia. Localized disease not uncommonly leads to fistula formation, particularly to the bladder and vagina. Diverticular disease does not predispose to malignancy.

Other Mechanical Disorders

These include strangulation of bowel in a hernia sac (see Figure 9.44) and volvulus. The latter is an apparently spontaneous twist in a loop of bowel (often small intestine or sigmoid colon). This may occur around a congenital or acquired fibrous adhesion or as a result of an unusually long mesentery. Volvulus and strangulation lead to luminal obstruction and eventually to infarction by venous thrombosis. Intussusception is an invagination of one bowel segment into another. There is usually a lesion at the apex of the invaginating bowel. This may be a polyp or an intramural tumour, or something as simple as a focus of lymphoid hyperplasia. The latter is usually the case in ileocolic intussusception, the most common type seen in clinical practice.

Intestinal Polyps and Neoplasms

As in the stomach, a number of discrete mucosal elevations ('polyps') are described in the intestines. Many are non-neoplastic, and most are more common in the large bowel. Thus, inflammatory polyps may be seen, often in association with Crohn's disease or ulcerative colitis. So-called hyperplastic (metaplastic) polyps are seen only in the large bowel, where they are the most frequently identified polyps. They are of uncertain cause. Hamartomatous polyps are spread (more or less evenly) though the stomach and intestines in the autosomal dominant inherited condition of Peutz–Jeghers syndrome, the main other feature of which is a characteristic circumoral skin pigmentation.

True neoplastic polyps are far more common in the large than small bowel. They are most often of epithelial origin, and are therefore termed adenomas. These lesions are common, being seen in about one-third of individuals at 70 years of age. There are two basic morphological varieties: one contains tubular crypts arising from a lobulated surface (the tubular adenoma); the other (less common) type has a small intestine-like velvety surface made up of numerous epithelial-lined projections (the villous adenoma; Figure 9.46). In practice, many adenomas show mixtures of both features and are called tubulovillous adenomas. Macroscopically, tubular adenomas are rounded, usually less than 15 mm in diameter, and are frequently attached to the bowel wall by a definite stalk. Villous adenomas are flatter and larger (often over 25 mm in diameter). In all adenomas the neoplastic cells are epithelial, and these show varying degrees of dysplasia.

Adenomatous polyps are important in their own right as causes of bleeding and anaemia due to traumatic surface ulceration by the passing faecal stream. Nonetheless, it is the association between these lesions and the development of invasive malignancy (adenocarcinoma) that is of greatest clinical concern.

The Adenoma–Carcinoma Sequence

It is thought that most – if not all – colorectal carcinomas develop in pre-existing adenomas. The evidence for this may be summarized as follows:

- adenomas and carcinomas share the same epidemiological spread in world populations (and the same topographical spread in the colon)
- patients with colorectal cancer have a higher incidence of adenomas than unaffected controls
- the risk of developing carcinoma increases markedly in patients with higher numbers of adenomatous polyps (e.g. familial adenomatous polyposis)

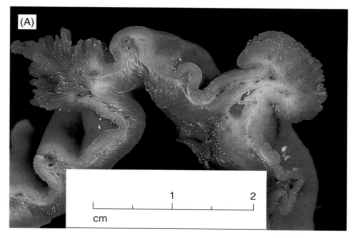

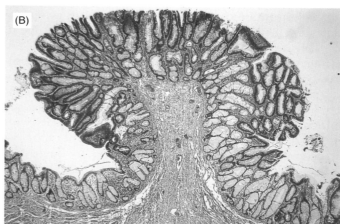

FIGURE 9.46 (A) Longitudinal section through resected bowel, showing two distinct adenomas. The lesion on the left shows the frond-like architecture of a villous adenoma, while that on the right shows the smoother lobulated outline of a tubular adenoma. (B) Low-power photomicrograph of a tubular adenoma, showing that the lesion is made up of distorted, elongated crypts. Even at this power the dark ('hyperchromatic') nuclei are visible. Note the raised stalk. This must be examined carefully for signs of early invasion.

- it is common to find residual adenomatous tissue on histological examination of cancers and, conversely, focal early invasive carcinoma can be seen arising in adenomatous polyps.

Colorectal Carcinoma

Cancers of the large bowel are among the most common neoplasms in Western society. There is a strong link with the lifestyle of developed countries which is confirmed in migrant studies. Diet is strongly implicated, particularly an intake which is rich in fat and poor in fibre. Antioxidant vitamins (A, D, E) are thought to be protective. Diet has an important effect on transit time through the gut, and also in modifying the resident flora. Fat-rich diets increase the bile acid content of faeces and also favour growth of clostridial species which are capable of generating carcinogenic compounds from the bile acids. Long-standing ulcerative colitis

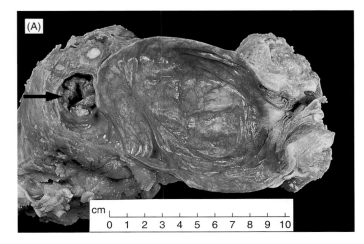

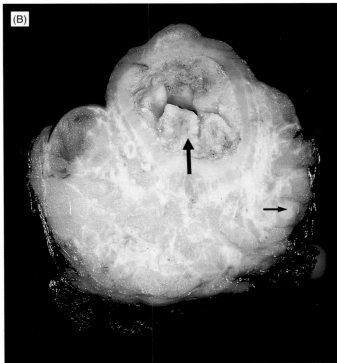

relatively more common. There are distinct macroscopic subtypes which show predilection for different regions of the bowel. Thus, rectal tumours are commonly seen as ulcerated raised plaques, while sigmoid, descending and transverse colon cancers most often present as a circumferential infiltrated 'napkin-ring' constriction (Figure 9.47). Carcinomas of the right colon characteristically appear as polypoid masses growing into the capacious lumen of this part of the gut. These macroscopic features underline differing modes of presentation with rectal tumours often presenting with fresh bleeding, annular constricting lesions as obstruction and right colonic tumours as an insidious anaemia.

Microscopically, the great majority of colorectal carcinomas are moderately differentiated adenocarcinomas (Figure 9.48). Some produce large amounts of mucin. By far the most important pathological parameter in clinical practice is the staging of the tumour on a surgical resection specimen using either Dukes' system (Figure 9.49) or, increasingly, the TNM system which has the advantage of subdividing Dukes' stage B tumours (the majority of surgically resected cases) into T3 and T4 (the latter defined as

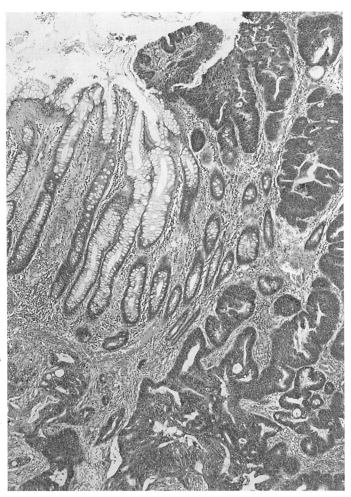

FIGURE 9.47 (A) Rectum opened up to give a view of a stenosing cancer (arrow) at the rectosigmoid junction. Note the enlarged white nodes in the adjacent fat. Microscopy showed these to be largely replaced by metastatic carcinoma. (B) Transverse section through a total mesorectal excision for rectal carcinoma. The tumour presents as a raised plaque (large arrow). There is extension through the wall into perirectal fat. Margin involvement was confirmed microscopically in the region indicated by the small arrow. The patient was therefore referred for radiotherapy.

(and to a lesser extent colonic Crohn's disease) carries a significantly increased risk of colorectal cancer.

Pathology of Large Bowel Carcinoma

The great majority of colorectal carcinomas are adenocarcinomas. About one-half are found in the rectum, a further one-third in the sigmoid, and the rest are spread equally across the remainder of the colon. There is some emerging evidence, however, that right-sided cancers are becoming

FIGURE 9.48 Invasive, moderately differentiated adenocarcinoma arising in large bowel mucosa.

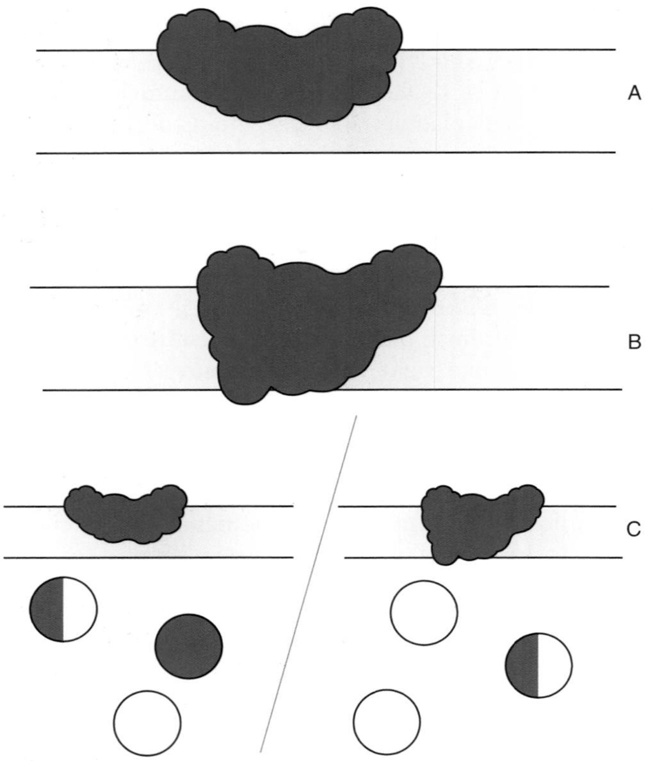

FIGURE 9.49 Dukes' staging system for large bowel carcinoma. Stage A tumours are confined to the bowel muscle wall. Stage B cancers show invasion completely through the muscle wall. Dukes' stage C is defined by the presence of lymph node metastases, irrespective of the depth of invasion of the primary tumour.

tumour through the bowel wall with peritoneal ulceration and/or invasion into other adjacent organs). T4 tumours have a worse prognosis and are usually considered for adjuvant chemotherapy.

Pathology in Clinical Practice

Recently, there has been considerable emphasis on assessing the completeness of excision of large bowel tumours, particularly in the case of the rectum which, unlike most of the intestine, is largely not covered by peritoneum but lies embedded in the deep pelvic soft tissues. The emphasis on assessing completeness of excision in the circumferential (soft tissue) margin has been instrumental in changing surgical practice, encouraging wider clearance in surgical resections of the rectum ('total mesorectal excision', see Fig. 9.47B). Pathological reporting of tumour stage and completeness of excision also has important implications in deciding on the use of adjuvant chemotherapy or radiotherapy. Identification by the pathologist of tumour invasion into veins in the pericolic/perirectal soft tissues is also of clinical importance, being predictive of future systemic metastatic disease.

Biology of Large Bowel Adenoma and Carcinoma

The strong clinical and epidemiological evidence in favour of a progression from normal through adenoma to carcinoma in the large bowel, together with the ready availability of tissue specimens, has made this system an ideal model for studying the genetic events involved in the development of a cancer. In this context, a number of crucial events have been defined:

- mutation and/or loss of the adenomatous polyposis coli (*APC*) gene is an early event in adenoma development
- mutational activation of the K-*ras* oncogene and loss of the long arm of chromosome 18 are important events in increasing growth of adenomas
- mutation and/or loss of the p53 tumour suppressor gene is associated with progression from adenoma to carcinoma.

Abnormalities in a number of other genes, notably those such as *hMLH1* and *hMSH2* involved in DNA repair, have also been noted in patients with hereditary non-polyposis colorectal cancer (see Special Study Topic 9.2) and in a proportion of sporadic carcinomas.

Adenoma and Carcinoma of the Small Intestine

Primary neoplasms of the small intestinal mucosa are very uncommon in comparison with the incidence of such neoplasms in the colorectum. An exception to this rule is the area of duodenum around the ampulla of Vater, where adenomatous lesions are well recognized. These may progress to invasive adenocarcinoma. These lesions are more common in patients with familial adenomatous polyposis (FAP). Adenomas and carcinomas of the small intestine have similar microscopic appearances to their large bowel equivalents.

Carcinoid Tumours

Cells of neuroendocrine type are seen admixed throughout the epithelial cell population of the intestines (also in the stomach and lung). These are defined by the presence of neurosecretory granules, and are also known as cells of the diffuse endocrine system or APUD (amine precursor uptake and decarboxylation) cells. Cells of this type produce a wide range of peptides which may be active either locally or systemically. Neoplasms of such cells are usually called carcinoids. The most common site of origin of such tumours is in the midgut-derived epithelium of the ileum and appendix (see below for details of appendiceal tumours). Ileal tumours are of low-grade malignancy, and not infrequently metastasize to local nodes or the liver. These neoplasms may present with local effects (e.g. obstruction, intussusception) or by systemic effects of active products produced by the tumour. Foregut carcinoids (including islet cell pancreatic neoplasms) may produce hormones such as gastrin or insulin. Midgut neoplasms more often produce smaller active products such as 5-HT. The latter is passed in the portal circulation to the liver where it is inactivated to 5-hydroxyindoleacetic acid (5-HIAA). Elevated 5-HIAA levels in urine can be used as an aid in diagnosing these tumours. Carcinoid syndrome is a systemic disorder characterized by flushing attacks, diarrhoea and, occasionally, endothelial thickening of the right side of the heart leading to tricuspid and pulmonary stenosis. This syndrome is usually seen when intestinal carcinoids have metastasized to the liver, and 5-HT is therefore released directly into the systemic circulation.

Intestinal Lymphoma

Malignant lymphomas in the gastrointestinal tract are most frequently seen in the stomach (55%), with most of the remaining cases arising in the intestines. Indeed, lymphoma is the most common form of small intestinal malignancy. The majority of tumours are of B-cell origin. T-cell lymphomas are rarer, but show a strong association with coeliac disease and are most commonly found in the small intestine. Clinically, lymphomas may present as bowel obstruction or as anaemia due to chronic blood loss. The prognosis and treatment depend on the grade and stage of tumour.

THE APPENDIX

The appendix is a vestigial narrow outpouching of the caecum that is of no important physiological utility, but is very important as a focus of intra-abdominal sepsis, being a major cause of the surgical 'acute abdomen'. It is an occasional site of primary neoplasia.

Acute Appendicitis

Although this disease is extremely common – particularly in the second and third decades of life – its aetiology is poorly understood. It is often thought to be due to luminal obstruction either by impacted hard faeces (a 'faecolith'), by enterobius worms, or by reactive hyperplasia of the lymphoid tissue in the wall of the appendix. However, in many cases of undoubted acute appendicitis there is no evident obstruction. The earliest morphological change is mucosal ulceration, perhaps reflecting increased intraluminal pressure. The inflammatory infiltrate spreads through the wall (acute suppurative appendicitis) rapidly causing a localized peritonitis (Figure 9.50). The blood vessels within the appendix become thrombosed, leading to ischaemic necrosis of the wall (gangrenous appendicitis). Unchecked, the appendix is then liable to spontaneous rupture with consequent disseminated peritonitis. This condition may be rapidly fatal through the development of septicaemia. Other complications include a localized inflammatory mass in the right iliac fossa (appendix abscess), subphrenic abscess and (by portal blood spread) hepatic abscess.

Less common causes of appendiceal inflammation include Crohn's disease, ulcerative colitis, tuberculosis and involvement in infection by *Yersinia pseudotuberculosis*.

Appendiceal Neoplasms

The appendix may become blocked and distended by mucus (mucocoele) due to the growth of a low grade mucinous tumour. When such a mucocoele ruptures, peritoneal

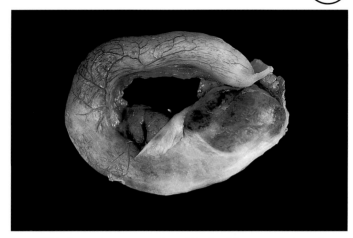

FIGURE 9.50 Appendicectomy specimen. The tip of the appendix is swollen, haemorrhagic, and partly covered by a purulent white exudate, typical of acute appendicitis.

dissemination of the mucus-producing tumour cells turns the abdomen into a gelatinous mass – a condition known clinically as pseudomyxoma peritonei. Frankly malignant adenocarcinomas, similar to these in the colon, do occur in the appendix, but are rare.

The appendix is a well-recognized site of development of carcinoid tumours. Most are identified incidentally at appendicectomy and have an excellent prognosis. One subtype, the goblet cell or adenocarcinoid, is more aggressive in its course.

THE ANUS

The anal canal is an ectodermal inpouching which typically measures 4 cm in length. It is lined by stratified squamous epithelium, and is continuous externally with the skin at the anal verge and internally with the rectum at the dentate (pectinate) line. The anus is susceptible to a number of disease conditions including fistulae and fissures. It is commonly involved in Crohn's disease. Cutaneous disease (dermatitis, psoriasis, etc.) may also involve the anal canal and perianal skin.

Haemorrhoids

These are prominent vascular cushions straddling the anorectal junction. In association with high intraluminal pressure they may become abnormally prominent, congested, and may even prolapse and ulcerate. Bleeding from haemorrhoids is common. The mere presence of these lesions does not exclude more significant pathology as they are not uncommonly associated with neoplasms or anal fissures.

Rectal Prolapse

Protrusion of part of the wall of the rectum into the anal canal is most commonly seen in women. If the mucosa alone is involved, the presentation may be as a solitary rectal ulcer which can be identified on biopsy by a characteristic pattern of crypt hyperplasia and congestion, fibrosis and muscularization of the lamina propria. These lesions may closely mimic malignant ulcers on clinical assessment.

Anal Neoplasms

Squamous carcinoma is the most common and important anal neoplasm. This disease shows a strong epidemiological association with human papillomavirus (HPV) infection and especially (as with carcinoma of the uterine cervix) with HPV types 16 and 18. Preinvasive disease can be identified as anal intraepithelial neoplasia (AIN), often in anal warts (condylomata). Much more rarely the anus may be the primary site of a malignant melanoma.

THE PERITONEUM

The peritoneum is a serous membrane lined by mesothelial cells. Like the pleura and pericardium, it has a parietal layer lining the abdominal wall and a visceral layer covering the organs (principally the gut) which protrude into the abdominal cavity.

Peritonitis

This term is normally used to describe acute inflammation of the peritoneum. The great majority of cases are due to perforation of a viscus (e.g. perforated peptic ulcer) or extension of inflammation from transmural inflammation of the gut (appendicitis, bowel infarction, diverticulitis). Commonly, peritonitis is diffusely spread across much of the peritoneal cavity, but may become localized (as in an appendicular, subphrenic or diverticular abscess). So-called primary bacterial peritonitis (i.e. not associated with underlying visceral disease) is rare.

Peritoneal Neoplasms

The peritoneum is a common site of secondary spread of neoplasms, often by direct spread of neoplastic cells from underlying organs (stomach, colon, pancreas, ovary). This occurrence may give rise to fluid accumulation (ascites). Occasionally, tumour cells may appear to migrate across the peritoneal cavity, forming distinct secondary deposits in other organs. The best example of this is the Krukenberg tumour, which involves the spread of diffuse-type gastric adenocarcinoma to the ovary.

Primary malignant mesothelioma may develop in the peritoneum. Like the more common pleural mesothelioma, there is a strong link to asbestos exposure.

 9.2 SPECIAL STUDY TOPIC

FAMILIAL PREDISPOSITION TO COLORECTAL CANCER

It has long been recognized that large-bowel cancers cluster in some families. This is most clearly manifest in familial adenomatous polyposis (FAP), a condition in which numerous adenomatous polyps develop from childhood. In untreated affected individuals, carcinoma is inevitable by the age of about 40 years. FAP is readily recognizable in affected patients because of its obvious phenotype. Although adenomatous polyps are the defining clinical feature in FAP, there are a number of other associated abnormalities, including abdominal desmoid tumours, osteomas and retinal abnormalities. Family studies showed that inheritance was clearly of the autosomal dominant type, with a high degree of penetrance. The gene responsible for the condition (called adenomatous polyposis coli, APC) was eventually mapped to a locus on the long arm of chromosome 5 (5q21). APC mutations have been identified in varying regions of this large gene, and there is a significant correlation between site of mutation and the familial phenotype. Some mutations are associated with particularly large numbers of adenomas while others are associated with some of the extraintestinal manifestations sometimes seen in FAP (e.g. abdominal desmoid tumours).

The protein product of APC has been characterized as a cytoplasmic protein the main function of which is to bind β-catenin. β-Catenin is involved in cell adhesion, and also acts as a nuclear signal, switching on a number of genes involved in cell proliferation. It may also have an effect in inhibiting cell death by the apoptotic pathway. Mutation of APC leads to loss of the β-catenin binding function. It is intuitively easy to see how the consequent deregulation of cell proliferation and disruption of cell–cell adhesion can contribute to the development of epithelial neoplasms. Increasing knowledge of the genetics of FAP has made a real contribution in the screening of affected families. In the past, all family members were regularly surveyed using colonoscopy, but now only those individuals who carry the mutation need be followed up. APC is a typical tumour suppressor gene in that both alleles normally need to be inactivated before a neoplasm develops. FAP patients carry the 'first hit' in the genome of all of their cells, and thus require just one acquired mutation or deletion to allow for clinical progression. In fact, APC mutations are a feature of many sporadic colorectal cancers. Indeed, mutations can be detected in the earliest stages of adenoma development, and inactivation of *APC* is probably the key first event in a common pathway of colorectal tumorigenesis.

A further important type of hereditary colorectal cancer has been defined in recent years – so-called hereditary non-polyposis colorectal cancer (HNPCC). This type was identified by looking at families in which there was an excessive incidence of large-bowel malignancies, particularly occurring at relatively young age. These families were initially defined on clinical grounds by the Amsterdam criteria:

- three or more relatives with colorectal cancer, one of whom is a first-degree relative of both of the others
- at least two generations affected
- at least one case diagnosed before the age of 50 years.

It was noted that such families manifested some unusual features. Some showed an excessive incidence of certain extracolonic tumours (e.g. carcinomas of endometrium, ovary, stomach). The colonic tumours themselves have certain definable features in HNPCC patients. They tend to arise in the proximal (right) colon, and to secrete more mucus than the majority of colonic tumours. Individual tumours also have a better prognosis than do sporadic cancers. Biologically, these neoplasms are also distinct from the usual in having a low incidence of *APC*, *ras* and *p53* mutations. They are characterized by a particular abnormality defined by variability in the sequences of the microsatellite regions of DNA within the tumour cells when compared with normal cellular DNA from the same patient (microsatellites are regions of non-coding DNA often containing long sequences of CA repeats). This 'microsatellite instability' was recognized as similar to that seen in bacteria and yeast deficient for DNA mismatch repair proteins. The genes responsible for the human condition (*hMSH2* and *hMLH1* among others) vary in different kindreds, but their products are known to be involved in this important mechanism of DNA repair.

HNPCC is more difficult to recognize than FAP because affected individuals do not have numerous polyps. At present, it seems prudent to look for mutations in younger patients in whom the tumours show microsatellite instability, and then to screen family members accordingly.

Large numbers of families remain wherein there is an undoubted predisposition to colorectal cancer but in which the genetic defect has not as yet been characterized. Ongoing developments in molecular genetics will undoubtedly increase our understanding of these issues and allow for increased opportunities for population screening.

Further Reading

Leslie A, Carey FA, Pratt NR, Steele RJ. The colorectal adenoma-carcinoma sequence. *Br J Surg* 2002; **89**: 845–860.

SUMMARY

Gastrointestinal disease includes many of the common congenital, inflammatory and neoplastic disorders of man. In the upper gastrointestinal tract, reflux of gastroduodenal contents into the oesophagus is associated with the increasingly frequent occurrence of Barrett's oesophagus and adenocarcinoma. *Helicobacter pylori* infection of the stomach is a very significant cause of disease, including gastric and duodenal ulceration, gastric adenocarcinoma and MALT lymphoma. Malabsorption of nutrients has numerous causes, including important small intestinal disorders, particularly coeliac disease. There are two major types of idiopathic inflammatory bowel disease; Crohn's disease is a granulomatous condition which may affect any part of the gastrointestinal tract, while ulcerative colitis is a mucosal disorder affecting only the large bowel. Colorectal carcinoma is one of the most common internal malignancies in man, arising most commonly on a background of adenomatous polyps. The prognosis is strongly dependent on tumour stage.

FURTHER READING

Day DW, Jass JA, Price AB, *et al. Morson and Dawson's Gastrointestinal Pathology*, 4th edn. Oxford: Blackwell Publishing, 2003.

Odze RD, Goldblum JR, Crawford JM. *Surgical Pathology of the GI Tract, Liver, Biliary Tract, and Pancreas*. Philadelphia: Saunders, 2004.

Rosai J. *Rosai and Ackerman's Surgical Pathology*, 9th edn. London: Mosby, 2004, Chapters 11 and 12, pp. 615–916.

10 THE LIVER, GALLBLADDER AND PANCREAS

David J Harrison, Alan K Foulis and Alastair D Burt

THE LIVER

Normal Structure

> **Key Points**
>
> - The liver is a large metabolically active organ involved in homeostasis and detoxification.
> - The predominant cell type is the hepatocyte.
> - Hepatocytes can be injured by a range of insults but have remarkable capacity for regeneration.

The liver is an important, multifunctional organ with major roles in the synthesis of plasma proteins, detoxification and excretion of exogenous and endogenous potentially toxic substances, and in digestion and absorption through the secretion of bile. It receives a dual blood supply from the hepatic artery and portal vein and drains through the sinusoids via the hepatic veins to the inferior vena cava. The portal venous system draws blood from the intestine and therefore everything that is absorbed from the gut passes through the liver before entering the systemic circulation. Failure of this metabolic guardian function in liver disease is an important determinant of clinical symptoms. Bile passes in the opposite direction to blood flow, from the canaliculus formed between two liver cells to the bile ducts. Three structures – the hepatic arteriole, portal venule and biliary duct – form the so-called portal triad that is embedded within loose connective tissue; this is one of the key structural landmarks at a microscopic level in the liver. The boundary between the portal tract (the fibrovascular connective tissue and the portal triad) and adjacent hepatocytes is called the limiting plate. The intrahepatic portal tree originates from the surrounding developing liver and this process involves complex control of cell proliferation, migration and programmed cell death. Failure of this process during intrauterine life can result in a spectrum of 'ductal plate malformations' causing failure of normal bile flow in infancy and later life. For example, mutation of the gene *Jagged-1* is associated with a failure of differentiation or survival of bile ducts resulting in atresia of ducts seen as part of Alagille syndrome (Figure 10.1).

It is convenient to think of the liver microanatomy in zones, loosely defined geographical areas corresponding to particular functions of the liver. Over the years a number of different systems have been developed, but there is still controversy over which is the best. In the acinar model the territory supplied by the blood vessels traversing the portal tracts is known as the acinar unit, and it in turn is divided into three zones (Figure 10.2). It is apparent that zone 1 is better oxygenated and this is where many synthetic processes, such as albumin production occur. By contrast zone 3 has many enzymes involved in phase 1 (oxidative) and phase 2 (conjugative) detoxification reactions. It experiences lower oxygen tensions and is thus more vulnerable to both toxic and ischaemic injury. Note that in this model some zone 3 hepatocytes actually lie very close to the portal tract. In the older lobular concept the terminal venule, draining blood from the parenchyma and returning it to the inferior vena cava, is the focus and is at the centre of the lobule. Thus blood flows from the corners of the lobule through the sinusoids into the terminal hepatic venules. This model is useful in explaining the haemodynamics of portal hypertension caused by obstruction to blood flow.

Within the parenchyma of the liver there is a complex network of cells. Although the predominant cell type is the hepatocyte a significant proportion of other cells, both resident and transitory are important. Hepatocytes are arranged in plates, lining the blood filled sinusoids. Sinusoidal endothelial cells are fenestrated allowing direct access of hepatocytes to blood. Lying on the endothelial and within

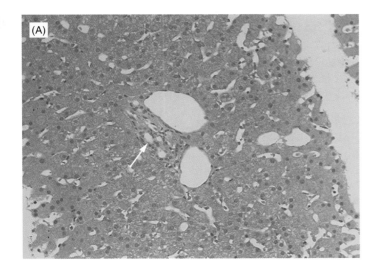

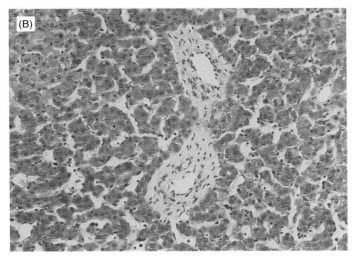

FIGURE 10.1 Comparison of normal liver (A) with biopsy from child with Alagille syndrome (B). In normal liver the portal tracts contain a bile duct (arrow), portal vein and hepatic artery but in Alagille the bile duct is missing.

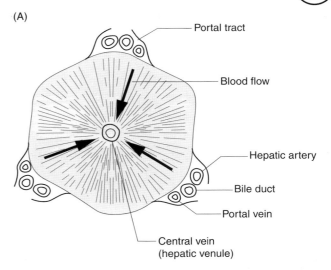

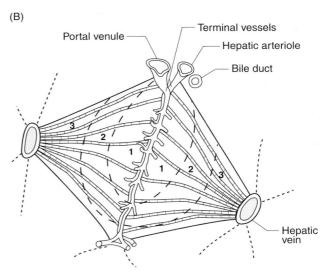

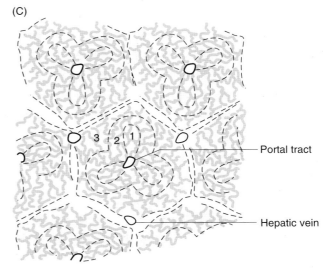

the sinusoidal space, the space of Disse, other cell types are found. These include the phagocytic Kupffer cell and the hepatic stellate cell, a precursor cell that is involved in liver fibrosis (Figure 10.3). When liver cells are injured regeneration is rapid and may be complete. Proliferation of hepatocytes can occur anywhere in the acinus although experimental studies suggest that there is a reserve of hepatic stem cells close to the portal tract.

Liver Function Tests

A set of biochemical investigations is commonly requested as part of the initial clinical workup of all patients with suspected liver disease. While the variables measured can give vital information to the clinician and to the pathologist interpreting a biopsy, a number of important caveats need to borne in mind to avoid overinterpretation of tests. First, the liver is frequently involved as a bystander in many cases of systemic illness. Do not assume that because liver function

FIGURE 10.2 Comparison of lobular and acinar models of liver microarchitecture: (A) Hepatic lobule arranged round a single central (hepatic) vein into which blood flows. (B) Simple acinus arranged around a hepatic artery branch. (C) Relationship between adjacent acini in liver.

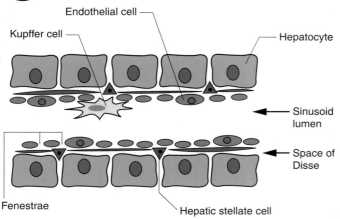

FIGURE 10.3 Schematic diagram of liver parenchyma and sinusoids.

tests are abnormal the liver is the main site of disease. Second, the tests are a package and should not individually be regarded as specific. Thus a raised bilirubin may not only indicate failure of liver excretory function but it may also indicate increased breakdown of red blood cells. Table 10.1 shows the major liver function tests and their usefulness.

TABLE 10.1 Routinely used liver function tests

Albumin	Synthesized exclusively by liver cells Reduction in serum levels in liver failure Low levels associated with oedema and ascites
Bilirubin	Serum levels increased in all forms of jaundice May be conjugated, unconjugated or mixed Normal levels <20 μm/L
Transaminases	Aspartate and alanine aminotransferases Released by injured hepatocytes Surrogate marker of liver cell necrosis but poor prognostic indicator
Alkaline phosphatase	Enzyme present in bile canaliculi Elevated levels in cholestatic liver disease (impaired bile flow) Other extrahepatic sources including bone
γ-Glutamyl transpeptidase	Also elevated in cholestatic disorders Enzyme induced by ethanol Surrogate marker of alcohol misuse
Prothrombin time	Reflects changes in levels of coagulation factors Prolonged in liver failure due to decreased synthesis of several clotting factors including those which are vitamin K dependent

Clinical Symptoms and Signs in Liver Disease

The liver capsule is innervated and so swelling or inflammation can cause pain. Major features alerting the clinician to the presence of significant liver disease all have a basis in pathophysiology and therefore may give important clues to the underlying liver problem. Thus itch may indicate retention of bile salts because of cholestasis, suggesting biliary disease. A tendency to bruise or bleed easily may indicate low platelet counts because portal hypertension associated with cirrhosis has caused splenic enlargement and increased destruction of platelets. Alternatively, hepatocyte necrosis caused by toxins, virus or drugs, may affect the synthetic function of the liver which normally produces most of the essential clotting factors (Figure 10.4). In broad terms the serious complications of liver disease can be divided into:

- manifestations of hepatic failure
- effects of portal hypertension (e.g. bleeding oesophageal varices)
- risk of liver cancer.

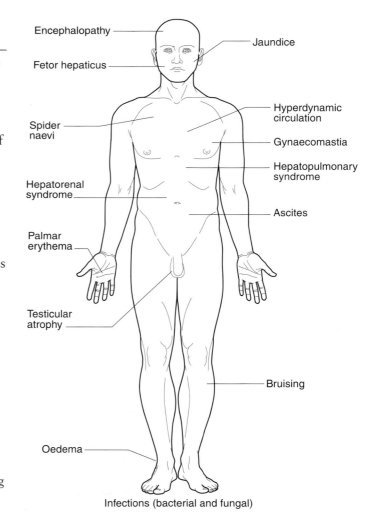

FIGURE 10.4 Features of hepatic failure.

Patterns of Injury and Causes of Liver Disease

The liver is susceptible to a wide range of insults and liver disease is an important cause of morbidity and mortality worldwide. The major causes of liver disease are outlined in Table 10.2. In broad terms, clinical disease can be regarded as either being acute or chronic. With acute liver injury the patient will either die of liver failure if the disease process is severe (or require liver transplantation) or will recover completely. By contrast, with chronic liver disease there is frequently progressive inflammation and scarring; this is accompanied by attempts at regeneration by surviving liver cells and cirrhosis develops. Patients with cirrhosis are then at risk of developing a malignant tumour, hepatocellular carcinoma.

TABLE 10.2 Major causes of liver disease

Toxic: alcohol and drugs
Viruses (hepatitis B and C)
Autoimmune disease (primary biliary cirrhosis; autoimmune hepatitis)
Cholestasis (e.g. biliary obstruction by gallstones)
Metabolic (haemochromatosis; Wilson's disease; α_1-antitrypsin deficiency)

Despite the many diverse causes of liver disease, the liver has a rather limited set of responses to injury. In some conditions the injury is manifest by accumulation of lipids within the hepatocytes: this is a central theme in alcoholic liver disease and in liver injury associated with the so-called metabolic syndrome (type 2 diabetes, hypertension, obesity) – the fatty liver diseases. In many disorders there is irreversible liver cell injury through either necrosis or apoptosis (pp. 52–53). Inflammation is a common feature, particularly in chronic conditions. The predominant inflammatory cell type is the T lymphocyte; these cells may have a key role in liver cell apoptosis. In response to liver cell loss, there is regeneration of surviving epithelial cells as noted above. In some situations there may be massive liver cell necrosis, where most of the parenchyma is lost; in such circumstances there may then not be sufficient critical mass of surviving cells to repopulate the liver. When there is persistent injury and inflammation there is stimulation of a repair process which involves the hepatic stellate cells; this leads to the development of fibrosis and is discussed more fully in Chapter 4.

Viral Hepatitis

Most clinically significant forms of viral hepatitis are caused by a disparate group of viruses known as hepatitis viruses (A, B, C, D or delta, E). In addition a number of other viruses including Epstein–Barr virus, cytomegalovirus, rubella and arboviruses (causing yellow fever) may at times be responsible for liver dysfunction. By convention, hepatitis is used to refer to diffuse liver injury although the severity of the injury may be heterogeneous within the liver. The clinical presentation is variable. Acute hepatitis A infection often presents with general malaise, anorexia and sometimes abdominal discomfort and liver tenderness. Only after this does the patient develop jaundice; thereafter recovery tends to occur. Sometimes presentation is with florid overwhelming liver failure. Other forms of viral hepatitis may present similarly with an acute hepatitis but more often the onset may be insidious with presentation only after evidence of chronic disease is present.

Hepatitis Viruses

Hepatitis A virus characteristically produces a mild illness and full recovery occurs. Hepatitis B and C virus infections frequently result in chronic hepatitis leading to cirrhosis and even hepatocellular carcinoma. Hepatitis D synergizes with hepatitis B to produce more severe disease. Hepatitis E infection generally resolves after a mild illness but pregnant women sometimes develop life-threatening liver failure. Hepatitis G virus is a more recent discovery but is unlikely to be a major pathogen in causing viral liver disease. A summary of the main hepatitis viruses is provided in Table 10.3.

Histology

Morphologically there is very little qualitative difference between the effects of the different hepatitis viruses although the severity may vary and the underlying mechanisms of hepatocyte death differ. Hepatitis A virus is thought to be directly cytopathic whereas hepatitis B and C viruses destroy liver cells by virtue of the cytotoxic T-cell response to virally infected cells. Many hepatocytes show sublethal injury in the form of cloudy swelling, or hydropic change but there is also programmed cell deletion (apoptosis). Shrunken, pyknotic cells are clearly visible in biopsies (Figure 10.5). In severe cases there may be bridging necrosis linking adjacent portal tracts and even massive widespread necrosis (Figure 10.5). This is associated clinically with fulminant liver failure. Associated with this is a lymphoid infiltrate in the sinusoids and portal tracts. Sinusoidal Kupffer cells are activated and are prominent; many contain ceroid pigment which represents phagocytosed debris from dead hepatocytes. In infection caused by hepatitis A virus plasma cells may be prominent in portal areas. Bilirubinostasis is common, with bile accumulated in hepatocytes and canaliculi.

As the liver can rapidly regenerate evidence of hepatocyte proliferation such as mitotic figures and binucleate cells can be seen, even during acute disease. Resolution results in structurally normal liver with no fibrosis, although a mild increase in chronic inflammatory cells may persist in portal areas for more than 6 months. Sometimes the viral hepatitis enters a chronic stage and may even progress to cirrhosis. This is particularly the case with hepatitis C in which some 85% of infected individuals fail to clear the virus; many of these patients develop progressive fibrosis and cirrhosis. With hepatitis B around 5% go on to become chronic carriers. In some parts of the world

TABLE 10.3 Viral hepatitides

	A	B	C*	D*	E*
Virus	RNA	DNA	RNA	Defective RNA	RNA
Spread	Faecal–oral	Blood products; sexually; intravenous drug use; mother-to-child	Blood products; intravenous drug use; sporadic	Probably as for hepatitis B	Faecal–oral
Incubation period	15–40 days	50–180 days	40–75 days	Coinfection with B or subsequent infection	30–50 days
Pathogenesis	Direct cytopathic	Triggers immune destruction	? Immune	Synergizes with B	? Direct
Chronicity	No	Yes	Yes	Yes	No
Geographical	Worldwide	Worldwide	Worldwide	?	Predominantly Asia
Diagnosis	IgM to virus	e antigen = infective; IgG to s antigen indicates previous infection	Antibody to HCV; HCV RNA detected by polymerase chain reaction	Protein present in hepatocyte nuclei	Antibody to hepatitis E virus

*Formerly grouped as 'non-A–non-B hepatitis'.

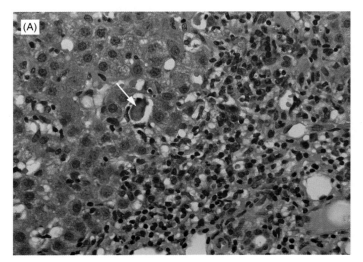
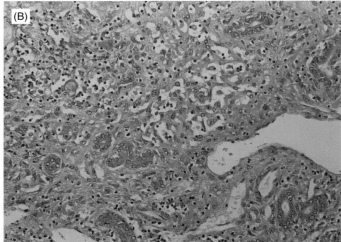

FIGURE 10.5 Liver cell necrosis in hepatitis. (A) An acidophil (apoptotic) body (arrow) – the dead hepatocyte – is surrounded by lymphocytes. (B) Massive necrosis where there are few remaining hepatocytes. The ductular structures seen here represent an attempt at regeneration.

individuals are infected early in life through infected mothers; many of these go on to get chronic disease with ultimately cirrhosis and hepatocellular carcinoma. It is estimated that some 350 million people worldwide are infected with hepatitis B.

Chronic Hepatitis

Liver inflammation persisting for greater than 6 months without sustained improvement is defined as chronic hepatitis. However, the disease may have a fluctuating course in terms of injury as assessed biochemically or by liver biopsy.

A spectrum of biopsy changes is seen depending on disease activity which itself may be modulated by immunosuppressive drugs and the underlying cause. The pathological features are summarized in Figure 10.6. The hallmark of chronic hepatitis is the presence of so-called interface hepatitis. This is a process of chronic inflammation leading to hepatocyte death and fibrosis, which occurs at the limiting plate of the portal tracts. If interface hepatitis is severe then bridging necrosis and fibrosis occur between adjacent portal regions leading to the rapid evolution of cirrhosis.

Chronic hepatitis is often perceived as being complicated and confusing. This is in part because the causes, clinical

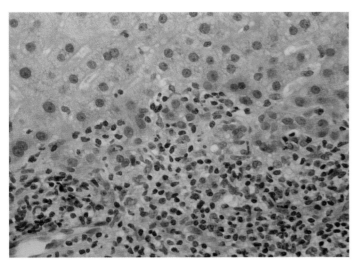

FIGURE 10.6 Chronic hepatitis: so-called interface hepatitis where there is inflammation and death of hepatocytes at the limiting plate between the parenchyma and the portal tract.

features, biochemical and immunological findings and morphological features overlap but are not interchangeable. In other words every case of chronic hepatitis should be regarded as a syndrome and the task of the investigating clinician is to discern as a much as possible about each of these components. For example, clinically a patient may have signs of liver disease. Immunologically there may be evidence of autoimmunity but this does not indicate whether or not there is cirrhosis. A biopsy may show cirrhosis but this does not necessarily give a reason for the underlying disease, and so on. Therefore it must be stressed that the biopsy diagnosis of chronic hepatitis is a morphological statement. Further clinical, imaging and serological investigation will be required to establish the aetiology in most cases (Table 10.4).

A number of attempts have been made to histologically 'score' the severity of liver disease on a liver biopsy. Each approach has its strengths and weaknesses, but it is valid and useful to comment on the amount of cell destruction and the extent of fibrosis. Both factors contribute to prognosis and inform on the benefits of therapeutic intervention.

TABLE 10.4 Aetiology and diagnosis of chronic hepatitis

Aetiology	Clinical features	Biochemical	Immunology	Additional biopsy features
Autoimmune	F > M Peak 15–20 and 45–55 years Other autoimmune diseases	–	Antinuclear Ab; antismooth muscle Ab	May be frequent plasma cells
Hepatitis B	M > F Any age More severe disease if hepatitis D virus is present	–	HBe and HBs antigens present	HBs antigen detected in hepatocytes by immunohistochemistry
Hepatitis C	Any age Often post-transfusion, homosexual, or drug misuser	–	Anti-HCV antibodies HCV RNA present	Steatosis and multinucleate hepatocytes by immunohistochemistry; lymphoid aggregates in portal tracts
Idiopathic and drug induced	Methyl dopa; isoniazid	–	Often have autoantibodies	Like autoimmune
α_1-Antitrypsin deficiency	Late childhood/young adult presentation May have emphysema Defect in α_1-antitrypsin secretion Homozygous ZZ phenotype causes disease	–	Low serum α_1-antitrypsin abnormal phenotype	Accumulation of α_1-antitrypsin, periodic acid-Schiff positive globules in hepatocytes
Wilson's disease	Kayser–Fleischer rings in cornea Lenticular degeneration in brain	Low serum caeruloplasmin	–	Excess copper and copper binding protein in liver

TABLE 10.5 Biliary disease

Disease	Clinical features	Biochemistry	Immunology	Biopsy	Other
Primary biliary cirrhosis	F > M 9:1 Itch Xanthelasma	Very high alkaline phosphatase	Antimitochondrial antibodies (AMA)	Granulomas; small bile duct destruction; chronic inflammation	Cirrhosis
Primary sclerosing cholangitis	M > F3: Two-thirds have ulcerative colitis	Very high alkaline phosphatase	Antibodies to neutrophil cytoplasmic antigens (ANCA)	Fibrous obliteration of larger ducts; chronic inflammation	Risk of cholangiocarcinoma
Obstruction (secondary)	Any age Gallstones Tumours Parasites	High alkaline phosphatase; very high bilirubin	–	Bile lakes; acute inflammation	Risk of ascending infection

Biliary Disease (Table 10.5)

Key Points

- The liver conjugates and excretes toxic substances in bile. Failure of this pathway leads to cholestasis, which in turn causes secondary damage to the hepatocytes.
- If prolonged cholestasis occurs then cirrhosis may ensue.
- Primary biliary disease (primary biliary cirrhosis and primary sclerosing cholangitis) is generally autoimmune.
- Secondary biliary disease is usually related to obstruction, either intrinsic such as tumour or gallstones or extrinsic such as liver flukes.

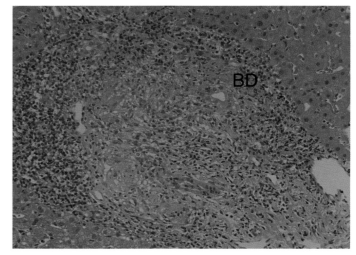

FIGURE 10.7 Primary biliary cirrhosis. An injured bile duct (BD) is surrounded by a granulomatous and lymphocytic infiltrate.

Primary Biliary Disease

In primary biliary disease there is destruction of bile ducts by immunological mechanisms. Damage to hepatocytes and subsequent fibrosis combined with hepatocyte regeneration lead to cirrhosis.

Primary Biliary Cirrhosis

In primary biliary cirrhosis there is a chronic inflammatory infiltrate in portal tracts, and lymphocytes can be seen migrating into the biliary epithelium that then degenerates and dies. This disease primarily affects small bile ducts. Approximately a quarter of biopsies contain epithelioid granulomas, sometimes in the hepatic parenchyma but often close to bile ducts (Figure 10.7). Patients are typically women in their sixth decade who may present with jaundice or itch (pruritus), due to retention of bile salts, and general feeling of malaise. Sometimes sequelae of cirrhosis such as ruptured oesophageal varices result in an accelerated and more dramatic presentation. The disease is often indolent and evidence may be found of abnormalities in liver function tests with the presence of antimitochondrial antibodies stretching back for some years if blood samples are available for testing.

Primary Sclerosing Cholangitis

This is usually associated with ulcerative colitis. There is fibrous obliteration of bile ducts (Figure 10.8). Larger ducts and even extrahepatic bile ducts may be affected. These patients are at risk of developing bile duct cancer – cholangiocarcinoma. In both primary biliary cirrhosis and primary sclerosing cholangitis periportal hepatocyte injury occurs and there is often proliferation of poorly formed ductular structures. This is probably a regenerative phenomenon (Figure 10.8).

Secondary Biliary Disease

This is usually the result of bile outflow obstruction as a result of gallstones. However, bile duct carcinoma, pancreatic

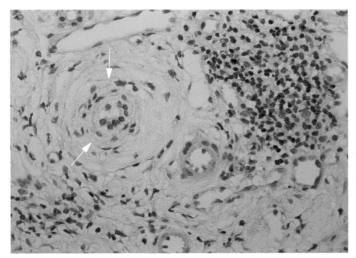

FIGURE 10.8 Sclerosing bile duct lesion in primary sclerosing cholangitis. A cuff of collagen is seen around a degenerate bile duct (arrows).

carcinoma, extrinsic compression of the bile duct by lymph nodes at the porta hepatis, or post-traumatic stricture may also cause obstruction. Bile accumulates in canaliculi between hepatocytes, and in Kupffer cells. It may extravasate to form bile lakes. These are more common in zone 3, perivenular hepatocytes. There is an inflammatory response, predominantly of acute inflammatory cells, which is most notable in the portal tracts. Oedema in portal tracts is often marked and there may be very extensive biliary reduplication, an increase in small, irregular duct-like structures. Prolonged obstruction leads to bridging between adjacent portal areas and eventual cirrhosis.

Alcoholic Liver Disease and Other Fatty Liver Diseases

Alcohol is one of the commonest causes of liver disease in developed countries. It can produce acute reversible injury (steatosis or fatty change) or irreversible changes characterized by hepatocyte death and fibrosis (alcoholic hepatitis and cirrhosis).

Pathogenesis

Habitual alcohol intake induces the microsomal ethanol oxidizing system (particularly the cytochrome P450 CYP2E1). This, in addition to alcohol dehydrogenases, produces acetaldehyde and depletes the cell of nicotinamide adenosine dinucleotide phosphate (reduced form) (NADPH). These changes directly cause triglyceride accumulation leading to fatty change as well as cell death. The inflammatory response to cell death includes cytokine production that triggers hepatic stellate cells to synthesize collagen.

Steatosis

Hepatocytes become swollen as cytoplasm accumulates globules of fat, particularly evident in zone 3 where alcohol metabolizing enzymes predominate. Steatosis is not specific to alcohol injury: it is also seen in obesity, diabetes, malabsorption syndromes and malnutrition. It is normally reversible but can in some cases cause massive enlargement of the liver (Figure 10.9).

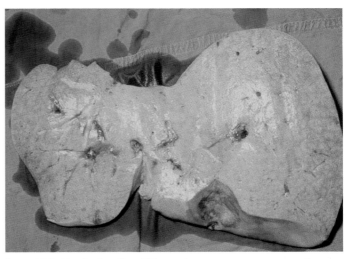

FIGURE 10.9 Massive fatty liver. This was the appearance at autopsy of a middle-aged woman with an 11-year history of alcohol misuse. The liver weighed 2890 g, over twice the normal weight.

Alcoholic hepatitis

Hepatocytes lose osmotic control and become ballooned and hydropic. Occasional cells undergo necrosis and elicit a focal neutrophil response (spotty necrosis). The cytoskeleton of cells is damaged and aggregates of prekeratin intermediate filaments are visible as Mallory's hyaline (Figure 10.10). Although not specific this is a useful diagnostic clue.

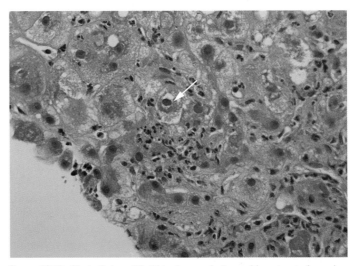

FIGURE 10.10 Alcoholic hepatitis. This shows a ballooned hepatocyte (arrow) containing a large Mallory body and surrounded by polymorphs.

Cirrhosis

Progressive injury and fibrosis leads to fibrous septa which join adjacent perivenular acinar zone 3 regions. Portal–venous bridging also occurs. Within these small delineated regions regenerative hepatocytes form nodules (micronodular cirrhosis). In the long term a significant proportion of patients with cirrhosis may develop hepatocellular carcinoma.

Non-alcoholic Fatty Liver Disease

A condition which is histologically similar to alcoholic steatosis and hepatitis is increasingly encountered in obese patients; in such patient populations there is a high incidence of type 2 diabetes mellitus. Patients are discovered as having abnormal liver function tests after blood testing for complaints of liver tenderness or tiredness. The underlying pathogenesis is thought to be related to an insulin-resistant state with altered metabolism of fatty acids. Whilst usually benign in course there are now well-documented instances of slow progression to cirrhosis. The importance of the condition is its increasing prevalence, its relationship to treatable or preventable conditions such as diabetes and obesity, and the necessity to ensure that patients are not falsely accused of secret excessive alcohol consumption and the attendant stigma associated with it.

10.1 SPECIAL STUDY TOPIC

NON-ALCOHOLIC FATTY LIVER DISEASE – A TWENTY-FIRST CENTURY CONDITION

Pathologists and clinicians have long appreciated that there is a spectrum of liver disease in chronic alcoholics. The earliest change is the accumulation of fat droplets within hepatocytes. This relates to a direct effect of alcohol metabolism on the handling of fat by liver cells. In chronic alcoholics, this change is exacerbated by there being a reduction in the carrier proteins that remove triglycerides from the liver cells. A proportion of chronic alcoholics progress to the next stage of disease, steatohepatitis. There is now, in addition to fat accumulation – simple steatosis, ballooning degeneration of the liver cells with cytoskeletal abnormality leading to Mallory body formation (p. 267), liver cell necrosis and apoptosis, and an accompanying inflammatory infiltrate. Classically, this is in the form of neutrophil polymorphs, and there is also a lymphocytic and macrophage component. This stage is also characterized by the presence of some fibrosis which is classically found encircling hepatocytes (so-called pericellular fibrosis).

In a proportion of patients with steatohepatitis there is then progression to cirrhosis which is generally of micronodular type. If the patient stops drinking at this stage there may be disappearance of the fat and the necroinflammation and the cirrhosis becomes modified moving from a micronodular to a macronodular pattern. In broad terms approximately 30–40% of chronic alcoholics will develop steatohepatitis and around 15% will develop cirrhosis. The factors which determine the individual susceptibility to progressive disease are not entirely known but there are a number of genetic polymorphisms of alcohol metabolizing enzymes and cytokines that appear to confer some degree of either increased risk or protection. Some ethnic groups are more susceptible to advanced disease than others (e.g. American Indians) and in broad terms females are more susceptible than males.

Approximately 30 years ago, cases of fatty liver disease with inflammation were described that resembled the steatohepatitis seen in alcoholic liver disease but were occurring in non-drinkers. This was referred to as non-alcoholic steatohepatitis (NASH) and over the ensuing time it has become apparent that there is a whole spectrum of disease in non-drinkers that resembles that in chronic alcoholics. This is now referred to as non-alcoholic fatty liver disease (NAFLD). The spectrum of this 'condition' also spans simple steatosis through steatohepatitis to active cirrhosis and in some a transition ultimately to an inactive cirrhosis. Some cases of cirrhosis that in the past were of unknown aetiology are now thought to be examples of end-stage 'burnt out' NAFLD (Figure 10.11).

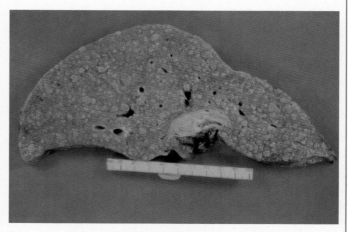

FIGURE 10.11 End-stage cirrhosis in a patient with fatty liver disease.

Early observations indicated that a number of therapeutic agents could give rise to NASH. Several of these are no longer used in clinical practice but drug-induced NASH is still observed in some patients treated for prolonged periods of time with high doses of amiodarone in the treatment of heart disease. Metabolites of amiodarone appear to interfere with a number of key metabolic processes in liver cells leading to ballooning degeneration, accumulation of fat and prominent Mallory body formation. It was also noted that some patients who were undergoing certain forms of weight reduction surgery (in particular jejunoileal bypass) developed severe necroinflammatory changes in the liver almost identical to that of alcoholic steatohepatitis; some of these progressed to cirrhosis. There is some intriguing evidence that even though such patients may be non-drinkers, alcohol may still play a part in this form of NASH. In patients in which there is some form of bowel diversion, there is commonly bacterial overgrowth in bowel loops. Such bacteria can generate alcohols; patients that develop severe liver disease after such surgery may be uniquely sensitive to small amounts of alcohol in the portal blood.

It also became apparent that patients with type 2 diabetes and the so-called metabolic syndrome developed the same spectrum of NAFLD. Indeed, over the past decade this has been recognized as an emerging and serious cause of liver disease that potentially has enormous public health implications. A large amount of epidemiological data indicates that there is a very high prevalence of NAFLD and NASH in North and South America, much of Asia-Pacific, the Middle East and Europe. It has now become the leading cause of referral to liver clinics in many parts of the world. It is regarded as a manifestation of the so-called insulin resistance syndrome in which there is an interplay between obesity, type 2 diabetes, cardiovascular disease and fatty liver disease.

Just how prevalent the disease is remains unclear because the data are based on tests that lack sensitivity and specificity. Studies from the USA using liver blood tests and abnormal liver ultrasound as surrogate markers of NAFLD have suggested that in the adult US population it may be as high as 30%. It is certainly a disease that appears to be becoming more prevalent, and this is undoubtedly related to the spiralling rates of obesity. More than 50% of adults in the USA are overweight and the rates in the UK are following suit. As noted above, some of these cases do progress to cirrhosis but the rate of progression remains controversial. In broad terms it appears to be slower than that seen in alcoholic liver disease. In some patients, however, with marked obesity and poorly controlled diabetes there may be more rapid progression. Estimates from epidemiological studies suggest that overall, cirrhosis may occur in around 5% of patients with NASH over a 10-year period.

The mechanisms behind the development of NAFLD are still poorly understood. From experimental animal work using short-term high fat feeding and genetically altered mice the first abnormality appears to be accumulation of fat in the hepatocytes. In humans there may also be a genetic basis for this with impairment of the metabolism (oxidation) of fatty acids. Fat accumulation in the liver appears to confer resistance to insulin by the hepatocytes. However, it also appears that peripheral insulin resistance, a central feature of the metabolic syndrome, is important in NAFLD. The relative significance of hepatic and peripheral insulin resistance is currently under intensive investigation. Such metabolic abnormalities might explain the accumulation of fat but do not satisfactorily address why some patients move from simple steatosis to steatohepatitis. It is now thought likely that this may be a multi-hit pathogenesis with steatosis being the first hit and the second and subsequent hits being related to the effects of oxidative stress in hepatocytes and/or cytokines such as tumour necrosis factor α. Finally there is emerging evidence that both steatosis and steatohepatitis may be due to the combined effects of severe peripheral insulin resistance and failure of circulating mediators that should combat the effects of high insulin levels (so-called adipokines). Levels of the adipokine, adiponectin are reduced in patients with progressive NAFLD.

Given the public health importance of NAFLD, there is now increasing attention paid to how this disorder may be controlled. Clearly the most logical (and probably most effective) are measures to prevent or reverse overeating and underactivity, thereby reducing the risk of central obesity, insulin resistance and as a consequence NAFLD. In addition, a number of new drugs which have been used in clinical trials, in particular the so-called glitazones, alter hepatic lipid storage and turnover.

Further Reading

Farrell GC, Larter CZ. Nonalcoholic liver disease: from steatosis to cirrhosis. *Hepathology* 2006; **43** (2 Suppl 1): S99–S112.

Liver Injury Caused by Drugs

This may be a predictable, dose-related toxic injury (e.g. paracetamol/acetaminophen) or an unpredictable, idiosyncratic reaction (such as the immunological injury present in halothane hepatitis). The injury may be primarily hepatotoxic (e.g. paracetamol) or cholestatic (e.g. chlorpromazine). The possibility of an adverse drug reaction should always be considered in patients taking medication who have abnormal liver function biochemistry.

Michelle was an 18-year-old woman studying design technology at college. She had always been in good health. She drank alcohol at weekends and intermittently smoked cigarettes but she did not use recreational drugs. She lived in a flat with her boyfriend who was an unemployed labourer. The couple had a difficult relationship and after one serious argument Michelle deliberately took an overdose of 24 paracetamol (acetaminophen) tablets. She was drunk at the time and her boyfriend was unaware that she had taken the tablets. She woke up the following day feeling unwell but put this down to a bad hangover. She did not seek any medical advice having taken the overdose. The following day she began to feel nauseous and sleepy and she went to bed. By the next day she felt very unwell and her boyfriend noticed that she was a strange colour. She was rushed to hospital; by this stage she was semi-comatose and unable to give any history. Following a detailed examination, it was established that she had no signs of chronic liver disease. She did, however, have jaundice (yellow pigmentation of the skin and sclera) and a peculiar smell to her breath (fetor hepaticus: see p. 262). Some bruising was also noted on her limbs.

The medical team involved in Michelle's care considered the possibility of an overdose and measured blood paracetamol levels; given the length of time since taking the tablets it is not surprising that the drug was undetectable in the blood. The team also used blood tests to assess liver and renal function. Serum albumin was reduced at 30 g/L. Serum transaminases (a measure of hepatocyte integrity – elevated levels indicate damage) were grossly elevated, serum alanine aminotransferase being 20 times the upper limit of normal whereas serum alkaline phosphatase (an indicator of cholestasis: impairment of bile flow) was only mildly elevated. Blood tests revealed no evidence of viral hepatitis and there was no evidence of an immunological problem. Renal function blood tests showed a serum urea of 48 mg/dL and creatinine of 564 μmol/L indicating renal failure. The precise cause of her problems remained a mystery to the medical team at this stage but it was clear that she now had developed liver and kidney failure (so-called hepatorenal syndrome) and they suspected that the underlying problem was a toxic injury.

Further evidence that Michelle had hepatic failure could be found by assessing her clotting times; this showed prolongation of the prothrombin time (see p. 262) and a markedly reduced factor V level in the blood. This explains the bruising noted on her limbs; by now she also showed bleeding of her gums. She had now developed deep coma and the decision was taken to put her on the urgent organ transplantation list. Fortunately a donor was identified within a matter of hours and she underwent a 5-hour operation in which a cadaveric liver was engrafted and the damaged liver removed. The liver that was removed was examined by the pathologists.

It weighed approximately 900 g (normal for this age and her body mass would be around 1400 g). It had a mottled appearance but no distinct masses were seen. Microscopically, sections of liver showed large areas of coagulative necrosis; this had a geographic pattern and could be seen around hepatic veins but not around portal tracts (Figure 10.12). This is described as zonal necrosis and is a classical appearance in toxin-induced liver injury such as that associated with paracetamol overdose. The distribution of damage can be explained by there being more drug metabolizing enzymes found normally in hepatocytes around the veins than elsewhere; more toxic metabolites are generated in these cells making them more susceptible to injury. After the transplant surgery Michelle became alert again and all blood tests

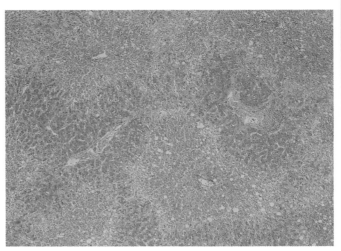

FIGURE 10.12 Histological changes in liver, removed at time of transplantation from patient in the case study. This shows zonal necrosis with coagulative necrosis involving all hepatocytes in the regions around hepatic veins and so-called midzones. There is some preservation of cells around the portal tracts.

showed that her liver function had essentially returned to normal. Furthermore her renal function also improved despite there being no specific intervention. The renal abnormalities in this situation were therefore secondary to the liver dysfunction and reversed when the hepatic function returned.

As noted elsewhere, the liver has a remarkable capacity for regeneration and after some acute insults can recover completely with a return to the normal structure and function. With Michelle however the degree of liver cell necrosis was such that it had exceeded the level beyond which such repair could occur and secondary effects on other organ systems had occurred. Had she not received a transplant she would certainly have died; fortunately she made good recovery after her operation. She admitted to the medical team that she had taken an overdose but she had not intended to take her life.

Storage Diseases

α_1-Antitrypsin deficiency and Wilson's disease have already been mentioned under chronic hepatitis. Many other lipid and glycogen storage diseases affect the liver but their precise description is beyond the scope of this book. Haemochromatosis is an autosomal recessive condition resulting in enhanced absorption of iron from the gut and a gross excess of iron stored in the liver (more than 10 times) normal. The gene responsible for this defect, *HFE*, is on chromosome 6 and in linkage disequilibrium with HLA A3. Two common mutations together explain more than 80% of cases. Recently other (non-*HFE*) genetic defects have been identified which may also lead to iron overload.

The excess iron is found in hepatocytes but as the severity of iron overload increases it is also found in the Kupffer cells and biliary epithelium (Figure 10.13). The presence of iron is directly fibrogenic and periportal fibrosis eventually leads to a predominantly macronodular cirrhosis. Treatment by venesection or with iron chelating drugs such as desferrioxamine prevent disease progression. This is a multisystem disease and iron is deposited in other organs. Excess accumulation in pancreatic islets can lead to diabetes; other endocrine effects include excess melanin production resulting in skin pigmentation: the syndrome of bronzed diabetes.

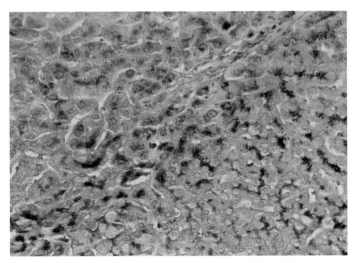

FIGURE 10.13 Genetic haemochromatosis. This shows staining of iron in hepatocytes using Perl's stain. The blue granules represent abnormal accumulation of haemosiderin; normal hepatocytes should be negative.

Secondary iron overload (secondary haemosiderosis) can occur in alcoholics, haemoglobinopathies and patients undergoing multiple transfusions. Iron is particularly prominent in Kupffer cells. Differentiation from primary genetic haemochromatosis may be impossible from a liver biopsy alone.

End-stage Cirrhosis

This is the end stage of many forms of liver injury and is defined as the presence of regenerative nodules separated by fibrous tissue septa, affecting the whole liver. Many clues to the aetiology of cirrhosis are not apparent in biopsies taken at this 'end stage'. If serological or biochemical evidence fails to reveal a cause then the cirrhosis is known as cryptogenic. Patients with cirrhosis may be symptom free for long periods of time but in many there will then be decompensation with the development of hepatic failure (see Figure 10.4).

Portal Hypertension

This is increased blood pressure in the portal vein, above 1 kPa (7 mmHg), reflecting the resistance to blood flow through grossly disturbed liver structure as occurs in cirrhosis. It is further compounded by intrahepatic arteriovenous shunting of blood. Portal hypertension is also caused by a variety of other conditions (Table 10.6). Portal hypertension leads to splenic enlargement and this may result in excessive removal of red cells and platelets from the blood – the syndrome of hypersplenism. There is also dilatation of the plexus of venous channels around the gastric fundus and oesophagus to form varices. These varices are thin walled and bleed readily, causing torrential and life-threatening haematemesis. Portal hypertension also contributes to the development of ascites.

TABLE 10.6 Causes of portal hypertension

Presinusoidal	Portal vein thrombosis
	Tumour
	Infection
	Portal tract fibrosis
	Biliary cirrhosis
	Sarcoidosis
	Schistosomiasis
Sinusoidal	Nodular regenerative hyperplasia
	Cirrhosis
	Sinusoidal fibrosis (some drugs)
Post-sinusoidal	Veno-occlusive disease (bush teas, some drugs)
	Budd–Chiari syndrome (hepatic vein thrombosis)

Congenital Malformations

Atresia of the extrahepatic ducts presents in neonates with signs of biliary obstruction. It may be partial or complete. As noted above there are some inherited disorders (e.g. Alagille syndrome) in which there is paucity or atresia of intrahepatic bile ducts. Solitary cysts, multiple cysts in association with some forms of renal cystic disease and congenital hepatic fibrosis are part of a spectrum of abnormal duct development. Von Meyenberg complexes are small nodules, often subcapsular, formed by groups of bile duct-like structures in a fibrous stroma. Focal nodular hyperplasia is a rare hamartoma sometimes associated with the contraceptive pill.

Tumours

Benign Tumours

Cavernous haemangiomas are found incidentally in the liver in about 2% of autopsies. Liver cell adenomas are associated with use of the contraceptive pill and anabolic steroids (Figure 10.14). They are well-defined nodules, vascular and well-differentiated. They lack biliary elements.

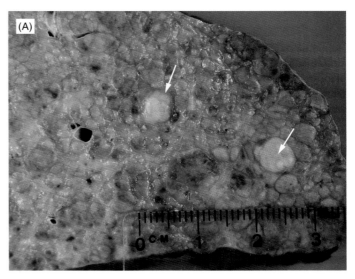

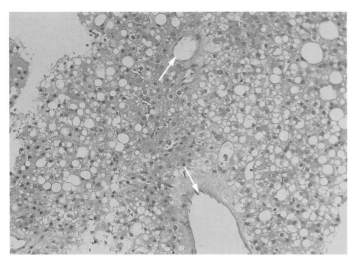

FIGURE 10.14 Histological appearances of a hepatic adenoma. This resembles non-tumorous liver and is composed of hepatocytes, but there are no portal tracts. Large atypical arteries are present (arrows).

Malignant Tumours

The commonest malignant tumour is metastatic carcinoma from lung, breast, gastrointestinal tract or pancreas. About four-fifths of primary tumours are hepatocellular carcinomas (Figure 10.15). The majority of cases arise in cirrhotic livers and may be multifocal. However, a small number arise in non-cirrhotic livers, including the fibrolamellar variant in young women which has a slightly better prognosis than the usual hepatocellular carcinoma if completely resected before metastasis has occurred. Histologically, the tumours vary from well to poorly differentiated, but the cells often resemble hepatocytes in their polygonal shape and granular cytoplasmon (see Figure 10.15). There may be evidence of bile secretion in well-differentiated tumours. Many less well-differentiated tumours produce and release α-fetoprotein (AFP), a useful serum marker for diagnosis and follow-up.

Worldwide the commonest aetiological factors are hepatitis B virus acting synergistically with aflatoxin B1, a mycotoxin product of *Aspergillus flavus*. Hepatitis C is probably also important and alcohol may have a promoter function, working synergistically with viral-induced damage and regeneration to promote the acquisition of mutations. All forms of cirrhosis increase the risk of hepatocellular carcinoma. Cholangiocarcinoma comprises about one-sixth of primary hepatic cancers. It is an adenocarcinoma which often

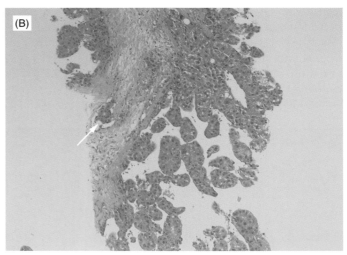

FIGURE 10.15 (A) Cirrhotic liver removed at time of transplantation. Several nodules (arrows) are larger and are either white or bile-stained; these are small hepatocellular carcinomas. (B) Biopsy appearances in hepatocellular carcinoma. The tumour has a trabecular arrangement and there is evidence of vascular invasion (arrow).

spreads by ramification of portal tracts through the liver. Its incidence is high in patients with primary sclerosing cholangitis and in southeast Asia where liver flukes are prevalent. There is some evidence that the disease is more common than previously thought, in part perhaps due to better recognition of the condition but perhaps also due to an underlying real increase in incidence that some have attributed to environmental factors, as yet undiscovered. Angiosarcomas are rare but important because they may be related to occupational exposure to vinyl chloride. Hepatoblastomas are very rare malignant tumours of infancy.

Non-viral Infections Causing Liver Disease

While viruses are the commonest cause of inflammatory liver disease a number of other important diseases can occur. Most of these are tropical but they can occur in anywhere with the increased movement of people now seen.

Weil's Disease

Caused by the spirochaete *Leptospira ictohaemorrhagica*, Weil's disease is contracted from water infected by rats. The spirochaete penetrates the skin and causes liver cell necrosis, presenting as jaundice and an increased tendency to bleeding.

Hydatid Disease

Caused by *Echinococcus granulosa* and contracted from a reservoir animal such as sheep this can result in cystic lesions within the liver. In addition to causing local problems by causing obstruction to bile flow the cysts may contain parasites that cause further disease if they rupture.

Amoebiasis

Encysted infection by *Entamoeba histolytica* may cause lesions that can cause compression of structures within the liver, for example leading to duct obstruction.

Flukes

Usually called liver flukes, organisms such as *Clonorchis sinensis* inhabit the bile ducts causing obstruction, inflammation, scarring and predisposing to cholangiocarcinoma.

Schistosomiasis

Schistosoma japonica and *S. mansoni* can migrate to liver. An inflammatory response to ova, particularly in portal tracts, may lead to scarring causing duct obstruction. Schistosome disease is a significant cause of secondary biliary cirrhosis.

Visceral Leishmaniasis

Parasitization of Kupffer cells may occur as part of a more generalized disease.

Malaria

Replication of malarial parasites may occur within hepatocytes and stuffing of Kupffer cells with red blood cells (erythrophagocytosis) can be seen.

Liver in Systemic Disease

The liver often shows non-specific reactive changes when intercurrent disease is present elsewhere, including mild inflammation and steatosis. Other more specific abnormalities include:

- amyloidosis
- sarcoidosis, in which granulomas may be found
- malignant infiltration by metastatic carcinoma or leukaemia
- tuberculosis, in miliary cases
- fungal infection, in cases of immunodeficiency such as acquired immune deficiency syndrome (AIDS) or immunosuppressive therapy
- cardiac failure, where perivenular congestion and atrophy may occur

- graft-versus-host disease following bone marrow transplantation
- fatty liver of pregnancy.

THE GALL BLADDER

Normal Function

The gall bladder is connected to the intrahepatic and extra-hepatic bile ducts by the cystic duct. It stores and concentrates bile from the liver and increases its viscosity by releasing mucus from the lining epithelium. The release of bile from the gallbladder is stimulated by food, especially fatty food, in the duodenum under the influence of cholecystokinin.

Gallstones (Cholelithiasis)

Although rare in developing countries, gallstones are extremely common in Western society. In many cases cholelithiasis remains undetected clinically and may be an incidental finding at autopsy. The primary problem is supersaturation of bile. Bile normally contains a suspension of cholesterol, held in suspension by phospholipid micelles containing lecithin, as well as bile acids and pigments derived from bilirubin. Nucleation occurs in the supersaturated, lithogenic bile and stones then enlarge (Figure 10.16). Stones may be single or multiple, small or large (Figure 10.17).

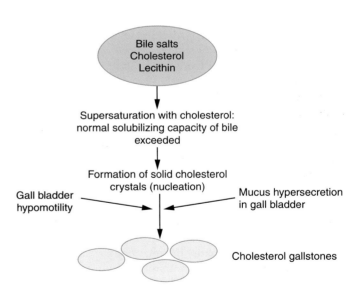

FIGURE 10.16 **Mechanisms of gallstone development.**

In some gall bladders excess cholesterol is phagocytosed by macrophages in the lamina propria. These aggregates of foamy macrophages produce yellow-stippling and protrusion of the gall bladder mucosa, an appearance known as cholesterolosis or 'strawberry' gall bladder. This is of no clinical significance.

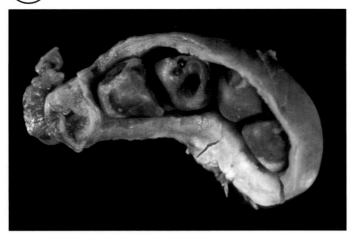

FIGURE 10.17 Macroscopic picture of gallbladder containing mixed stones.

Cholecystitis

Acute Cholecystitis

Initially acute cholecystitis is usually the result of an injury to the gallbladder mucosa caused by gallstones, perhaps by obstruction of the cystic duct. However, in fully developed cases there is often superimposed infection by bowel commensal bacteria which further amplifies the acute inflammatory response. Histologically there is ulceration of mucosa with vascular congestion, oedema and exudation. The neutrophil polymorph infiltrate may extend throughout the entire thickness of the gall bladder wall. A dilated, pus-filled gall bladder is known as empyema and there is a danger of rupture. Obstruction of the cystic duct with no infection may result in accumulation of sterile mucus which distends the gall bladder to produce a mucocoele.

Chronic Cholecystitis

This is generally associated with gallstones and may follow acute cholecystitis or develop insidiously. Features of acute cholecystitis may be superimposed on it. The gallbladder is thickened and fibrotic muscle fibres are hypertrophied. The mucosal epithelium may be atrophic or hyperplastic, sometimes forming diverticula which can reach the serosal surface (these diverticula are often called Rokitansky–Aschoff sinuses). The presence of cholesterol and bile in damaged diverticula stimulates a xanthogranulomatous response, with large numbers of foamy histiocytes and multinucleated foreign body giant cells containing cholesterol crystals. Severe chronic cholecystitis often causes fibrosis of the gall bladder bed so that the inflamed organ is firmly adherent to the liver and difficult to remove.

Tumours

All tumours of the gall bladder are rare, but adenocarcinoma is the most frequent. This tends to arise in fundus, and infiltrate diffusely without causing any symptoms until it is at an advanced stage. More than three-quarters of cases have gallstones. Occasional squamous carcinomas have been described, presumably arising from metaplastic squamous epithelium. Gallstones are invariably found in these cases.

THE PANCREAS

Normal Structure and Function

> **Key Points**
> - The exocrine pancreas secretes digestive enzymes.
> - The endocrine cells are grouped together in islets of Langerhans.
> - The principal hormones secreted by the islets are insulin and glucagon.

The pancreas is often thought of as two separate organs – an exocrine one concerned with digestion, and an endocrine one concerned with the metabolism of carbohydrate, fat and protein. Their association within one gland is simply regarded as fortuitous. However, knowledge of the anatomy, physiology and pathology of the pancreas militates against this simplistic approach.

Structure

Connective tissue septa divide the pancreas into lobules. Within the lobule the secretory unit is the acinus. The secretory products pass into the acinar lumen and drain to the main pancreatic duct. In 85% of cases the pancreatic duct joins the common bile duct to form the ampulla of Vater which then enters the duodenum. In 15% of cases the two ducts do not join to form an ampulla and they enter the duodenum separately. Endocrine cells are grouped together into islets. Most of the islet endocrine cells are insulin-secreting B cells and glucagon-secreting A cells. Somatostatin-secreting D cells and pancreatic polypeptide secreting PP cells also exist.

The anatomy of the pancreatic blood supply is significant. Within lobules much of the circulation passes by arterioles to the islets, the exocrine tissue being supplied by a portal system of capillaries which drains the blood from the sinusoids of the islets (Figure 10.18). The pancreatic acini around islets are thus exposed to very high levels of islet hormones – possibly several hundred times higher than the levels in the systemic circulation.

Functional Aspects

The exocrine pancreas secretes about 1–2 L/day of an alkaline fluid containing about 20 enzymes. Bicarbonate is secreted by the duct epithelium. The enzymes include proteases – trypsin and chymotrypsin – lipases, phospholipases, elastase and amylase. Protease inhibitors are also present within acinar cells and in the pancreatic secretion. Most enzymes are secreted in precursor forms which are activated in the duodenum, a process in which trypsin has a key role.

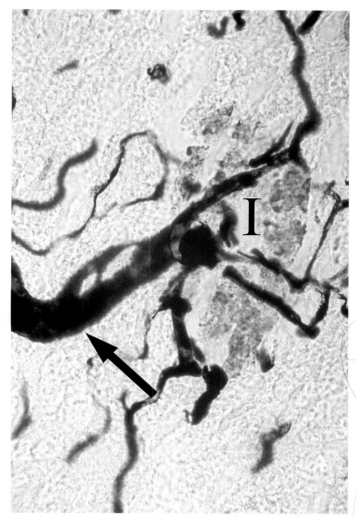

FIGURE 10.18 Islet blood supply. The vasculature in this pancreas has been injected with India Ink. The islets have been immunostained to show insulin-containing B cells. An arteriole (arrowed) enters the islet (I) and divides into intra-islet sinusoids which leave the islet and supply the surrounding exocrine tissue.

In addition to its anabolic systemic effects insulin is a major trophic hormone for the exocrine pancreas, increasing the rate of DNA and protein synthesis in acinar tissue. Weight for weight the exocrine pancreas synthesizes considerably more protein (mainly enzymes) than any other tissue in the body (eight times more than the liver, for example). Since one of the main actions of insulin in all cells of the body is to stimulate protein synthesis, it is interesting to speculate that the islets, with their distinct blood supply that ensures very high levels of insulin in the exocrine capillaries, have evolved to aid the massive protein-synthesizing requirements of the exocrine pancreas. Thus the pancreas, in some respects, functions as a single organ.

Pancreatitis

Pancreatitis is classified clinically and pathologically into acute and chronic forms.

Acute Pancreatitis

> **Key Points**
> - Pancreatitis is associated with gall stones or alcohol misuse.
> - There is upper abdominal pain.
> - Serum amylase is raised.
> - There is autodigestion, causing fat necrosis.
> - Systemic complications include shock.
> - Local complications are pseudocyst and abscess.

Acute pancreatitis is defined as an acute inflammatory process within the pancreas usually associated with necrosis of intrapancreatic acini and adipose tissue. If there is macroscopic haemorrhage the term acute haemorrhagic pancreatitis is used, but this probably simply represents the most severe form of acute pancreatitis.

Clinical Features

The onset is sudden with abdominal pain, vomiting and collapse and may easily be confused clinically with perforation of a peptic ulcer. The diagnosis is confirmed by demonstrating a serum amylase level greater than 1200 IU/L. Two-thirds of patients admitted to hospital have a mild illness which settles readily with nasogastric suction and intravenous fluids. Severe pancreatitis, characterized by shock, hypocalcaemia, hypoxaemia and hyperglycaemia, is less common and has 50% mortality.

Pathogenesis

The initiating event in gallstone-associated pancreatitis appears to be temporary impaction of a gallstone at the ampulla of Vater. If this results in retrograde reflux of bile into the pancreatic duct, acute pancreatitis may be triggered. Reflux will only occur if there is a common channel between the pancreatic duct and common bile duct and if the stone is of the right size (usually about 3 mm in diameter). Thus not everyone with gallstones will have acute pancreatitis.

The initial damage in the pancreas in gallstone acute pancreatitis appears to be to the pancreatic duct epithelial cells. This results in duct inflammation and periductal necrosis, seen microscopically (Figure 10.19). Normal bile alone does not damage the pancreatic duct, but infected bile or bile preincubated with trypsin causes ductal inflammation and necrosis when infused into the pancreatic duct at physiological pressure. Both infection and trypsin convert primary bile salts into secondary bile salts which are toxic to pancreatic duct epithelium. Bile is infected in at least 40% of cases of gallstone pancreatitis and, in the presence of an obstructing stone, bile which has refluxed into the pancreas can be altered by pancreatic trypsin. Although in alcohol-associated acute pancreatitis the pancreatic ducts are also thought to be the initial site of damage, the mechanism causing this is not known, and is likely to be different from that involved in gallstone pancreatitis.

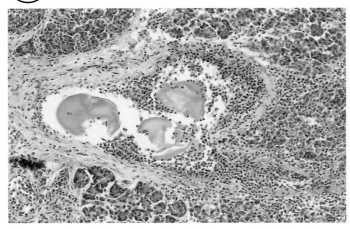

FIGURE 10.19 Duct inflammation and perilobular necrosis. An inflamed interlobular duct is present which contains proteinaceous concretions and polymorphs. An acute inflammatory infiltrate extends into the surrounding exocrine parenchyma.

Wherever the process starts, necrosis causes release of digestive enzymes into the substance of the pancreas. These enzymes are thought to damage further pancreatic parenchymal cells and blood vessels by a process of autodigestion. Necrotic blood vessels, particularly veins, are liable to thrombose causing ischaemic damage to further areas of pancreas, thus initiating a vicious cycle of further enzyme release which may result in extensive coagulative necrosis of entire lobules and intervening ducts and blood vessels (panlobular necrosis) – this corresponds to the macroscopic appearance of acute haemorrhagic pancreatitis (Figure 10.20). Release of pancreatic enzymes into the tissues surrounding the pancreas causes fat necrosis of the adipose tissue (Figure 10.21) and peritonitis, which initially is likely to be sterile.

Defence Mechanisms

Plasma contains the antiproteolytic enzymes α_1-antitrypsin and α_2-macroglobulin and pancreatic juice contains

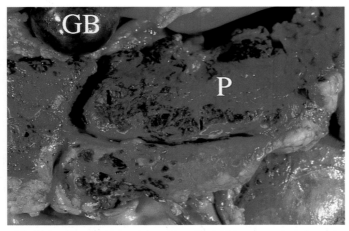

FIGURE 10.20 Acute haemorrhagic pancreatitis. In this autopsy the pancreas (P) and gallbladder (GB) have been exposed. The pancreas is haemorrhagic and necrotic.

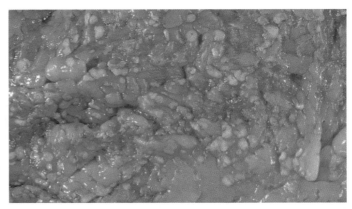

FIGURE 10.21 Fat necrosis of the omentum. Dark yellow flecks of fat necrosis can readily be seen.

pancreatic secretory trypsin inhibitor. These combine with active proteolytic enzymes such as trypsin to inactivate them. Release and activation of these antiproteolytic enzymes in the inflammatory exudate in acute pancreatitis may help inhibit the autodigestive process.

Complications of Acute Pancreatitis

Systemic

Severe acute pancreatitis is complicated by chemical peritonitis which, even in the absence of superadded bacterial peritonitis, can cause death from endotoxic shock due to escape of intestinal endotoxin into the circulation. Release of pancreatic enzymes into the blood may also contribute to the shock syndrome complex, in which adult respiratory distress syndrome and acute renal failure are serious, life-threatening, additional complications.

Local

Sepsis in a necrotic pancreas may result in widespread suppuration or a pancreatic abscess. The causal organisms are *E. coli* and other gut commensals. Another local effect is the formation of a pseudocyst – a localized collection of pancreatic juice and necrotic debris resulting from disruption of the pancreatic ductal drainage. It is lined by granulation tissue and commonly forms in the lesser sac.

Chronic Pancreatitis

Key Points

- Chronic pancreatitis is associated with alcohol misuse.
- There is severe long-lasting upper abdominal pain.
- There is pancreatic calcification.
- Eventually there is pancreatic exocrine and endocrine insufficiency.

Clinical Features

Most patients present with episodes of severe, erratic abdominal pain which may persist for years and lead to analgesic addiction. The pain may be exacerbated by food and thus weight loss may ensue. Some patients develop intermittent jaundice due to stenosis of the common bile duct. Steatorrhoea and diabetes (exocrine and endocrine pancreatic failure) are usually later manifestations, but may be the presenting features in the few patients in whom the disease process has been painless. Plain abdominal radiographs may show diffuse pancreatic calcification and endoscopic retrograde pancreatography shows the presence of intraductal calculi plus areas of stenosis and dilation of the main pancreatic duct.

Aetiology and Pathogenesis

Most cases of chronic pancreatitis occur in patients who abuse alcohol. The disease is not associated with gallstones. Epidemiologically, it is common in wine drinking countries where a high alcohol intake is accompanied also by a diet rich in protein. Alcohol increases the protein concentration in pancreatic juice with subsequent precipitation of concretions in the ducts: when calcified these form stones which can be seen on plain abdominal radiographs. The stones ulcerate the ductal epithelium leading to periductal inflammation and fibrosis (Figure 10.22). The fibrous tissue contracts and causes ductal strictures with secondary dilatation of the duct behind the stricture and acinar atrophy.

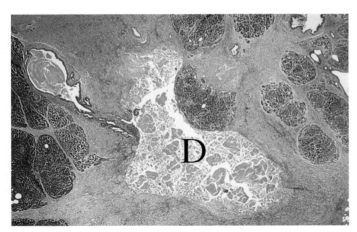

FIGURE 10.22 Chronic pancreatitis. The main pancreatic duct (D) is ulcerated and contains concretions. Scar tissue surrounds the duct and pancreatic lobules.

Hereditary chronic pancreatitis is a rare disorder with an autosomal dominant transmission. It is caused by a mutation in the cationic trypsinogen gene and patients present before the age of 20 years. The mutation interferes with a trypsin inactivation mechanism allowing active trypsin within the pancreatic duct to trigger pancreatic autodigestion.

It will be appreciated that the site of initial damage in the pancreas in both alcohol-related acute pancreatitis and chronic pancreatitis is the pancreatic duct. Not surprisingly therefore, there is some overlap clinically and pathologically between these two conditions in affected alcoholics. Thus, a patient may present with typical acute pancreatitis and this may be the prelude to continuing chronic pain and the development of chronic pancreatitis. In turn patients

with chronic pancreatitis may have particularly severe episodes of pain which clinically and biochemically are indistinguishable from an attack of acute pancreatitis.

Carcinoma of the Pancreas

Key Points
- Histologically pancreatic carcinomas are adenocarcinomas.
- Commonest in head of pancreas.
- It usually presents as obstructive jaundice.
- Prognosis is very poor, even in those patients treated surgically.

Carcinoma of the pancreas has doubled in incidence in the UK during the past 50 years. The increase in the USA has been even higher and there it now ranks second only to colorectal carcinoma among alimentary tract cancers. It is commoner in males than females and increases progressively in incidence after the age of 50 years. Epidemiologically, it has been linked to smoking and a high-fat/high-protein diet. There is an increased risk of pancreatic carcinoma in patients with chronic pancreatitis and particularly those with hereditary chronic pancreatitis.

Sixty-five per cent of tumours are situated in the head of the pancreas where they usually obstruct the common bile duct, causing obstructive jaundice. Carcinoma arising in the body or tail of the pancreas is usually clinically silent until there are multiple metastases. Pancreatic cancer may also present with bizarre clinical effects due to unexplained venous thrombosis (migrating thrombophlebitis), peripheral neuropathy or myopathy.

Histologically, the tumour is an adenocarcinoma. Ninety per cent of tumours have Kirstin-*ras* gene mutations at codon 12 leading to activation of this oncogene. This suggests that Kirstin-*ras* mutations are an early event in the development of this cancer. Diagnosis is made by imaging and brush cytology of the pancreatic or common bile duct at endoscopy (if the tumour is in the head of pancreas). Ultrasound-guided percutaneous fine needle aspiration cytology or biopsy can also be done. The prognosis in carcinoma of the pancreas is extremely bad, 90% of patients not surviving more than 6 months. Patients with carcinoma in the immediate region of the ampulla often present relatively early with obstructive jaundice. Survival following surgery in these patients is usually better than that following surgery for carcinoma of the head of pancreas, but even here the 5-year survival rate is only approximately 25%.

Endocrine Tumours of the Pancreas

An islet cell tumour is usually a solitary discrete nodule embedded in the pancreas. Microscopically, the tumour cells closely resemble normal islet cells, and form cords or clusters separated by fibrous stroma.

A 68-year-old woman presented with a 1-week history of epigastric pain, anorexia and light stools. She was noted to be jaundiced (bilirubin 270 μmol/L, alkaline phosphatase 768 IU/L, aspartate aminotransferase 116 IU/L, alanine aminotransferase 149 IU/L, γ-glutamyl transferase 417 IU/L). Abdominal ultrasound showed markedly dilated intra- and extrahepatic ducts. The common bile duct was 20 mm diameter at its upper end. There was no evidence of gallstones. Pancreas, liver, spleen and kidneys were unremarkable on the scan. Endoscopic retrograde choledocho-pancreatography was performed and a bulging tumour was seen at the ampulla prior to cannulation of the ducts. Bile drainage was achieved with a sphincterotomy and multiple biopsies were taken of the ampullary tumour. Microscopy of the biopsies showed the presence of an ulcerated moderately differentiated adenocarcinoma (Figure 10.23). CT scan of the abdomen showed no evidence of tumour in the head of pancreas or liver. Whipple's operation was performed (removal of duodenum, common bile duct, gall bladder and head of pancreas *en bloc*). There was a 15 mm diameter tumour at the ampulla (Figure 10.24). The tumour invaded the duodenal wall, the common bile duct and a small area of the head of the pancreas. All the resection margins were free of tumour as were the lymph nodes in the specimen. The patient was well and tumour-free 2.5 years later.

COMMENT

The anatomical site of this adenocarcinoma, the ampulla of Vater, ensured a relatively early clinical presentation due to biliary obstruction. The tumour appears to have been removed before it had metastasized. Carcinomas arising at clinically more silent sites, for example the body or tail of pancreas, have usually metastasized by the time of clinical presentation.

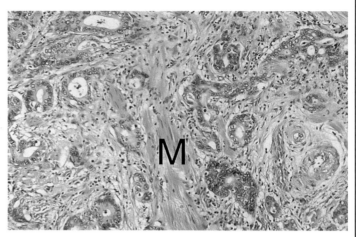

FIGURE 10.23 Periampullary tumour. This is a moderately differentiated adenocarcinoma which is invading through smooth muscle (M).

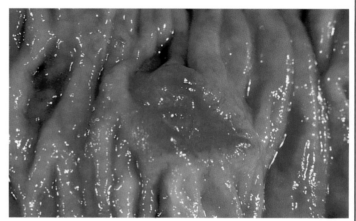

FIGURE 10.24 Periampullary tumour in the duodenum. It is forming a raised ulcer, 15 mm in diameter.

Insulinoma

This is the commonest islet cell tumour, although still very rare. It is associated clinically with recurrent attacks of hypoglycaemia – which may result in confusion, mania, dizziness or coma. These effects are reversed by taking glucose or by excision of the tumour. Ninety per cent of insulinomas are benign.

Gastrinoma

Gastrin is normally produced only by G cells in the stomach and duodenum. Most gastrinomas occur in the submucosa of the duodenum or the gastric antrum but the pancreas is the most common site for an ectopic gastrinoma. Gastrinomas are associated with Zollinger–Ellison syndrome in which persistent hypersecretion of acid gastric juice causes duodenal and even jejunal peptic ulceration. Most pancreatic gastrinomas are malignant.

SUMMARY

- The liver is a metabolically active tissue which can be subjected to a wide range of insults including viral infections, toxins and chemicals (in particular alcohol), autoimmune processes and inherited metabolic diseases.
- Distinct patterns of injury are seen with different agents (e.g. viruses – chronic hepatitis; biliary disease – cholestatic injury; alcohol excess and metabolic syndrome – fatty liver disease).
- Acute liver injury is associated with hepatocyte necrosis; if extensive this may be associated with liver failure

but where there is less damage the liver may undergo marked regeneration with a return to normal structure.

- Chronic liver injury is generally associated with fibrosis; when accompanied by nodular regenerative change there may be transformation of the liver architecture to cirrhosis.
- The key clinical complications of liver disease are: (i) failure of normal liver function (synthetic, detoxifying etc.); (ii) portal hypertension; and (iii) risk of hepatic malignancy.
- Gallstones (cholelithiasis) are common in Western countries.
- Acute and chronic cholecystitis are important and sometimes serious complications of gallstone disease.
- Acute pancreatitis is a life-threatening condition which is associated with gallstone disease and alcohol excess.
- Chronic pancreatitis may also be caused by excess alcohol and can lead to pancreatic exocrine and endocrine insufficiency.
- Carcinoma of the pancreas, an important form of solid organ malignancy of increasing incidence, commonly presents with obstructive jaundice.

FURTHER READING

Burt AD, Portmann BC, Ferrell LD. *MacSween's Pathology of the Liver*, 5th edn. Edinburgh: Churchill Livingstone, 2006.

Iacobuzio-Donahue CA, Montgomery EA. *Gastro-intestinal and Liver Pathology*. Edinburgh: Churchill Livingstone, 2005.

Odze RD, Goldblum JR, Crawford JM. *Surgical Pathology of the GI Tract, Liver, Biliary Tract and Pancreas*. Philadelphia: Saunders, 2004.

11 THE NERVOUS SYSTEMS AND THE EYE

David I Graham, James AR Nicoll and Fiona Roberts

NORMAL STRUCTURE AND FUNCTION

The central nervous system (CNS), i.e. the brain and the spinal cord, is composed of two types of tissue, both involved in disease processes. The first consists of the highly specialized nerve cells (neurons) and the neuroglial cells, all of which are of neuroepithelial origin. The second comprises the meninges, the blood vessels and their supporting connective tissue, all derived from mesoderm and the microglia (phagocytic cells).

APPLIED ANATOMY

The dura mater acts as the periosteum to the skull and spine. Extensions of the dura – the falx cerebri and the tentorium cerebelli – subdivide the cranial cavity into three spaces, two supratentorial and one infratentorial (the posterior fossa). The subdural space lies between the dura and the outer surface of the arachnoid, and blood or pus can spread widely throughout it (Figure 11.1). The arachnoid lies in contact with the dura; the pia is closely attached to the brain. The subarachnoid space is filled with cerebrospinal fluid (CSF). It is widest in the basal cisterns and within sulci. It contains the major cerebral arteries and veins; arterial branches pass into the brain.

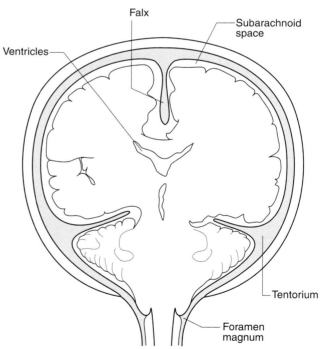

FIGURE 11.1 The intracranial compartments: see text. (From Adams JA and Graham DI. *Introduction to Neuropathology*. London: Churchill Livingstone, 1988.)

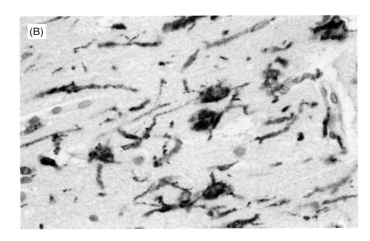

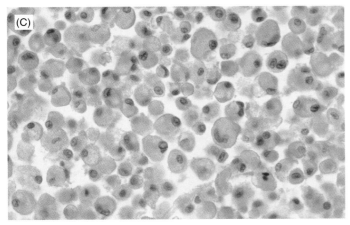

FIGURE 11.6 (Continued)

Blood Vessels

Proliferation of capillaries is seen around infarcts and abscesses, and in relation to rapidly growing cerebral tumours. Dysfunction of the blood–brain barrier may result in vascular oedema and swelling of the brain (see below).

RAISED INTRACRANIAL PRESSURE, BRAIN SWELLING AND OEDEMA AND HYDROCEPHALUS

After the fontanelles close in late infancy, the intracranial contents of the brain (about 70% of the intracranial volume), CSF (about 15%) and blood (about 15%) are enclosed in a rigid bony container. Any increase in the volume of one component will lead to an increase in intracranial pressure (ICP) unless compensated by a corresponding reduction of the others. Thus, pathological processes such as tumour, haematoma or a massive recent cerebral infarct ultimately cause an increase in ICP (Table 11.2). There is, however, a period of spatial compensation during which the ICP remains within normal limits brought about principally due to a reduction in the volume of CSF within the ventricles and the subarachnoid space and by a reduction in the volume of

TABLE 11.2 Definitions of raised intracranial pressure (ICP)

Normal upper limit of ICP is about 2.7 kPa (20 mmHg)
High ICP is above 5.4 kPa (40 mmHg)
Raised ICP is usually due to an intracranial expanding mass
A pressure gradient forms between supratentorial and infratentorial compartments, or between the intracranial and spinal subarachnoid spaces

blood within the intracranial veins. When all available space has been used a critical point is reached beyond which a further slight increase in the volume of the intracranial contents will cause an abrupt increase of ICP and rapid deterioration in the patient's condition. Arteriolar vasodilation due to increased arterial $PaCO_2$, or the use of some anaesthetic agents, may be sufficient to produce this effect. The compensatory mechanisms fail more quickly when the lesion is expanding rapidly. Intracranial expanding lesions (Tables 11.3 and 11.4) also cause distortion and displacement of the brain and the associated increase in ICP is often of greater prognostic significance than the nature of the lesion itself.

TABLE 11.3 Neurological features associated with progressive elevation of intracranial pressure due to a unilateral supratentorial intracranial expanding lesion

Reduction in level of consciousness
Dilation of pupil ipsilateral to mass lesion and papilloedema
Bradycardia, increase in pulse pressure and increase in mean arterial blood pressure
Cheyne–Stokes respiration

TABLE 11.4 Principal changes in the intracranial compartment due to a unilateral mass lesion

Narrowing of sulci and flattening of gyri
Reduction in size of ipsilateral ventricle
Midline shift
Supracallosal (subfalcine) hernia
Tentorial hernia
Compression of ipsilateral ocular nerve
Tonsillar hernia
Brainstem haemorrhage/infarction including Kernohan notch
Calcarine infarction

In a tentorial hernia the medial part of the ipsilateral temporal lobe is squeezed through the tentorial opening (Figure 11.7) and compresses and displaces the midbrain against the contralateral rigid edge of the tentorium (Figure 11.8). This pressure may produce a distinct groove on the contralateral surface of the midbrain: the Kernohan notch. The tentorial opening is plugged, CSF is continuously produced, and a pressure gradient develops, the supratentorial

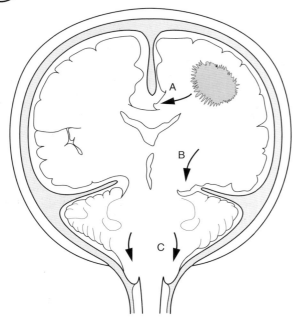

FIGURE 11.7 Raised intracranial pressure, showing the intracranial compartments and the result of a mass lesion on the right hand side. In addition to a shift of the midline structures and distortion of the ventricular system, there is (A) a supracallosal (subfalcine) hernia; (B) a tentorial hernia; (C) a tonsillar hernia.

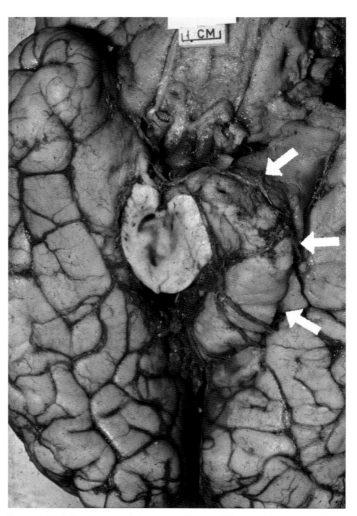

FIGURE 11.8 Raised intracranial pressure. The medial part of the temporal lobe has pushed medially and downwards to form a tentorial hernia. The deep groove (arrows) indicates the position of the edge of the tentorium. There is also secondary haemorrhage into the brainstem.

pressure exceeding the infratentorial. This is associated with a rapid deterioration in the patient's conscious level.

A tonsillar hernia (cerebellar cone), i.e. impaction of the cerebellar tonsils in the foramen magnum, is most common with infratentorial expanding lesions. The tonsils compress the medulla and produce apnoea by distorting the respiratory centre. By obstructing the flow of CSF through the fourth ventricle, such herniation may further increase the ICP so that a vicious circle is set up.

In a patient with an intracranial expanding lesion lumbar puncture can precipitate internal herniation with serious consequences. Even if only a small amount of CSF is withdrawn, more may leak into the spinal extradural space via the puncture wound in the meninges. Lumbar puncture is therefore contraindicated in a patient thought to have a raised ICP until the presence of an intracranial expanding lesion has been excluded by computed tomography (CT) or magnetic resonance imaging (MRI).

Brain Swelling and Oedema

An increase in the volume of the brain due to oedema or increased cerebral blood volume contributes to raised ICP. Vasodilation leading to an increase in cerebral blood volume may occur due to hypoxia or hypercapnia, or as a result of loss of vasomotor tone which may complicate acute brain damage.

Cerebral oedema is classified as vasogenic or cytotoxic. The vasogenic type corresponds to oedema elsewhere in the body resulting from an increased filtration pressure and/or increased permeability of the capillaries and venules. It is often prominent in the tissue around cerebral contusions, recent infarcts, a brain abscess and very frequently in association with a brain tumour. In the less common cytotoxic oedema, usually seen in some metabolic derangements, intracellular fluid accumulates. This is a disturbance of cellular osmoregulation, the blood–brain barrier to proteins remaining intact.

Hydrocephalus

The term hydrocephalus means an increased volume of CSF within the cranial cavity (Table 11.5). The commonest cause of enlargement of the ventricles is cerebral atrophy (see p. 304) in which ICP is not increased. Acute hydrocephalus with increased ICP is most often due to obstruction to the free flow of CSF. The ventricles enlarge and there is a reduction in the bulk of the white matter in the

TABLE 11.5 *Major forms of hydrocephalus*

Internal hydrocephalus is increased volume of CSF within the ventricular system
External hydrocephalus is an excess of CSF in the subarachnoid space
Communicating hydrocephalus is when CSF can flow freely from the ventricular system to the subarachnoid space
Non-communicating hydrocephalus is when CSF cannot flow from the fourth ventricle to the subarachnoid space
Compensatory hydrocephalus is an increased volume of CSF after loss of brain tissue

cerebral hemispheres. In obstructive hydrocephalus it is the site of the lesion rather than its nature which is of importance. Thus, even a small lesion in a critical site adjacent to an interventricular foramen of Monro or the aqueduct in the midbrain will rapidly produce hydrocephalus. Any process such as previous meningitis or subarachnoid haemorrhage that results in partial obliteration of the subarachnoid space will also obstruct the flow of CSF.

The ventricular system proximal to the obstruction enlarges. If it is at a foramen of Monro, one lateral ventricle enlarges: if it is in the third ventricle or the aqueduct, both lateral ventricles enlarge; if it is at the exit foramina of the fourth ventricle, the entire ventricular system enlarges; if the obstruction is in the subarachnoid space, the entire ventricular system enlarges but on this occasion the hydrocephalus is communicating in type because CSF can flow out of the exit foramina in the fourth ventricle into the subarachnoid space.

Normal Pressure Hydrocephalus

This is characterized by ventricular enlargement and a clinical syndrome of progressive dementia, disturbance of gait and urinary incontinence or urgency. Routine measurements of CSF pressure may be normal but continuous monitoring of ICP can demonstrate episodes of moderate intracranial hypertension. It has been suggested that a more appropriate term might be intermittent hydrocephalus. A ventriculoperitoneal shunt may cause clinical improvement. In most cases the cause is not known, but there may be a history of previous subarachnoid haemorrhage after a head injury or a previous haemorrhagic stroke, leading to partial obliteration of the subarachnoid space.

HEAD INJURY

There are two principal types of head injury – missile and blunt. In blunt head injury the two main causes of damage to the brain are acceleration/deceleration and contact. Sudden deceleration or acceleration of the head causes the brain to move within the cranial cavity producing shear strains within the brain or contact between brain and the

bony irregularities at the base of the skull. Damage is particularly severe when there is a rotational element in the acceleration/deceleration. Nothing needs to strike the head nor the head to strike anything to produce brain damage – what matters is the acceleration/deceleration conditions that exist at the moment of injury. The various features of brain damage are classified as primary and secondary according to whether they occur at the moment of injury or occur as a subsequent reaction to the injury and are therefore potentially preventable.

Missile injuries are produced by various types of object which fall or are propelled through the air. The object often enters the cranial cavity producing focal brain damage. See Table 11.6 for a summary of the key epidemiological features of head injury.

TABLE 11.6 *Epidemiology of traumatic brain injury*

Trauma is the commonest cause of death under 45 years old
Brain damage after head injury is the most important factor contributing to death or serious incapacity
About 300 per 100 000 of the population require hospital admission per year
Principal causes of head injury include road traffic accidents, falls, assaults and injuries at work, in the home and during sports
Head injuries from road traffic accidents are most common in young men: alcohol is frequently involved

Blunt Injury: Primary Damage

The major elements in blunt injury are fracture of the skull, contusions/lacerations usually with subarachnoid haemorrhage, intracranial haematomas and diffuse traumatic axonal injury.

Fracture of the Skull

Many patients with a fracture do not sustain significant brain damage while about 25% of fatal head injuries are not associated with a fracture; in patients with a fracture, however, there is a high incidence of intracranial haematoma. The fracture may be depressed causing local pressure on the brain. If there is a scalp laceration the fracture is compound and a potential source of intracranial sepsis. Any fracture of the base of the skull provides a potential source of infection from the nose, the paranasal sinuses or middle ear; there may be CSF rhinorrhoea or otorrhoea. Tearing of a meningeal artery may produce an extradural haematoma.

Cerebral Contusions and Lacerations

These are the commonest form of brain damage directly attributable to injury. They may occur at the site of contact particularly if there is a depressed fracture, but in any blunt head injury they tend to involve the frontal poles, the orbital

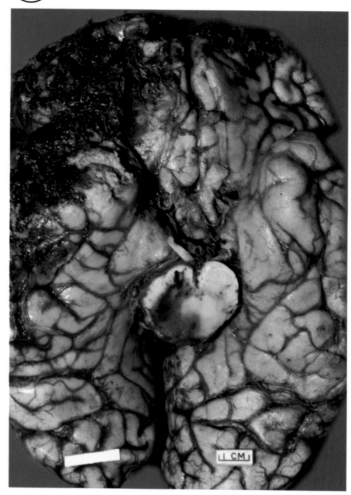

FIGURE 11.9 Cerebral contusions. The frontal and temporal lobes are affected by haemorrhagic contusions.

gyri, the temporal poles and the inferior and lateral surfaces of the anterior halves of the temporal lobes (Figure 11.9).

Haematoma

Intracranial Haematoma

This is a frequent complication of a head injury and is the commonest cause of deterioration and death in patients who have been conscious immediately after their injury. The incidence of haematoma is high in patients with a fracture of the skull. Traumatic intracranial haematomas may be extradural, subdural, subarachnoid or intracerebral.

Extradural Haematoma

This results from haemorrhage from a meningeal blood vessel, usually the middle meningeal artery damaged by a skull fracture. The haematoma gradually strips the dura from the skull to form a large ovoid mass that progressively compresses the adjacent brain. The initial injury may seem mild as the patient experiences a lucid interval of some hours before developing headache and becoming drowsy. As the

haematoma enlarges, the ICP increases and the patient lapses into coma and may die unless the haematoma is evacuated.

Subdural Haematoma

A subdural haematoma results from rupture of bridging veins which drain into the superior sagittal sinus, or from haemorrhage into the subdural space from severe surface contusions. The blood spreads diffusely throughout the subdural space.

Acute subdural haematoma

This is a common autopsy finding if death has occurred soon after the injury. The haematoma may be large and act as an acute intracranial expanding lesion, or it may only be a thin film of blood. Some patients with acute subdural haematoma experience a lucid interval similar to that associated with extradural haematoma.

Chronic subdural haematoma

Chronic subdural haematoma presents weeks or months after an apparently trivial head injury; some patients deny any history of injury. The haematoma is organized and becomes encapsulated in a fibrous membrane. Chronic subdural haematoma is particularly common in old people who already have some cerebral atrophy; because the haematoma expands very slowly, probably as the result of repeated small haemorrhages into it, it may become quite large before symptoms appear. In untreated cases, however, death is usually attributable to brain damage secondary to a high ICP. Chronic subdural haematoma is frequently bilateral.

Intracerebral Haematoma

Intracerebral haematoma tends to be associated with contusions and occurs principally in the frontal or the temporal lobe. The term 'burst lobe' is used to describe the combination of an intracerebral haematoma in continuity with a subdural haematoma through surface contusions. Small, deeply seated intracerebral haematomas – often referred to as 'basal ganglia haematomas' also occur and have a higher incidence in patients with diffuse traumatic axonal injury (see below).

Diffuse Traumatic Axonal Injury

Nerve fibres are torn at the moment of injury as a result of shear strains produced by acceleration/deceleration forces, particularly rotational. This may occur in the absence of contusions and the only abnormalities observed at autopsy may be haemorrhagic lesions in the corpus callosum (Figure 11.10) and in the rostral brainstem: the diagnosis can only be made after histological examination. The striking abnormality is the presence of axonal varicosities and bulbs in many regions of the brain (Figure 11.11). In patients who survive for weeks or months – usually in a severely disabled or vegetative state – there is enlargement of the ventricular system due to a reduction in the bulk of the white matter. There are often also small, shrunken, cystic lesions in the corpus callosum and in the rostral brainstem. Microscopy at

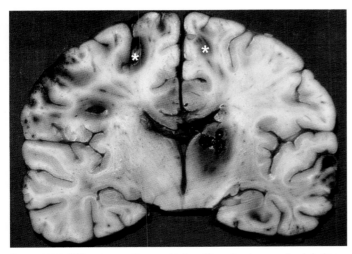

FIGURE 11.10 Diffuse traumatic axonal injury. There is a haemorrhagic lesion in the corpus callosum to the right of the midline. There are also gliding contusions (*) in the dorso-medial sectors of the hemispheres and a haematoma in the right thalamus. Note relative absence of superficial contusions.

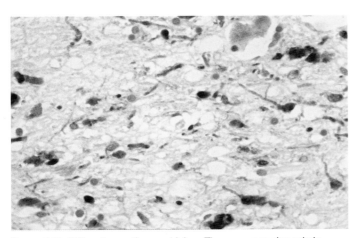

FIGURE 11.11 Diffuse traumatic axonal injury. There are many irregularly shaped axons and some bulbs in the corpus callosum. (Immunohistochemistry βAPP.)

this stage shows widespread Wallerian degeneration secondary to the axonal disruption.

Blunt Injury: Secondary Damage

The main features are raised ICP, ischaemia and infection. Secondary damage after a head injury with brain swelling often causes an increase in ICP and distortion and herniation of the brain (see p. 285). Particularly in children there may be acute swelling of both hemispheres soon after injury.

Ischaemic Brain Damage

This is a frequent occurrence. Some of the causes are recognized, for example cardiorespiratory arrest or status epilepticus. The pathogenesis of other types of ischaemic damage is not understood but it is probably attributable to some acute haemodynamic instability soon after injury.

Infection

Infection brought about by bacteria entering the skull through a compound fracture of the vault or through a basal skull fracture, usually presents as meningitis and mainly in the early post-traumatic period. A small traumatic fistula from the subarachnoid space to one of the sinuses may result in late-onset sepsis. Intracranial abscess is rare and is usually secondary to a penetrating injury.

Clinical aspects of the pathogenesis of brain damage due to a head injury are complex and the primary damage may be the beginning of an evolving process which may range from progressive improvement – as in most patients with so-called concussion – to death. Diffuse brain damage is probably the most important with regard to the clinical outcome since, unlike intracranial haematoma, much of it is not amenable to treatment. An internationally recognized method of describing unconsciousness is the Glasgow Coma Score and outcome the Glasgow Outcome Scale.

Head injury is a major cause of disability and death. Of patients who survive the initial injury and remain in coma for at least 6 hours, one-third die within 6 months, a third recover, a third are moderately or severely disabled; around 3% are vegetative. Residual disabilities include mental (impaired intellect, memory and behavioural problems) and physical defects (hemiparesis and dysphasia). Most recovery occurs within the first 6 months after injury. There is an accumulating population of disabled survivors from head injury, 1 in 300 families having a member with such a disability.

Head injury is an important cause of epilepsy. About 5% of patients admitted to hospital after blunt head injury develop seizures. These tend to occur in the first week after injury (early epilepsy) or are delayed for 2–3 months (late epilepsy). With penetrating head injuries the incidence of epilepsy is about 45%.

CIRCULATORY DISTURBANCES: VASCULAR DISEASE AND HYPOXIC BRAIN DAMAGE

Cerebrovascular disease (stroke) is a sudden disturbance of brain function of vascular origin. The annual incidence in Western countries varies between 150 and 200 per 100 000 population. Strokes account for 10% of all deaths; about 50% of new strokes are fatal and of those who survive about 50% are permanently disabled and only 10% return to normal activity. A distinction is made between transient ischaemic attacks – a fully reversible neurological deficit usually lasting for a few minutes but occasionally up to 24 hours in which it is assumed that no structural brain damage has occurred – and a completed stroke where permanent brain damage of varying severity has developed. The numerous risk factors for strokes due to infarction and haemorrhage include those for atheroma (p. 112) and hypertension.

Arterial Supply to Brain

The arterial supply to the cerebral hemispheres is derived from branches of the circle of Willis, an anastomotic channel between the major cerebral arteries of the base of the brain (Figure 11.12). Potential anastomoses between the vertebral and internal carotid arteries are important if the blood flow through the internal carotid or vertebral arteries is compromised. There is an increased risk of infarction if these potential anastomoses are deficient due to an anomaly in the circle of Willis or acquired disease such as atheromatous stenosis.

The spinal cord is supplied from the spinal branches of the vertebral, deep cervical, intercostal and lumbar arteries which arise from the aorta in a segmental manner and feed into an anterior spinal artery which supplies the anterior two-thirds of the spinal cord and two smaller posterior spinal arteries. Structural damage resulting from ischaemia usually takes the form of an infarct but in less severe ischaemia only neurons undergo necrosis (selective neuronal necrosis).

necrosis. Infarcts range from small discrete lesions to necrosis of large parts of the brain: they may occur in any part of the brain but most commonly in the distribution of the middle cerebral artery. All or only part of the arterial territory may be affected (Figure 11.13).

The structural changes depend upon the size of the lesion and the survival time. A cerebral infarct may be pale or haemorrhagic. An intensely haemorrhagic infarct may resemble a haematoma, but the architecture of the necrotic tissue is preserved (Figure 11.14). A pale infarct less than 24 hours old is difficult to identify macroscopically, but thereafter the dead tissue becomes soft and swollen and there is a loss of the normal sharp definition between the grey and white matter. Swelling of the necrotic tissue and oedema of the surrounding brain may cause a large infarct to act as an acutely expanding mass lesion with raised ICP (Figure 11.15). Within a few days the infarct becomes soft as the dead tissue disintegrates.

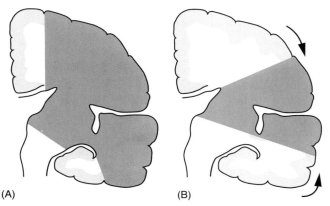

(A)   (B)

FIGURE 11.13 Diagrammatic representations of infarcts in the territory supplied by a middle cerebral artery. (A) infarct involving the entire territory, (B) infarct restricted to the central territory. Arrows in (B) indicate collateral flow from the anterior and posterior cerebral arteries. (From Adams JH and Graham DI. *Introduction to Neuropathology*. London: Churchill Livingstone, 1988.)

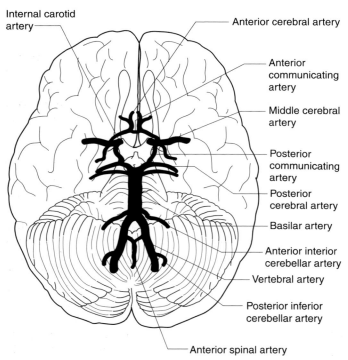

Internal carotid artery —
Anterior cerebral artery

Anterior communicating artery

Middle cerebral artery

Posterior communicating artery

Posterior cerebral artery

Basilar artery

Anterior interior cerebellar artery

Vertebral artery

Posterior inferior cerebellar artery

Anterior spinal artery

FIGURE 11.12 Circle of Willis. The anterior part of the circle is derived from the internal carotid arteries which divide into the proximal portions of the paired middle and anterior cerebral arteries, and the posterior part of the circle is derived from the vertebral and basilar system which gives origin to the paired posterior cerebral arteries. The circle is completed anteriorly by the anterior communicating artery which joins the anterior cerebral arteries and posteriorly by the posterior communicating arteries, which join the posterior cerebral and internal carotid arteries.

Cerebral Infarction

Following a local arrest or reduction of cerebral blood flow (CBF) cellular elements of an area of brain may undergo

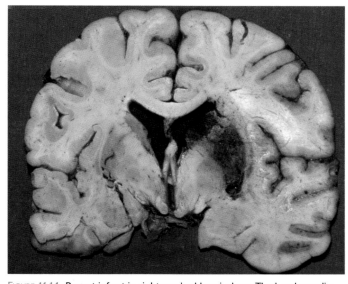

FIGURE 11.14 Recent infarct in right cerebral hemisphere. The basal ganglia show the features of haemorrhagic infarction (reperfusion injury).

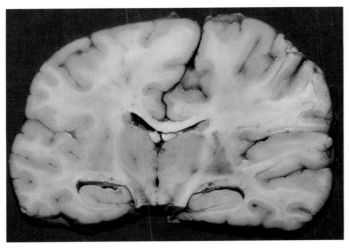

FIGURE 11.15 Cerebral infarction. There is a large infarct in the right cerebral hemisphere due to occlusion of the ipsilateral internal carotid artery. There are internal herniae and some asymmetry of the ventricles due to midline shift.

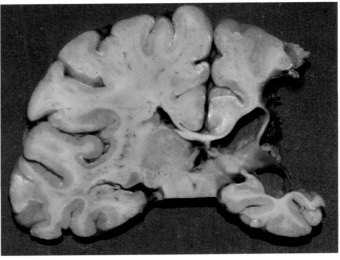

FIGURE 11.16 Cerebral infarction of several years' duration. The necrotic tissue has been removed and the ipsilateral lateral ventricle is enlarged (compensatory hydrocephalus).

During the following weeks the dead tissue is removed and there is gliosis. The lesion ultimately becomes shrunken and cystic and, if there has been haemorrhage, brown due to haemosiderin within macrophages. Shrinkage of a cerebral infarct is usually accompanied by enlargement of the adjacent ventricle (Figure 11.16). Wallerian degeneration of the interrupted nerve fibres occurs; thus, if the infarct involves the internal capsule, there is progressive shrinkage of the pyramidal tract in the brainstem and spinal cord.

The pathogenesis of cerebral infarction includes embolism, atheroma and many other causes. Cerebral embolism accounts for between 30% and 60% of strokes. Most emboli pass into the middle cerebral artery, and many produce only transient occlusion. The major sources are the heart (p. 107), and atheroma of the extracranial neck arteries and arch of aorta. Atheromatous narrowing or occlusion may occur in any part of the carotid or vertebral arteries. Stenosis does not necessarily lead to infarction because at normal blood pressure the internal cross-sectional area of an artery must be reduced by up to 90% before blood flow is impaired; a combination of systemic circulatory insufficiency and stenosis results in many cases of infarction. The commonest site is at the origin of an internal carotid artery, but infarction results only if the collateral circulation is inadequate. In some cases, thrombosis extends along the internal carotid artery into the middle and anterior cerebral arteries to produce infarction of a large part of the cerebral hemisphere. The commonest intracranial site of thrombosis is a middle cerebral artery, usually due to embolism, thrombosis formed on atheroma, or basal vasospasm after rupture of an adjacent saccular aneurysm. Occlusion of the extracranial neck arteries may also follow embolism, dissecting aneurysm and trauma. The vertebral artery may be occluded due to deformation by osteophytes, by certain neck movements, for example hyperextension during intubation for anaesthesia, or by rheumatoid arthritis with subluxation of atlanto-occipital joint.

Primary thrombosis of the veins and venous sinuses (noninfectious or marantic) occurs most frequently in poorly nourished and dehydrated children during the course of acute infections; it may occur in adults with congestive cardiac failure, or during pregnancy and the puerperium. Thrombosis may be secondary to pyogenic infection (septic thrombosis).

Brain Damage due to Cardiac Arrest

Neurons require a continuous adequate supply of oxygen and glucose which depends on cardiorespiratory function and on cerebral blood flow, which is determined by the cerebral perfusion pressure (the difference between the systemic arterial blood pressure and the cerebral venous pressure). An autoregulatory mechanism maintains a relatively constant cerebral blood flow in spite of changes in perfusion pressure even when systemic arterial pressure falls as low as 50 mmHg provided the subject is in the horizontal position. At arterial pressures lower than this, cerebral blood flow falls rapidly. Autoregulation may be impaired in hypertension, in hypoxia or hypercapnia, or in many acute conditions producing brain damage, for example head injury and strokes.

Patients who sustain severe diffuse brain damage after cardiac arrest often die within a few days. The brain may appear normal macroscopically, but if the patient has survived for more than 12 hours, microscopy shows widespread and severe neuronal necrosis with a distinctive pattern of selective vulnerability. Worst affected are the neocortex and hippocampus with greatest involvement of the Ammon's horn. There is diffuse necrosis of the Purkinje cells of the cerebellum and loss of the sensory nuclei of the brainstem. In general, brain damage is more severe in young children than adults. A similar pattern of damage may be seen in carbon

11.1 SPECIAL STUDY TOPIC

(written by I Bone, Emeritus Professor of Neurology, University of Glasgow)

THROMBOLYTIC THERAPY IN ACUTE ISCHAEMIC STROKE

The management of patients with ischaemic strokes in specialized stroke units has greatly improved outcomes. In part this has been through good general management of blood pressure (avoiding hypotension), maintaining adequate oxygenation, anticipating dysphagia with the risk of aspiration, prophylaxis of venous thrombosis in the immobile, and suppressing fever, if present.

An increasing part of acute management involves the consideration of methods that may re-canalize the occluded blood vessel thus permitting reperfusion and salvage of ischaemic non-necrotic tissue. Natural fibrinolysins normally released by the injured endothelium may not work sufficiently quickly to be clinically effective. Thrombolytic agents speed up the conversion of plasminogen to plasmin, a potent natural fibrinolytic, thus promoting early clot lysis. Several different thrombolytic agents have been developed and trialled in ischaemic stroke.

Streptokinase

Clinical trials of intravenous streptokinase have failed to show benefit in patients with acute ischaemic stroke though it is uncertain whether this difference from tissue plasminogen activator (tPA) trial results (see below) reflects a longer time window from onset (<6 hours), the dose used or the specific properties of streptokinase itself. Intra-arterial streptokinase, urokinase and prourokinase are undergoing clinical trials.

Tissue Plasminogen Activator

The results of the National Institute of Neurologic Disorders and Stroke (NINDS) tPA trial were published in December 1995 and resulted in approval by the US Food and Drug Administration for clinical uses. The NINDS study showed that the use of intravenous tPA within 3 hours of ischaemic stroke onset substantially improved long-term functional outcome when compared with placebo, even with the risk of symptomatic intracerebral haemorrhage included. The trial showed that for every 100 patients given IV tPA, 12 more experience complete neurological recovery when compared with placebo. Symptomatic intracranial haemorrhage occurred in 6%. The risk of intracerebral haemorrhage increased significantly in patients treated with tPA where the computed tomographic (CT) scan showed obvious evidence of early infarction as well as in those with more marked clinical deficit (as measured by the NIH Stroke Scale) at baseline.[1]

The European Cooperative Acute Stroke Study (ECASS) randomized trial of IV tPA[2] with a 6-hour time limit to treatment and using a higher dose of tPA did not demonstrate benefit, largely due to the high rate of brain haemorrhage. A follow-up trial from the European investigators (ECASS II) tested a lower dose of IV tPA (0.9 per kg) in the 3–6-hour window and excluded patients with early extensive infarction visible on CT. This study showed no significant benefit.[3]

From these studies a maximum time from stroke onset to treatment of 3 hours is recommended. A CT scan must be carried out prior to treatment to exclude intracranial bleeding or extensive infarction evidenced by sulcal effacement, mass effect and oedema. Caution is advised before giving intravenous tPA to patients with severe stroke (NIH Stroke Scale >23). This treatment should not be given to those who are severely hypertensive (systolic pressure greater than 185 mmHg or diastolic pressure greater than 110 mmHg), have a recent history of head injury or blood loss, are rapidly recovering or have experienced seizure at presentation. Treating patients who do not fulfil protocol guidelines results in excessive risk with no observable benefit. Debate persists as to how specialist the provisions of a stroke centre offering such treatment should be. Combined intravenous and intra-arterial regimens remain under study as do other modes of clot lysis (glycoprotein 11b/111a inhibitors) and fragmentation (ultrasound).

References

1 Adams HP Jr, Brott TG, Furlan AJ, *et al.* Guidelines for thrombolytic therapy for acute stroke: a supplement to the guidelines for the management of patients with acute ischemic stroke. A statement for healthcare professionals from a Special Writing Group of the Stroke Council, American Heart Association. *Circulation* 1996; **94**: 1167–1167.

2 Hacke W, Kaste M, Fieschi C, *et al.* Intravenous thrombolysis with recombinant tissue plasminogen activator for acute hemispheric stroke. The European Cooperative Acute Stroke Study (ECASS). *JAMA* 1995; **274**: 1017–1025.

3 Hacke W, Kaste M, Fieschi C, *et al.* Randomised double-blind placebo-controlled trial of thrombolytic therapy with intravenous alteplase in acute ischaemic stroke (ECASS II). Second European-Australasian Acute Stroke Study Investigators. *Lancet* 1998; **352**: 1245–1251.

4 The NINDS t-PA Stroke Study Group. Intracerebral haemorrhage after intravenous t-PA therapy for ischemic stroke. *Stroke* 1997; **28**: 2109–2118.

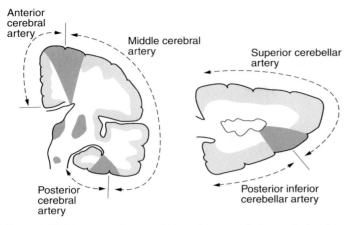

FIGURE 11.17 Diagram to show arterial boundary zones in the cerebral and cerebellar hemispheres. They lie between the territories supplied by the major arteries.

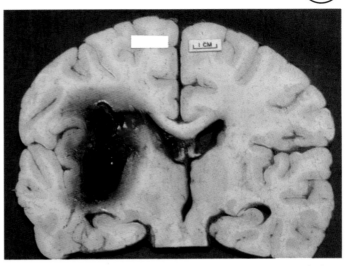

FIGURE 11.18 Intracerebral haemorrhage. There is a large haematoma in the basal ganglia due to chronic hypertension.

monoxide intoxication, and status epilepticus. Severe hypoglycaemia may also cause widespread brain damage.

Brain damage due to hypotension is concentrated in the boundary zones between the main cerebral and cerebellar arterial territories (Figure 11.17). The lesions tend to be largest in the parieto-occipital regions where the territories of the anterior, middle and posterior cerebral arteries meet. There is variable involvement of the basal ganglia. The hippocampi, despite their vulnerability to cardiac arrest, are usually not involved. This type of brain damage is seen most commonly in shock and in fatal head injury and is caused by a major episode of hypotension; autoregulation fails and cerebral blood flow falls most in the boundary zones, those regions most remote from the parent arteries.

Spontaneous (Non-traumatic) Intracranial Haemorrhage

The major types are intracerebral and subarachnoid haemorrhage. Intracerebral haematomas develop in late middle age due to rupture of one of the numerous microaneurysms found in hypertensive individuals, most commonly in the basal ganglia and the internal capsule (Figure 11.18): other sites are the pons and the cerebellum. The haematoma rapidly increases in size and produces a sudden rise in ICP with distortion and herniation of the brain. Blood may rupture into the ventricles or into the subarachnoid space. The onset is sudden, and patients with large haematomas rarely survive for more than a day or two.

The autopsy appearances vary with time; a recent haematoma is composed of dark red clot, but after a week the periphery is brownish and there are early reactive changes in capillaries and astrocytes. Gliosis leads eventually to the formation of a poorly defined capsule and the clot is ultimately completely removed by macrophages and replaced by yellow fluid to form a cyst.

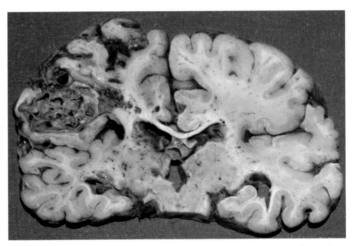

FIGURE 11.19 Arteriovenous malformation. There is a large plexus of vascular channels of varying size in the upper part of the left cerebral hemisphere. (Reproduced from Graham DI, Nicoll JAR, Bone I. *Adams & Graham's Introduction to Neuropathology*, 3rd edn. London: Hodder Arnold, 2006.)

Another common cause of spontaneous intracranial haemorrhage is rupture of a vascular malformation which may range from a small capillary angioma to a massive lesion composed of large, often thick walled vascular channels (Figure 11.19). Many of these lesions are compatible with long survival, sometimes punctuated by episodes of subarachnoid haemorrhage. Spontaneous intracranial haemorrhage may be due to bleeding into a tumour or to haemorrhagic diseases, for example acute leukaemia, coagulation disorders.

Subarachnoid Haemorrhage

In about 65% of patients with spontaneous (nontraumatic) subarachnoid haemorrhage this is due to rupture of a saccular aneurysm on one of the major cerebral arteries and in about 5% due to rupture of a vascular malformation. In a further 10–15% it is due to some other disease, such as a blood dyscrasia or extension of either an intracerebral or an intraventricular haemorrhage into the subarachnoid space. In up to 5% of patients a cause is not found.

Saccular aneurysms occur on the arteries of the base of the brain in about 12% of the adult population and rupture occurs in 6–12 per 100 000 population per year. About 10–15% of patients are found to have multiple (usually two or three) lesions. The common sites are the upper end of internal carotid artery (40%), the anterior communicating artery (30%), the middle cerebral artery (20%), the basilar and vertebral arteries (5–10%). Aneurysms occur more commonly in women, and between 40 and 60 years of age. While often called congenital aneurysms, the developmental abnormality is a defect in the media of the artery at a division. Early atheroma and hypertension contribute to the development of the aneurysm. Most aneurysms that rupture measure 5–10 mm in diameter. Some 10% of patients die before reaching hospital, and a further 30% within the next few days. A further 35% re-bleed and die within the first year, most of these within the first 2 weeks.

When a saccular aneurysm ruptures, the haemorrhage may be limited to its immediate vicinity, but more often it spreads extensively through the CSF in the subarachnoid space (Figure 11.20). Blood may track into the brain to produce an intracerebral haematoma with an acute expanding lesion which often ruptures into the ventricles. If the aneurysm is embedded in brain tissue, intracerebral haemorrhage may occur without subarachnoid haemorrhage. Anterior communicating artery aneurysms tend to burst into the frontal lobe, posterior communicating aneurysms into the temporal lobe. Late complications include cerebral infarction in the distribution of the affected artery, probably attributable to arterial vasospasm, and hydrocephalus.

Fusiform atheromatous aneurysms of major cerebral arteries occur, but rarely rupture. Mycotic aneurysms produced by infected emboli may also occur. Dissecting aneurysms of the aorta (see p. 123) may extend into the carotid arteries thus restricting blood flow.

INFECTIONS OF THE NERVOUS SYSTEM

The brain and spinal cord are relatively well protected against invasion of microorganisms by the skeleton, by the dura, the blood–brain barrier, the microglia and the systemic immune system. However, microorganisms which have gained access may spread rapidly, particularly by the CSF pathways, and many relatively non-pathogenic microorganisms can in various circumstances cause serious infections of the nervous system (Table 11.7).

Clinical features of acute CNS infection include headache, neck stiffness, photophobia, pyrexia, malaise and

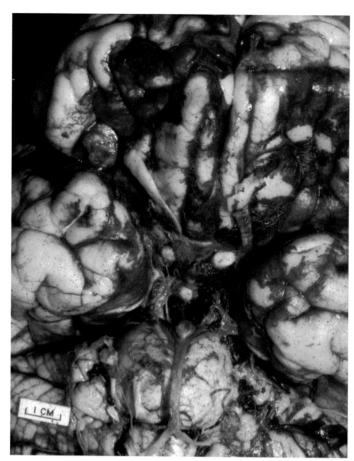

FIGURE 11.20 Subarachnoid haemorrhage. Due to rupture of a saccular aneurysm there are large amounts of recent haemorrhage in the basal cisterns. Dissection showed an aneurysm arising from the upper end of the basilar artery.

TABLE 11.7 Risk factors for infection of the nervous system

Trauma (particularly with compound fractures)
Congenital malformations (e.g. spina bifida)
Iatrogenic (e.g. neurosurgical procedures or lumbar puncture)
Local foci of infection, e.g. mastoid and middle ear
Blood-borne infection
Immunodeficiency states

impaired consciousness. Relevant enquiries include the patient's occupation, recent travel and risk factors for HIV infection. Investigation includes examination of the CSF, usually by lumbar puncture, although the risks of this procedure in the presence of raised ICP must be borne in mind. The key features of the CSF in infections and opportunistic infections of the brain are summarized in Tables 11.8 and 11.9.

TABLE 11.8 Cerebrospinal fluid in infections

	Glucose (mmol/L)	Protein (g/L)	Cells
Normal	2.7–4.1	0.15–0.45	<5 lymphocytes/mm^3
Bacterial meningitis	Increased	Increased	+++ polymorphs
Abscess	Normal	Increased	+ polymorphs and lymphocytes
Viral meningitis	Normal	Increased	++ lymphocytes
Tuberculosis	Decreased	Increased	++ polymorphs early, lymphocytes late

TABLE 11.9 Opportunistic infections

Viruses	Papova virus (progressive multifocal leucoencephalopathy)
	Cytomegalovirus encephalitis/myelitis/retinitis
	Herpes simplex (type 2) meningitis or myelitis
	Herpes simplex (type 1) encephalitis
	Immunosuppressive measles myelitis or encephalitis
	Varicella zoster encephalitis/myelitis
Bacteria	*Mycobacterium avium intracellulare*
	Nocardia (abscesses)
	Syphilis
Fungi	*Cryptococcus neoformans*
	Candida albicans
	Aspergillus fumigatus
	Mucormycosis
	Coccidioidomycosis
	Histoplasmosis
Protozoa	Toxoplasmosis (*Toxoplasma gondii*)

Bacterial Infections

Key Points

- Spread to CNS may be haematogenous, from bone infection or trauma.
- Bacterial infections cause meningitis and brain abscess.
- In bacterial meningitis the CSF is turbid and contains polymorphs and bacteria.
- Brain abscess presents as a space-occupying lesion.
- Tuberculosis causes a subacute meningitis or abscess (tuberculoma).

Acute Bacterial Meningitis

Bacterial meningitis, characterized by spread of bacteria and inflammatory cells through the subarachnoid space, is an emergency requiring rapid diagnosis and treatment. The commonest causative organisms are *Escherichia coli* in infants, *Haemophilus influenzae* in children, *Neisseria meningitidis* in young adults and *Streptococcus pneumoniae* in the elderly.

Most cases of meningitis are of haematogenous origin. Infection with *N. meningitidis* (meningococcal meningitis) is spread by droplet infection from nasopharyngeal carriers and may occur as an epidemic. The meningococci pass to the meninges by the bloodstream and fatal meningococcal septicaemia can occur before meningitis develops; a purpuric rash is an important early sign. Early antibiotic therapy may be given on clinical suspicion but the precise diagnosis depends on examination of the CSF (see Table 11.8). The causal organisms are often apparent in stained films but sometimes they can be detected only by culture. Immunization reduces the risk of infection.

Meningitis may also be brought about by spread from infection in the bones of the skull or after a compound fracture of the skull. Iatrogenic infection occasionally follows surgery or lumbar puncture. In meningitis, pus is found in the intracranial and spinal subarachnoid spaces, and is thickest at the base of the brain. In rapidly fatal cases there may be no more than an excess of turbid fluid in the sulci and histological examination is required to confirm the presence of acute inflammation. The ventricles may contain turbid CSF. Mild hydrocephalus is common because the exudate interferes with the flow of CSF.

Long-term effects are common in survivors and include hydrocephalus due to obliteration of the exit foramina of the fourth ventricle and/or subarachnoid space. Involvement of cranial nerves traversing the subarachnoid space may result in cranial nerve palsies.

Brain Abscess

The clinical features include fever and those of raised ICP. The abscess consists of pus surrounded by oedematous brain containing reactive astrocytes, and, within 2–3 weeks, a collagenous capsule. The causative organisms include streptococci, *Bacteroides*, *Proteus*, staphylococci, *E. coli* and *H. influenzae*, and there may be mixed infections. There are several possible routes of infection. Local spread from infection in the skull (chronic otitis media, chronic mastoiditis, penetrating injury or surgery) usually results in a single abscess (Figure 11.21), while multiple brain abscesses often follow haematogenous spread from infection in lung (bronchiectasis, pneumonia, empyema) or heart (infective endocarditis). Haematogenous spread is also associated with congenital heart disease with a right-to-left shunt.

Clinical diagnosis is by recognition of a focal lesion in the brain with a necrotic centre by CT or MR scan and by aspiration of abscess contents and microbiological culture.

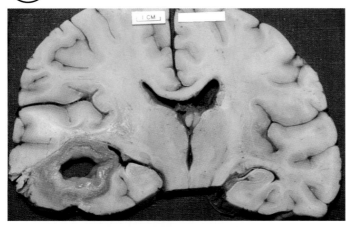

FIGURE 11.21 Cerebral abscess. There is an encapsulated abscess in the left temporal lobe secondary to chronic suppurative otitis media. (Reproduced from Graham DI, Nicoll JAR, Bone I. *Adams & Graham's Introduction to Neuropathology*, 3rd edn. London: Hodder Arnold, 2006.)

Treatment comprises antibiotic therapy and may include therapeutic aspiration of pus.

Tuberculosis

Infection of the CNS by *Mycobacterium tuberculosis* is always secondary to disease elsewhere; its frequency is therefore related to the incidence of tuberculosis in a given population. There are two principal forms – tuberculous meningitis and tuberculomas.

Tuberculous Meningitis

The bacilli almost always reach the subarachnoid space by the bloodstream, either as a component of miliary tuberculosis or spread from a tuberculous focus elsewhere in the body. Occasionally infection spreads to the subarachnoid space from tuberculosis of a vertebral body. Tuberculous meningitis has a subacute or chronic course. A gelatinous or caseous exudate, which is most abundant in the basal cisterns (Figure 11.22A), within sulci and around the spinal cord, obstructs the flow of CSF with almost invariable hydrocephalus. Small tubercles measuring 1–2 mm in diameter may be seen in the pia arachnoid. Lymphocytes, plasma cells and macrophages are seen but Langhans'-type giant cells are uncommon (Figure 11.22B). Obliterative endarteritis causes small infarcts in the brain or in the cranial nerve roots leading to focal neurological signs. Mycobacteria are rarely seen on examination of the CSF (Ziehl–Nielsen stain) but may be demonstrated by culture, fluorescence of rhodamine auramine or by polymerase chain reaction.

Tuberculoma

In countries where tuberculosis is rife, tuberculoma (tuberculous abscess) is a common cause of an intracranial

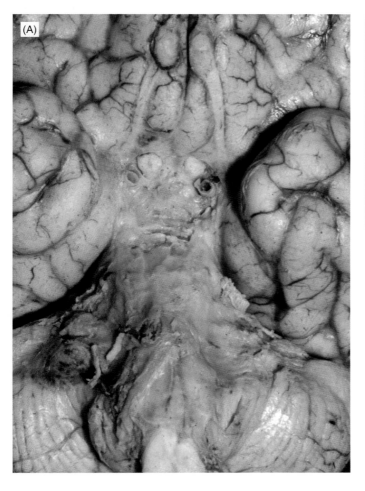

(A)

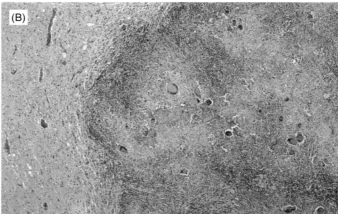

(B)

FIGURE 11.22 Tuberculous meningitis. (A) There is thick exudate at the base of the brain. (B) Within the meninges is a caseating granulomatous inflammatory process with Langhans' giant cells.

expanding lesion. In adults they usually occur in the cerebral hemispheres but in children particularly affect the cerebellum. A tuberculoma has a core of caseous material surrounded by granulomatous inflammation with lymphocytes, epithelioid histiocytes (macrophages) and Langhans'-type giant cells.

Syphilis

Syphilis, caused by *Treponema pallidum*, is now uncommon. It may cause a transient meningoencephalitis (secondary stage), a subacute meningitis (tertiary stage) with cranial nerve palsies, gummas in the meninges and a subacute encephalitis causing progressive dementia many years after the primary infection (general paralysis of the insane). Degeneration of the posterior spinal columns results in the *syndrome of tabes dorsalis*.

Fungal Infections

Fungal infections of the CNS are uncommon and usually arise by haematogenous spread from the lungs or by direct spread from the nose and sinuses. As lesions at the portal of entry may be small and readily overlooked, the brain may appear to be the only organ involved. In other cases infection of the nervous system may be a manifestation of generalized infection. Immunocompromised patients are particularly vulnerable to fungal infections.

Brain abscesses, often multiple, may be caused by *Aspergillus*, *Candida* and *Histoplasma*. Accurate identification depends on culture. Colonization of the walls of blood vessels by fungi and associated thrombosis result in infarction. The inflammatory response is predominantly chronic. *Mucormycosis*, a rare opportunistic infection with a particular predilection for poorly controlled diabetic patients, starts in the paranasal regions and spreads directly into the anterior fossa of the skull to produce selective involvement of the frontal lobes. *Cryptococcosis* infection usually presents as a subacute meningitis; the exudate in the subarachnoid space is gelatinous and contains masses of encapsulated cryptococci.

Viral Infections

Key Points

- Spread of virus to the CNS is usually via the haematogenous route.
- Viral meningitis is usually mild.
- Viral encephalitis (e.g. due to herpes simplex virus) is uncommon but severe.
- Persistent viral infections occur (subacute sclerosing panencephalitis and progressive multifocal leucoencephalopathy).
- In acquired immune deficiency syndrome (AIDS) the CNS is affected by human immunodeficiency virus (HIV) encephalitis, opportunistic infection and lymphoma.

Patients with acute viral infections present with aseptic meningitis or encephalitis. Most viruses reach the nervous system by the bloodstream often after primary replication of the virus in lymphoid tissue. The viruses enter the body by various routes, for example infections of the skin or mucous membranes (herpes simplex virus), by the alimentary tract (enteroviruses), or by the bite of an arthropod (arboviruses). The rabies virus reaches the CNS by travelling along the peripheral nerves.

Aseptic Meningitis

This common but usually not severe acute infection of the CNS occurs particularly in children and is most often due to enteroviruses or the mumps virus. Since aseptic meningitis is rarely fatal, little is known about its pathology which probably amounts to infiltration of the subarachnoid space by lymphocytes, plasma cells and macrophages.

Acute Viral Encephalitis

Many types of acute viral encephalitis have similar histological features with lymphocytes forming cuffs around blood vessels and extending into the brain parenchyma (Figure 11.23). Viral inclusion bodies may be seen (Figure 11.24) in neurons or glial cells and viral antigens can be demonstrated by immunocytochemistry. The causal virus can usually be isolated from brain tissue (biopsy or autopsy) but rarely from the CSF. There may be necrosis, ranging from selective neuronal necrosis in poliomyelitis to frank infarction of grey and white matter in herpes simplex encephalitis. After tissue destruction astrocytosis and lipid-containing macrophages appear. There may be a diffuse hyperplasia of microglia with the formation of rod cells (see Figure 11.6 on pp. 284–285) and small clusters of microglia.

Herpes Simplex Encephalitis

This often rapidly fatal necrotizing encephalitis is almost always due to herpes simplex type I and is the commonest viral encephalitis encountered in western Europe. There is extensive asymmetrical necrosis in the temporal lobes, in the

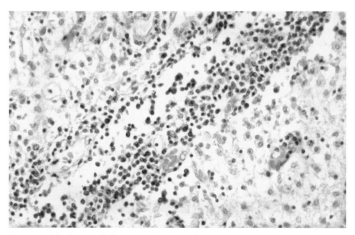

FIGURE 11.23 Acute viral meningitis. The inflammatory cells (mainly around small blood vessels) are lymphocytes and plasma cells.

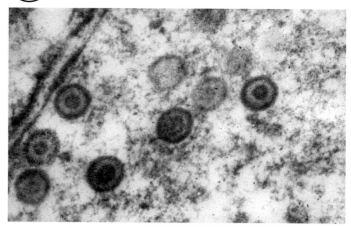

FIGURE 11.24 Acute viral encephalitis. Intracellular herpes simplex viral particles. (Electron microscopy.)

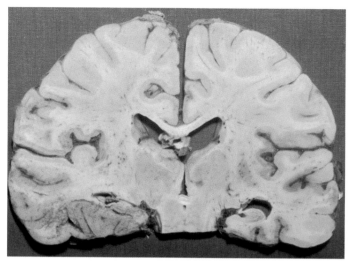

FIGURE 11.26 Encephalitis due to herpes simplex virus. This patient survived for several weeks, severely brain damaged. The affected regions are now shrunken and focally cystic. The left temporal lobe is more severely affected than the right one.

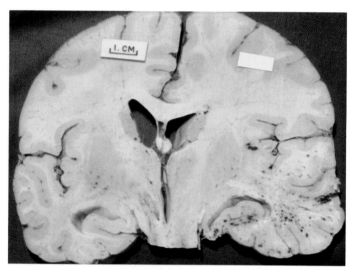

FIGURE 11.25 Encephalitis due to herpes simplex virus. Within the swollen right temporal lobe there are many small haemorrhagic foci. There is also a shift of the midline structures to the left.

insulae and in the cingulate gyri. Swelling of the more severely affected temporal lobe is often sufficient to produce a shift of the midline structures and a tentorial hernia (Figure 11.25). If the patient survives the acute stage, the necrotic tissue becomes shrunken and cystic (Figure 11.26). Despite the selective distribution of the necrosis, histological examination discloses a diffuse meningoencephalitis. Appropriate antiviral treatment should be given as soon as the diagnosis is considered. Confirmatory biopsy from the temporal lobe is now rarely performed as drug therapy is non-toxic.

Varicella Zoster

Asymptomatic latent infection is established in sensory ganglia after chickenpox in childhood. Re-activation of the virus occurs episodically with ageing and in the immunosuppressed. There is inflammation of the ganglion and a painful cutaneous rash in the appropriate dermatome, most commonly in the thoracic and trigeminal distribution.

Cytomegalovirus

Cytomegalovirus CNS infection may be acquired *in utero*. In the neonate it presents as an acute disseminated necrotizing encephalomyelitis with selective involvement of periventricular tissue. Cytomegalic inclusions ('owl's eye' inclusions) may be found in various types of cell. Survivors almost always have learning difficulties, the principal abnormalities in the brain being hydrocephalus and periventricular calcification. Infection early in pregnancy may lead to malformations such as microgyria. Periventricular encephalitis is also seen in opportunistic infection with cytomegalovirus in patients with AIDS.

Infections with Enteroviruses

Polioviruses, coxsackie and ECHO viruses are small RNA viruses that are frequent causes of aseptic meningitis. Enteroviruses are ingested then multiply in the pharynx and gastrointestinal tract. Within a few days, virus is present in adjacent lymphoid tissue and, if the antibody response is inadequate, virus reaches the CNS by the bloodstream. Faecal excretion of virus continues long after the acute infection.

Acute Anterior Poliomyelitis

This disease is classically due to polioviruses but is occasionally caused by other enteroviruses. The virus selectively attacks neurons in the ventral horns of the spinal cord, particularly in the lumbar and cervical enlargements, leading to paralysis of the limb muscles. If the motor nuclei in the brainstem are affected – bulbar polio – there may be involvement of the respiratory centre. In the acute stage the CNS usually appears normal macroscopically but there may be foci of haemorrhage in the brainstem and ventral horns. Microscopy discloses the typical features of a generalised acute viral encephalitis with selectively severe involvement of the spinal cord or brainstem. After the acute stage of the disease, there is loss of neurons in the affected ventral horns, atrophy of the related nerve roots and neurogenic atrophy of the affected muscles (p. 369).

Infections with Arboviruses

These RNA viruses are transmitted from host to host by bloodsucking insects and multiply in both vertebrate and invertebrate hosts. Man is not a natural host for any arbovirus but may become infected during periods of epizootic spread among the natural hosts (usually wild birds and small mammals). Severe forms of encephalitis in man include St. Louis encephalitis, which is mosquito borne, and louping ill, due to a tick borne virus.

Rabies

Rabies remains a major problem in many countries. Most human cases follow the bite of a rabid dog although the major reservoirs are the fox, the skunk and the jackal. The rhabdovirus enters the body from the saliva and reaches the CNS by retrograde transport along peripheral nerves from the bite. The incubation of the disease varies according to the distance of the bite from the CNS; sometimes it is as short as 2 weeks but more commonly is 13 months or even longer. As the old name of *hydrophobia* implies, spasm of the muscles of swallowing on attempting to drink water may be an early symptom. The pathognomonic histological feature is the Negri body, an intracytoplasmic inclusion 1–7 μm in diameter within which virus can be identified.

Persistent Virus Infections

Subacute Sclerosing Panencephalitis (SSPE)

This rare form of encephalitis occurs mainly between the ages of 4 and 20 years and has a prolonged clinical course. It occurs some years after an apparently uncomplicated bout of measles and appears to be due to re-activation of latent measles virus. There are high levels of both IgM and IgG antibodies in the blood and CSF. Microscopic examination shows a subacute meningoencephalitis. Neuronophagia is common, and residual neurons may contain intranuclear and/or cytoplasmic inclusion bodies. There is considerable gliosis in the white matter.

Progressive Multifocal Leucoencephalopathy (PML)

This disease, caused by viruses of the polyoma subgroup of papovaviruses, is virtually restricted to immunocompromised patients. Distributed throughout the white matter are multiple small grey foci of demyelination which can coalesce to form large often cystic areas. Demyelination is accompanied by large bizarre astrocytes, macrophages and abnormal oligodendrocytes whose large nuclei contain inclusion bodies which consist of pseudocrystalline arrays of virions.

Acquired Immunodeficiency Syndrome

Key Points

- About 60% of patients with AIDS have clinical neurological abnormalities.
- Neuropathological abnormalities are identified at autopsy in almost 90%.
- The CNS may be affected in three ways: direct effects of HIV itself, opportunistic infection secondary to the immunosuppression, and lymphoma.
- Often a patient with AIDS may have more than one CNS pathology.
- Antiretroviral treatment enables patients to live relatively healthy lives.

A mild self-limiting meningitis is common in early HIV infection. An encephalitis occurring in later stages in 15–60% of patients is thought to underlie the clinically defined AIDS-related dementia; it is characterized by multinucleated giant cells seen particularly around blood vessels (Figure 11.27) in the white matter often associated with diffuse degeneration of the white matter. Replication of HIV occurs within these giant cells. Some patients develop HIV-associated myelopathy ('vacuolar myelopathy') analogous to HIV encephalitis.

Opportunistic infections

The commoner opportunistic infections to involve the CNS in AIDS include toxoplasmosis, progressive multifocal leucoencephalopathy, cryptococcosis, cytomegalovirus encephalitis and fungal infections. These are described in more detail in Chapter 19.

Lymphoma

Primary or secondary lymphomas may occur. Most are high-grade B-cell non-Hodgkin's lymphomas. Many are associated with Epstein–Barr virus infection.

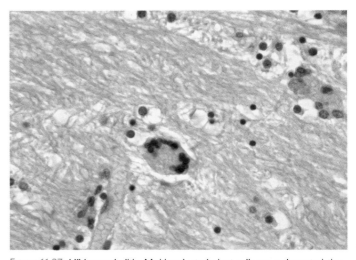

FIGURE 11.27 HIV encephalitis. Multinucleated giant cells are a characteristic feature.

Opportunistic Infections in Immunocompromised Patients

Immunocompromised patients including those with AIDS, transplant recipients, patients with haematological or lymphoid disorders, diabetics and patients undergoing chemotherapy or radiotherapy are particularly vulnerable to infection. They are at risk of severe disease from organisms which often result in only mild or asymptomatic infection in the immunocompetent (see Table 11.9); these are described in Chapter 19.

DEMYELINATING DISEASES

Myelin is formed from the cell membrane of oligodendrocytes and wraps axons to facilitate saltatory conduction of action potentials. Demyelinating disorders of the CNS are characterized by destruction of myelin sheaths with relative preservation of axons (primary or selective demyelination). They are distinct from genetic disorders of myelin formation (dysmyelination) and from diseases causing breakdown of myelin secondary to neuronal destruction (Wallerian degeneration). See Table 11.10 for classification of demyelinating diseases.

TABLE 11.10 Classification of demyelinating diseases

Primary	Multiple sclerosis
	Acute disseminated (perivenous) encephalomyelitis
	Acute haemorrhagic leucoencephalitis
Secondary	
Viral	Progressive multifocal leucoencephalopathy
Toxic/metabolic	Central pontine myelinolysis
	Marchiafava–Bignami disease

Multiple Sclerosis

Key Points

- It is the commonest demyelinating disorder.
- It is a chronic disease with onset in early adulthood.
- There are usually multiple focal lesions in the brain and spinal cord.
- Selective loss of myelin with preservation of axons.

Clinical Features

Multiple sclerosis is the commonest demyelinating disorder and is characterized by multifocal demyelination and gliosis in the brain and spinal cord. It is slightly more common in females than males and the peak age of onset is in the 20s and 30s. Clinical signs and symptoms reflect the distribution of demyelination in the brain and spinal cord. Presentation is usually with a focal neurological deficit such as optic neuritis, limb weakness, diplopia, paraesthesia, bladder dysfunction, vertigo and nystagmus; these often resolve spontaneously. The disease is characterized by relapses and remissions in early years but recurring episodes tend to result in increasing disability. The intervening periods of remission may extend over years, and the rate of progress and severity vary considerably. In some cases, the disease becomes relentlessly progressive in the later stages, often leading to paraplegia due to extensive involvement of the spinal cord. Occasionally the presentation is acute and rapidly progressive, or there is slow chronic progression from the start. Clinical diagnosis may be difficult especially in the early stages (Table 11.11). The lifespan may be normal, but severely disabled patients are at risk from bronchopneumonia, urinary tract infections and bed sores.

TABLE 11.11 Diagnosis of multiple sclerosis

Clinical evidence of lesions disseminated in space and time
Magnetic resonance imaging or computed tomography scan showing multiple focal CNS lesions particularly in white matter
Visual evoked responses – electrophysiological evidence of slowed conduction
Oligoclonal bands of IgG in cerebrospinal fluid

Pathology

In multiple sclerosis foci of primary demyelination (plaques) are distributed widely throughout the CNS. These well-circumscribed firm, grey lesions vary greatly in number, size and location. They are commonly found in cerebral white matter, especially adjacent to the lateral ventricles, optic nerves and chiasm, brainstem, cerebellar white matter and spinal cord. The appearances of the plaques vary with their age.

In acute plaques, in which there is a substantial amount of active demyelination, there is selective destruction of myelin sheaths with sparing of axons. A prominent inflammatory cell infiltrate of lipid-laden macrophages containing myelin breakdown products, lymphocytes and plasma cells is seen. Magnetic resonance imaging studies suggest that localized breakdown of the blood–brain barrier is a very early, possibly initiating, event in the formation of a plaque. Chronic plaques, in which the demyelination occurred many years before are commonly seen at post-mortem examination (Figure 11.28). Histologically there is complete loss of myelin (Figure 11.29) with a reduction in the number of oligodendrocytes. Axons in the lesion, which are normal or only slightly reduced in density, therefore have no myelin sheaths. Astrocytes are increased in numbers and are hypertrophic. There is often a scanty infiltrate of T lymphocytes. Re-myelination can occur in multiple sclerosis and is recognized by areas of myelin staining intermediate in intensity between normal white matter and complete demyelination.

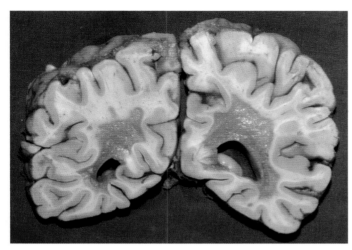

FIGURE 11.28 Multiple sclerosis. There are large grey plaques of demyelination in relation to the occipital horns of the ventricles.

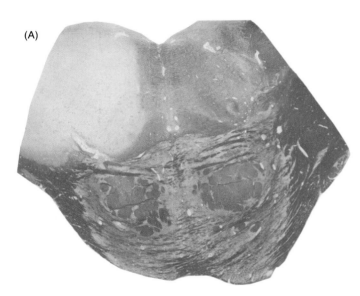

(A)

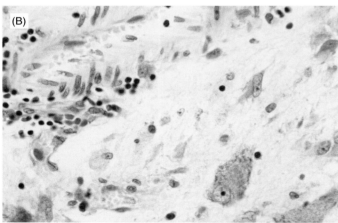

(B)

FIGURE 11.29 Multiple sclerosis. (A) There is a plaque of demyelination in one dorsolateral sector of the pons. (B) Within the area of demyelination there is preservation of neurons and variable cuffing of blood vessels by lymphocytes. (Luxol fast blue/cresyl violet.)

Electron microscopy demonstrates axons with characteristic abnormally thin myelin sheaths.

The pathological basis of clinical remission in multiple sclerosis is not known but may include re-myelination, resolution of oedema and restoration of conduction in demyelinated axons, for example by re-distribution of the membrane ion channels on which the action potential relies.

Aetiology

Familial aggregation of multiple sclerosis and twin studies which show a higher level of concordance among monozygotic than dizygotic twins suggest that genetic factors may be important. Multiple sclerosis is not inherited in a simple genetic fashion, but patients have over-representation of certain histocompatability antigens (A3, B7, DW2 and DR2) suggesting that genetic variation in control of the immune response may be important. The variation in the prevalence of multiple sclerosis with latitude is unexplained: there is a gradient in each hemisphere with high disease rates at high latitudes, for example in northeast Scotland (1 in 500 of the population) and virtual absence at the equator. Environmental factors, particularly in childhood, appear to be important. People who migrate from one area to another after the age of 15 years retain the incidence of their childhood locality. Before the second world war, multiple sclerosis was unknown in the isolated communities of the Faroe islands but with increased contact with the rest of the world has come a high prevalence of multiple sclerosis. While these studies suggest an infective aetiology, none of the numerous candidate organisms studied has been consistently implicated. Oligoclonal bands of IgG in CSF indicate that IgG is produced by plasma cells derived from a small number of B-lymphocyte clones. These observations may indicate a reaction to an infective agent or an autoimmune response to a neural component (e.g. myelin). Demyelinating antibodies have been detected in the serum of patients with multiple sclerosis, but these are not specific as they are found in patients with other disorders.

This evidence can be combined into a hypothesis: immune-mediated demyelination is triggered in genetically susceptible individuals by an infective organism acquired in childhood. Despite our ignorance about the pathogenesis of multiple sclerosis, drugs which target specific facets of the immune system (e.g. interferon β) appear to slow progression of disease in some cases.

Other Demyelinating Disorders

Acute Disseminated (Perivenous) Encephalomyelitis

This self-limiting disease of older children and young adults is an unusual sequel to various acute viral diseases such as mumps, measles, chicken pox or rubella (post-infectious encephalitis) and primary vaccination against smallpox and rabies (post-vaccinial encephalitis). Onset is rapid, occurring between 5 and 14 days after the start of the initial infection or immunization. Diffusely distributed throughout the brain and spinal cord are characteristic areas of perivenular demyelination associated with inflammatory oedema and infiltrated mainly by neutrophil polymorphs in the acute state and later by lymphocytes and macrophages. The disease is due to an autoimmune response directed against CNS antigen such as myelin basic protein.

Acute Haemorrhagic Leucoencephalitis

This uncommon disease has a rapid onset, a short clinical course and usually a fatal outcome. It may occur as a sequel to viral infections, septic shock, drug treatment and hypersensitivity reactions. At autopsy the brain is swollen and there are numerous petechial haemorrhages, particularly in the white matter. Microscopic examination shows focal necrosis of the walls of venules and arterioles, perivascular haemorrhages and perivascular demyelination, often with infiltration first by neutrophil polymorphs and later by lymphocytes and macrophages. The condition is thought to be a hyperacute variant of acute disseminated perivenous encephalomyelitis and to be caused by the deposition of immune complexes and the activation of complement.

Progressive multifocal leucoencephalopathy is described on p. 299.

Central Pontine Myelinolysis

This is characterized by a symmetrical area of demyelination in the centre of the tegmentum of the pons. It occurs most often in middle-aged or elderly alcoholics and seems to be associated with rapid therapeutic correction of hyponatraemia.

METABOLIC DISORDERS

Primary Metabolic Disorders

This group of disorders usually develop in early life; although uncommon, they make a considerable contribution to morbidity and mortality in children. They may present with neurological symptoms alone or with other systemic abnormalities. Different diseases may share a common phenotype such as a cherry-red spot of the macula. Many are inherited as autosomal recessive diseases and a few show X-linked recessive inheritance. In most a critical enzyme system is absent or inactive. Many of these disorders are due to deficiencies of particular lysosomal enzymes which play an essential role in the degradation of normal metabolites or cell-breakdown products, for example lipids, carbohydrates, mucopolysaccharides (Figure 11.30), amino acids. As a result the undegraded material accumulates in and enlarges the lysosomes of certain cells, the distribution depending on the particular enzyme deficiency. Some disorders affect neurons which become enlarged with a ballooned appearance (neuronal storage disorders); others affect white matter (leucodystrophies). Diagnosis by assay of the relevant lysosomal enzymes in blood, urine, leucocytes or cultured fibroblasts is now often possible. The lipid storage disorders (sphingolipidoses) are probably

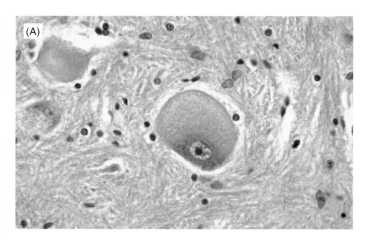

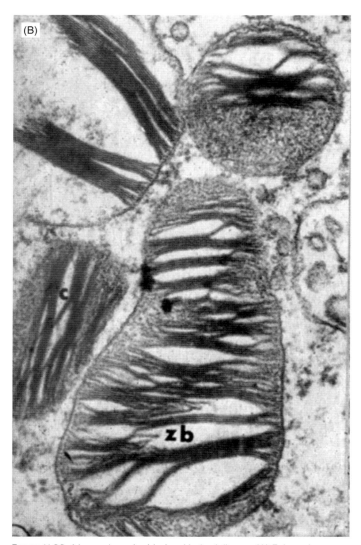

FIGURE 11.30 Mucopolysaccharidosis – Hurlers' disease. (A) Enlarged neurons due to accumulation of periodic acid-Schiff (PAS)-positive cytoplasmic material that has displaced the nucleus. (B) Membrane-bound collections of lipid lamellae. zb = zebra bodies. (Electron microscopy.) (Reproduced from Graham DI, Nicoll JAR, Bone I. *Adams & Graham's Introduction to Neuropathology*, 3rd edn. London: Hodder Arnold, 2006.)

the most important group. The sphingolipids include gangliosides, cerebrosides, sulphatides and sphingomyelins. One of the commonest storage disorders affecting especially the neurons is Tay–Sachs disease, the classic infantile type of amaurotic family idiocy.

The leucodystrophies, a complex group of uncommon disorders, have in common diffuse symmetrical demyelination and astrocytosis of the white matter of the cerebral hemispheres, and sometimes also of the cerebellum, the brainstem and the spinal cord. Most types are genetically determined and occur in childhood. They are therefore regarded as dysmyelinating diseases in the belief that the myelin is biochemically abnormal before it degenerates, in contrast to the primary demyelinating disorders in which myelination is thought to be normal prior to the onset of the demyelination.

Other Inborn Errors of Metabolism

Neonatal hypothyroidism, phenylketonuria and galactosaemia are the most important of these because they can be detected by screening tests in infants, and brain damage can be prevented or reduced either by replacement therapy or by exclusion of the precursor substances from the diet.

Hepatolenticular Degeneration

Hepatolenticular degeneration (Wilson's disease) is an autosomal recessive disorder of copper metabolism in which cirrhosis of the liver is accompanied by brain changes, mainly in the putamen and caudate nucleus, which become soft, shrunken and ultimately cystic. Neuronal loss is accompanied by large astrocytes with strikingly vesicular swollen nuclei (Alzheimer type II astrocytes). A greenish-brown discoloration of the cornea near the limbus (known as the Kayser–Fleischer ring) is also due to the deposition of copper.

Secondary Metabolic Disorders

The metabolic complexity of the CNS makes it dependent on the functional integrity of other systems in the body. Therefore, it is not surprising that secondary metabolic effects on the CNS are an early manifestation of systemic disease. In many instances the clinical features are reversible and there are minimal morphological changes. It is only when the metabolic disorder has been profound and prolonged that structural changes occur.

These disorders include brain damage due to hypoxia after cardiac arrest, carbon monoxide poisoning and hypoglycaemia.

Hepatic Encephalopathy

Hepatic encephalopathy invariably accompanies severe liver failure. In massive hepatic necrosis acute hepatic encephalopathy is characterized by rapidly developing coma. In cirrhosis, particularly when there is portal systemic shunting of blood, chronic hepatic encephalopathy develops. Hepatic encephalopathy is due to an accumulation of neurotoxic substances in the blood which have an origin in the gastrointestinal tract and are normally metabolized from the portal vein by the liver.

Kernicterus

Kernicterus is a metabolic disorder in the perinatal period also known as bilirubin encephalopathy. Severe jaundice in infancy carries the risk of brain damage, particularly when the plasma level of unconjugated bilirubin exceeds $250\,\mu mol/L$. In premature infants functional immaturity of the liver is responsible, but in full-term infants haemolytic anaemia due to fetal–maternal Rh incompatibility or glucose 6-phosphate dehydrogenase (G6PD) deficiency are important causes.

DEFICIENCY DISORDERS AND INTOXICATIONS

Deficiencies of vitamins and protein are responsible for various neurological disorders. In 'developed' countries many cases of vitamin deficiency are due to alcohol misuse, less commonly to malabsorption from gastrointestinal tract disease and rarely to food fads. In contrast, the deficiency syndromes that are common in 'underdeveloped' countries are usually due to an inadequate food supply. Malnutrition may cause irreparable brain damage at critical periods of prenatal and postnatal development.

Deficiency Disorders

Vitamin B₁ (Thiamine) Deficiency

Vitamin B_1 deficiency, in addition to causing a peripheral neuropathy, sometimes presents as the Wernicke–Korsakoff syndrome (Wernicke's encephalopathy). The deficiency may be chronic as in alcoholism or prolonged malnutrition, or acute, for example as a complication of persistent vomiting. The clinical onset is acute or subacute: features include disturbances of consciousness, ophthalmoplegia, nystagmus and ataxia and, if untreated, terminal coma. The blood pyruvate level is raised. In acutely fatal cases there are petechial haemorrhages in the mamillary bodies, in the floor and walls of the third ventricle, the thalami, around the aqueduct in the midbrain, and in the floor of the fourth ventricle. Improvement following the administration of the vitamin B group may be dramatic, but a full recovery is unlikely if structures are already damaged before treatment is started. Such patients usually have a persistent psychosis of Korsakoff type.

Ethanol consumption during pregnancy can cause a variety of CNS abnormalities which range from macroscopic changes with mental impairment (fetal alcohol syndrome) to more subtle cognitive and behavioural disorders (fetal alcohol effects).

Vitamin B₁₂ (Cyanocobalamin) Deficiency

Vitamin B_{12} deficiency particularly affects haemopoietic tissue, epithelial surfaces and the nervous system, with structural abnormalities in the spinal cord and in the optic and peripheral nerves. In subacute combined degeneration

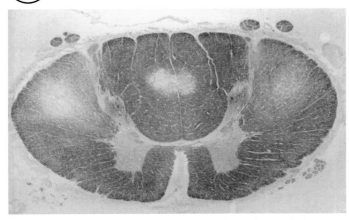

FIGURE 11.31 Subacute combined degeneration of the spinal cord. There is vacuolar degeneration in the posterior and lateral columns. (Luxol fast blue/cresyl violet.) (Reproduced from Graham DI, Nicoll JAR, Bone I. *Adams & Graham's Introduction to Neuropathology*, 3rd edn. London: Hodder Arnold, 2006.)

of the spinal cord there are degenerative changes in the lateral and posterior columns, particularly in the thoracic region (Figure 11.31).

Intoxications

Interest in the effect of toxins on the nervous system has been growing rapidly. Some disorders may occur after exposure to substances including alcohol/ethanol, therapeutic drugs, pest control products, industrial chemicals, chemical warfare agents, food additives, heavy metals and narcotics.

Key Points

Key neurological features of alcohol misuse:

- increased incidence of head injury
- withdrawal induced epilepsy (this is the most common cause of late onset epilepsy)
- cerebral atrophy, particularly of the frontal lobes
- delerium tremens; Wernicke's encephalopathy/Korsakoff psychosis
- partial atrophy of superior vermis of cerebellum
- peripheral neuropathy
- fetal alcohol syndrome
- muscle disease
- central pontine myelinolysis.

AGEING AND DEMENTIA

Ageing and the Brain

The mean adult brain weight is 1450 g for males and 1350 g for females, with a range of ±100 g about these means, in keeping with differences between the sexes in body mass. After about the age of 65 years the brain becomes smaller as a result of atrophy, losing up to 100 g in weight, and the cerebral hemispheres shrink away from the skull. Atrophy of the brain is shown by narrowed gyri and widened sulci, particularly at the frontal and temporal poles. The cerebral cortex is thinned, there is a reduction in the amount of white matter and compensatory enlargement of the ventricular system. Microscopic changes may include gliosis, a slight loss of neurons and a few senile plaques in the cerebral cortex. Mild cerebrovascular pathology is very common including arteriosclerosis in the basal ganglia and cerebral white matter and amyloid deposition in the walls of small cortical and meningeal blood vessels; these changes are not necessarily associated with any intellectual impairment.

Dementia

Dementia can be defined as an acquired and persistent generalized disturbance of higher mental functions in an otherwise alert person. Dementia is rare before the age of 60 years, but becomes increasingly common with age, affecting 5% of those over 65 years and 25% of those over 80 years. The commonest causes of dementia are Alzheimer's disease, cerebrovascular disease and Lewy body disease; there are many rarer causes. It is important to establish the underlying cause of the dementia as effective treatment is available for some of the disorders, and may be soon for others as our knowledge is rapidly increasing. Counselling is appropriate for those disorders with a genetic component, for example Huntington's disease. The causes of dementia are summarized in Table 11.12.

TABLE 11.12 Causes of dementia

Neurodegenerative disorders	
Common	Alzheimer's disease
	Dementia with Lewy bodies
Rare	Huntington's disease
	Pick's disease
	Creutzfeldt–Jakob disease
	Dementia of frontal type
	Progressive supranuclear palsy
Cerebrovascular disease	Multi-infarct dementia
	Arteriosclerotic dementia
	Global hypoxia/hypoperfusion
	Vasculitis
Infections	HIV/AIDS
	Neurosyphilis
	Herpes simplex encephalitis
	Subacute sclerosing panencephalitis
	Progressive multifocal leucoencephalopathy
Trauma	Traumatic brain damage
	Dementia pugilistica (boxers)
	Chronic subdural haematoma
Metabolic, toxic and nutritional deficiency	Chronic alcoholism
	Hepatic failure
	Renal failure

(*Continued*)

TABLE 11.12 (*Continued*)

	Hypothyroidism
	Vitamin deficiencies: thiamine (Wernicke–Korsakoff syndrome)
Myelin disorders	Multiple sclerosis
	Leucodystrophy
Neoplasia	Primary or secondary tumours (especially frontal lobe)
	Paraneoplastic syndromes
Miscellaneous	Hydrocephalus

Alzheimer's Disease

> **Key Points**
>
> - This is a progressive condition, fatal within 5–10 years.
> - It is usually sporadic, rarely there is autosomal dominant inheritance.
> - Apolipoprotein E (*ApoE*) ε4 allele is a genetic risk factor.
> - There is cerebral atrophy.
> - Histological features include plaques, neurofibrillary tangles, loss of neurons and synapses.

Alzheimer's disease accounts for about 70% of cases of dementia and is the fourth commonest cause of death in developed countries after heart disease, cancer and stroke. There are approximately 4 million with the disease in the USA with an annual cost of $100 billion; the figures for the UK are 600 000 patients and £5.5 billion annual cost. Most patients are cared for in the community within families or in nursing homes. This represents an enormous social and economic burden which will increase in the coming decades with the predicted increasing lifespan in most countries throughout the world. Some liken Alzheimer's disease to an acceleration of the normal ageing process, others consider it to be a separate entity. Presentation is frequently with memory impairment due to involvement of the temporal lobes. The course is invariably progressive and fatal, typically within 5–10 years. Most patients die from bronchopneumonia or inanition. In a very small proportion of cases (<1%), the disease is inherited in an autosomal dominant manner.

Pathology

At post mortem the brain is atrophied, sometimes weighing less than 1000 g. The atrophy is accentuated in the frontal and temporal lobes and there is compensatory enlargement of the ventricles (Figure 11.32). A definite diagnosis of Alzheimer's disease requires histological examination of the brain. The microscopic features found in the cerebral cortex are:

- Plaques: small focal deposits in the cerebral cortex of amyloid β-protein. Some plaques contain dystrophic neuronal processes (neuritic plaques) (Figure 11.33).

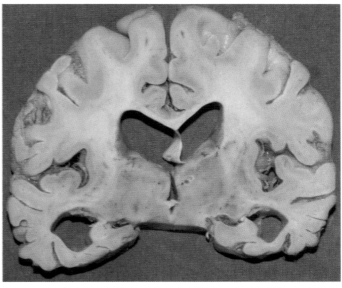

FIGURE 11.32 Alzheimer's disease. There is selective atrophy of the medial parts of each temporal lobe with associated compensatory hydrocephalus.

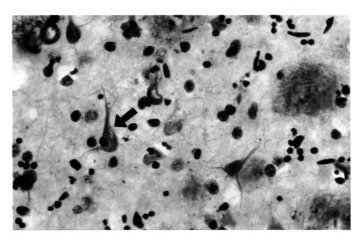

FIGURE 11.33 Alzheimer's disease. There is a typical senile plaque composed of filamentous and granular material. A neurofibrillary tangle is seen in a neuron (arrow). (Kings amyloid stain.)

- Neurofibrillary tangles: abnormal aggregates of cytoskeletal filaments within a neuron (termed paired helical filaments and largely composed of *tau* protein) (Figure 11.33).
- Amyloid angiopathy: accumulation of amyloid β-protein in the walls of cerebral and meningeal blood vessels.
- Loss of neurons.
- Loss of synapses.

Aetiology

The pathogenesis of Alzheimer's disease is still unclear although there has been intense focus on the deposition of amyloid β-protein in the cortex as a putative initiating event. A small number of familial cases have a point mutation in the amyloid precursor protein (*APP*) gene (located on chromosome 21), from which amyloid β-protein is derived.

Additional autosomal dominant disease-causing point mutations include presenilin 1 and 2. Individuals with Down syndrome, who have trisomy 21 and therefore three copies of the *APP* gene, all develop Alzheimer's disease by the age of 40 years. Deposition of amyloid β-protein has been identified as one of the earliest features of Alzheimer pathology to appear in those with Down syndrome dying at an younger age. However, a causal role for extracellular deposition of this protein in the pathogenesis of AD has not yet been established with certainty, and there is also evidence for a mechanism involving disturbance of the neuronal cytoskeleton.

Neurochemical studies have shown impairment of the cholinergic system, with decreased choline acetyl transferase activity in the cerebral cortex. Although this is not the only neurotransmitter system affected, current attempts at therapy are aimed to reverse this deficit. There is also evidence that anti-inflammatory medication, manipulation of the sex hormones and peripheral immunization with the Aβ protein may influence the course of the disease.

Dementia with Lewy Bodies

This disorder is now known to account for 10–20% of all cases of dementia. Clinical distinction from other forms of dementia is challenging but characteristic features include fluctuating cognitive function, visual hallucinations and a Parkinsonian movement disorder. Indeed, there is a considerable overlap with Parkinson's disease. Macroscopically, there is atrophy of the cerebrum similar to that seen in Alzheimer's disease but, in addition, there is loss of pigmentation of the substantia nigra. Microscopically, in addition to depletion of pigmented neurons in the substantia nigra and Lewy bodies in residual neurons, as seen in Parkinson's disease, Lewy bodies are also present in the cerebral cortex. There is a poorly understood overlap with Alzheimer's disease as many of the patients also have plaques and tangles. α-Synuclein has recently been implicated and point mutations in the gene encoding this protein have been identified in familial cases of Parkinson's disease: the protein is a component of both cortical and brainstem Lewy bodies.

Vascular Dementia

The term vascular dementia implies that the cognitive dysfunction is due to cerebrovascular disease. Clinical clues to a vascular cause for dementia include abrupt onset and a stepwise deterioration, a fluctuating course, a history of stroke and imaging evidence of cerebrovascular pathology. There is increasing recognition that vascular pathology may contribute to the dementia associated with Alzheimer's disease and Lewy body dementia. Large regional cerebral infarcts are unlikely to present with dementia.

Multi-infarct Dementia

This is dementia associated with multiple small infarcts typically scattered widely throughout the cerebral hemispheres.

It is relatively common, accounting for 10–15% of all cases of dementia. Most patients are elderly and hypertensive. Widespread atheroma of the major cerebral arteries results in repeated cerebral infarction. Some studies have suggested that there is a critical volume of infarction (50–100 mL) which acts as a threshold above which the development of dementia is likely. Assessment of the distribution of the infarcts has not clearly demonstrated specific brain regions implicated in this disorder. However, it seems likely that cognitive function is associated with involvement of the limbic system and association cortex.

Other Causes of Dementia

Huntington's Disease

In this autosomal dominant disorder progressive dementia is accompanied by involuntary choreiform movements. Huntington's disease (HD) usually begins in the 40s or 50s and has an incidence of about 47 per 100 000 population. The cause of Huntington's disease is an increased number of trinucleotide repeats (CAG), which encode glutamine, in the *huntingtin* gene on chromosome 4. The normal gene contains 9–37 CAG repeats, whereas in patients with HD there may be in the region of 37–100. This knowledge allows prediction of susceptibility in as yet unaffected family members and antenatal testing. The mutation is unstable and the phenomenon of anticipation may occur: in succeeding generations the disease occurs with an earlier age of onset and with increasing severity as the number of CAG repeats increases. On examination of the brain the most striking feature is selective atrophy of the caudate nucleus (Figure 11.34). There may also be cortical atrophy. Histological examination reveals loss of small neurons and

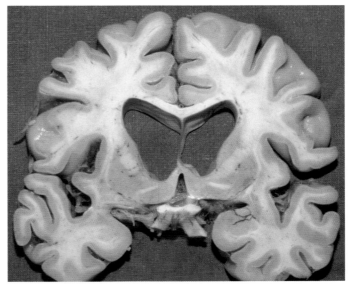

Figure 11.34 Huntington's disease. The basal ganglia are markedly atrophied with a flattened outline compared with age-matched control. The cerebral cortex is also atrophied and compensatory hydrocephalus is a feature.

gliosis in the caudate nuclei with variable involvement of other nuclei in the basal ganglia and the cerebral cortex. Several neurotransmitter systems are affected, but probably the most important is a reduction in γ-aminobutyric acid (GABA), together with enzymes associated with it such as glutamic acid decarboxylase.

AIDS Dementia

AIDS dementia is discussed on p. 299 and p. 518.

Pick's Disease

This is typically associated with severe and relatively selective atrophy of the frontal and/or temporal lobes and may be inherited as an autosomal dominant trait. Histologically, there may be spherical neuronal cytoplasmic inclusions (Pick bodies) and swollen neurons.

Creutzfeldt–Jakob Disease

Creutzfeldt–Jakob disease (CJD) is unusual in that it may be acquired by transmission, inherited as an autosomal dominant trait (about 10% of cases) or occur sporadically. Iatrogenic transmission has rarely occurred via contaminated neurosurgical instruments, cadaveric dural and corneal grafts and cadaveric pituitary extracts (used for growth hormone and gonadotrophin replacement). It can also be transmitted to experimental animals. The incubation period may vary from several years to decades. The incidence of CJD in most countries is about 1 case/million per year. It is characterized clinically by rapidly progressive dementia, myoclonus (repeated jerking movements of the limbs) and a typical appearance on electroencephalography (EEG). Macroscopically, the brain appears normal with little or no atrophy. At present the diagnosis can only be made with certainty by histological examination. The microscopic features are vacuolation of grey matter (spongiform encephalopathy) with neuronal loss and gliosis (Figure 11.35).

Creutzfeldt–Jakob disease is due to an unconventional transmissible agent which is very resistant to normal disinfecting procedures such as standard autoclaving. It appears to have no nucleic acid but to be composed only of protein, hence the term prion. The disease process is characterized by the conversion of a normal cellular protein (PrP^c)

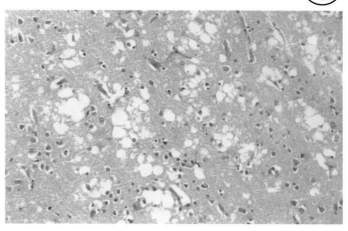

FIGURE 11.35 Creutzfeldt–Jakob disease. There is spongiform change in the cortex that is characterized by many vacuoles which become coalescent. Neuronal loss and astrocytosis are accompanying features.

into an abnormal isoform (PrP^{sc}) by a change in conformation. The PrP^{sc} which accumulates in affected tissue is derived from the host PrP gene and can be detected by immunohistochemistry. The relationship between transmissibility and genetic factors is not yet entirely clear. However, there are thought to be two ways in which PrP^{sc} can form. First, by a point mutation in the *PrP* gene – this occurs in the familial form of CJD. Secondly, the presence of PrP^{sc} induces the conversion of PrP^c into more PrP^{sc} – this occurs when the disorder is transmitted. Homozygosity at codon 129, which codes for either methionine or valine, of the host *PrP* gene appears to represent a genetic susceptibility factor.

New Variant CJD

This disorder described in the UK is thought to be caused by ingestion of products from cattle infected with bovine spongiform encephalopathy. Presentation is with psychiatric symptoms (anxiety and depression), cerebellar ataxia and dementia in patients under the age of 40 years. The clinical time course is more protracted than for classic CJD. Pathologically, there is abundant deposition of PrP with numerous 'florid plaques', composed of amyloid cores surrounded by vacuoles, in the cerebral cortex and cerebellum.

11.1 CASE HISTORY

VARIANT CREUTZFELDT–JAKOB DISEASE

A 16-year-old boy with learning difficulties was referred with a 4-week history of slurred speech, personality change and urinary incontinence. There was no known family history of adolescent-onset neurological disease. Detailed investigations ruled out obvious metabolic disease and spinocerebellar ataxia. He continued to deteriorate with declining behaviour, and became incontinent of urine and faeces, wheelchair bound and malnourished.

A year after disease onset he was admitted to a regional neurology service and re-investigated.

On examination he was mute, opened eyes spontaneously, had positive jaw jerk and snout reflex and spontaneous myoclonus. A clinical diagnosis of variant CJD (vCJD) was made. CSF showed an increase in the brain specific protein 14-3-3. Magnetic resonance imaging showed bilateral high signal change in the posterior thalamic nuclei or pulvinar region (Figure 11.36). The electroencephalogram (Figure 11.37) was non-specific with slow-wave changes.

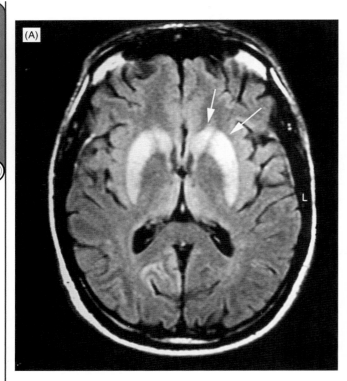

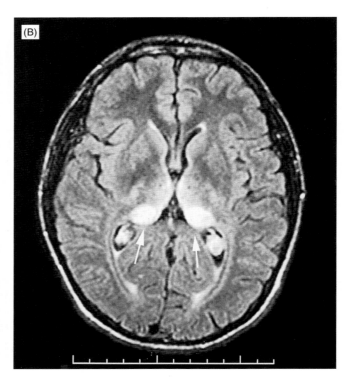

FIGURE 11.36 (A) Sporadic Creutzfeldt–Jakob disease (CJD). Axial fluid attenuated inversion recovery (FLAIR) magnetic resonance (MR) image at level of basal ganglia in a patient with pathologically confirmed sporadic CJD showing symmetrical hyperintensity of the caudate head and anterior putamen (arrows). (B) New variant CJD. Axial FLAIR MR image at the level of the basal ganglia in a patient with pathologically confirmed variant CJD demonstrating bilateral hyperintensity of the pulvinar nucleus of the thalamus (arrows). (Courtesy of Professor I Bone, Department of Neurology, Southern General Hospital, Glasgow and Professor J W Ironside, Department of Neuropathology, Western General Hospital, Edinburgh.)

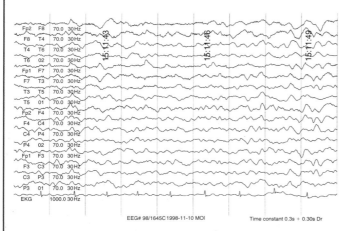

FIGURE 11.37 vCJD. Electroencephalogram. Non-specific slow wave activity. (Courtesy of Professor I Bone, Department of Neurology, Southern General Hospital, Glasgow and Professor J W Ironside, Department of Neuropathology, Western General Hospital, Edinburgh.)

Clinical Course

Initially, following initiation of percutaneous endoscopic gastrostomy (PEG) feeding, he was discharged home to his family. However escalating care needs eventually led to hospice admission. He died 18 months after the onset of his initial symptoms.

Neuropathological examination confirmed the diagnosis of vCJD showing spongiform change, florid plaques, neuronal loss and gliosis in the thalamus (most marked in the pulvinar) and extensive accumulation of abnormal prion protein (PrP) within the cerebral (Figure 11.38) and cerebellar cortex. Abnormal PrP was also present in lymphoid tissues throughout the body, including the tonsil, lymph nodes and spleen. Prion protein genotyping showed him to be methionine homozygous at codon 129, with no mutations detected.

Learning Points

- CSF examination is essentially normal though brain specific protein analysis can be a useful aid. Protein 14-3-3 is elevated in 50% of vCJD, being more sensitive in CJD.
- Increased MRI signal change in the pulvinar is highly supportive (sensitive) but not specific.
- EEG is generally non-specific. The triphasic complexes seen in CJD do not seem to occur in vCJD.

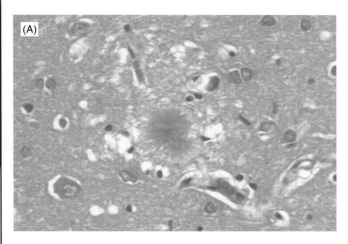

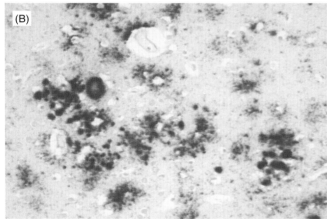

FIGURE 11.38 CJD. (A) A florid plaque in the cerebral cortex formed of amyloid fibres of PrP. (B) Extensive accumulation of PrP in cortex. (A: H&E; B Immunohistochemistry PrP.) (Courtesy of Professor I Bone, Department of Neurology, Southern General Hospital, Glasgow and Professor J W Ironside, Department of Neuropathology, Western General Hospital, Edinburgh.)

- Florid plaques are the neuropathological hallmark of vCJD and do not occur in other forms of CJD. Likewise, abnormal PrP is detectable in lymphoid tissues only in vCJD.
- All cases (to date) of vCJD are homozygous for methionine at codon 129. This is also true for 70% of sporadic CJD (only 30% of the general population show this genotype).

Further Reading

Green AJE, Thompson EJ, Stewart GE, *et al*. Raised concentrations of brain specific proteins in patients with sporadic and variant CJD. *J Neurol Neurosurg Psychiatry* 2000; **69**: 419.

Ironside JW, Head MW, Bell JE, *et al*. Laboratory diagnosis of variant Creutzfeldt–Jakob disease. *Histopathology* 2000; **37**: 1–9.

Zeidler M, Sellar RJ, Collie DA, *et al*. The pulvinar sign on magnetic resonance imaging in variant CJD. *Lancet* 2000; **355**: 1412–1418.

DISORDERS OF MOVEMENT

This diverse group of disorders is characterized by a progressive degeneration of neurons and their associated pathways within anatomically or functionally defined regions or systems. Patients may present therefore with the clinical features of dysfunction of the motor or sensory systems, cerebellar ataxia, involuntary movements, alone or in combination with other neurological abnormalities. Dementia may be a feature if neuronal degeneration is widespread. These disorders can occur in isolation or there may be overlap, both clinically and pathologically. The conditions described here are relatively discrete and well-defined examples of this group of disorders and are summarized in Table 11.13.

Parkinsonism

Parkinsonism refers to the clinical syndrome of disturbed motor function characterized by tremor, rigidity and slowing of movement (bradykinesia). It is brought about by damage to, or malfunction of, the nigral system which may have many causes including drugs and toxins (e.g. phenothiazines, manganese), vascular disease, viral infections (e.g. encephalitis lethargica), trauma (e.g. dementia pugilistica) and multiple system atrophy (striatonigral degeneration). Most cases are idiopathic, known as Parkinson's disease. It occurs most often in elderly patients with a prevalence of about 1% over the age of 60 years.

The clinical syndrome is caused by selective and progressive destruction of the pigmented neurons in the substantia nigra, accompanied by deposition of granules of neuro-melanin pigment. Residual pigmented neurons contain large intracytoplasmic inclusions known as Lewy bodies (Figure 11.39B). In advanced cases, depigmentation of the substantia nigra is readily apparent macroscopically (Figure 11.39A). The neurons of the substantia nigra project to the corpus striatum (globus pallidus and putamen) where they release the neurotransmitter dopamine. Treatment with a dopamine precursor (L-dopa)

TABLE 11.13 Principal disorders of movement

Disorder	Location of neurodegeneration	Clinical features
Parkinson's disease	Substantia nigra	Parkinsonism: tremor, rigidity, bradykinesia
Motor neuron disease	Lower and/or upper motor neurons	Weakness, atrophy of muscles, fasciculation
Multiple system atrophy	Variable including: cerebellum and connections, autonomic neurons of spinal cord, striatonigral system	Cerebellar and autonomic dysfunction, Parkinsonism
Friedreich's ataxia	Posterior columns of the spinal cord and spinocerebellar tracts	Ataxia, dysarthria, sensory abnormalities

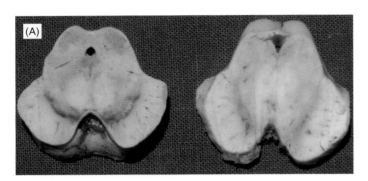

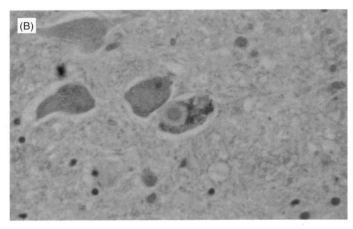

FIGURE 11.39 Parkinson's disease. (A) Compared with the normally pigmented substantia nigra on the left there is depigmentation of the substantia nigra on the right. (B) The Lewy body consists of a rounded eosinophilic inclusion which classically comprises a dense core surrounded by a pale halo.

may relieve the symptoms of the disease but does not slow the progress of the underlying neuronal degeneration. Most cases of Parkinson's disease occur sporadically but, rarely, it is inherited as an autosomal dominant trait with mutations in the *park 1* gene on chromosome 4 encoding α-synuclein, a component of Lewy bodies. There is a poorly understood overlap with dementia with Lewy bodies.

Motor Neuron Disease

In this disorder there is a relentless and progressive degeneration of motor neurons. It tends to occur in middle and late adult life and is more common in males and is usually fatal in 4–5 years from respiratory failure. Motor neuron disease occurs worldwide and accounts for approximately 1 per 1000 deaths. It is usually sporadic and the aetiology is unknown. However, some pedigrees have been identified in which motor neuron disease is inherited as an autosomal dominant trait due to mutations in the gene encoding superoxide dismutase, a free radical scavenger on chromosome 21. Three variants of motor neuron disease are recognized according to the distribution of the disease process:

- *Progressive muscular atrophy:* selective involvement of the lower motor neurons of the spinal cord (anterior horn cells) results in weakness, fasciculation and atrophy affecting limb muscles.
- *Progressive bulbar palsy:* selective involvement of the cranial nerve motor nuclei in the brainstem which causes wasting and fasciculation affecting the tongue, dysarthria and dysphagia.
- *Amyotrophic lateral sclerosis:* upper motor neurons are affected leading to degeneration of the corticospinal tracts and a spastic paraparesis.

No sharply dividing line can be drawn between these variants and their names merely emphasize that in any one case the early stages of the disease may have a particular distribution. In the terminal stages there is often widespread involvement of motor neurons in the brainstem and spinal cord.

Pathologically, there is atrophy of the anterior horns with loss of motor neurons and astrocytosis, particularly in the cervical and lumbar segments of the spinal cord. There may be degeneration of the pyramidal tracts resulting from involvement of the primary motor cortex. The hypoglossal nuclei in the brainstem are usually conspicuously involved by neuronal depletion. Affected muscles show severe neurogenic atrophy.

DEVELOPMENTAL ABNORMALITIES

Serious developmental abnormalities affect between 2% and 3% of all infants at birth, and of these approximately a third are malformations of the CNS. In over half, the aetiology remains undetermined, but genetic factors, maternal infections such as rubella and cytomegalovirus, the fetal alcohol syndrome and exposure to pharmaceutical drugs, tobacco and possibly vitamin deficiencies are implicated. The teratogenic effects of an agent depend on its nature, the gestational stage at which it acts and the genetic background of the individual.

The clinically important disorders in which there are chromosomal abnormalities include trisomy 21, 18 and 13, Klinefelter's syndrome (XXY) and Turner's syndrome (XO). Down's syndrome (trisomy 21) has an incidence of 1.4 per 1000 live births. The incidence in babies born to women over the age of 40 is about 1% and increases with age. The brain is usually small and the characteristic feature in cases more than 30 years of age is the presence of a large number of Alzheimer neurofibrillary tangles and plaques.

Defects in the Neural Tube

These are among the most common congenital malformations. The incidence in the UK varies from 0.1% to 1% of live births: there is a familial tendency and the risk of recurrence after one affected child is about 5%. Defects of the neural tube may be diagnosed prenatally in 90% of cases by the presence of raised α-fetoprotein levels in blood and amniotic fluid and by ultrasonography. Defects arise from failure of closure of the neural tube and are induced by damage occurring during the fourth week of fetal development from a combination of genetic and environmental factors.

Anencephaly is more common in female infants than male. The head is retroflexed, the cranial vault is missing, and the base of the skull is flattened. The brain is represented by a small disorganized mass of glia, malformed brain and choroid plexus which sits on the base of the skull and is usually covered by a thin smooth membrane.

Spina Bifida

Spina bifida is a result of failure of fusion of the neural arches (Figure 11.40). The majority occur in the lumbosacral region.

Spina Bifida Cystica

Some 80–90% of cases have a myelomeningocoele in which the abnormal cord is exposed by a defect in skin, the vertebral arches and meninges: there are often associated abnormalities such as syringomyelia or diastematomyelia. In the remaining 10–20% of cases, the lesion is a meningocoele which involves only meninges, the vertebral arches and skin. The cord is virtually normal. Most patients who survive with myelomeningocoele are paraplegic with absence of sphincter control; many have learning disabilities. There is an increased risk of meningitis and urinary tract infections. Hydrocephalus occurs in cases with an associated Arnold–Chiari malformation.

Spina Bifida Occulta

This is said to occur in around 10% of normal adults as determined by the absence of one or more spinous processes within the lumbosacral region on radiology. The overlying skin may be abnormally pigmented or there may be a hairy patch or dermal sinus. It is normally asymptomatic but neurological disturbances may develop in adult life.

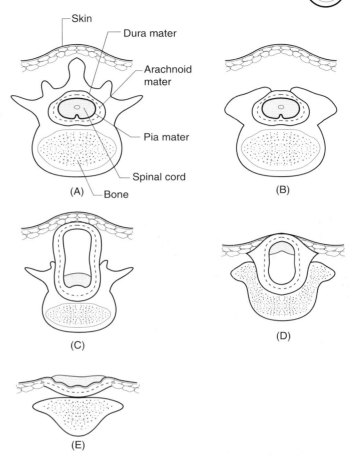

FIGURE 11.40 Defects of the neural tube: diagrammatic representation of spina bifida. (A) normal; (B) spina bifida occulta; (C) meningocoele; (D) myelomeningocoele; (E) myelocoele. (From Adams JH and Graham DI. *Introduction to Neuropathology*. London: Churchill Livingstone, 1988.)

Hydrocephalus

Hydrocephalus is commonly seen in severe abnormalities. The principal causes are spina bifida, Arnold–Chiari malformation, aqueduct stenosis, intrauterine infections and intrauterine CNS haemorrhage.

Chiari Malformations

Chiari malformations affect the cerebellum, the brainstem and the base of the skull. The commonest (Arnold–Chiari malformation) is second in frequency to anencephaly among severe CNS malformations. In it an abnormality of the hindbrain and cerebellum is associated with a lumbar myelomeningocoele and hydrocephalus.

Microcephaly

Microcephaly denotes a brain that weighs less than 1000 g in adults and more than two standard deviations below the mean normal weight for the age and sex of the patient.

Phacomatoses

This group of mainly familial disorders is characterized by malformations of the neuraxis together with multiple small tumours which involve neuroectodermal structures. The skin, the eyes and some internal organs such as the kidneys are also commonly involved.

Neurofibromatosis

Type 1 (von Recklinghausen's disease) is a relatively common (1 in 3000) autosomal dominant disease characterized by cutaneous *café-au-lait* pigmentation and neurofibromas. In the central form of the disease (type 2) tumours are common, the most characteristic being bilateral schwannomas of the VIII cranial nerve, and tumours of spinal nerve roots.

Tuberous Sclerosis (Bourneville's Disease)

This is a Mendelian dominant condition that occurs in 1/100 000. It is characterized by seizures, learning difficulties and various skin manifestations. Rhabdomyomas of the heart occur in a third of cases. The brain may be small, normal or of increased size, the most characteristic feature being the presence of pale, firm tubers in the cerebral cortex.

THE SPINAL CORD

The spinal cord extends from the base of the skull where it is continuous with the medulla to the first lumbar vertebra below which it becomes the filum terminale. The major ascending tracts carry sensation to the cerebellum, thalamus and cerebral cortex.

The tissue of the spinal cord is similar to that of the brain, but the relative frequencies of various lesions are very different. Specific diseases of the spinal cord are described elsewhere, but so-called transverse lesions, various types of spinal injury and the consequent ascending and descending Wallerian degeneration within the cord, and vascular lesions will be dealt with here. Spinal cord disease tends to result in a combination of motor, sensory and autonomic dysfunction.

Applied Anatomy

The spinal cord in transverse section is shown in Figure 11.41. Descending fibres are motor, ascending fibres sensory. The descending fibres associated with higher control of sphincter function are in the lateral white matter of the cord just in front of the lateral corticospinal tracts. Ascending fibres associated with bladder function are in the more superficial part of the lateral white columns.

Transverse Lesions

These occur when partial or complete interruption of the cord is produced by local disease or trauma.

Causes of Slowly Progressive Effects

- Extrinsic tumours in the extradural space, e.g. metastatic carcinoma (Figure 11.42) or lymphoma, or in the subdural space, for example meningioma or Schwannoma.
- Intrinsic tumours, for example astrocytoma or ependymoma, are rarer causes.
- Tuberculosis is still a common cause in various parts of the world. It leads to angular curvature of the spine, 'cold' abscesses and granulomatous masses, any of which can cause pressure on the cord: this may be so severe that infarction of the cord may occur at this level.
- Lesions in the vertebral column, for example prolapsed intervertebral disc, cervical spondylosis, kyphoscoliosis.

Causes of Acute Transverse Lesions

- Trauma, usually a fracture-dislocation of the vertebra.
- Infarction when the circulation of the anterior spinal artery is impaired.
- Haemorrhage usually from a vascular malformation.
- Transverse myelitis. This is a clinical rather than a pathological term and is used to describe an acute transverse

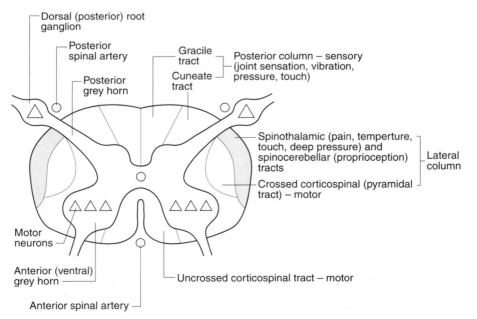

FIGURE 11.41 Normal spinal cord.

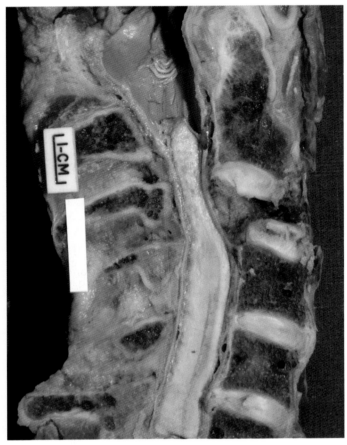

FIGURE 11.42 Compression of the spinal cord. Metastatic carcinoma in the vertebral bodies is compressing the spinal cord.

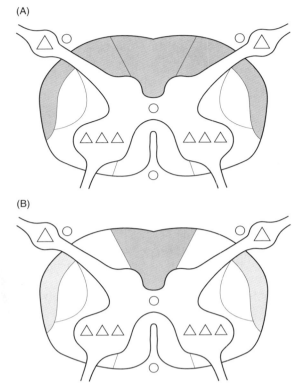

FIGURE 11.43 The spinal cord above a transverse lesion. (A) Immediately above there is degeneration of the posterior columns and the spinocerebellar and the spinothalamic tracts. (B) Well above there is preservation of the cuneate tracts and there is less severe degeneration of the spinothalamic and spinocerebellar tracts.

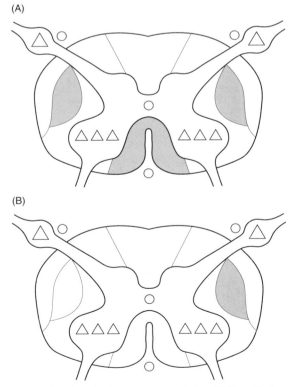

FIGURE 11.44 Spinal cord below a transverse lesion. (A) There is degeneration in the corticospinal tracts. (B) There is degeneration in one corticospinal tract due to an old infarct in the internal capsule.

lesion in the spinal cord in the absence of a compressive lesion. Causes include infarction, demyelination, caisson disease, infection or haemorrhage.

● Acute demyelination.

The inevitable consequence of a total or partial transverse lesion of the cord, besides the local damage, is the development of ascending (Figure 11.43) and descending (Figure 11.44) Wallerian degeneration in the interrupted tracts of the spinal cord. Degeneration occurs in those fibres that are separated from their cell bodies by the lesion.

Spinal Injury

Non-missile injuries result from subluxations and fracture/dislocations of the vertebral column, and are usually brought about by acute flexion or extension. Missile injuries are caused by bullets or by stab wounds. The clinical outcome depends on the severity of irreversible damage at the level of injury where there are varying degrees of haemorrhagic necrosis. The affected cord is soft, swollen and there is often a haematoma within the cord (traumatic haematomyelia) (Figure 11.45). This often extends above and below the level of injury. Eventually the dead tissue is removed and the cord becomes greatly narrowed. A delayed result of

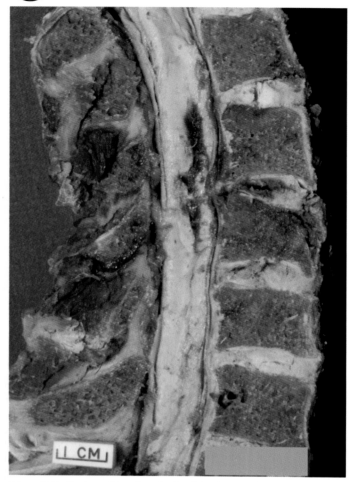

FIGURE 11.45 Fracture-dislocation of spine. Note haemorrhage into the intervertebral disc and associated spinal cord.

trauma, often after many years, is the development of post-traumatic syringomyelia.

Spina Bifida

See p. 311.

Syringomyelia

Syringomyelia is a cyst-like space (syrinx) that develops within the cervical cord (syringomyelia) or lower brainstem (syringobulbia). The cavity usually extends through several segments of the cervical cord and as it enlarges the cord becomes swollen and soft. Occasionally, syringomyelia occurs in association with tumours affecting the spinal cord. The effects are due to destruction of the cord by the enlarging cavity. The first fibres to be affected are the decussating sensory fibres conveying the sensations of heat and pain: the resulting defect, known as dissociated anaesthesia, is a selective insensitivity to heat and pain in the region corresponding to the involved segments of the spinal cord. A neuropathic arthritis affecting the joints of the upper limbs often occurs.

Prolapsed Intervertebral Disc

This is a common cause of compression of the nerve roots and more rarely causes compression of the cord. The intervertebral disc consists of a central nodule of semifluid matrix, the nucleus pulposus, surrounded by a ring of fibrous tissue and fibrocartilage, the annulus fibrosus. The posterior segment of the annulus is thinner and less firmly attached to bone and, following unusual stress, part of the matrix of the nucleus pulposus may herniate through it. This lesion, often termed 'slipped disc', usually tracks posterolaterally and compresses the nerve root in the intervertebral foramen (Figure 11.46). Disc protrusions almost always occur in the lumbar spine and L5/S1, L4/L5 and L3/L4 discs are affected in that order of frequency: they also occur occasionally in the cervical spine. A small protrusion may produce localized pain by irritation of the posterior longitudinal ligament, a larger one may give sciatica root pain due to pressure on nerves leaving the spinal column. The rarer central protrusions may compress the cauda equina, causing paraparesis and sphincter dysfunction.

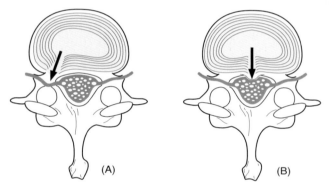

FIGURE 11.46 Prolapsed intervertebral disc. (A) Posterolateral protrusion compressing a nerve. (B) Central protrusion compressing the cauda equina. (From Adams JH and Graham DI. *Introduction to Neuropathology*. London: Churchill Livingstone, 1988.)

Cervical Spondylosis

Cervical spondylosis results from degeneration of intervertebral discs in the cervical region. The disc spaces are narrowed, osteophytes form and, in addition to compression of nerve roots, there may be interference with the blood supply to the spinal cord where the vertebral canal is narrowest. The importance of cervical spondylosis is uncertain as it can be demonstrated radiologically in some 50% of adults over the age of 50 and in some 75% over 65. It may be therefore that secondary ischaemic damage in the spinal cord – cervical myelopathy – occurs only in individuals with congenital narrowing of the vertebral canal.

Vascular Damage to the Spinal Cord

This is usually due to pathology in the anterior spinal artery. The blood supply to the ventral portion of the cord may be affected in neurosyphilis, collagen disorders, compression of the segmental artery by tumour, dissecting aneurysm of the aorta and surgery on the aorta.

TUMOURS OF THE NERVOUS SYSTEM

Key Points

- CNS tumours may be intrinsic (neuroepithelial) or extrinsic to the neuraxis, or metastatic.
- Metastatic tumours, in adults, are far commoner than primary tumours.
- Most patients present with headache, seizures or focal neurological deficits.
- Most intrinsic tumours are derived from glial cells ('gliomas').
- Gliomas are regarded as low or high grade rather than truly benign or malignant.
- The commonest primary brain tumour is glioblastoma – a rapidly growing high grade tumour.

Primary brain tumours are uncommon with an annual incidence of 5–10/100 000 of the population. Although rare in childhood, in this age group they are the second commonest form of neoplasm, exceeded only by leukaemia. Intracranial tumours behave as expanding intracranial lesions leading to raised ICP. The effective size of the tumour is frequently contributed to by oedema in the adjacent brain; this usually responds dramatically to corticosteroid therapy. Magnetic resonance imaging or CT allows the tumour to be located and biopsied to provide a histological diagnosis. Treatment options include surgery, radiotherapy and chemotherapy.

The aetiology of primary CNS tumours is largely unknown. Immunosuppression, whether due to AIDS, drug therapy (e.g. in patients with renal transplants) or leukaemia is associated with the development of lymphomas. Development of neoplasms is increasingly recognized to be associated with specific genetic alterations in the tumour cells: for example, *p53* mutations and *PDGFR* gene amplification in low-grade astrocytomas; *EGFR* gene amplification and loss of one copy of parts of chromosomes 10 and 19 in glioblastomas; loss of heterozygosity of 1p and 19q in oligodendrogliomas; chromosome 22 alterations in meningiomas. A number of genetic syndromes, although rare, have a well-documented association with CNS tumours (Table 11.14).

An abbreviated version of the current World Health Organization classification of tumours of the nervous system is given in Table 11.15. The classification is based mainly on the histological appearance of the tumour. Diagnosis is often

TABLE 11.14 Familial tumour syndromes

Genetic syndrome	Associated tumours
Neurofibromatosis type 1	Neurofibromas, gliomas, malignant peripheral nerve sheath tumours
Neurofibromatosis type 2	Schwannomas, meningiomas, gliomas
von Hippel–Lindau	Haemangioblastoma
Li–Fraumeni (*p53* germline mutations)	Gliomas
Tuberous sclerosis	Subependymal giant cell astrocytoma

TABLE 11.15 Simplified World Health Organization classification of tumours of the central nervous system

Astrocytic tumours	Astrocytoma
	Anaplastic astrocytoma
	Glioblastoma
	Pilocytic astrocytoma
	Pleomorphic xanthoastrocytoma
	Subendymal giant cell astrocytoma
Oligodendroglial tumours	Oligodendroglioma
	Anaplastic oligodendroglioma
Ependymal tumours	Ependymoma
	Anaplastic ependymoma
	Myxopapillary ependymoma
	Subependymoma
Mixed gliomas	
Choroid plexus tumours	Choroid plexus papilloma
	Choroid plexus carcinoma
Neuronal and mixed neuronal-glial tumours	Gangliocytoma
	Ganglioglioma
Primitive neuroectodermal tumours	Medulloblastoma
	Neuroblastoma
Tumours of cranial and spinal nerves	Schwannoma
	Neurofibroma
	Malignant peripheral nerve sheath tumour
Tumours of the meninges	Meningioma
	Anaplastic meningioma
	Haemangioblastoma
	Hemangiopericytoma
Haemopoietic neoplasms	Primary lymphoma
Germ cell tumours	Germinoma
	Embryonal carcinoma
	Yolk sac tumour (endodermal sinus tumour)
	Choriocarcinoma
	Teratoma
	Mixed germ cell tumours
Cysts and tumour-like lesions	Epidermoid cyst
	Dermoid cyst
	Colloid cyst of the third ventricle
Tumours of the sellar region	Pituitary adenoma
	Pituitary carcinoma
	Craniopharyngioma
Local extensions from regional tumours	Paraganglioma
	Chordoma
Metastatic tumours	Focal deposits
	Malignant meningitis

facilitated by immunocytochemistry. For example glial tumours express GFAP and neuronal tumours express specific neuronal antigens. Tumours may be conveniently categorised as intrinsic when arising in the substance of the brain or spinal cord, extrinsic when arising in adjacent structures and compressing the brain or spinal cord, and metastatic.

Intrinsic Tumours

Most primary brain tumours, known collectively as 'gliomas', are derived from glial cells, i.e. astrocytes, oligodendrocytes and ependymal cells. The corresponding tumours are astrocytoma, oligodendroglioma and ependymoma. Some are low grade and composed of well differentiated cells without mitotic figures. High-grade glial tumours are composed of poorly differentiated pleomorphic cells; features including mitoses, endothelial cell hyperplasia and tumour necrosis are likely to be present. As in other tissues, the general rule usually applies that the more primitive or undifferentiated the cells are, the more rapid is the tumour growth. The terms 'benign' and 'malignant' do not readily apply to glial tumours. No matter how well differentiated or benign a glioma appears, it almost invariably infiltrates into the adjacent brain, rendering complete surgical excision impossible and recurrence almost certain. On the other hand, no matter how rapidly growing and poorly differentiated the glioma appears, metastasis outside the CNS is very unlikely. Occasionally, glial tumour cells spread diffusely throughout the subarachnoid space (meningeal gliomatosis).

Astrocytoma

Astrocytoma is a low-grade tumour that occurs most frequently in the cerebrum of young adults. Computed tomography or MR scans show an ill-defined low density lesion without contrast enhancement. Macroscopically, the tumour may be difficult to distinguish from the surrounding brain. It is homogeneous, abnormally firm, may contain cysts and diffusely infiltrates surrounding brain structures. Histologically, the tumour is composed of cells resembling astrocytes. Mitoses, endothelial cell hyperplasia and necrosis are not present. The mean survival is 8 years, most eventually transforming to a high-grade tumour (anaplastic astrocytoma or glioblastoma). The rare pilocytic variant occurs in children and young adults typically in the cerebellum or optic nerves; unusually among gliomas it is very low grade and may be regarded as benign. Anaplastic astrocytoma has a peak incidence in the fifth decade. Mitotic figures are identified but there is no endothelial hyperplasia or necrosis. Mean survival is 2–3 years.

Glioblastoma

Glioblastoma is by far the commonest glial tumour and usually arises in patients over the age of 50 years. It may derive by evolution of an astrocytoma or arise *de novo* as a glioblastoma. Imaging typically shows a central low density area with a ring of surrounding enhancement. Macroscopically it is firm, white or yellow in colour with areas of haemorrhage

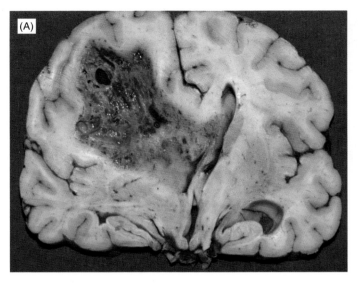

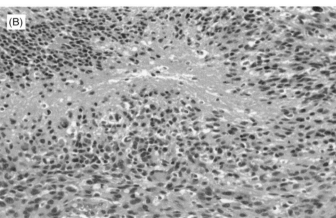

FIGURE 11.47 Glioblastoma. (A) There is a partly cystic necrotic tumour in the posterior frontal lobe that has remarkably well-defined margins. Associated brain swelling has produced internal herniation, ventricular asymmetry and a shift of the medial structures. (B) There are serpiginous foci of necrosis with surrounding nuclear pseudopalizading. The tumour is pleomorphic and multinucleate tumour giant cells, vascular endothelial cell hyperplasia and mitotic figures are present.

and necrosis; although it may appear well circumscribed, histologically there is infiltration of surrounding brain structures by tumour cells (Figure 11.47). Mitoses, endothelial cell hyperplasia and tumour necrosis are present. The prognosis is very poor with a mean survival of less than a year.

Oligodendroglioma

This is a slowly growing, relatively circumscribed and commonly calcified tumour. The cells are uniformly small and round, resembling normal oligodendroglial cells, with clear cytoplasm and distinct cell membranes. Anaplastic change is less common than in astrocytomas. In comparison with astrocytic tumours there is a poor correlation between the histological features and biological behaviour. Prolonged survival may occur.

GLIOBLASTOMA

Presentation

A 65-year-old woman presented with a history that in recent weeks her family complained her driving had become quite erratic and on occasions she had been unable to change lanes when driving on the motorway. More recently, she described a 'heavy feeling in her head' when waking up in the morning, which would clear up after a few hours. This 'headache' had become more intense in the past few days, and she had vomited on one occasion. She had a history of previous surgery for breast carcinoma some 15 years earlier. On examination, she was found to have bilateral papilloedema, a homonymous left hemianopia and slightly increased tone on the left side. There was also a degree of left-sided inattention.

Investigations

A CT scan was done and this showed a large space-occupying lesion in the right hemisphere, extending from the temporal into the parietal lobe (Figure 11.48A, B). There was significant mass effect, with distortion and effacement of the ventricular system on that side and midline shift from right to left (Figure 11.48B). After the administration of contrast, there was irregular, inhomogeneous enhancement (black arrow), with areas of hypodensity within the lesion (white arrow), probably representing

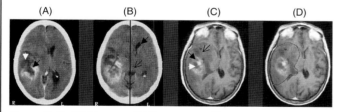

FIGURE 11.48 Glioblastoma. (A) Post-contrast CT scan, showing enhancement (black arrows), necrotic centre (white arrow) and mass effect. (B) Post-contrast CT scan, showing midline shift (black line is the midline of the cranial cavity, with the right frontal horn (black arrow) and the third ventricle (open arrow) on the left of the midline. (C) Post-contrast MRI scan, showing enhancement (black arrow), necrosis (white arrow) and swelling (open arrow). (D) Post-contrast MRI scan, showing probable extent of tumour cells. (Courtesy of Mr Papanastassiou, Department of Neurosurgery, Southern General Hospital, Glasgow.)

necrosis, and surrounding vasogenic oedema (Figure 11.48A). An MRI scan was also taken, partly in view of her previous history of breast carcinoma to exclude the presence of multiple lesions. The post-gadolinium enhanced T1 images demonstrate rather better the features of this tumour (Figure 11.48C, D). There were no other visible lesions.

Her family's comments about her driving are typical of somebody with peripheral hemianopic visual field loss, which initially goes unnoticed, until a traffic accident or near-miss occurs. Her headaches were indicative of raised ICP with their diffuse, 'heavy' nature and their early morning occurrence. This was confirmed by the presence of papilloedema on funduscopy. The scan appearances are those of an intra-axial malignant brain tumour, most likely primary (intrinsic), but in view of her previous history of breast carcinoma a secondary or metastatic lesion could not be totally excluded.

Management

The patient was started on high-dose steroids (dexamethasone 4 mg four times daily), which helped resolve her headaches within a couple of days. She then underwent craniotomy and tumour resection, as the most efficient way of reducing the tumour mass effect, as well as obtaining tissue for histological diagnosis. The tumour was confirmed as a primary brain tumour and classified as a glioblastoma, grade 4 (WHO classification). This is the most aggressive malignant brain tumour, with a reported median survival of 9–12 months, despite maximum therapy involving surgery, radiotherapy and often chemotherapy. She received post-operative external beam radiotherapy (60 Gray in 30 fractions) and remained well and active for the next 8 months, until she had signs of tumour recurrence. She received no other therapy and she died 10 months from diagnosis.

Despite the often clear delineation of the enhancing part of the tumour on imaging, glioblastoma is a diffuse tumour with malignant cells spreading out from the main tumour mass, usually along white matter pathways. Biopsy and post-mortem studies have shown that the extent of tumour cell spread will quite often include the area of surrounding oedema (open arrow in Figure 11.48C and outlined in Figure 11.48D) and on occasions even spread to the other hemisphere through the corpus callosum.

Ependymoma

Ependymoma occurs in relation to the ventricles, the central canal of the spinal cord or filum terminale, in keeping with its origin from ependymal cells. A common site is in the fourth ventricle in children. The tumour cells are characteristically orientated around small blood vessels to form perivascular pseudorosettes. A high-grade variant (anaplastic ependymoma) has a marked tendency to seed through the CSF pathways. Myxopapillary ependymoma arises at the lower end of the spinal cord from the filum terminale. It is a very slowly growing, gelatinous tumour that ensheathes the nerve roots of the cauda equina. The tumour consists of papillary structures comprising a central vascular core surrounded by mucoid connective tissue and covered by ependymal cells.

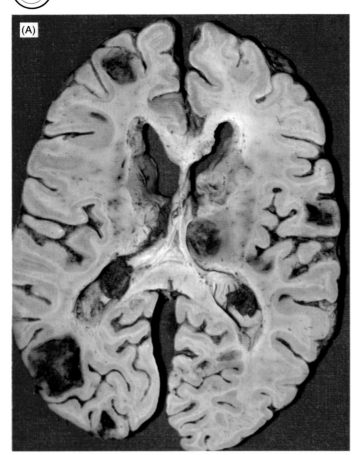

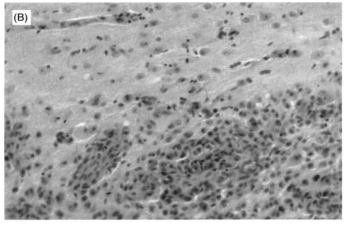

FIGURE 11.51 Metastatic tumour. (A) Horizontal slice of brain in which there are multiple metastases. (B) Interface between brain tissue and deposit of metastatic melanoma.

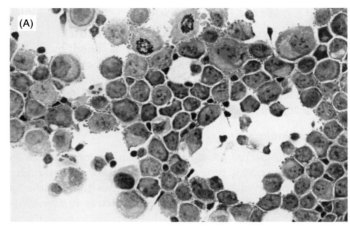

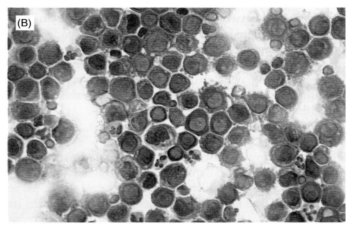

FIGURE 11.52 Malignant meningitis. (A) Cytospin preparation that shows many large malignant cells with nuclear pleomorphism and multiple nucleoli and a mitosis. (B) Cytospin preparation immunoreacts with epithelial marker confirming metastatic carcinoma (same case as A). (A: Leishman; B: immunohistochemistry cytokeratin.)

Non-metastatic (Remote Paraneoplastic) Effects of Carcinoma

Various indirect neurological syndromes develop in about 3% of all patients with carcinoma, without a constant relationship between the course of the neurological disorders and that of the carcinoma (Table 11.16). They may develop concurrently or the neurological disorder may antedate evidence of tumour. The commonest disorders are peripheral neuropathy,

the brain or spinal cord. Patients often present with cranial nerve palsies. Malignant cells may be identified in CSF (Figure 11.52). The neoplastic cells may be secondary (e.g. carcinoma, melanoma) or primary (e.g. medulloblastoma, ependymoma, glioblastoma).

TABLE 11.16 Commonest non-metastatic neurological effects of carcinoma

A peripheral neuropathy which may be predominantly motor or sensory, or of mixed type

A myasthenic syndrome, diffuse encephalomyelitis affecting particularly the medial parts of the temporal lobes – limbic encephalitis

Subacute cerebellar atrophy characterized by a severe loss of Purkinje cells and degeneration of the long motor and sensory tracts in the spinal cord a myasthenic syndrome (p. 371), encephalomyelitis and subacute atrophy of the cerebellum.

The pathogenesis of these syndromes is incompletely understood. A likely explanation is that of an antigen–antibody reaction following the discovery of specific circulating antibodies against neural tissue, anti-YO (paraneoplastic cerebellar degeneration) and anti-HU (paraneoplastic encephalomyelitis/sensory neuropathy) being the best characterized.

THE PERIPHERAL NERVOUS SYSTEM

Normal Structure and Function

The peripheral nervous system (PNS) comprises the paired cranial nerves, with the exception of the olfactory and the optic nerves, which join the CNS at different parts of the brain stem, the 31 pairs of spinal nerves and their endings, the fibres of the autonomic nervous system (sympathetic and parasympathetic) and the associated ganglia.

Most peripheral nerves are mixed, comprising somatic motor and sensory, visceral sensory and autonomic fibres. The nerve fibres are either myelinated (3–12 µm in diameter) or unmyelinated (average diameter of 1.5 µm). Fibre density alters with disease and decreases with age.

Histologically, a peripheral nerve consists of longitudinally orientated nerve fibres running in a fascicle. Each fibre is surrounded by collagenous tissue called the endoneurium, each fascicle by perineurium and all of the fascicles in a given nerve by the epineurium. Within the endoneurium the myelinated axons are supported by Schwann cells which manufacture and maintain the myelin sheaths between nodes of Ranvier. Unlike the oligodendrocyte of the CNS which supports the internodal myelin of many axons, the Schwann cell supports the internodal myelin of only one segment of an axon. The thickness of the myelin sheath is proportional to the diameter of the axon.

By electron micrography (EM) an axon of the PNS consists of a plasma membrane, the axolemma, and axoplasm which contains 25-nm microtubules and 10-nm neurofilaments, mitochondria and various types of vesicles and granules. There is continuous movement of the various components of the axon both away from (anterograde transport) and towards (retrograde transport) the neuronal cell body. The speed of transport varies between 4 and 400 mm/day.

Applied Anatomy and Nerve Conduction

Biopsy of a peripheral nerve is an invasive procedure and therefore is only undertaken after full consideration of the clinical history including information about family, occupation, drugs, systemic disease, the physical examination, electrophysiology and the results of any laboratory tests.

Nerve conduction studies consist of placing a bipolar stimulator to measure latency, amplitude and speed of the electrical impulse along a sensory or motor nerve. Slowing of conduction is indicative of a demyelinating disorder,

whereas the amplitude of the electrical response indicates the number of functioning axons in the nerve. Conduction studies can also be used to investigate nerve function of the brachial and lumbosacral plexus or nerve roots, and the neuromuscular junction in myasthenia gravis and the Eaton Lambert syndrome (see p. 371).

The sural nerve, which is purely sensory, is usually chosen: if a motor nerve is required then the musculocutaneous nerve and associated muscle are sampled. In the laboratory routine examination includes paraffin histology, resin-embedded semithin sections and EM. Morphometry and teasing after osmification may also be carried out.

Reactions to Injury and Disease

Peripheral nerves undergo three main types of degeneration: axonal (Wallerian), distal axonal and segmental demyelination. They are also capable of regeneration. Features of more than one of these changes may be seen in an individual case, although one type tends to predominate. Determining the nature of the change is important as recovery is quicker if Schwann cells can remyelinate a fibre rapidly, whereas recovery would be greatly delayed if Wallerian degeneration occurred.

Axonal (Wallerian) Degeneration

The changes are similar to those seen in the CNS (see p. 283). They may follow death of neuronal cell bodies in the spinal cord, or injury to nerve roots or peripheral nerves. Distal to the site of injury there is degeneration of the axon and its myelin sheath. The debris is removed by macrophages and Schwann cells proliferate to form new myelin if axonal regeneration (i.e. sprouting) has occurred. If the continuity of the endoneurial tubes is preserved then the chance of recovery is greater. Axons regenerate at the rate of about 2 mm/day. However, many sprouts may not reach the distal stump, and will proliferate in the dense tissue scar to form a painful swelling called an amputation or traumatic neuroma. Proximal to the lesion the neuronal cell body may undergo central chromatolysis a feature that is now recognized as a metabolic response to the attempt at regeneration.

Distal Axonal Degeneration

In the 'dying back' of distal neuropathies, which present typically with sensory loss in a 'glove and stocking' distribution, degeneration of axons occurs first, the process then extending backwards towards the neuronal cell body; this in turn results in secondary loss of myelin.

Segmental Demyelination

This occurs when there is damage to Schwann cells and the myelin sheath of a previously healthy myelinated nerve. The result is an axon that shows patchy loss of internodal myelin. With recovery the damaged internodal myelin is usually replaced by the myelin from several adjacent Schwann cells, leading to a decrease in the internodal length. In a segment with repeated demyelination and attempts at healing, there is hyperplasia of Schwann cells with concentric wrapping of their cell processes and the formation of 'onion bulbs' along the nerve fibres. This type of change is typically seen in the chronic neuropathies.

Clinical Presentation and Classification of Peripheral Neuropathies

Patients may present with sensory, motor or mixed features depending on the cause, the diameter of the affected fibres, and whether the fibres were myelinated or not. In general there are two broad categories of neuropathy *viz.* the polyneuropathies, which may be acute or chronic in onset and manifest as widespread symmetrical involvement, and the plexus syndromes and mononeuropathies.

Classification may be by (i) speed of onset (acute, subacute or chronic); (ii) functional disturbance (motor, sensory, autonomic or mixed); (iii) distribution (proximal, distal, symmetrical or asymmetrical); (iv) pathological process (axonal degeneration, 'dying back' or segmental demyelination); or (v) causation (infections, metabolic, inflammation, vascular, carcinomatous, etc.) – see Table 11.17. Disease of a single peripheral nerve is termed a mononeuropathy.

TABLE 11.17 **Principal features of the neuropathies**

Onset	Cause	Clinical	Pathology
Acute (days–weeks)	Inflammatory		
	post infectious (Guillain-Barré)	Motor, distal, autonomic	Demyelination
	vasculitis	multiple mononeuropathy	Axonal
	Infections		
	herpes zoster	Dermatomal	Axonal
	herpes simplex	Oral/genital	Axonal
	HIV	Variable	Variable
	diphtheria	Mixed cranial nerve	Demyelination
	Metabolic		
	porphyria	Motor, autonomic	Axonal
Subacute (weeks)	Drugs		
	isoniazid	Sensorimotor	Axonal
	vincristine	Sensorimotor, distal	Axonal
	cis-platinum		
	Environmental	Usually sensory	Axonal
	lead	Motor	
	solvents		
	acrylamide		
	Nutritional	Distal sensory	Axonal, demyelination
	alcohol abuse		
	vitamin B deficiency		
Chronic (months–years)	Infection		
	leprosy	Distal	Axonal
	HIV	Variable	Variable
	Malignancy		
	paraneoplastic	Sensory or sensorimotor	Axonal
	Connective tissue	Often multiple	
	disorders	mononeuropathy	Vascular
	Metabolic	Variable	Axonal
	diabetes mellitus		
	uraemia		
	Chronic inflammatory demyelinating polyneuropathy (CIDP)	Sensorimotor	Demyelination
	Hereditary motor and sensory neuropathy (HMSN)	Variable, distal	'Onion bulbs'

When many single nerves are damaged one after the other, this is referred to as mononeuritis multiplex. A knowledge of the anatomy and muscle innervation of the plexuses and peripheral nerves is essential to localize the site of the lesion and deduce its likely cause.

Polyneuropathies

Guillain-Barré syndrome

This is the most common cause of acute onset neuromuscular paralysis starting within 1–2 weeks of a febrile illness; there is also an association with immunization, surgery and malignancy. It has an incidence of about 2 per 100 000 and presents with rapid onset of numbness, paraesthesiae and an ascending paralysis. There may be involvement of the IIIrd cranial nerve and autonomic involvement may present as sphincter disturbance and cardiac arrhythmia. CSF changes are typical with a high protein in absence of or few lymphocytes.

There is a severe inflammatory polyneuropathy with a morality of 5–10%; ventilation is required in up to 20% of cases. Most cases recover over many months/years: however, a few develop a chronic relapsing/remitting disease with 'onion bulb' thickening of peripheral nerves.

The principal pathology is segmental demyelination secondary to a T-cell mediated immune response. There is a strong relationship with *Campylobacter jejuni* (about 25% of UK-based cases), mycoplasma pneumoniae and HIV, all of which have ganglioside-like epitopes as the postulated mechanism initiating the autoimmune response.

Diabetes Mellitus

This is the most common metabolic cause of a neuropathy that may present as a symmetrical predominantly sensory polyneuropathy occurring in some 10–30% of all diabetics, with autonomic neuropathy, proximal painful motor neuropathy or cranial mononeuropathy affecting principally the IIIrd, IVth and VIth nerves. All types and sizes of nerve may be affected. The sensory and autonomic neuropathies are due to axonal and segmental demyelinative changes, where as the motor and cranial neuropathies are probably vascular in origin as many of the perineurial and endoneurial capillaries are narrowed by thickened basal lamina.

Uraemia

Symptoms and signs parallel renal function tending to resolve as kidney function improves.

Paraneoplastic

This is one of the remote effects of malignancy on the nervous systems. Usually there is a sensory or mixed sensorimotor neuropathy in association with small cell carcinoma of the bronchus, but also with lymphoma. There may be anti-Hu antibodies in serum.

Paraproteinaemia

May occur in association with myeloma, lymphoma and Waldenstrom's macroglobinaemia. In about 10% of the late-onset chronic cases there is a specific IgM antibody to myelin-associated glycoprotein. There is both axonal loss and demyelination.

Toxins

There are many substances that may damage either the neuronal cell body or its myelinated axon. Principal among these are alcohol abuse and the associated nutritional and vitamin B deficiencies, recreational (e.g., heroin) and prescription drugs (e.g. isoniazid, vinca alkaloids, dapsone), and occupational exposure to chemicals such as lead, arsenic, solvents and acrylamide. Characteristically cases present with a 'drying back' neuropathy.

Infections

The two most common causes are herpes zoster and leprosy. In zoster the virus lies dormant in the dorsal root ganglia and if reactivated passes down the nerve to the associated sensory dermatome manifesting as shingles. In the tuberculoid form of leprosy there is destruction of peripheral nerves by granulomatous inflammation resulting in skin ulceration and loss of digits.

Hereditary Diseases

The hereditary motor sensory neuropathies (HMSN) are a heterogeneous group of disorders with a prevalence of about 1:2500 characterized clinically by distal wasting, the lower limbs having an 'inverted wine bottle' appearance. Principal among this group is HMSN 1 (Charcot-Marie-Tooth disease) which is an autosomal dominant disorder in about two-thirds of whom there is duplication of PMP-22 (17p11.2) which encodes a Schwann cell protein. Histologically, a characteristic feature of the pathology is demyelination with thickened 'onion bulbs' reflecting repeated remyelination.

Vascular Disease

Atheroma and arteriosclerosis are common causes of peripheral neuropathy. The result is ischaemia which may amount to infarction of nerve roots or peripheral nerve. Involvement of the lower limbs is common especially in diabetics. Multiple mononeuropathy due to vasculitis may also be a presenting feature of polyarteritis nodosa, SLE and rheumatoid arthritis.

Plexus Syndromes and Mononeurophathies

Patients with brachial plexus involvement may present with a thoracic outlet syndrome, brachial 'neuritis' or with a Pancoast tumour. Lumbosacral plexus syndromes usually result from surgical trauma after hysterectomy, lumbar sympathectomy from compression by an abdominal mass, infiltration by tumour or after radiotherapy.

Trauma with fractures, compression and entrapment are common causes of a mononeuropathy. There is also an association with certain systemic diseases that include diabetes mellitus, vasculitis, sarcoidosis and leprosy.

Commonly affected sites are nerve roots compressed in intervertebral foramina of the spine by intervertebral disc prolapse or osteophytes, the median nerve in the carpal tunnel at the wrist, the ulnar nerve in the flexor carpal tunnel at the elbow, and the common personeal nerve at the neck of the fibula. The nerve distal to the site of injury undergoes axonal (Wallerian) degeneration.

Disorders of the Neuromuscular Junction

These include myaesthenia gravis and the Eaton Lambert syndrome both of which are described elsewhere (see p. 371).

Nerve Sheath Tumours

Schwannomas and neurofibromas may develop anywhere is the peripheral nervous system including within the cranial cavity or spinal canal (see p. 319). Similar lesions are also seen in the skin.

THE EYE

The pathological changes that occur in the eye and in the orbit are in many respects identical to those described in other systems of the body. However, owing to the particular anatomical and functional properties of the eye, there are some important specific disease processes. The structure of the eye is shown in Figure 11.53.

Genetic Disease

Retinitis Pigmentosa

This is a group of inherited diseases in which there is progressive loss of photoreceptors from the peripheral retina to the macula resulting in tunnel vision. This is associated with secondary proliferation of the retinal pigment epithelium causing scattered pigmentation of the fundus. One of the autosomal dominant forms of the disease appears to be due to a mutation in the gene coding for rhodopsin, the rod photoreceptor pigment.

Ocular Inflammation

Inflammation of the Conjunctiva and Cornea

Conjunctivitis is commonly associated with allergies. However, there are several other causal agents including bacterial and viral infections, *Chlamydia trachomatis* and dry eyes (conjunctivitis sicca). Adenoviruses of various types cause hyperplasia of lymphoid tissue – follicular conjunctivitis. Adenovirus type 8 causes epidemic haemorrhagic conjunctivitis.

Both adults and neonates may develop conjunctivitis caused by C. *trachomatis* (types D–K). In neonates the infection may be severe and is contracted on passage through the

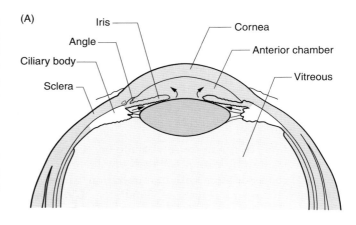

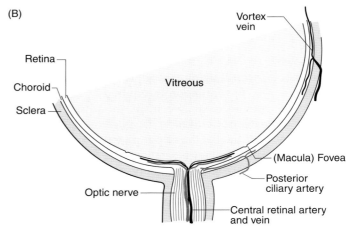

FIGURE 11.53 (A) Structures of the anterior segment of the eye, and the principal route of aqueous flow. (B) Structures of the posterior segment of the eye, and vascular supply to the choroid, retina and optic disc.

birth canal. On microscopy characteristic intracytoplasmic inclusions are seen in smears of conjunctival epithelium. Infection caused by C. *trachomatis* (types A–C) is the commonest cause of blindness in tropical zones due to conjunctival scarring, eyelid distortion and abrasion of the cornea by in-turned lashes.

Ulceration of the cornea is common and is usually viral or bacterial. The cornea is particularly involved in herpes simplex infection, the epithelium being destroyed in a fingerlike or dendritic pattern. Herpes simplex keratitis is often recurrent and the resulting corneal scarring may require corneal transplantation.

Intraocular Infections

Pyogenic Bacterial Infection

Traumatic penetration of the cornea or sclera leads to the introduction of bacteria usually staphylococci, streptococci or Gram-negative rods. Alternatively organisms may reach the eye via the bloodstream from a distant source of infection – *metastatic endophthalmitis*. Abscesses may form in any chamber of the eye.

Other Infections

Candida spp. are the most common fungal pathogen in the eye and are most frequently reported in immunosuppressed patients and in intravenous drug misusers where they cause metastatic endophthalmitis. Herpes simplex and cytomegalovirus attack the retina and lead to haemorrhagic necrotizing retinitis particularly in immunocompromised patients.

The protozoan parasite *Toxoplasma gondii* is acquired by eating poorly cooked meat or from soil contaminated by cat faeces. It causes a progressive, recurring retinochoroiditis particularly in congenitally infected individuals. Dogs are the natural host for the nematode worm *Toxocara canis*. Contamination of soil and grass by ova can result in accidental ingestion particularly in young children. The ocular manifestations include a unilateral granulomatous endophthalmitis.

Granulomatous Inflammation

Tuberculosis, syphilis and brucellosis are rare ocular infections that result in granulomatous inflammation usually located in the uveal tract (iris, ciliary body and choroid). The ocular manifestations of sarcoidosis include noncaseating granulomas in the iris, choroid, retina and optic nerve. Lens induced uveitis occurs when degenerate antigenic lens protein escapes through the lens capsule. Leakage of lens protein into the anterior chamber, either spontaneously or as a result of trauma, may induce a giant cell granulomatous reaction.

Sympathetic ophthalmitis, a bilateral granulomatous uveitis can occur after injury to one eye. The injury usually includes uveal incarceration within the sclera. Sympathetic ophthalmitis is considered an autoimmune disease, possibly induced by exposure of retinal antigens to the immune recognition system of the uveal tract. It can usually be prevented if the injured eye is enucleated within 3 weeks.

Rheumatoid Disease

The ocular complications of this connective tissue disease include corneal ulceration and spontaneous perforation (rheumatoid melt) and a necrotizing scleritis. Severe collagen destruction in the sclera may result in perforation (scleromalacia perforans).

Non-specific Non-granulomatous Uveitis

In many cases the cause of chronic uveitis is unknown, despite intense investigation. In early stages there is lymphocytic infiltration of the uveal tract. However, in most cases of uveitis the globe is enucleated during the chronic stage of the disease when the inflammatory process is complicated by loss of vision and pain. The end stage of any chronic inflammatory disease is a striking shrinkage of the eye with massive subretinal fibrosis and secondary ossification – phthisis bulbi (Figure 11.54).

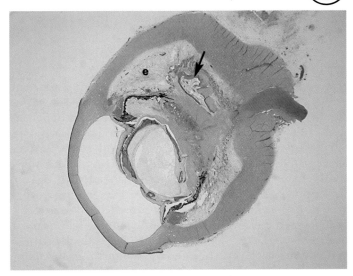

FIGURE 11.54 Shrinkage and disorganization of the eye following inflammation (phthisis bulbi). The retina is detached and entrapped within fibrous tissue. There is osseous metaplasia (arrow). Low pressure has resulted in an exudate (E) in the suprachoroidal space.

Vascular and Degenerative Diseases

Retinal Vascular Disease

Important changes occur when there is focal occlusive disease (diabetes, malignant hypertension) in the retinal arterioles: the subsequent ischaemia leads to exudation through damaged capillary endothelium. The clinical and pathological changes of retinal ischaemia include soft exudates, hard exudates, haemorrhage and neovascularization. A soft exudate or cotton-wool spot represents a microinfarction of the retina due to acute arterial occlusion and appears rapidly. Conversely, hard exudates take several years to form and appear as discrete pale yellow areas in the retina due to accumulation of plasma rich exudates leaking from capillaries in the outer plexiform layer of the retina. When small arterioles rupture, the blood tracks within the nerve fibre layer to produce flame-shaped haemorrhages. Blot or dot haemorrhages are seen when blood accumulates in the outer plexiform layer after rupture of capillaries. Haemorrhages are most prominent when venous outflow is partially impaired by thrombosis in the central retinal vein. Circular haemorrhages with white centres (Roth's spots) are classically seen in bacterial endocarditis.

One of the most important responses to focal retinal ischaemia is the release of vasoformative factors from surviving neural tissue: this causes proliferation of endothelial cells into the ischaemic area – neovascularization. Although this process is potentially beneficial, the delicate newly formed vessels tend to penetrate the vitreous where they stimulate the formation of membranes that cause retinal detachment and blindness. Vasoproliferative retinopathy is a common complication of the later stages of diabetes mellitus, so-called diabetic retinopathy; this can now be controlled by laser treatment.

Age-related Macular Degeneration

Age related macular degeneration is the most important cause of untreatable visual loss in the ageing Western population. The pathogenesis is poorly understood but recent studies have implicated local inflammation and activation of complement amongst the processes involved. In particular, a specific polymorphism (Y402H) in the gene encoding complement factor H is strongly associated with disease susceptibility. The disease results in atrophy of photoreceptors at the macula and is accompanied by degenerative changes in the retinal pigment epithelium (senile macular degeneration). This degeneration in the retinal pigment epithelium may be complicated by haemorrhage and fibrosis (senile disciform degeneration of the macula). The overlying photoreceptor tissue is destroyed with loss of central vision. Early senile disciform degeneration may now be treated by intraocular injection of vascular endothelial growth factor inhibitors.

Cataract

The biconvex lens substance is formed by cells that contain transparent crystalline lens proteins. A cataract is any opacity of the crystalline lens. The cells of the lens are enclosed in an elastic membrane, the lens capsule. Metabolism of the lens is maintained by diffusion of nutrients from the aqueous. Any change in the biochemical composition of the aqueous fluid as occurs in metabolic diseases, for example diabetes mellitus or hypocalcaemia, may result in formation of abnormal, opaque proteins in the damaged lens cells. Other insults such as uveitis, ionizing radiation or trauma may also result in opacities. Congenital cataracts may form if there is damage to the developing lens fibres *in utero*, for instance as a result of rubella infection. The most common form of cataract, however, is senile cataract, which is due to degradation of lens proteins in the oldest, central part of the lens. Most cases of cataract are treated by removal of the opaque lens matter by 'phacoemulsification' and the insertion of a plastic lens implant into the residue of the lens capsule behind the iris.

Glaucoma

Glaucoma is a generic name for a group of diseases in which the intraocular pressure increases to a level that impairs the vascular perfusion of the neural tissue and causes blindness. The most serious effects on visual function are due to ischaemic atrophy of the axons in the nerve fibres of the disc and secondary atrophy of the nerve fibre layer of the retina. Excavation or cupping of the disc may become so advanced that it extends into the optic nerve (Figure 11.55). The rise in pressure is due to obstruction to the outflow of aqueous, which can occur (i) as the result

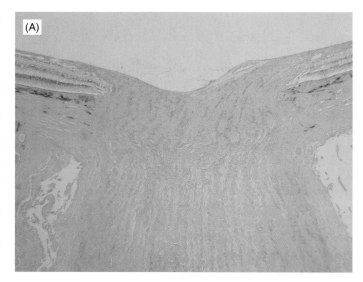

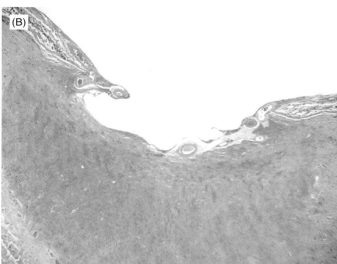

FIGURE 11.55 Optic nerve in glaucoma. (A) Normal optic disc for comparison. (B) Atrophic nerve head giving rise to 'cupping' seen in advanced glaucoma.

of closing of the chamber angle; (ii) as the result of an abnormality within the outflow system; or (iii) due to a developmental failure in modelling of the trabecular meshwork and the chamber angle.

Closed-angle Glaucoma

In the primary form the iridocorneal angle is narrow and the anterior chamber is shallow. In such individuals the iris and lens may come into contact when the iris is in mid-dilatation: this prevents the flow of aqueous through the pupil and pressure builds up behind the iris, which becomes further bowed anteriorly and causes further occlusion of the angle. This form of glaucoma is of acute onset, with ocular congestion, corneal oedema and severe pain. If untreated, blindness occurs due to pressure on the blood vessels in the optic disc.

Secondary closed-angle glaucoma has many causes, but the most common is due to fibrovascular adhesion between iris and cornea following ischaemic retinal disease and uveitis.

Open-angle Glaucoma

The primary type is an insidious disease of the elderly and the condition may go unnoticed in the early stages. It is presumed that the abnormally high intraocular pressure is due to an abnormal resistance in the outflow system. However, no cause for this has yet been established. In secondary open-angle glaucoma there is mechanical obstruction of the outflow system by inflammatory cells, tumour cells or particulate matter from a degenerative lens cortex.

Congenital Glaucoma

In infants and children, glaucoma can result from developmental abnormalities in which there is a failure in modelling of the trabecular meshwork and the chamber angle in the early stages of intrauterine life. Increasing intraocular pressure causes the malleable infant eye to expand uniformly, and it may become so large that it resembles an ox eye – buphthalmos.

Tumours

The tumours of the eyelid, conjunctiva and orbital tissues do not differ significantly in morphology and behaviour from those occurring elsewhere. Intraocular tumours are rare, but are important because of the serious effect on vision and their unusual patterns of behaviour. The most common intraocular tumours are malignant melanoma and metastases in adults, and retinoblastoma in children.

Malignant Melanoma

Malignant melanoma may occur in any part of the eye, but is most common in the choroid. The tumour adopts a collar-stud or nodular mass and may be pigmented or non-pigmented (Figure 11.56A). Microscopically the tumour cells are either spindle-shaped or round-epithelioid (Figure 11.56B). Growth within the eye can lead to retinal detachment, cataract, and secondary closed-angle glaucoma due to lens–pupil block or neovascularization. Extension outwith the eye usually takes place through intrascleral vascular and neural channels and the choroidal (vortex) veins.

The prognosis is best for small tumours (less than 7 mm in diameter) of spindle cell type which carry a 95% 5-year survival. Conversely, large tumours (greater than 15 mm in diameter) of epithelioid cell type have a 50% 5-year survival rate. Clinical course is not always predictable and this tumour is notorious for producing multiple, rapidly enlarging liver metastases as long as 20 years after enucleation of the affected eye (the big liver and glass-eye syndrome). More recently certain cytogenetic abnormalities, including monosomy 3, have been shown to be better predictors of metastatic disease than clinical or histological criteria.

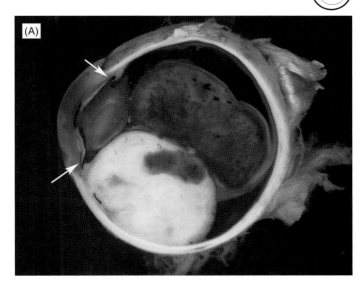

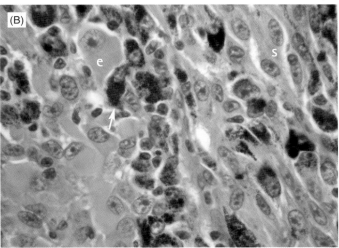

FIGURE 11.56 Malignant melanoma of the choroid. (A) This large tumour shows both pigmented and non-pigmented areas and has pushed the lens forward causing closure of the chamber angle (arrow) with secondary glaucoma. (B) Histology of this tumour shows large epithelioid cells (e) and spindle cells (s). Some of the cells contain brown melanin pigment (arrow).

Retinoblastoma

This is a malignant tumour of the retina, which occurs in infants and children: the incidence is approximately 1 in 23 000 live births. It affects both sexes equally and in 40% of cases other relatives are affected. The familial cases are inherited in an autosomal dominant manner although penetrance is variable. These familial cases are at an increased risk of a second malignancy, especially in bone or soft tissue. Spontaneous, non-familial tumours are usually unilateral and present at a later age.

The retinoblastoma gene occurs on the long arm of chromosome 13(13q14). It codes for the RB nucleoprotein, which normally suppresses cell division. In order for a tumour to develop, both copies of the retinoblastoma gene must be lost (the 'two-hit' hypothesis). In familial cases the first hit occurs

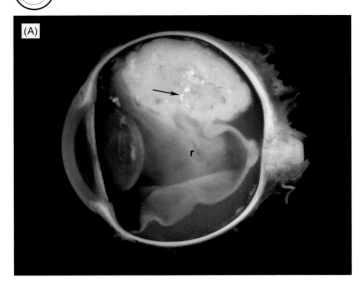

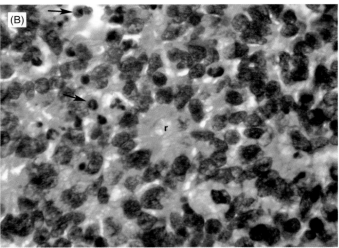

FIGURE 11.57 Retinoblastoma. (A) This large white tumour is in continuity with the retina (r). There is focal calcification within the tumour (arrow). (B) Histology of this tumour shows typical rosettes (r) as well as numerous apoptotic bodies (arrows).

through inheritance of a mutant allele and affects every cell in the body. The second hit occurs as a somatic mutation. In non-familial cases two acquired somatic mutations occur such that these tumours are usually unilateral and unifocal. Clinically the child may present with a squint due to poor vision in the affected eye. When the tumour is large and fills the vitreous or detaches the retina, a white mass is seen behind the lens giving a white pupil (leucocoria).

A retinoblastoma forms a solid white partially calcified and partially necrotic mass (Figure 11.57A). The tumour is composed of small, round cells with scanty cytoplasm and a high mitotic rate. Differentiation is seen as circular rosettes of tumour cells (Figure 11.57B). Extraocular extension occurs either by spread along the optic nerve into the brain or through the sclera into the orbit. Involvement of the choroid may result in metastases to visceral organs. With modern forms of management including surgery, systemic chemotherapy and radiotherapy cure rates in excess of 90% are the rule.

SUMMARY

- Cerebrovascular disease is the third most common cause of death.
- Disease of the CNS is a major cause of mortality and morbidity in childhood.
- 75% of patients who die in a neurosurgical intensive care unit, do so as a result of an expanding intracranial mass lesion.
- Head injury is the most common cause of death in patients under the age of 30 years.
- Infections of the CNS are not uncommon, and even in the context of AIDS and other diseases in which the immune system is impaired, they are treatable.
- Neurodegenerative diseases are usually progressive, associated with ageing, and characterized by abnormal accumulation of proteins that result in dysfunction and cell death. The causes of some rare familial types are known, but the great majority are considered to be due to an interaction between genetic susceptibility and environmental factors.
- Most cases of dementia result from neurodegenerative disease.
- Alzheimer's disease is the most common cause of dementia being responsible for about 70% of cases; dementia with Lewy bodies accounts for 15%.
- Several years after the peak of bovine spongiform encephalopathy, cases of vCJD were identified in the UK.
- Myelin is unique to the nervous system (CNS and PNS) and in health is required for normal salutatory conduction of action potentials. Multiple sclerosis (of the CNS) and neuropathy (of the PNS) are common forms of demyelination.
- Intrinsic tumours of the brain are uncommon; more common are metastatic tumours from the bronchus, breast and gastrointestinal tract.
- Corneal ulceration is usually caused by viruses or bacteria.
- Following injury to one eye, both eyes may be affected by sympathetic ophthalmitis.
- Intraocular vascular proliferation is a common complication of late-stage diabetes mellitus.
- Age-related macular degeneration is an important cause of untreatable blindness in the Western world.
- Primary open-angle glaucoma is a common cause of insidious visual loss in the elderly.
- Malignant melanoma is the commonest primary intraocular tumour in adults.
- Retinoblastoma is the commonest primary intraocular tumour in children.

FURTHER READING

Ellison D, Love S, Chimelli L, *et al. Neuropathology. A Reference Text of CNS Pathology*, 2nd edn. London: Mosby, 2004.

Graham DI, Bell JE, Ironside JW. *Color Atlas and Text of Neuropathology*. London: Mosby-Wolfe, 1995.

Graham DI, Lantos PL. *Greenfield's Neuropathology*, 7th edn. London: Arnold, 2002.

Graham DI, Nicoll JAR, Bone I. *Adams & Graham's Introduction to Neuropathology*, 3rd edn. London: Hodder Arnold, 2006.

Gray F, de Girolami U, Poirier J. *Escourolle and Poirier. Manual of Basic Neuropathology*, 4th edn. Philadelphia: Butterworth Heinemann, 2004.

Lee WR. *Ophthalmic Histopathology*. Berlin: Springer-Verlag, 2002.

Lindsay KW, Bone I, Callendar R. *Neurology and Neurosurgery Illustrated*, 4th edn. Edinburgh: Churchill Livingstone, 2004.

Spencer WH (ed). *Ophthalmic Pathology*, Vol 1–4. Philadelphia: WB Saunders, 1996.

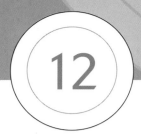

THE LOCOMOTOR SYSTEM

12

Robin Reid

INTRODUCTION

Disorders of the locomotor system are not among the most important diseases in terms of mortality, but they are of enormous social and economic significance in terms of their morbidity. For example, they are responsible for about 20% of general practitioner consultations. Osteoporosis, rheumatoid arthritis, osteoarthritis and backache are particularly important in this regard.

NORMAL BONE STRUCTURE AND FUNCTION

Bone has two main functions. It forms a rigid endoskeleton and has a central role in mineral homeostasis, principally of calcium and phosphate, and also of sodium and magnesium.

Bone is composed of cells, a protein matrix and mineral. There are two main cell types: bone-forming cells, principally osteoblasts, and bone-resorbing cells called osteoclasts (Figure 12.1D). Osteoblasts are derived from primitive bone marrow stromal cells known as osteoprogenitor cells under the influence of growth factors such as bone morphogenic proteins (BMPs). Osteoblasts lie in sheets on the surface of bone trabeculae and during active bone synthesis are large cells whose cytoplasm contains abundant rough endoplasmic reticulum and Golgi apparatus for protein synthesis and processing, and is rich in alkaline phosphatase for mineralization of the matrix. They express numerous receptors including those for oestrogen and androgens, vitamin D, parathyroid hormone (PTH), growth factors and cytokines. After completing a cycle of activity osteoblasts undergo apoptosis or mature into osteocytes, relatively inactive cells which lie in lacunae within bone. Long cytoplasmic processes run within canaliculi through bone and interconnect osteocytes and osteoblasts by intercellular junctions. Osteocytes may be sensitive to electric currents produced by deformation of crystals in bone (piezo-electricity), and so may be involved in control of bone remodelling in response to mechanical stress.

Osteoclasts are large multinucleated cells derived, under the influence of colony-stimulating factors and tumour necrosis factor, from haemopoietic stem cells of granulocyte-macrophage lineage. Stimulated by interleukins such as interleukin 1 (IL1) and IL6, they closely attach to bone at their periphery (sealing zone), and secrete acid, generated by carbonic anhydrase, and lysosomal enzymes including acid phosphatase and collagenase to remove mineral and matrix simultaneously. Measurement of urinary collagen degradation products such as deoxypyridinoline (DPD) and terminal peptide fragments from type I collagen provides an indication of osteoclastic activity. Their plasma membrane is thrown into folds forming a 'ruffled border' with abundant surface area adjacent to bone. Osteoclasts lie in the shallow depressions (Howship's lacunae) so formed on the surface of bone.

The protein matrix of bone consists largely of type I collagen, with small amounts of non-collagenous proteins produced mainly by osteoblasts. These include calcium-binding proteins such as osteonectin and bone sialoprotein, those involved in mineralization such as osteocalcin, whose synthesis is vitamin K dependent, and serum levels of which reflect osteoblastic activity. Cell adhesion proteins, including osteopontin and growth factors including transforming growth factor β (TGFβ) are also present.

Bone is initially laid down as a non-mineralized protein-rich form known as osteoid. Over the next 10 days or so, osteoid becomes mineralized to form bone. The mineral

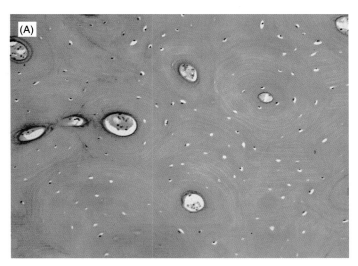

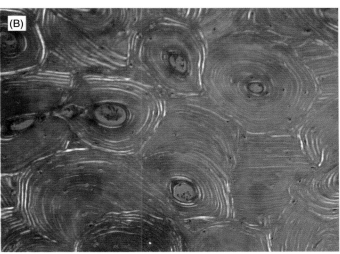

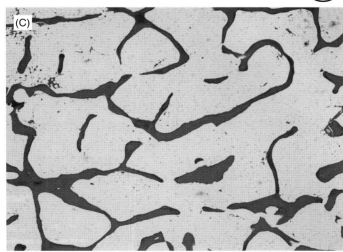

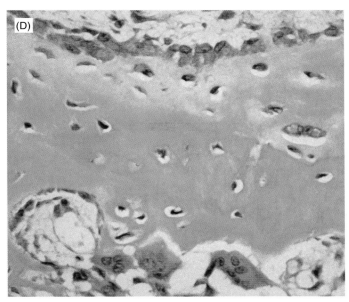

FIGURE 12.1 Normal bone structure and function. (A) Cortical bone is arranged in concentric cylindrical structures – Haversian systems – here seen in cross-section. (B) Polarization microscopy shows the lamellar structure well. (C) Bone within the medulla forms a meshwork of trabeculae, this is known as cancellous bone; this is also lamellar in type. (D) The cellular composition of bone shown in this photomicrograph is of rapidly formed woven bone with a random arrangement of the collagen fibres. A row (or sheet in three dimensions) of osteoblasts covers the upper surface of the bone: the perinuclear vacuoles are the prominent Golgi apparatus of protein synthesizing and exporting cells. Osteocytes are seen within their lacunae within the bone trabecula. Three active multinucleated osteoclasts lie within resorption cavities on the lower surface.

matrix accounts for two-thirds of bone mass; its main component is hydroxyapatite $(Ca_{10}(PO_4)_6(OH)_2)$. Substantial amounts of sodium, potassium, magnesium, carbonate and citrate are also present.

Types of Bone

Bone is found in two patterns, woven and lamellar (Fig. 12.1). Woven bone is formed where bone is laid down rapidly as in fetal growth, during healing of a fracture and in bone-forming tumours. It contains numerous plump osteocytes and collagen fibres are arranged randomly.

Lamellar bone is slowly laid down, is structurally strong and forms the adult skeleton. The collagen lies in parallel sheets whose fibres run in different directions, resulting in a laminated structure. The osteocytes are small and relatively sparse. Adult lamellar bone is arranged in two forms. Compact bone forms the cortex of bones. Between the subperiosteal and endosteal plates of circumferential bone, lie Haversian systems (osteons) (see Figure 12.1A), concentric arrays of bone surrounding a central artery and vein. Cancellous (spongy) bone, found between the cortices of bones and at the ends of long bones, is composed of plates or trabeculae separated by marrow spaces. Compact bone accounts for about 80% of the adult skeleton and cancellous bone about 20%.

Bone Turnover

Bone is constantly being formed and resorbed; approximately 10% of the adult skeleton is replaced annually. Bone remodelling is carried out by osteoclasts and osteoblasts coupled together by chemical mediators in bone modelling units (BMUs) so that adult bone mass is kept fairly constant. Imbalance of formation and resorption can cause disease: it may lead to a decreased bone mass, for example in osteoporosis (p. 333). Bone turnover is a complex process which is gradually becoming understood and is illustrated in Figure 12.2 and discussed in more detail in Special Study Topic 12.1.

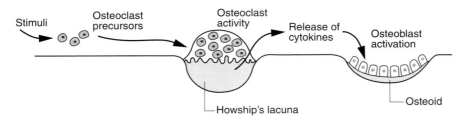

FIGURE 12.2 The cycle of bone turnover. Various agents promote bone resorption by stimulating osteoclast formation and maturation. As these cells resorb bone, cytokines are released which in turn promote osteoblastic activity, thus completing the cycle.

12.1 SPECIAL STUDY TOPIC

CONTROL OF BONE TURNOVER

In recent years considerable advances have been made in our understanding of the mechanisms which control bone turnover and in particular of the factors regulating osteoclast formation and bone destruction. This may lead to targeted therapies for the common metabolic bone dis-orders of osteoporosis and Paget's disease, and the bone destruction which is a feature of metastatic tumours in the skeleton.

Osteoclast Formation

As has been indicated earlier, osteoclasts are multinucleated cells derived from precursors of monocyte/macrophage lineage. These cells fuse to form non-functioning osteoclasts (Figure 12.3), which are then activated, resorb bone and eventually undergo apoptosis, thus stopping the phase of bone resorption. The cycle of bone turnover starts with activation of bone resorption.

Osteoclast formation is promoted by two main substances – macrophage colony-stimulating factor (M-CSF), derived from bone marrow stromal cells and osteoblasts, and a more recently identified factor known as RANK ligand (receptor activator of nuclear factor κB ligand) or as TRANCE (tumour necrosis factor related activation induced cytokine). This molecule is produced by and expressed on the surface of marrow stromal cells. RANK ligand acts through a cell surface receptor, RANK, on the surface of osteoclast precursors. It appears that most factors which stimulate osteoclast formation, for example vitamin D, PTH-related peptide (PTHrP) and interleukin 11 (IL11) do so by upregulating RANK ligand expression.

Unsurprisingly, as in any biological system, there is an antagonistic mechanism which in health ensures homeostasis. This inhibitory substance is known as osteoprotegerin

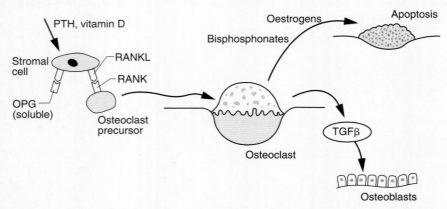

FIGURE 12.3 Osteoclast precursors (monocyte/macrophage lineage cells) are stimulated to become osteoclasts by receptor activator of nuclear factor κB ligand (RANKL). This molecule is upregulated on the surface of marrow stromal cells by vitamin D (Vit D), parathyroid hormone (PTH) and other factors. Overactivity of RANK L is normally prevented by the soluble protein osteoprotegerin (OPG). In the process of removing bone, osteoclasts produce cytokines such as transforming growth factor β (TGFβ) which both stimulate osteoblasts to produce new bone and inhibit osteoclasts. Unwanted osteoclasts undergo apoptosis under the influence of oestrogens and bisphosphonates.

(OPG) and is a soluble protein which competes with the cell-bound RANK ligand. OPG is a member of the TNF superfamily and is produced by a wide variety of cell types. Effectively, the ratio of RANK ligand to OPG at any site will determine the extent of bone resorption. As osteoclastic activity removes bone, in the process cytokines such as TGFβ are released which both inhibit osteoclasts and stimulate osteoblasts. Thus, when the phase of resorption ceases, osteoblasts start to synthesize newly formed uncalcified matrix (known as osteoid), which becomes mineralized approximately 7 days later. A very thin layer of osteoid covering up to 20% of the trabecular surface area is therefore a normal finding.

Much work has been carried out in animal models. Transgenic mice deficient in RANK ligand and those overexpressing OPG both develop osteopetrosis (p. 340); in contrast, animals lacking OPG develop osteopenia (osteoporosis).

Regulation of Bone Destruction in Malignant Disease

Bone destruction is a major problem in patients with metastatic carcinoma and those with myeloma. Although cancer cells can resorb bone directly in tissue culture, there is no doubt that *in vivo* bone destruction is primarily due to the action of osteoclasts. Thus anti-osteoclast therapies such as bisphosphonates are often effective. It appears that PTHrP is the most important of the many factors produced by tumour cells which can stimulate osteoclastic activity. Growth factors such

as TGFβ, fibroblast growth factor and insulin-like growth factors are released as the bone matrix is resorbed and these in turn promote further tumour growth. In this way a vicious cycle is established (Figure 12.4). Tumour necrosis factor β appears to be the major osteoclast-stimulating factor in multiple myeloma.

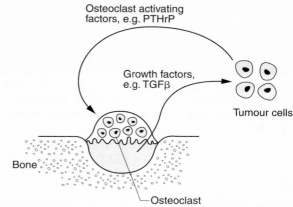

FIGURE 12.4 The vicious cycle of bone destruction. Osteoclasts produce growth factors that stimulate tumour cells in the marrow to grow and proliferate. More tumour cells produce more osteoclast activating factors and the vicious cycle is completed. TGFβ = transforming growth factor β; PTHrP = parathyroid hormone-related peptide.

Further Reading

Graham R, Russell G, Espina B, Hulley P. Bone biology and the pathogenesis of osteoporosis. *Curr Opin Rheumatol* 2006;18(Suppl 1):S3–S10.

DISEASES OF BONE

Metabolic Bone Disease

Metabolic bone diseases are a group of generalized skeletal disorders which result from abnormal formation, resorption or mineralization of bone.

Osteoporosis

> **Key Points**
>
> - Bone mass is reduced, but chemical composition remains normal.
> - Symptoms commonest in post-menopausal women, but may also occur in elderly men and in all age groups.
> - It may result in fractures of long bones and vertebral collapse (Figure 12.5).

Osteoporosis occurs when bone strength is reduced below the level required for its normal structural function. Bone

strength is determined by two factors: bone mass and bone quality. The term osteoporosis is usually applied to the common generalized disorder which predisposes to fractures, especially in the elderly. The localized form that occurs following immobilization is a form of disuse atrophy. In both forms of osteoporosis the bone, although reduced in amount, is of normal chemical composition and is fully mineralized.

The concept of osteoporosis has changed greatly in recent years. Traditionally, it had been viewed as a disorder of post-menopausal women with fractures. Now, it is regarded as a clinically silent disorder which affects all ages. Furthermore, it is now possible to detect presymptomatic osteoporosis and to prevent its progression. Generalized osteoporosis has two main subgroups:

- primary osteoporosis – which usually affects women after the menopause and men later in life
- secondary osteoporosis – when the reduced bone mass is caused by other diseases or drug effects.

TABLE 12.4 Major causes of osteomalacia and rickets

Vitamin D deficiency	
Dietary insufficiency	
Malabsorption	Coeliac disease, gastric and bowel surgery, biliary disease
Reduced skin synthesis	Low UV light exposure, skin pigmentation, low skin exposure
Abnormal vitamin D metabolism	
Increased degradation	Drugs, e.g. anticonvulsants
Diminished 25 hydroxylation	Chronic liver disease
Decreased 1α hydroxylation	Renal failure, type 1 vitamin D dependent rickets,
Normal vitamin D levels	
End organ resistance	Type 2 vitamin D dependent rickets
Low serum phosphate	Renal tubular disorders, e.g. Fanconi syndrome, x-linked hypophosphataemic rickets
Abnormal bone mineralization	
Low bone alkaline phosphatase	Hypophosphatasia
Chemicals, drugs	Aluminium toxicity

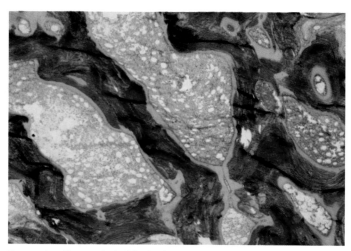

FIGURE 12.7 Osteomalacia. Histological examination of undecalcified sections shows that most of the bone (purple) surfaces are covered by a thick layer of unmineralized osteoid (pale blue), reflecting the delay in mineralization. (Toluidine blue.)

and leads to a thickened and irregular hypertrophic zone. The woven bone laid down on the surface of cartilage is also not mineralized and so there is failure to remodel the metaphysis. Treatment of the underlying cause (e.g. oral vitamin D in dietary deficiency) is rapidly followed by mineralization of matrix and the radiological appearances of the epiphyses revert to normal, but bone deformity may remain.

Hyperparathyroidism

Key Points

- Hyperparathyroidism may be primary, secondary or tertiary.
- There is increased bone resorption with osteoporosis and fractures.
- It has renal, muscular and gastrointestinal effects.

Parathyroid hormone is important in the regulation of calcium metabolism and bone turnover and has effects on both osteoblast and osteoclastic activity. Overactivity of the parathyroid glands is classified as primary, secondary or tertiary (p. 467). Primary hyperparathyroidism is usually due to the presence of a parathyroid adenoma but in less than 5% of cases there is diffuse hyperplasia of all four glands, especially in patients with multiple endocrine neoplasia (MEN I and IIA), or a parathyroid carcinoma. Primary hyperparathyroidism affects 1 in 1000 people and is the commonest cause of hypercalcaemia in asymptomatic individuals; early diagnosis due to routine measurement of serum calcium means that bone disease is now found in under 5% of cases. Secondary hyperparathyroidism is a physiological response of hyperplasia and increased PTH secretion to hypocalcaemia. The most common cause is chronic renal failure, the bone changes of which are discussed below. Tertiary hyperparathyroidism may occur in long-standing secondary hyperparathyroidism when an autonomous nodule develops in a hyperplastic gland, resulting in hypercalcaemia.

Clinical Features

The bone changes are the same in each form, but depend on the duration and severity of the hyperparathyroidism. Some patients complain of bone pain. Radiographs may be normal or show generalized osteopenia and there may be subperiosteal cortical resorption, particularly affecting the phalanges and sometimes the outer ends of the clavicles. Rarely, especially in secondary hyperparathyroidism, there is an increase in bone density (osteosclerosis). Occasionally, one or more localized areas of radiolucency, so-called brown tumours, are seen. In hyperparathyroidism there is an increased incidence of pseudogout and gout (pp. 359–361). Surgical removal of a parathyroid adenoma or of hyperplastic glands is followed by a rapid fall in serum levels of parathyroid hormone, and diminution of osteoclastic activity. Normal bone structure is usually rapidly restored.

Pathology

Due to increased parathyroid hormone levels, there is increased bone resorption produced by increased numbers of osteoclasts. These are seen on the surface of and within trabeculae of cancellous bone and in Haversian systems of cortical bone. As resorption is accompanied by increased bone formation osteoblasts are found lined up on the surfaces, but overall there is loss of bone. As the disease progresses much bone may be resorbed and replaced by small irregular trabeculae of woven bone, with loss of the normal bony architecture. Fibrous tissue forms around sites of resorption and in longstanding cases the marrow spaces become filled with fibrous tissue in which cystic degeneration occasionally occurs. In the past, these features led to the descriptive term 'osteitis fibrosa cystica'. In 'brown tumours' (Figure 12.8) bone is replaced by numerous osteoclasts, fibrous tissue and haemorrhage with abundant haemosiderin resulting in a destructive lesion which may simulate giant cell tumour of bone (p. 347).

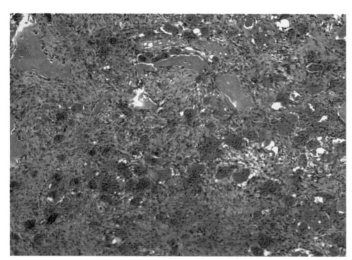

FIGURE 12.8 Brown tumour of hyperparathyroidism. The patient was a middle-aged woman with a past history of two malignant tumours who developed a destructive lesion of the distal humerus. Biopsy shows numerous osteoclasts among fibrous stroma and some reactive new bone formation. She was also known to have chronic renal failure. The lytic lesion rapidly filled-in following removal of an enlarged parathyroid gland.

Renal Osteodystrophy

Key Points

- Hyperparathyroidism, osteomalacia and adynamic bone disease.
- However, modern management of renal failure has altered the patterns of disease.

Renal osteodystrophy refers to the complex group of bone changes seen in patients with chronic renal failure (p. 375). Renal osteodystrophy is a combination of secondary hyperparathyroidism and osteomalacia, although the latter is less common. In the past 20 years new treatments have emerged which have altered the pattern of disease seen.

Pathophysiology of Renal Osteodystrophy

The pathophysiology of renal osteodystrophy is summarized in Figure 12.9. Diminished glomerular filtration and reduced tubular excretion lead to retention of phosphate which causes a reciprocal fall in serum calcium and also impairs renal 1α-hydroxylase causing a reduction in vitamin D synthesis. Both these factors stimulate parathyroid hormone secretion and parathyroid hyperplasia so that serum calcium and phosphate levels return to normal. The lower renal mass produces less 1α-hydroxylase, and less synthesis of $1,25(OH)_2D_3$ results leading to osteomalacia. In the past a severe form of osteomalacia seen in dialysis patients with bone pain, pathological fracture and muscle weakness was shown to be due to inhibition of normal mineralization by deposition of aluminium derived from dialysis fluid or orally administered aluminium-containing phosphate-binding gels.

The aim of modern treatment is to maintain normal serum calcium and phosphate levels, to lower parathyroid hormone levels and to correct any vitamin D deficiency. Hyperparathyroid bone disease has become less frequent and less severe, while osteomalacia is now uncommonly seen. As these forms decrease, there has been an increase in adynamic bone disease, a state of low bone turnover leading to reduced bone mass and an increased risk of fracture, seen especially in those on continuous peritoneal dialysis. This is thought to be due to inhibition of osteoblastic activity.

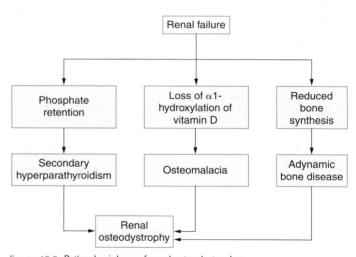

FIGURE 12.9 Pathophysiology of renal osteodystrophy.

Pathology

The histological changes vary between high and low turnover forms. In the former, the appearances include those of hyperparathyroidism as described above. In keeping with a high turnover state there is frequently an increase in trabecular surface area covered by osteoid, but the seams are of normal thickness and the mineralization front is normal. When coexistent osteomalacia develops, there are thickened osteoid seams and a reduced mineralization front. In adynamic bone disease the bone surfaces are inactive with little osteoblastic or osteoblastic activity.

Osteosclerosis, increased density of bone due to extensive formation of woven bone, may be seen, usually in the axial skeleton. Areas of sclerosis adjacent to the vertebral end plates give a striped radiological appearance known as a 'rugger jersey spine'. In patients undergoing long-term haemodialysis accumulation of β_2-microglobulin leads to deposition of amyloid especially in the bones, joints and periarticular structures.

Renal transplant recipients are at risk of developing osteonecrosis, particularly of femoral heads and condyles (p. 341) and osteoporosis. As steroid therapy is implicated in both conditions, the use of cyclosporin as an immunosuppressive agent and consequent reduction of steroid dosage resulted in a lower incidence of these complications.

Paget's Disease of Bone

Key Points
- Paget's disease is a common disease in elderly people, especially among those of Anglo-Saxon origin.
- Increased bone resorption leads to increased turnover.
- The abnormal bone is structurally weak.
- The thickened bone may compress nerves or spinal cord.

Paget's disease is a disorder of excessive turnover of bone which results in disorganization of bone architecture. Although commonly discussed with metabolic bone diseases it is not a generalized skeletal disorder, but may affect part or all of one bone, several or many bones. Most frequently vertebrae, pelvis, skull and femur, tibia and humerus are involved. The incidence of Paget's disease shows considerable geographical variation. Almost unknown in Japan and rare in Scandinavia and the tropics, it is common in Britain and in people of Anglo-Saxon origin. Occasionally found in young adults, Paget's disease can be detected at autopsy or by radiology in about 3% of patients over 40 years, rising to 10% of those over 80. There is a slight male preponderance. There is a significant hereditary predisposition.

Clinical Features

Of the large number of people with Paget's disease only about 5% have symptoms. The common complaints are:

- Bone pain.
- Deformity. Even when thickened, the bone in Paget's disease is structurally weak due to destruction of cortical Haversian systems; this leads to bowing of long bones.

- Pathological fractures, often transverse, result from structurally weakened bone.
- Osteoarthritis occurs more commonly due to stresses thrown on the joints by bone deformity.
- Deafness is caused by compression of the eighth cranial nerve whose exit foramen is narrowed through the thickened skull.
- Spinal cord compression may follow enlargement, or less commonly, collapse of an involved vertebra.
- Paget's sarcoma. This most serious complication is fortunately rare, affecting less than 1% of patients. The sarcoma usually arises in long bones, especially the femur and humerus and is usually an osteosarcoma or high grade undifferentiated sarcoma. The prognosis in Paget's sarcoma is poor; most patients develop early pulmonary metastases and die within 2 years.
- Rarely, patients with extensive Paget's disease have high cardiac output and compromised cardiac function due to increased blood flow through the affected bones.

Pathology

Paget's disease starts at one site in a bone and gradually extends with a lytic advancing front. Radiographs of long bones may show a sharply defined flame-shaped area of bone resorption, while localized rarefaction of the skull is known as osteoporosis circumscripta. In early Paget's disease there is intense activity of very large osteoclasts; in response plump osteoblasts rapidly lay down new bone, some of which is woven rather than lamellar. The marrow spaces contain vascular fibrous tissue. As the disease progresses, resorption lessens and bone formation becomes more prominent with increasing sclerosis. The shafts of long bones are thickened on the periosteal and endosteal surfaces so that the bone is enlarged and the marrow cavity narrowed. The weakened bones may be bowed. The skull enlarges and is sometimes three to four times thicker than normal (Figure 12.10). Histologically, the trabeculae become thickened, and show a 'mosaic' or 'jigsaw' pattern of cement lines indicating previous phases of bone resorption and formation (Figure 12.11). Normal cortical Haversian systems are replaced by irregularly arranged trabeculae. Eventually the marrow becomes densely fibrosed and the bone surfaces become inactive.

Aetiology

The aetiology is uncertain. One theory is that Paget's disease is due to viral infection of osteoclasts and their precursors. Intranuclear inclusions found in the osteoclasts of patients with Paget's disease resemble those of myxoviruses, while immunohistochemical techniques and some nucleic acid hybridization studies support this theory. As indicated above, there is a genetic predisposition to Paget's disease. Mutations of the sequestosome 1 gene (*SQSTM1*) are found in some cases.

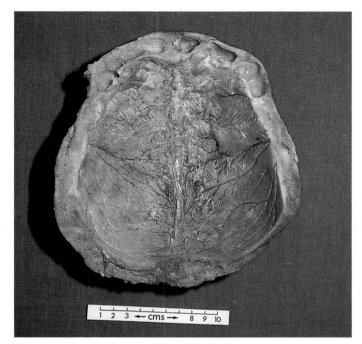

FIGURE 12.10 Paget's disease of bone. Characteristic thickening of the skull with loss of distinction between the tables.

Generalized Developmental Abnormalities of Bone

Key Points

- Generalized developmental abnormalities of bone are rare conditions, usually presenting in childhood.
- There is abnormal growth or structure of bone.
- Underlying molecular mechanisms are increasingly understood.
- There is potential for genetic screening.

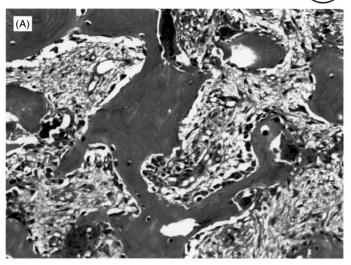

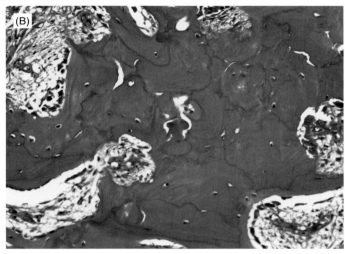

FIGURE 12.11 Paget's disease of bone. (A) The active phase is characterized by numerous large osteoclasts eroding bone, followed by new bone formation by sheets of osteoblasts. The marrow is replaced by vascular fibrous tissue. (B) Repeated episodes of irregular resorption and synthesis result in a jigsaw or mosaic pattern of cement (reversal) lines.

Osteogenesis Imperfecta (Brittle Bone Syndrome)

This is a rare (1–5 in 100 000 births) inherited disease characterized by bone fragility and repeated fractures. There are several subtypes which vary in the severity of the disease and the age of onset; in some there are extraskeletal abnormalities, such as abnormal dentine (dentinogenesis imperfecta), cardiac valvular disease and blue sclerae (the choroid pigment may be seen through the thinned sclerae). The current classification and the underlying molecular mechanisms that explain the clinical variations are summarized in Table 12.5.

Pathogenesis

Osteogenesis imperfecta results from mutations in the structural genes for type I collagen. Type I collagen is composed of two proteins, pro-α_1 and pro-α_2 encoded by two genes *COL-1-A1* and *COL-1-A2*, which are located on chromosomes 17 and 7 respectively. Two pro-α_1 and one pro-α_2 chains twist together to form a triple helix. Numerous mutations including gene deletions, insertions and duplications have been described, but most cases are caused by single-point mutations. In the mild form of osteogenesis imperfecta (type 1) the collagen is of normal type, but is present in reduced amounts. This is often due to mutations which knock out one copy of the *COL-1-A1* gene leading to diminished production of the collagen α_1 chain. Thus, although the amount of bone is reduced, it is structurally normal. In contrast, in the more severe forms mutations within the collagen genes result in abnormal collagen protein chains which combine to form an abnormal triple helix. The resulting collagen is structurally weaker, and also turns over more rapidly. In the more severe forms the commonest

TABLE 12.5 Osteogenesis imperfecta: major subtypes

Type	Clinical features	Inheritance
I	Mild: fractures, little deformity, normal stature, blue sclerae, joint laxity, deafness, ± dentinogenesis imperfecta	Autosomal dominant
II	Perinatal lethal: severe disease, usually lethal in perinatal period, short limbs	New dominant mutations
III	Progressive deforming: severe progressive disease, short stature, deformity, sclerae blue in infancy, white later	Heterogeneous: majority autosomal dominant
IV	Moderate deformity, short stature, normal sclerae, ±dentinogenesis imperfecta (intermediate between I and III)	Autosomal dominant

defects are single base mutations which result in substitution of a glycine amino acid by a larger amino acid such as asparagine. Glycine is essential in the formation of the collagen triple helix. The closer the mutation is to the carboxy-terminal end of the chain, from which the helix winds up, and the larger the substituting amino acid, the more badly affected is the collagen formed.

The pathological appearances vary depending on the severity of the clinical disease. In general, osteoblast activity is defective with a reduction in bone formation, so that osteocytes appear crowded. The more severely affected the patient, the higher the proportion of woven to lamellar bone. The shafts of long bones are thin while the epiphyses are broad and often disorganized. Multiple fractures may result in bowing of limb bones. Hyperplastic fracture callus may simulate the development of a sarcoma.

The radiological appearance of multiple healing fractures of varying ages may be misinterpreted as evidence of 'non-accidental injury', with serious medicolegal implications for the parents.

Achondroplasia

Achondroplasia is the commonest skeletal dysplasia (1 in 15 000 to 40 000 live births) and is characterized by short stature; failure of enchondral ossification leading to diminished growth of the limbs. Achondroplasia is inherited in an autosomal dominant manner, and is due to a mutation of the fibroblast growth factor receptor 3 (FGFR3) gene on chromosome 4. This gene has a very high mutation rate; thus over 80% of affected children are born to normal parents. The mutation causes the receptor to be switched on, suppressing cartilage growth. Other mutations of this gene give rise to other rarer bone dysplasias. Patients with achondroplasia have distinctive features: the head appears large, the forehead bulging and the root of the nose sunken. The limbs are disproportionately short compared with the trunk and cranium. The hands are broad with fingers of equal length (trident hands). The spinal canal is narrowed and spinal cord compression is common in adults. These changes

are a consequence of the abnormal enchondral ossification. At the epiphyseal line the cartilage cells form short rows or are irregularly arranged, with little or no ossification, resulting in reduced bone growth.

Some affected infants die, usually from neurological complications such as hydrocephalus due to maldevelopment of the skull base, but most survive into adult life with normal intellect.

Osteopetrosis (Marble Bone Disease, Albers-Schönberg Disease)

Key Points

- There are dense bones due to reduced osteoclastic activity.
- There are pathological fractures.
- There is obliteration of marrow cavity leading to anaemia.
- There is nerve compression leading to blindness, deafness.

Osteopetrosis is a heterogeneous group of disorders characterized by increased bone density due to defective osteoclastic activity. Broadly, there is a severe form of infancy, usually inherited as an autosomal recessive condition, in which there is failure of resorption of the fetal cartilaginous model of bones so that the marrow cavities fail to form. Severe anaemia with a peripheral blood leucoerythroblastic reaction develops which, with infections due to leucopenia, may be life-threatening. The bones are radio-opaque and show evidence of abnormal remodelling. Despite the increased bone density the bones are structurally abnormal and are subject to pathological fracture. Skull involvement with narrowing of exit foramina may result in deafness or blindness. Patients with severe disease may be treated by bone marrow transplantation. Donor osteoclasts derived from marrow precursors resorb the cartilaginous matrix and allow remodelling. Milder forms inherited as autosomal dominant traits are often not recognized until adult life, typically following a fracture. The precise pathogenetic mechanisms in humans remain uncertain in most cases: in one mild form, an absence of osteoclast carbonic anhydrase activity is responsible.

Osteonecrosis

> **Key Points**
>
> - Osteonecrosis involves death of bone due to loss of blood supply.
> - There are major causes: trauma, metabolic disorders, steroids.
> - Juxta-articular necrosis leads to destruction of joints.

Osteonecrosis (aseptic necrosis, avascular necrosis) refers to death of bone due to interference with its blood supply, by definition not associated with infection. The most common cause is a fracture that disrupts the major blood supply to an area of bone; the femoral head and scaphoid are two sites where the distribution of vessels is especially likely to cause clinically important osteonecrosis.

A large number of non-traumatic conditions are associated with osteonecrosis (Table 12.6) and sometimes no clear cause can be found (idiopathic). In some cases the pathogenesis seems clear: in compressed air workers nitrogen bubbles form during decompression and block small blood vessels, while in sickle cell anaemia sludging of red cells has the same effect. In contrast, the mechanisms responsible for the osteonecrosis complicating steroid therapy and alcohol excess are speculative.

Necrosis may involve the cancellous bone of the shaft of a long bone. The resulting infarct is sometimes seen as an area of increased density on radiographs due chiefly to calcification of dead marrow. Such lesions are asymptomatic, although rarely may be complicated by a sarcoma. In contrast, in juxta-articular sites such as the femoral head

TABLE 12.6 **Cause of osteonecrosis**

Trauma, e.g. fracture of neck of femur
Dysbarism (Caisson disease)
Sickle cell disease
Gaucher's disease
Alcohol excess
Steroid therapy
Radiotherapy
Connective tissue disorders, e.g. systemic lupus erythematosus

(Figure 12.12) or condyles, a wedged-shaped segment of necrotic bone may eventually collapse with deformity of the joint surface and secondary osteoarthritis. The histological features are of necrosis of haemopoietic marrow followed by loss of osteocytes from their lacunae. Initial steps

in repair consist of revascularization of dead marrow followed by deposition of live bone on the surface of necrotic trabeculae (appositional new bone).

Osteonecrosis is seen in several disorders of childhood. Perthes' disease affects the hips in children, particularly boys, who present with pain and a limp. About 10% of cases are bilateral. Pathologically there is osteonecrosis of the femoral epiphysis which may heal without significant deformity or

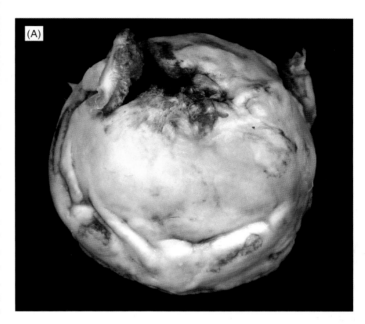

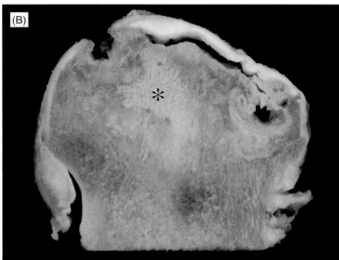

FIGURE 12.12 Osteonecrosis (avascular necrosis) of the femoral head. The articular surface of the femoral head shows a crescent-shaped depression (A) which, on the cut section (B) is seen to be due to a subchondral fracture. The yellow tissue (*) is necrotic bone.

may collapse, often resulting in osteoarthritis in later life. In other conditions bone necrosis follows an episode of trauma. In osteochondritis dissecans a wedge-shaped area of bone and its attached articular cartilage separate from the articular surface leaving a well demarcated defect. The bone undergoes necrosis. This commonly involves the lateral aspect of the medial femoral condyle; the loose body (p. 362) may cause locking and damage to the articular cartilage. Similar conditions may affect the tarsal navicular (Köhler's disease), the lunate (Kienböck's disease) and the second metatarsal (Freiberg's disease).

Infection of Bone and Joints

Osteomyelitis

> **Key Points**
>
> - It may be due to bloodborne microorganisms or direct inoculation.
> - Causative organisms are pyogenic organisms, especially *Staphylococcus aureus.*
> - It is characterized by bone necrosis and reactive bone formation.
> - There is a risk of chronic osteomyelitis.
> - Early diagnosis is important.

Osteomyelitis occurs in several circumstances. Classic acute osteomyelitis affects mainly children and adolescents; organisms reach bone by blood spread from a focus elsewhere such as a boil. Frequently, no source can be found and it is assumed that there is a minor lesion which is clinically inapparent or has healed. Any bone may be affected but the metaphyses of long bones (distal femur, proximal tibia and humerus) adjacent to actively growing epiphyses, and the vertebral column are most often involved. The incidence of this disease has fallen in recent decades. Intravenous drug misusers and those with genitourinary infections are at risk of haematogenous

osteomyelitis often due to coliforms. More common is spread from an adjacent site of infection: examples include compound fractures or following orthopaedic surgery, especially where metallic implants such as nails, plates and screws and prosthetic joints are inserted. Another important cause is diabetes mellitus, particularly with peripheral vascular disease and skin ulcers. Awareness of the disease is important as delay in diagnosis and failure to institute antibiotic treatment may lead to considerable morbidity.

The causative organism of most serious infections is coagulase-positive *Staphylococcus*, although streptococci, coagulase-negative *Staphylococcus*, Gram-negative bacilli and anaerobes are sometimes isolated. Sickle cell anaemia predisposes to infection by salmonellae.

Typically, the patient with acute osteomyelitis is unwell with a high fever, and complains of severe pain and tenderness aggravated by any movement. The erythrocyte sedimentation rate, the white blood count and acute phase reactants such as C-reactive protein are usually elevated. Changes on conventional radiographs frequently do not appear for 7 days or so, but magnetic resonance scanning shows abnormal signal much earlier. If acute osteomyelitis is suspected blood cultures should be taken and large doses of antibiotics given immediately to avert septicaemia. A high index of suspicion is required to make the diagnosis in immunosuppressed patients who frequently have few symptoms or signs.

Pathology

The following description refers to untreated acute haematogenous osteomyelitis (Figure 12.13). Most cases involve the metaphysis of long bones where dilated vascular sinusoids with sluggish blood flow provide an ideal site for multiplication of bacteria. Bacteria pass into the marrow spaces and provoke an acute inflammatory response. Pus

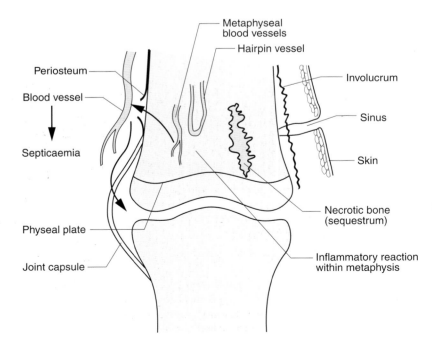

FIGURE 12.13 Osteomyelitis is often due to haematogenous spread from foci elsewhere. The bacteria lodge within metaphyseal (hairpin) blood vessels and set up an inflammatory reaction in the medullary canal, which spreads through the cortex, elevates the periosteum and may spread locally into an adjacent joint, causing septic arthritis, or into blood vessels leading to bacteraemia or septicaemia. Interference with blood supply leads to bone death, with formation of a 'sequestrum'; meantime, the periosteum lays down a shell of new bone, the involucrum. Pus may track to the skin surface forming a discharging sinus.

spreads rapidly throughout the medullary cavity and the cortex, elevates the periosteum and forms a subperiosteal abscess. Pus may track into the surrounding soft tissues, ultimately reaching the skin surface to form a sinus. Vascular thrombosis leads to bone necrosis, the piece of dead bone being known as a sequestrum. Meanwhile cytokines released by the inflammatory cells activate osteoclasts causing bone destruction. As infection becomes less acute, subperiosteal new bone may form an incomplete shell (involucrum) around the dead bone.

Complications

- Septicaemia – spread of infection, particularly when due to staphylococci, may lead to septicaemia with abscesses in lung, kidney or myocardium and acute endocarditis. This accounted for a mortality of 25% before antibiotic therapy was available.
- Septic arthritis – direct spread of infection occurs in joints such as the hip and shoulder in which the metaphysis lies within the joint capsule.
- Alteration in growth rate – damage to the epiphyseal plate, particularly in infants, may lead to growth retardation, while occasionally increased blood flow causes accelerated growth.
- Chronic osteomyelitis – acute osteomyelitis, particularly in adults, may become chronic with recurrent exacerbation of infection with abscesses, discharging sinuses and increasing patchy bone sclerosis. Secondary amyloidosis and occasionally squamous carcinoma arising in a sinus may complicate longstanding chronic osteomyelitis.

Subacute Pyogenic Infection

Many patients develop a subacute pyogenic infection with an insidious onset and little fever or malaise. Most cases affect the spine, but other bones may be involved.

Vertebral osteomyelitis

Infection of the vertebral column occurs mainly in adults; spread is usually haematogenous, either arterial or by retrograde spread through the vertebral venous plexus which communicates directly with pelvic veins. In about two-thirds of patients the lumbar spine is involved. *Staphylococcus aureus* is the commonest organism; infection with coliforms often follows genitourinary surgery. In most patients the onset is insidious with intermittent attacks of backache and little fever. The initial focus is in or close to the vertebral endplate; infection spreads to involve the adjacent disc and cancellous bone of the vertebral body, both of which undergo necrosis. Pressure on the spinal cord may lead to paraplegia. Some collapse of bone occurs with loss of the disc space; reactive new bone formation may cause spontaneous fusion of adjacent vertebrae.

Brodie's abscess

This is a form of localized subacute or chronic osteomyelitis which is usually situated in the metaphysis of a long bone, especially the upper end of the tibia and usually in adolescents.

A central cavity containing pus, which may be sterile, is lined by granulation tissue and surrounded by reactive bone sclerosis.

Septic Arthritis

> **Key Points**
>
> - It may be caused by haematogenous spread or direct inoculation.
> - *Staphylococcus aureus* is the main causative organism.
> - There is rapid destruction of joints unless treated early.

Joint infection may result from haematogenous spread to synovium, from direct extension from acute osteomyelitis, or follow penetrating injury or surgery especially joint replacement or arthroscopy. *Staphylococcus aureus* is the commonest causative organism, but *Neisseria gonorrhoeae* (p. 509) is a common cause in young adults and *Haemophilus influenzae* in infancy. Patients with rheumatoid arthritis and those on steroid therapy are at increased risk from joint infection, which often gives rise to few local symptoms. Classically, children and young adults present with high fever and a swollen, hot, painful joint. While an inflamed knee is obvious clinically, inflammation of the hip, common in infancy, may be readily missed. Elderly patients frequently show few signs of systemic upset.

Gonococcal arthritis is now a major cause of bacterial arthritis especially in healthy young adults. Most patients complain of flitting pain in many joints particularly the knees, ankles, wrists and elbows. Tenosynovitis and a skin rash are often present. It is thought that joint involvement follows a bacteraemic phase after genital infection. Culture of gonococci from inflamed joints is often difficult. Permanent joint damage rarely results.

Pathology

The synovium is acutely inflamed with large numbers of neutrophils which cause destruction of the articular cartilage (Figure 12.14). Effective early treatment is likely to

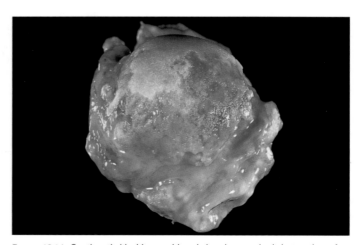

FIGURE 12.14 Septic arthritis. Humeral head showing marked destruction of the articular cartilage by acute inflammation.

preserve joint function, while loss of articular cartilage is followed by osteoarthritis.

Tuberculosis of Bone and Joints

In recent years the overall incidence of tuberculosis in developed countries has risen due to the emergence of acquired immune deficiency syndrome (AIDS), immigration from developing countries and emergence of drug-resistant strains. Skeletal tuberculosis is almost always due to haematogenous spread from infection elsewhere, usually lung or urinary tract; the patient should be investigated to find this source of infection. *Mycobacterium tuberculosis* is responsible for most infections but atypical mycobacteria are important in the immunocompromised. Early diagnosis and treatment are important to minimize tissue destruction.

About half of the infections involve the spine (tuberculous spondylitis; Pott's disease), usually the lower thoracic and lumbar vertebrae (Figure 12.15). Initially one vertebral body is affected with early involvement of the intervertebral disc. Bone destruction leads to vertebral collapse. A local paraspinal abscess develops and infection may extend along the anterior spinal ligaments to other vertebrae, or track

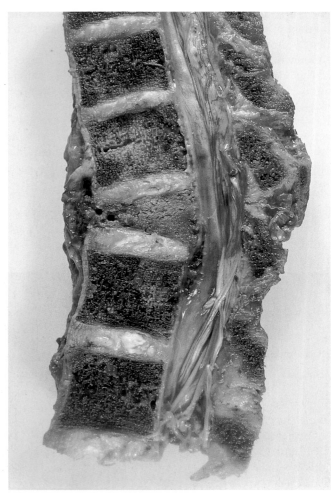

FIGURE 12.15 Tuberculosis of spine: there is involvement of at least two vertebrae, one of which has collapsed. The discs are better preserved than is typically seen. The differential diagnosis includes metastatic carcinoma.

anteriorly along tissue planes. In the lumbar spine infection may spread along the sheath of the psoas muscle to point in the groin as a 'cold' or 'psoas' abscess. Angulation of the spine may occur with a severe kyphosis (tuberculous gibbus). Patients with vertebral tuberculosis may develop spinal cord compression, either early in the disease due to pressure from an extradural abscess or bone or disc material, or late when the cord may be stretched over the apex of a severe kyphosis.

Tuberculous arthritis results from haematogenous spread of infection to synovium or by extension from an affected intracapsular portion of bone. The hip and knee are most commonly involved. Inflammation of the synovium invades the subchondral bone and dissects it from the articular cartilage leading to destruction of the joint surface. Less commonly, bone involvement occurs in the absence of joint disease, typically with destructive lesions in the metaphysis of long bones, for example the knee, femoral neck and greater trochanter. The tubular bones of the hands may be affected (dactylitis).

The histological appearances are typical of tuberculosis elsewhere; alcohol and acid-fast bacilli may be identified in histological sections, but are often difficult to find; for this reason, tissue should also be submitted for bacteriological examination including culture. Polymerase chain reaction to detect the bacterial DNA is a rapid and sensitive technique.

Other Infections of Bone and Joints

Brucellosis

Brucellosis is transmitted to humans from infected animals or animal products. Infection of bone and joints is common in chronic brucellosis, and less so in the acute form. Typically one or a few peripheral joints, especially the hip and knee, are involved; sacroiliitis is also seen. The organism is difficult to culture but positive serological tests allow diagnosis. Histologically the synovium or bone contains non-caseating granulomas.

Lyme Disease

This is a multisystem infection caused by the spirochete *Borrelia burgdorferi*, which is transmitted by ticks of the genus *Ixodes*, particularly in areas with large deer populations. (The name derives from Lyme, Connecticut, where a cluster of children with arthritis led in 1975 to recognition of the disease.) A skin rash (erythema chronicum migrans), cardiac, nervous system and osteoarticular involvement have all been described.

Joint manifestations include migratory joint pains, intermittent attacks of acute arthritis and chronic erosive arthritis which, in about 10% of patients may cause permanent disability. Large joints, particularly the knee, are affected. Lyme arthritis responds to treatment with high-dose penicillin, although irreversible damage may have occurred.

Viral Arthritis

Many common viral infections, for example hepatitis C, mumps, rubella and its vaccine and parvovirus are associated with transient arthritis or arthralgia. In all instances the arthritis is non-destructive and does not lead to chronic joint disease.

Infections related to prosthetic joint replacements are discussed on p. 361.

TUMOURS IN BONE

Key Points

- Metastatic carcinoma is far commoner than primary bone tumours.
- Breast, lung, prostate, kidney and thyroid are common primary sites.
- Myeloma is by far the commonest primary tumour (p. 218).
- Osteosarcoma and Ewing's sarcoma particularly affect adolescents and are highly malignant.
- Chondrosarcoma is usually a tumour of middle aged to elderly and of fairly low grade.

Metastatic Tumours

Metastatic tumours far exceed primary bone tumours in frequency, and may be found at autopsy in at least 50% of patients dying with disseminated tumour. Almost all are carcinomas, particularly those arising from bronchus, breast, prostate, kidney and thyroid, which account for 80% in adults. In children neuroblastoma and rhabdomyosarcoma often spread to bone. Metastases occur most commonly in areas where haemopoietic marrow is present, in adults the vertebral column, ribs, proximal femur and humerus (Figure 12.16). Retrograde spread to the spine occurs along the prevertebral venous plexus. Metastases distal to the knee and elbow (acral metastases) are rare, and are usually due to bronchial carcinoma. Metastatic tumours in bone occasionally present as solitary lesions, but usually multiple further metastases rapidly develop. Surgical removal of a primary renal or thyroid carcinoma and a solitary metastasis may result in long survival.

Many bone metastases are asymptomatic; the clinical effects are of pain, and bone destruction (osteolysis) leading to pathological fracture of long bones, and vertebral collapse or spinal cord compression. Rarely carcinomas, typically of prostate and sometimes of breast, may induce reactive new bone formation giving rise to osteosclerotic metastases. Hypercalcaemia is usually due to the production by tumour cells of PTHrP, which has functional similarity to PTH (humoral hypercalcaemia of malignancy). The mechanisms of bone destruction are discussed in Special Study Topic 12.1.

Primary Bone Tumours

Although much less common than metastases, primary tumours are an important cause of disability and death, particularly in the young. As they are rare, expertise in management is concentrated in regional centres. A summary of the typical anatomical locations and age ranges is given in Table 12.7.

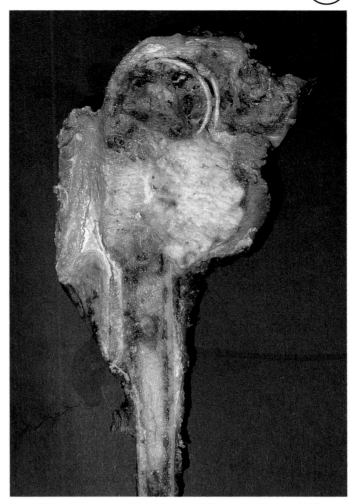

FIGURE 12.16 Metastatic carcinoma in bone. This proximal humerus with adjacent shoulder joint and glenoid was resected for metastatic renal carcinoma. A large tumour mass occupies the medulla and has extended into adjacent soft tissue particularly medially.

Benign Bone Tumours

Osteoid Osteoma

This lesion commonly occurs in the shafts of long bones of adolescents and young adults, who complain of persistent pain, worse at night, often relieved by aspirin. Lesions in the spine often cause scoliosis, whereas those close to joints may simulate arthritis. Radiographs show a small lucent nidus, usually less than 1 cm in diameter, which is often surrounded by a mass of sclerotic bone; computed tomography (CT) and magnetic resonance imaging (MRI) are superior to plain radiographs in demonstrating the nidus. Isotope bone scans show a 'hot' area of increased uptake.

The lesion consists of a well-defined, highly vascular nidus of trabeculae of woven bone and benign osteoblasts. The nidus is surrounded by a variable amount of reactive bone (Figure 12.17). Symptoms may recur if the lesion is incompletely removed. Most cases are now treated by radiofrequency ablation. Benign bone forming lesions greater than 1 cm are known as osteoblastoma, and commonly affect the

TABLE 12.7 Primary bone tumours

Tumour	Main age group (years)	Major site(s)
Osteoma	Adults	Skull, sinuses
Osteoid osteoma	10–30	Long bones, spine
Osteoblastoma	10–30	Spine, long bones
Enchondroma	Wide range	50% hands, feet
Osteochondroma	10–20	Metaphysis of long bones
Chondroblastoma	10–20	Epiphysis of long bones
Chondromyxoid fibroma	5–30	Metaphysis of long bones
Aneurysmal bone cyst	5–20	Spine, metaphysis of long bones
Simple bone cyst	5–15	Metaphysis of long bones
Fibrous dysplasia	5–30	Any, especially femur, ribs, skull
Non-ossifying fibroma	5–15	Metaphysis of long bones
Adamantinoma	10–50	Diaphysis of tibia
Giant cell tumour	20–45	Epiphysis of long bones
Osteosarcoma	10–25	Metaphysis of long bones, knee
Parosteal osteosarcoma	20–50	Surface, metaphysis of long bones, 60% femur
Chondrosarcoma	40–70	Pelvis, femur, humerus, rib
Malignant fibrous histiocytoma	Adults	Metaphysis of long bones
Chordoma	40–70	Sacrum, skull base, spine
Ewing's tumour	5–20	Long bones, pelvis

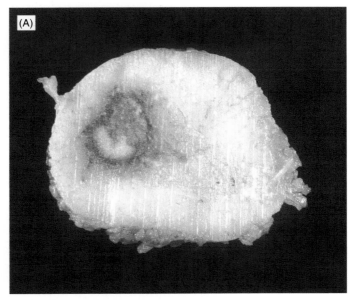
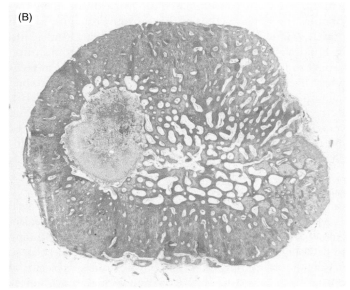

FIGURE 12.17 **Osteoid osteoma.** This shows a transverse section of an excised length of fibula containing a nidus of an osteoid osteoma both on naked eye (A) inspection and histology (B). The nidus is well defined and is surrounded by sclerotic bone.

spine. They tend not to be surrounded by sclerotic bone and pain is less of a feature than with osteoid osteoma; large lesions may cause spinal cord compression.

Enchondroma

This is a benign intramedullary tumour of cartilage. Over half occur within the tubular bones of the hands and feet, although long bones such as the humerus and femur may be affected. Many enchondromas are asymptomatic incidental radiological findings of lytic lesions often with spotty calcification. Lesions in the hand may cause swelling or pain following injury, sometimes with a pathological fracture. Chondromas are composed of lobules of blue grey cartilage consisting of a hyaline matrix containing uniform chondrocytes with small darkly staining nuclei. In multiple enchondromatosis the hands are almost invariably affected, but there may be involvement of long bones with deformity. When predominantly unilateral the condition is referred to as Ollier's disease. The combination of multiple enchondromatosis and soft tissue haemangiomas is known as Maffucci's syndrome. Both conditions are usually not inherited.

Malignant transformation of solitary enchondromas is rare. In contrast 20% of patients with enchondromatosis develop chondrosarcoma, whereas the risk is higher still in those with Maffucci's syndrome. In addition these patients appear to be at increased risk of non-skeletal malignancies such as primary brain tumours and pancreatic carcinoma.

Osteocartilaginous Exostosis

Osteocartilaginous exostosis (osteochondroma) is a common bony outgrowth covered by a proliferating cartilage cap (Figure 12.18) attached to the metaphyses of long bones, especially the femur, humerus and tibia. Although previously regarded as a developmental anomaly arising from the epiphyseal growth plate, it is now thought to be a benign neoplasm. The lesions are usually noticed in childhood; growth commonly ceases in adult life, and sometimes the cartilaginous cap is completely replaced by bone.

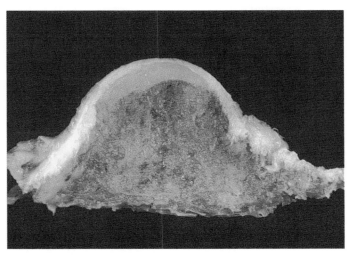

FIGURE 12.18 Osteocartilaginous exostosis. This small exostosis consists of a thin cartilaginous cap with underlying cancellous bone.

Exostoses are usually single; hereditary multiple exostoses (diaphyseal aclasis) is inherited as an autosomal dominant trait and is usually due to mutation of one of two genes, *EXT1* and *EXT2*, which encode enzymes involved in the synthesis of the cartilaginous extracellular matrix. Malignant change is rare in solitary exostoses and less than 2% of those patients with multiple lesions develop chondrosarcoma, which is usually of low grade. Pain, not associated with fracture of the stalk of the exostosis or with bursitis, or resumption of growth raise suspicion of malignancy.

Subungual exostosis is a painful mass of bone and cartilage which usually involves the distal phalanx of the great toe and commonly arises as a reaction to infection or trauma. It never becomes malignant.

Giant Cell Tumour (Osteoclastoma)

Giant cell tumour principally affects individuals between 20 and 40 years of age. Most tumours occur in long bones with

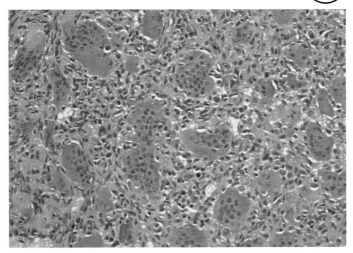

FIGURE 12.19 Giant cell tumour of bone. The tumour consists of large multinucleated osteoclasts of reactive nature interspersed with ovoid mononuclear tumour cells.

half in the distal femur and proximal tibia. Almost all arise in the bone end, although extension into the metaphysis is often seen. Giant cell tumours rarely occur at the site of an open epiphyseal plate. Giant cell tumour is a lytic lesion which often causes eccentric expansion and may be covered by a shell of subperiosteal bone or extend into the soft tissue. Pathological fracture often occurs. Grossly the tumour is soft and red with areas of haemorrhage and necrosis. On microscopy, ovoid mononuclear tumour cells are interspersed with very large reactive osteoclasts (Figure 12.19).

Giant cell tumour is a benign but locally aggressive tumour. The incidence of local recurrence depends on the extent of surgery: around 20% of cases treated by curettage recur locally, often with soft tissue involvement. A very small number metastasize or undergo sarcomatous transformation, usually after treatment and recurrence, particularly after radiotherapy, and then spread to the lungs.

Malignant Primary Bone Tumours

Osteosarcoma

Key Points

- Osteosarcoma is a malignant tumour whose cells form bone.
- Peak age is 10–25 years.
- Over half arise around knee.
- Metaphysis of long bones is affected.
- There is early bloodborne metastasis.

Other than multiple myeloma (p. 218), osteosarcoma is the commonest primary malignant tumour of bone, with approximately 150 new cases (3/1 000 000 population) diagnosed in Britain each year. Three-quarters of patients are between 10 and 25 years old with males more frequently affected. In more than half of patients over 40 years the tumour complicates Paget's disease, whereas some tumours arise in previously irradiated bone. Patients present with increasing pain and swelling; pathological fracture is unusual. Most osteosarcomas arise in the medullary cavity of the metaphysis of long bones, with over half around the knee, at the site of maximum skeletal growth. The proximal humerus and femur and distal radius are other common sites. Most osteosarcomas arise sporadically, but some occur in families with the Li–Fraumeni syndrome and familial retinoblastoma (p. 97). Parosteal osteosarcoma is a low-grade tumour which forms a well-defined lobulated mass often on the posterior aspect of the distal femur or on the proximal humerus. Metastatic spread is less frequent and the prognosis is much better than in conventional osteosarcoma.

Pathology

By definition, osteosarcoma is a malignant tumour where osteoid or bone is formed directly by the tumour cells (Figure 12.20). The gross appearances vary greatly. Some tumours are densely sclerotic, whereas others are fleshy. Telangiectatic osteosarcomas contain large blood-filled spaces. The naked eye appearances are modified by the response to preoperative chemotherapy which gives rise to large areas of necrosis and haemorrhage. The histological appearances also vary. Some tumours containing abundant 'tumour bone'; in others, only small foci of bone or osteoid are present and much of the tumour consists of malignant cartilage or sheets of malignant spindle-shaped cells.

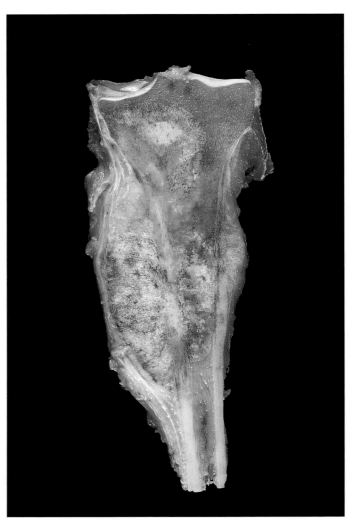

FIGURE 12.21 Osteosarcoma. This large tumour has arisen in the metaphysis of the proximal tibia and has penetrated the cortex to extend through the periosteum forming a circumferential soft tissue extension. The growth plate is closed, but the tumour has penetrated through its scar to involve the epiphysis.

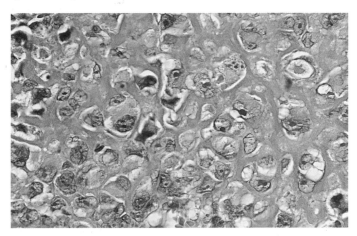

FIGURE 12.20 Osteosarcoma. A delicate meshwork of eosinophilic osteoid matrix has been formed directly by large ovoid malignant cells.

Osteosarcoma spreads within the medulla then penetrates and partially destroys the cortex to extend beneath the periosteum and sometimes later into soft tissue (Figure 12.21). In rapidly growing tumours the periosteum is raised and lays down spicules of new bone perpendicular to the cortex (sunray spiculation), whereas at the junction between raised and normal periosteum Codman's triangle of reactive bone may develop.

Prognosis and treatment

Osteosarcoma is an aggressive tumour with early bloodborne pulmonary metastases, which are evident at presentation in 15% or so. In most patients undetectable pulmonary micrometastases are also already present when the primary tumour is discovered. In an attempt to deal with these silent metastases modern therapy combines preoperative and postoperative chemotherapy with surgery. Many patients can be treated by local resection and endoprosthetic replacement, rather than by amputation. Of patients treated by surgery alone only 20% or so survived 5 years. With modern combination chemotherapy approximately 65% of patients survive for 5 years. Osteosarcoma arising in Paget's disease has a worse prognosis.

Chondrosarcoma

Chondrosarcoma usually arises *de novo*, though about 10% of cases are due to malignant change in a pre-existing benign cartilage tumour. The tumour may occur within the medullary cavity (central) or on the surface of bone (peripheral) usually in relation to an exostosis. Chondrosarcoma normally affects

A 13-year-old girl complained of increasing pain in her left knee over a 3-month period. In the past month she had also been aware of the development of swelling in her distal thigh. A radiograph (Figure 12.22) showed a destructive lesion in the metaphysis of the distal femur with periosteal reaction and MR scanning confirmed the presence of a large tumour with a soft tissue extension. A needle biopsy was carried out and showed a highly malignant tumour (Figure 12.23). Despite the poorly differentiated nature of this tumour, the presence of a small amount of osteoid formation in this clinical and radiological context helped to establish a diagnosis of osteosarcoma. A chest radiograph and CT showed no evidence of metastases.

The patient was treated with three courses of neoadjuvant chemotherapy (doxorubicin and platinum based). After this, the distal femur was excised with

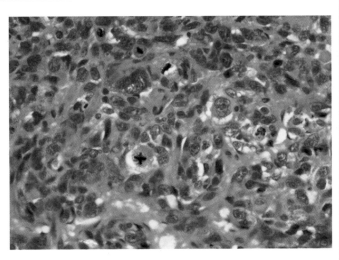

FIGURE 12.23 Biopsy of femur. The tumour shows large cells with pleomorphic nuclei, and numerous mitotic figures including one abnormal one. Although osteoid is not present in this biopsy, it was seen elsewhere and the features are those of an osteosarcoma.

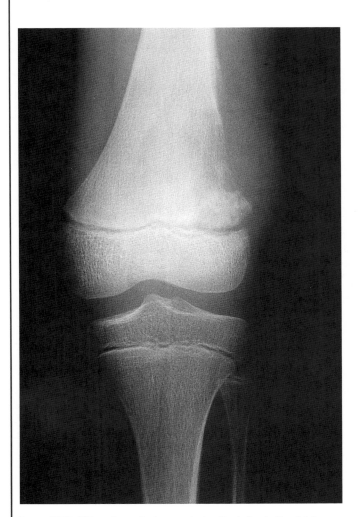

FIGURE 12.22 This radiograph shows a destructive lesion in the distal femoral metaphysis with cortical destruction and soft tissue extension. A periosteal reaction is present (Codman's triangle). The features are of a malignant tumour and in this age group osteosarcoma is the likeliest diagnosis.

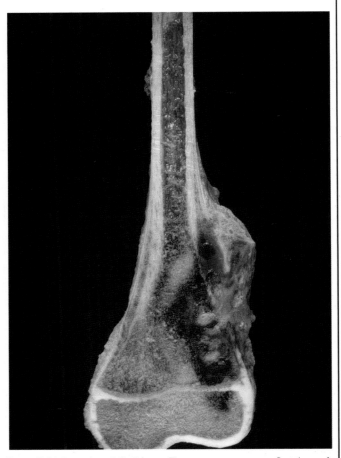

FIGURE 12.24 Resection of distal femur. The gross appearances reflect those of the radiograph in Figure 12.22. There is a large tumour occupying much of the medullary canal; it has penetrated through the cortex into soft tissue. This extraosseous mass has shrunk, representing a good response to preoperative chemotherapy. Tumour has also penetrated the physeal plate to extend into the epiphysis, indicating this is an incomplete barrier to tumour spread.

insertion of a custom-made prosthesis. The resected femur was examined pathologically (Figure 12.24) and it was noted that almost all of the tumour had undergone necrosis, with only small areas containing damaged tumour cells (Figure 12.25).

Three more courses of chemotherapy were given, and the patient remains well several years later.

The main learning points from this case are:

● this is the typical age and a typical site for an osteosarcoma

● osteosarcomas can be histologically highly malignant and are usually clinically aggressive

● such tumours respond well to chemotherapy, which permits limb-sparing surgery

● the diagnosis of bone tumours requires their discussion at multidisciplinary team meetings where clinical, radiological and histopathological evidence is correlated.

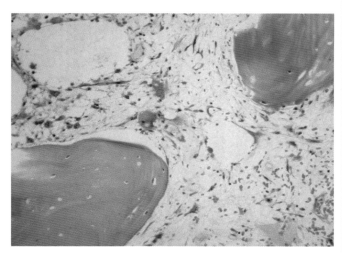

FIGURE 12.25 This section from the medullary canal shows two large bony trabeculae separated by loose fibrovascular tissue. Compared with Fig 12.23 almost all the tumour cells have been killed and there are only occasional residual cells which have been severely damaged by chemotherapy.

the middle aged and elderly. Most tumours arise in the axial skeleton, especially the pelvis, shoulder girdle and ribs, or in the proximal femur and humerus (Figure 12.26), and is rare in the tubular bones of the hands and feet. Most patients with chondrosarcoma complain of swelling or pain. Indeed, pain associated with a cartilage tumour in the absence of pathological fracture or other mechanical cause is highly suggestive of malignancy.

Pathology

Central tumours consist of lobules or sheets of cartilage which may permeate throughout the marrow spaces and erode the bone cortex. More aggressive tumours destroy the cortex and form a subperiosteal mass. Focal calcification is a distinct radiological finding. A greatly thickened cartilaginous cap with nodules of proliferating cartilage on the surface indicates that malignant change in an exostosis has occurred.

Most chondrosarcomas do not show the classic cytological features of malignancy. The finding of many chondrocytes with a plump nucleus and moderate numbers of binucleate cells in a cartilage tumour of the axial skeleton allows a diagnosis of malignancy if the clinical and radiological features are also compatible. Only rare high-grade chondrosarcomas contain pleomorphic cells and moderate numbers of mitoses (Figure 12.27).

Prognosis and treatment

Most chondrosarcomas are slow-growing tumours which often run a prolonged course with repeated local recurrences. Tumours of the pelvis or chest wall may be surgically irresectable and eventually lead to death by involvement of vital structures. Only around 15% of chondrosarcomas metastasize, usually to the lungs. Successful management of

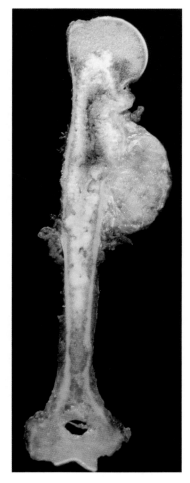

FIGURE 12.26 Chondrosarcoma. This advanced tumour of the proximal humerus has arisen within the medullary canal, but has extended through the medial humeral cortex to form a large soft tissue mass.

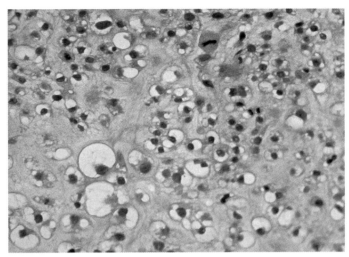

FIGURE 12.27 Chondrosarcoma. This tumour is clearly cartilaginous as the cells lie within lacunae in a chondroid matrix, but there is considerable variation in nuclear size and three mitotic figures are present. This is therefore a high-grade tumour.

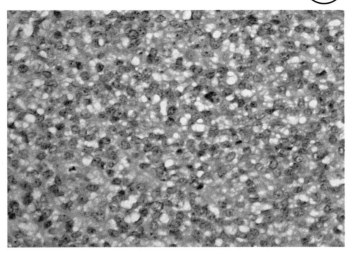

FIGURE 12.28 Ewing's sarcoma. This is a malignant round cell tumour whose cells have clear cytoplasm due to the presence of glycogen. The nuclei are regular and mitotic figures are sparse for such an aggressive tumour.

chondrosarcoma is best achieved by adequate wide surgical excision at the first operation; chondrosarcoma is rarely sensitive to chemotherapy or radiotherapy.

Ewing's Sarcoma

This highly malignant tumour typically affects the long bones and flat bones of the pelvis, scapulae and ribs of children and adolescents. The tumour originates within the medullary cavity but rapidly penetrates the cortex, elevates the periosteum and forms a large soft tissue mass. Radiographs show a moth-eaten pattern of bone destruction, often with parallel layers of reactive periosteal new bone giving a so-called onion skin appearance. Patients present with pain and swelling; in some, fever and elevation of white cell count and erythrocyte sedimentation rate may simulate osteomyelitis.

Aetiology

Ewing's sarcoma is a primitive tumour of neuroectodermal origin. Cytogenetic analysis has shown a characteristic rearrangement of the *EWS* gene on chromosome 22 with the FLI-1 gene on chromosome 11 in a reciprocal translocation t(11; 22)(q24;q12). This hybrid gene produces a chimeric protein which acts as an activated transcription factor. Other translocations have been found in a minority of Ewing's tumours.

Pathology

Ewing's sarcoma consists of sheets of small round cells with uniform pale nuclei and sparse mitotic activity (Figure 12.28). There is often intracellular glycogen and the cells usually express a cell surface antigen CD99. Ewing's tumour must be distinguished from other round cell tumours, for example lymphoma of bone and metastatic neuroblastoma

in young children, in which urinary catecholamine levels are usually elevated.

Prognosis and treatment

Ewing's tumour is highly aggressive with early metastases to lung and other bones. The prognosis is especially poor in those patients with systemic symptoms, and large tumours especially those in the pelvis. Like osteosarcoma, combined therapy with chemotherapy and surgery or radiotherapy has significantly improved the prognosis so that over 50% of patients now survive.

Malignant Fibrous Histiocytoma

This group of tumours includes spindle cell tumours of bone whose cells do not form bone. A wide age range of patients usually present with pain, swelling or pathological fracture. Typically a destructive lesion is seen in the metaphysis of a long bone. About a third of cases arise in association with pre-existing lesions such as Paget's disease or previous irradiation. Malignant fibrous histiocytoma is an aggressive tumour, early bloodborne metastases being common. The cells of malignant fibrous histiocytoma are typically arranged in short bundles radiating from a central point – a 'storiform' pattern like rush matting or the spokes of a wheel. The tumour is probably best regarded as a primitive sarcoma of fibroblast origin. Metastatic carcinoma, especially of bronchus and kidney, may have a spindle cell appearance which can be confused with malignant fibrous histiocytoma.

Non-Hodgkin Lymphoma of Bone

Although disseminated non-Hodgkin lymphoma commonly involves bone, primary malignant lymphoma is relatively rare. Most tumours are diffuse non-Hodgkin lymphomas of large B-cell type. In contrast with disseminated lymphoma involving bone, primary bone lymphoma has a relatively good prognosis; between 50% and 80% of patients survive 5 years, especially those who are young.

Chordoma

This rare tumour arises from notochordal remnants and affects the sacrum, base of skull and less commonly the vertebrae of the middle aged or elderly. Chordomas are slow-growing tumours with symptoms due to pressure on adjacent organs. Sacrococcygeal tumours give symptoms from sacral nerve compression and a large palpable mass may be felt on rectal examination. Chordomas tend to kill by local invasion, but around 10% eventually metastasize. They are lobulated gelatinous tumours which infiltrate bone and extend into adjacent tissues. Microscopy shows cords of vacuolated (physaliferous) cells which express epithelial antigens such as cytokeratin which helps in the distinction from chondrosarcoma.

Tumour-like Lesions of Bone

Fibrous Dysplasia

This benign abnormality of bone may affect one or several bones. Most patients present in childhood, although new lesions may develop after puberty. Rib, jaw, femur and tibia are common sites. Increasing deformity and multiple fractures may occur, although lesions usually cease to grow at puberty. Malignant change is rare in the absence of radiation therapy. Fibrous dysplasia often expands the bone and consists of white gritty fibrous tissue, occasionally with cysts and nodules of cartilage. Histologically, loose spindle celled fibrous stroma contains scattered curving 'lobster-claw' trabeculae of woven bone (Figure 12.29). These are not arranged along stress lines and sometimes give rise to a 'ground glass' appearance on radiology. Osteoblasts are not present on the surfaces of trabeculae which are formed by metaplasia from the stroma. The triad of polyostotic fibrous dysplasia (multiple bone

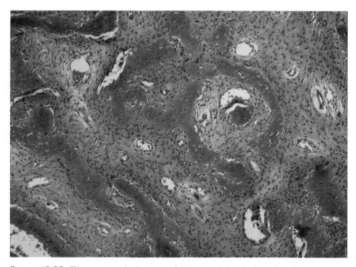

FIGURE 12.29 Fibrous dysplasia. Irregularly orientated trabeculae of woven bone are formed from a vascular fibroblastic stroma.

involvement), patchy skin pigmentation and precocious puberty is referred to as Albright's syndrome, a condition commoner in girls. It is due to mutation of the *GNAS1* gene which codes for an ADP-dependent G protein.

Langerhans' Cell Histiocytosis (Eosinophil Granuloma)

Langerhans' cell histiocytosis may occur at any age or site, but most commonly arises in children and young adults with one or more lesions in skull, long bones, vertebrae and pelvis. Well-defined lytic lesions are seen, although in long bones cortical erosion and pathological fracture may occur suggesting malignancy. Vertebral involvement may lead to bony collapse and a flat dense vertebra (vertebra plana). Histologically, groups of pale-staining Langerhans' cells are mixed with numerous eosinophils. Patients with solitary or few lesions may be cured by surgery or low doses of radiotherapy or the lesions may heal spontaneously. It is important to ascertain whether there is systemic involvement for this worsens the prognosis.

Metaphyseal Fibrous Defect

This is a common developmental abnormality with a distinctive radiological appearance; a scalloped radiolucent area with a sclerotic margin is seen in the metaphyseal cortex of long bones of children. These lesions may disappear spontaneously or enlarge to involve the medullary cavity, when they are known as non-ossifying fibromas, and which may cause pathological fracture. The lesion has a bright orange colour due to the presence of many lipid laden macrophages, which lie in whorled fibrous tissue which contains small osteoclasts.

Cysts of Bone

Aneurysmal bone cysts may affect any bone but typically the posterior elements of vertebrae and the metaphysis of long bones. Patients, usually children and young adults, complain of pain and swelling which often increases rapidly. Radiographs show a well-circumscribed area of bone lysis, often with very marked eccentric expansion sometimes described as a 'blow out'. Anastomosing blood-filled spaces are seen (Figure 12.30), separated by fibrous septa containing bony trabeculae and osteoclastic giant cells. Although aneurysmal bone cysts may simulate a malignant tumour clinically and radiologically, they are benign. Recent evidence indicates that they are benign neoplasms and not simply reactive conditions. A variety of benign and malignant tumours may contain areas of secondary aneurysmal bone cyst change, so the pathologist must examine the entire specimen for any pre-existing lesion.

Simple (unicameral) bone cysts are common findings in children and adolescents and affect the metaphyses of the humerus, femur and tibia. The patient typically presents with a pathological fracture. Radiological examination shows a slightly expanded cyst with a thinned cortex. The cyst is smooth walled and contains clear fluid unless there has been a fracture. The wall consists of a thin layer of fibrous tissue, sometimes containing osteoclasts and haemosiderin. Injection of steroids into the cyst promotes healing.

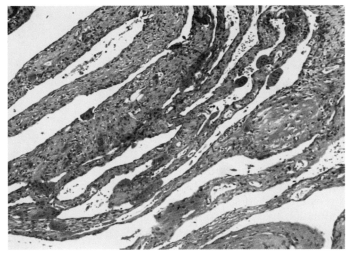

FIGURE 12.30 Aneurysmal bone cyst. The lesion consists of septa containing some osteoclasts, fibroblasts and osteoid, but there is no endothelial lining, indicating that this is not a haemangioma.

Subchondral cysts are frequently seen in osteoarthritis. Similar fibrous walled cysts containing mucoid fluid may occur near the bone end in the absence of degenerative joint disease and are referred to as intraosseous ganglia. Hydatid cysts (p. 541) may occur in bone.

DISEASES OF JOINTS

Normal Joint Structure

There are two main types of joint. Synovial (diarthrodial) joints have a synovial lining and usually allow large amounts of movement. Synarthroses are joints where the bones are joined by fibrous tissue, for example the cranial sutures, or by cartilage, for example pubic symphysis. In these, movement is very limited; they will not be discussed further.

The basic structure of a synovial joint (Figure 12.31) is that the two bone ends are covered by articular cartilage and have a synovial lining which produces fluid which nourishes and lubricates the cartilage. Joint stability is maintained by the joint capsule, a dense fibrous sheath which encloses the joint, and ligaments, localized bands of fibrous tissue which limit joint movement. Some joints contain fibrocartilaginous structures, such as the menisci of the knee, which aid movement by improving the fit of the articulating surfaces.

Articular Cartilage

The hyaline cartilage (Figure 12.31B) which covers the bone ends is an avascular tissue which provides a smooth, low friction surface. It resists compressive forces by deforming under mechanical loading but recovers its shape on removal of the load. Normal articular cartilage is a smooth, bluish, translucent material composed of chondrocytes, proteoglycans, collagen and water.

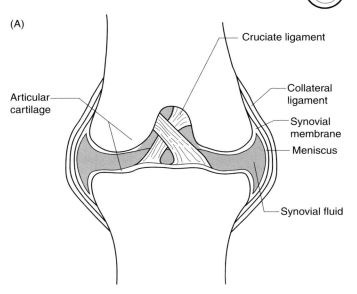

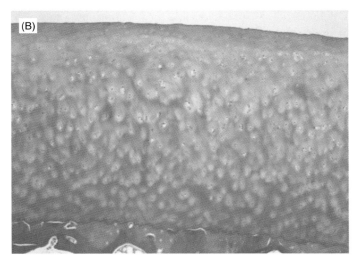

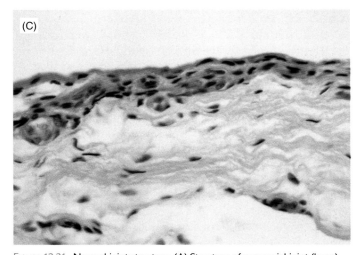

FIGURE 12.31 Normal joint structure. (A) Structure of a synovial joint (knee). (B) Articular cartilage is a smooth-surfaced material covering the bone ends. Small uniform chondrocytes lie in lacunae within a hyaline matrix. (C) In health, the synovial membrane consists of fibrovascular tissue covered by a thin layer of flattened cells, which on ultrastructure can be shown to be a mixture of fibroblasts and histiocytes.

Collagen is responsible for much of the tensile strength of cartilage. Around 90% of collagen in articular cartilage is type II, while other types (V, VI, IX, X, XI) are also found in specific zones, for example type VI is located chiefly around chondrocytes. Other proteins such as chondronectin and anchorin may link collagen and chondrocytes. In the deep and intermediate zones collagen fibres are orientated perpendicular to the articular surface, while in the superficial zone the fibres lie parallel to the surface forming the 'lamina splendens' a poorly cellular layer. The intracellular matrix of cartilage contains proteoglycan core proteins, link proteins, hyaluronic acid and glycosaminoglycans (largely keratan sulphate and chondroitin sulphate). These macromolecules are capable of binding large amounts of water. The numerous anionic groups on glycosaminoglycan chains cause mutual repulsion. Together these factors endow cartilage with the ability to resist compression. Proteoglycans are not evenly distributed in cartilage, being present in larger amounts in deeper zones and around chondrocytes.

Chondrocytes are responsible for the continuing turnover of the extracellular matrix of articular cartilage. They synthesize matrix components (e.g. collagen, proteoglycans) as well as enzymes (e.g. collagenase) capable of degrading them. The 'lacunae' seen around chondrocytes by light microscopy are artefacts caused by shrinkage of cytoplasm during fixation.

Joint motion and mechanical loading appear to be essential for the maintenance of normal articular cartilage; immobilization rapidly leads to atrophy.

Synovium

The synovial membrane (Figure 12.31C) covers all intra-articular structures except articular cartilage and fibrocartilaginous menisci. It consists of a layer of fibrous or adipose tissue supporting the intima, a surface of synovial lining cells, which broadly fall into two subtypes: macrophage-like cells which are phagocytic and fibroblast-like cells that secrete hyaluronic acid into the synovial fluid. In health this viscous fluid is present in small amounts, acts as a lubricant and is of importance in the nutrition of articular cartilage.

Arthritis

Disorders of the joints are disabling conditions which cause serious morbidity to the affected individual. They are of major economic importance both to the patients, who may have long periods off work, and to society as a whole. Joint replacement is a very common and expensive operation in terms of professional time, bed occupancy and prosthetic materials. Over 40 000 total hip replacements and a similar number of knee replacements are carried out each year in the UK, mostly for osteoarthritis and rheumatoid arthritis. In this section, osteoarthritis, the most common form of joint disease and rheumatoid arthritis, one of the autoimmune diseases, and many other less common forms of inflammatory arthritis will be described. Infections of joints have already been discussed.

Osteoarthritis (Degenerative Joint Disease)

Key Points

- This is the commonest form of arthritis.
- It mainly affects middle-aged and elderly people.
- Weightbearing joints are worst affected.
- It is a disorder of articular cartilage.
- Final common pathway of joint damage.

Osteoarthritis is the commonest chronic joint disease affecting over 2 million people in the UK. It is largely a disease of the elderly affecting at least one joint in two-thirds of the population over 75. It principally affects the large weight-bearing joints (hip, knee) and the joints of the cervical and lower lumbar spine. Osteoarthritis in the young is usually seen only when there is a predisposing cause (Table 12.8). Primary generalized osteoarthritis, often familial and more common in females, affects multiple joints including the interphalangeal joints of the hands. Palpable osteophytes of the distal and proximal interphalangeal joints are known as Heberden's and Bouchard's nodes respectively. Although unsightly, these cause little disability.

TABLE 12.8 Conditions that predispose to osteoarthritis

Underlying joint disorders	Metabolic/endocrine
Intra-articular fracture	Ochronosis (alkaptonuria)
Previous infective arthritis	Haemochromatosis
Rheumatoid or other inflammatory arthritis	Gout
Osteonecrosis including Perthe's disease	
Congenital dislocation of the hip	
Intra-articular corticosteroids in excess	
Abnormal stresses	**Neuropathic disorders**
Malaligned fracture	Peripheral neuropathy
? Chronic over use	Spinal cord disorders e.g. syringomyelia

Clinical Features

Patients complain of pain, relieved by rest, stiffness and sometimes crepitus on movement. Osteoarthritis of the hip often results in a characteristic limp (antalgic gait). Spinal involvement, principally of the intervertebral discs and the posterior apophyseal joints is very common, and gives rise to stiffness, and pain due to compression of nerve roots, particularly in the cervical spine. Bony spurs may compress the vertebral arteries compromising cerebral blood flow.

Pathology

In osteoarthritis changes are seen within the articular cartilage, the underlying bone and, secondarily, within the synovium. An early change is loss of proteoglycan from the superficial zone of articular cartilage. Disruption of the smooth surface of cartilage follows, initially tangential to the surface (flaking) and then extending vertically into the deeper zones (fibrillation); this pattern conforms to the arrangement of collagen fibres previously described. Proliferation of chondrocytes, forming clusters around fissures, and increased proteoglycan synthesis may be regarded as unsuccessful attempts at healing. Progressive loss of articular cartilage occurs by abrasion, with eventual exposure of the underlying bone, which becomes greatly thickened and polished smooth like ivory (eburnation; Figure 12.32). Cystic spaces containing loose fibrous tissue appear in the subchondral bone. Bone remodelling alters the shape of the joint surface. This is particularly obvious in osteoarthritis of the femoral head where the superior weight-bearing surface is flattened. At the margin of the articular cartilage outgrowths of cartilage develop and undergo ossification to become osteophytes. These may cause deformity and limitation of movement.

The synovium may be normal, but is often hypertrophied with mild chronic inflammation. Abraded fragments of bone and cartilage become embedded in the synovium.

Aetiology and Pathogenesis

Osteoarthritis is not a single disease, but is the end result of joint damage from many causes. In the past, osteoarthritis was considered to be a degenerative disease. A more modern approach is to regard it as an active disease process – as the response of a joint to injury. There is both synthesis of new components and loss of existing tissue in the process of remodelling. It is most likely that the primary change in osteoarthritis is an alteration of the chondrocyte activity with a resulting change in the composition of the articular cartilage, in particular of proteoglycans. Local low-grade inflammation appears to be important and there is evidence that cytokines such as IL1 and TNFα act on the chondrocyte causing it to release metalloproteinases which degrade the matrix. Genetic factors are also important: mutations of type II collagen genes are found in some families with osteoarthritis and mutation of the ADAM12 gene (encoding a protease enzyme) also appears to be important.

The reasons for joint destruction in many of the secondary forms of osteoarthritis are easy to understand. Thus, loss of articular cartilage due to previous septic or rheumatoid arthritis or an incongruity of the articular surface due to an intra-articular fracture can readily be accepted as leading to further cartilage damage. Chronic overuse, for example in the knees and ankles of footballers, does appear to contribute to the subsequent development of osteoarthritis.

Neuropathic Arthropathy (Charcot's Joint)

This accelerated form of osteoarthritis occurs in a joint which has lost proprioceptive and pain sensation, for example in diabetes or similar sensory neuropathy, syphilis and syringomyelia (p. 314). The cartilage is destroyed and the bone ends become distorted with formation of very large osteophytes. These and the joint surface may fracture with hyperplastic callus formation. Progressive disorganization of the joint results, the florid changes contrasting with the relative lack of pain.

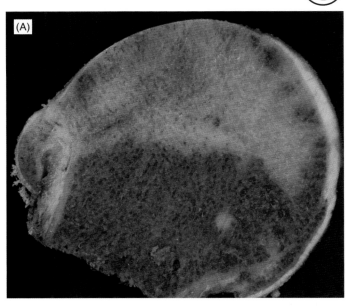

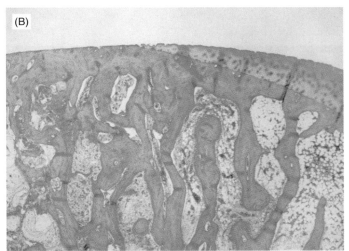

FIGURE 12.32 Osteoarthritis. (A) The articular cartilage is lost from the weightbearing surface of this femoral head; if the acetabular cartilage is similarly lost, then it is easy to see why the joint space becomes narrowed on radiology. The underlying bone so exposed becomes thickened and polished. Osteophytes, protruding pieces of cartilage and bone have formed at the joint margin. (B) The articular cartilage is progressively thinned from right to left and is finally lost completely. To the left of this, bone provides the articular surface and it is noticeably thicker (sclerotic) in this area.

Rheumatoid Arthritis

Key Points

- It an autoimmune disorder with genetic and environmental aetiology.
- Rheumatoid arthritis particularly affects young to middle-aged females.
- It is a multisystem disease.
- It involves primarily inflammation of synovium with secondary joint damage.

In contrast with osteoarthritis, rheumatoid arthritis is a systemic inflammatory disease, the brunt of which usually falls on the joints. It is common, affecting 1% of the adult population, and occurs more often in females. Any age from childhood to old age may be affected, but the onset is typically in the fourth to sixth decades.

Rheumatoid arthritis may involve any synovial joint, but is usually a symmetrical polyarthritis affecting principally the metacarpophalangeal and proximal interphalangeal joints, the wrist, shoulder and knee. Patients complain of pain and stiffness especially in the morning. The affected joints are warm and swollen due to joint effusion and synovial hyperplasia. The onset is usually insidious over weeks or months, but rarely symptoms may develop more acutely over days. In most cases the disease follows a course of repeated, partial or complete remissions and relapses, with further loss of function during each relapse. Less commonly, the disease progresses rapidly with joint destruction and severe disability. Some patients have one episode of arthritis which resolves, and have no further problem.

In 75% of patients, rheumatoid factors (p. 358) can be identified in the serum and synovial fluid. These are antibodies, usually of IgM, IgG and IgA type, which react with the Fc compartment of IgG to form immune complexes. Patients whose serum contains these antibodies are known as seropositive. This is associated with more aggressive disease than those without rheumatoid factors (seronegative). More recently, antibodies against cyclic citrullinated proteins (CCP) appear to be equally sensitive but far more specific than rheumatoid factors for the diagnosis of rheumatoid arthritis.

Pathology

Joint involvement in rheumatoid arthritis is characterized by inflammation and hyperplasia of the synovium followed by destruction of articular structures (Figure 12.33). The synovium is thrown into villous folds often matted together by fibrin; hyperplasia of synovial lining cells occurs. The synovium is infiltrated by lymphocytes and plasma cells; lymphoid aggregates with germinal centres are often seen. Fibrin exudes onto the synovial surface, sometimes forming loose

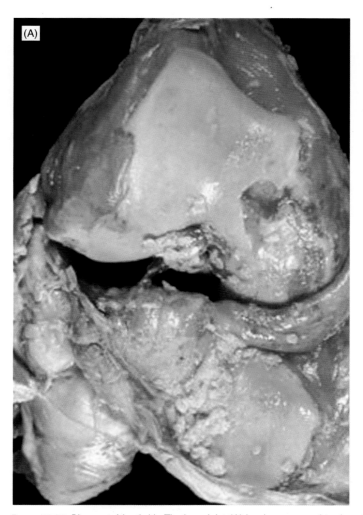

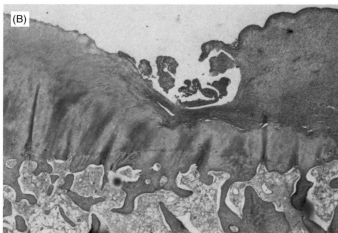

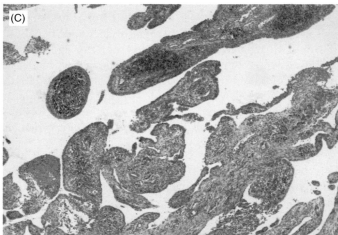

FIGURE 12.33 Rheumatoid arthritis. The knee joint (A) has been opened to show the distal femur whose articular cartilage has been eroded from the periphery by haemosiderin-stained pannus. Low-power microscopy (B) demonstrates that the pannus grows over and erodes the cartilage. The synovium (C) shows a villous architecture, the fronds are densely infiltrated by chronic inflammatory cells and there is fibrinous exudate.

bodies known as rice bodies. Neutrophil polymorphs are present in synovial fluid from inflamed joints but are seen in the superficial synovium in significant numbers only during acute exacerbations.

These changes in the synovium are reversible; however when granulation tissue grows over the surface of the articular cartilage the pannus so formed interferes with the nutrition of cartilage and causes degradation of its matrix. Permanent joint damage now results. Resorption of the subchondral bone gives rise to radiological 'erosions'. If much articular cartilage is lost, granulation tissue from both sides of the joint forms adhesions, followed sometimes by fibrous union (fibrous ankylosis).

Destruction of the joint capsule and tendons, which are eroded by inflamed synovium of tendon sheaths, leads to striking deformities. Ulnar deviation of the fingers is common and dislocation and subluxation lead to characteristic boutonnière and swan-neck deformities. There is atrophy of muscles surrounding the joints (e.g. interossei in the hand), while a combination of disuse atrophy and local hyperaemia leads to loss of bone close to the bone ends (juxta-articular osteoporosis). Involvement of the cervical spine may lead to atlantoaxial subluxation and spinal cord compression. Hyperextension during intubation for general anaesthesia may precipitate neurological damage.

Extra-articular Manifestations

It must be re-emphasized that rheumatoid arthritis is a multisystem disease; although its effects on the joints give rise to much morbidity, there are many extra-articular complications which may be severe and life threatening:

- Vascular and cardiac disease – patients with rheumatoid disease are at much increased risk of vascular disease including atheroma and ischaemic heart disease. Myocarditis and endocarditis are seldom seen.
- Vasculitis – arteritis with fibrinoid necrosis of the vessel wall (p. 120), although uncommon in rheumatoid arthritis, usually affects seropositive patients with severe disease. Immune complex deposition with complement activation is responsible for the damage to the vessel wall. The effects are usually mild with splinter haemorrhages in the nail folds, but gangrene of digits and infarction of viscera occasionally occur. Vasculitis may lead to peripheral neuropathy (p. 322).
- Rheumatoid nodules – these nodules consist of a central area of fibrinoid necrosis surrounded by macrophages (Figure 12.34). Rheumatoid nodules are found in 20–35% of patients with rheumatoid arthritis and are typically located in the subcutaneous tissues over extensor surfaces such as the olecranon process. They may also be seen in the viscera. Rheumatoid nodules develop in patients who are usually seropositive; their presence often indicates a more aggressive course.
- Pulmonary disease (p. 170) – diffuse pulmonary fibrosis may occur in RA. Rheumatoid nodules are occasionally found in the lung. Rarely, patients with rheumatoid arthritis and pneumoconiosis develop large rheumatoid nodules with central breakdown and widespread fibrosis. This is known as Caplan's syndrome. The incidence of this complication has diminished with that of pneumoconiosis.
- Serosal inflammation – pericarditis and pleurisy are common.
- Amyloidosis – rheumatoid arthritis is one of the most common causes of secondary amyloidosis (p. 389).
- Anaemia – like many chronic diseases, rheumatoid arthritis is often complicated by microcytic hypochromic anaemia (anaemia of chronic disease p. 209), while non-steroidal anti-inflammatory drugs may produce acute erosive gastritis, repeated minor episodes of gastrointestinal blood loss and iron deficiency.
- Felty's syndrome – less than 1% of patients with rheumatoid arthritis, usually those with other extra-articular manifestations, develop splenomegaly with hypersplenism and leucopenia which may lead to infections.
- Eye involvement – keratoconjunctivitis sicca as part of Sjögren's syndrome (p. 229) is the commonest ocular complication of rheumatoid arthritis. Inflammation of the sclera (scleritis) may lead to perforation of the globe (scleromalacia perforans). Histologically, this is characterized by fibrinoid necrosis of collagen with surrounding histiocytes, a reaction similar to rheumatoid nodules (p. 357).

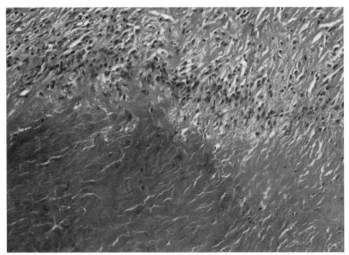

FIGURE 12.34 Rheumatoid nodule. The lower half of the illustration consists of necrobiotic collagen with basophilic (blue) staining. Above, and surrounding this, is a reaction of histiocytic cells whose nuclei are oriented in a parallel manner known as palisading.

Aetiology and Pathogenesis

Despite much research, the cause of rheumatoid arthritis remains unknown. This is a complex problem and only a simplified account can be given. Rheumatoid arthritis is an autoimmune disorder affecting individuals with a genetic predisposition who are exposed to an appropriate antigenic stimulus. Once initiated, the disease appears to

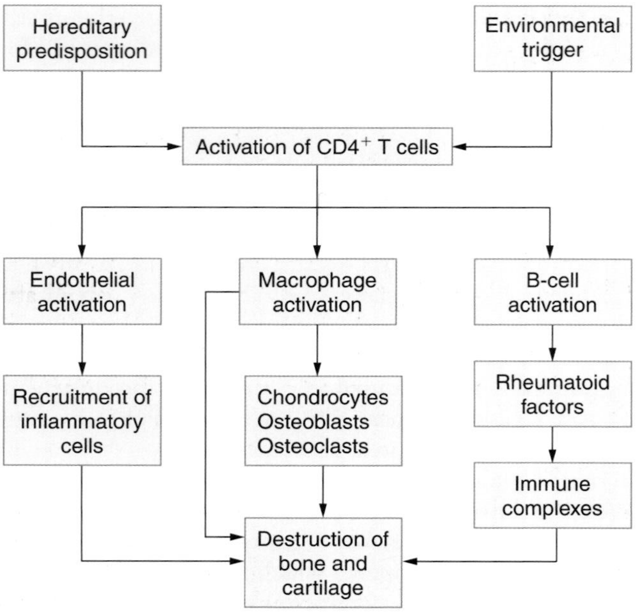

FIGURE 12.35 Pathogenesis of rheumatoid arthritis.

be self-perpetuating, usually resulting in joint destruction. A summary of the mechanisms thought to be responsible is given in Figure 12.35.

Genetic Predisposition

It has long been known that rheumatoid arthritis has a familial tendency, but that not all members of a family are affected. Susceptibility to rheumatoid arthritis is associated with certain alleles of the class II major histocompatibility complex (MHC) (see p. 24) particularly human leucocyte antigen (HLA)-DRB1. Class II MHC molecules are expressed on the surface of antigen presenting cells and are essential for recognition of antigen by T cells.

Initiating Factors

The trigger for the development of rheumatoid arthritis has not been identified. It is possible that a variety of different antigenic stimuli may be responsible. The prime suspects have been infective agents, in particular viruses such as Epstein–Barr virus and human parvovirus B19, but evidence that rheumatoid arthritis is started by an infection is circumstantial. Endogenous antigens may be responsible for triggering rheumatoid arthritis. Autoantibodies directed against IgG (rheumatoid factors) and type II collagen are found in the serum and synovial fluid of many patients with rheumatoid arthritis, but there is no convincing evidence that these initiate the disease.

Development of Synovitis

The earliest pathological change found in rheumatoid synovium is a perivascular accumulation of T lymphocytes (principally CD4 positive). Synovial lining cells and macrophages process antigen and present it to T lymphocytes which then proliferate. T cells activate macrophages, stimulate proliferation of endothelial cells (angiogenesis) and

also activate B cells. These differentiate into plasma cells, which produce antibodies including rheumatoid factors. In this way the synovial membrane mass is greatly increased with an extensive network of new blood vessels, an accumulation of T cells, B cells, plasma cells and macrophages.

Destruction of Joint Structures

The irreversible destruction of the joint occurs when the proliferating synovium invades articular cartilage, subchondral bone, tendons and joint capsule. Synovial cells and macrophages produce proteolytic enzymes such as collagenase and stromelysin, which are capable of destroying the matrix proteins of cartilage and bone. They also produce cytokines such as TNFα and IL1, which appear to be particularly important in joint damage; anticytokine therapies are now widely used. Under cytokine influence chondrocytes reduce their production of intercellular matrix and secrete enzymes which break down existing matrix. Immune complexes formed by rheumatoid factors and IgG activate complement (p. 22) which contributes to tissue damage. Chemotactic factors such as C5a and leukotriene B4 attract neutrophil polymorphs into the synovial fluid. These cells degranulate with the release of proteinases, which participate in the destruction of articular cartilage. Erosion of subchondral bone, is largely attributable to activation of osteoclasts by cytokines such as RANK ligand (p. 332) rather than by direct proteolytic action.

Juvenile Rheumatoid Arthritis (Still's Disease)

This disease differs in several ways from adult rheumatoid arthritis. By definition the disorder commences below the age of 16, most commonly between 1 and 3 years. Patients often present with involvement of a few joints, or with severe systemic disease which may precede development of arthritis. These patients have a high spiking fever, often with daily or twice daily elevations of temperature, accompanied by a distinctive macular rash seen on the trunk, proximal limbs and over pressure areas. There may be hepatosplenomegaly, lymphadenopathy or serosal inflammation, especially pericarditis.

Juvenile rheumatoid arthritis generally involves the knees, wrists, elbows and ankles. Involvement of the cervical spine and sacroiliac joints are common. Most patients are seronegative. Other features include growth retardation and chronic uveitis which may lead to blindness. The pathological features resemble those seen in adult rheumatoid arthritis. The disease often persists into adult life or it may go into spontaneous remission.

Seronegative Arthritis

Key Points

- There is sacroiliac and spinal involvement as well as the peripheral joints.
- Patients often have uveitis and aortitis.
- There is a strong association with HLA-B27.

This term is applied to a group of inflammatory poly-arthritides in which tests for rheumatoid factor are negative and which tend to involve the sacroiliac joints and the spine (spondylitis) as well as peripheral joints. The group includes ankylosing spondylitis, psoriatic arthropathy, reactive arthritis and arthritis associated with Crohn's disease and ulcerative colitis, but excludes cases of seronegative rheumatoid arthritis.

Association with HLA-B27

There is a strong association between seronegative arthritis with sacroiliac involvement and the histocompatability antigen HLA-B27. About 8% of a general Caucasian population possess this antigen, whereas over 90% of patients with ankylosing spondylitis, 70–90% with Reiter's syndrome and 50–70% with psoriatic arthropathy are positive. Patients homozygous for HLA-B27 tend to have more severe disease.

Ankylosing Spondylitis

This is now recognized to be a common disorder with a prevalence of 0.5–1% in Western populations, although in many cases, especially in women, symptoms are mild and recognition depends on radiological changes. Patients, often with a family history and typically in their early twenties, complain of persistent sacroiliac and lumbar pain with limitation of movement. The onset is usually insidious. As many as 20% of patients present with symptoms of pain and swelling relating to asymmetrical involvement of the peripheral joints especially of the lower limbs; during the course of the disease a further 15% develop similar problems. The condition is usually self-limiting but in a minority progresses until the spine is fused (bamboo spine). When the cervical spine is involved, atlanto-axial dislocation may occur and care must be exercised during anaesthesia.

Pathology

Ankylosing spondylitis is characterized by inflammation occurring at the sites of insertion of ligaments into bone, the joint capsule and fibres of the annulus fibrosus. The site of ligamentous insertion is the enthesis, and the resultant disease is known as enthesopathy. Inflammation is followed by fibrosis and ossification, particularly around intervertebral discs, with the formation of bridging spurs of bone (syndesmophytes), the apophyseal and sacroiliac joints, and sometimes the costovertebral joints. The synovitis histologically resembles that seen in rheumatoid arthritis. Bony ankylosis is more common than in rheumatoid arthritis, and may affect large joints, particularly the hips.

Extra-articular manifestations

Patients with ankylosing spondylitis may lose weight and develop low-grade fever with a high erythrocyte sedimentation rate (ESR). Uveitis (p. 325) occurs in a quarter of cases, and a similar proportion develop aortitis with aortic incompetence (p. 148). Although chest expansion is often restricted, pulmonary ventilation is usually well maintained. Diffuse bilateral upper lobe fibrosis, of uncertain aetiology, is a well-recognized late complication.

Other Sero-negative Arthritides

Reactive arthritis

This term describes non-infective arthritis which follows infections elsewhere. Reiter's syndrome was defined as the triad of arthritis, conjunctivitis and urethritis, but the spectrum of reactive arthritis is broader and may follow infections with *Shigella*, *Salmonella*, *Yersinia* and *Campylobacter*. Post-venereal reactive arthritis associated with non-specific urethritis due to *Chlamydia* or *Mycoplasma* is much more common in males. The arthritis typically affects the large weightbearing joints, the hands, feet and spine, and is often persistent or recurrent. Insertional tendonitis affecting the Achilles tendon and plantar fascia are common.

Psoriatic arthropathy

Approximately 10% of patients with psoriasis (p. 479) develop an associated arthritis, typically affecting a few joints with an asymmetrical distribution. The distal interphalangeal joints of the hands and feet, knees, hips, ankles and wrists are commonly involved. In a few patients inflammation is restricted largely to the distal interphalangeal joints, commonly associated with pitting of the nails due to psoriasis, and rarely progressing to osteolysis of the affected phalanges (arthritis mutilans). Sacroiliac and spinal involvement occurs in up to 40% of patients. Pathologically the changes in the synovium resemble those of rheumatoid arthritis.

Arthritis in inflammatory bowel disease

Peripheral and spinal arthritis can be found in patients with Crohn's disease and ulcerative colitis.

Haemophilic Arthropathy

Patients with haemophilia (p. 39) are at risk of repeated episodes of intra-articular haemorrhage (haemarthrosis) and ultimately chronic destructive arthritis. The knees, ankles, elbows, shoulders and hips are most often affected. The joint becomes chronically swollen, with limitation of movement.

Pathologically, the synovium becomes grossly hyperplastic and laden with haemosiderin. There is invasion and erosion of articular cartilage from the margin, and changes of osteoarthritis develop. Many chondrocytes contain haemosiderin; it appears that accumulation of iron is of major importance in the pathogenesis of haemophilic arthropathy, both by its effect on chondrocyte metabolism and also by stimulating synovial proliferation.

Arthritis due to Deposition of Crystals

Gout

Key Points

- The cause is excess levels of uric acid.
- There may be acute or chronic arthritis.
- Crystals are identified on joint aspiration.
- There is accumulation of urates, known as tophi.

Gout is an arthritis resulting from deposition of uric acid crystals. Gout particularly affects middle-aged men; less than 10% of patients are women, usually post-menopausal women. It is usually associated with hyperuricaemia, defined as an elevated serum urate concentration greater than 7 mg/dL (0.5 mmol/L), but occasionally the serum urate level may be normal during an attack. Most hyperuricaemic patients remain asymptomatic; the proportion developing clinical gout increases with the serum urate level. Gout may cause an acute arthritis, or in longstanding cases may lead to a chronic destructive arthritis. Asymptomatic hyperuricaemia is strongly associated with hypertension, cardiovascular disease and the insulin resistance syndrome.

Acute gout

One or more joints are affected and are exquisitely painful, red and swollen. In over half of patients the metatarsophalangeal joint of the big toe is the first joint to be affected (podagra); this is probably explicable on the grounds that the lower temperature of the extremities reduces the solubility of urates. Dietary or alcoholic excess, drugs, trauma or surgery often precipitate attacks, usually starting at night and lasting for a few days or weeks. Examination of fluid aspirated from an involved joint shows many inflammatory cells, particularly neutrophil polymorphs and large numbers of needle-shaped crystals within and outside cells. Neutrophils phagocytose urate crystals and release lysosomal enzymes. Complement is activated and other mediators of inflammation such as leukotrienes and prostaglandins are released, with further chemotaxis for neutrophils. Macrophages are also involved: they release cytokines such as IL1, TNFα and IL8.

Chronic 'tophaceous' gout

Chronic 'tophaceous' gout is associated with the formation of crystalline deposits (tophi) of sodium biurate particularly in fibrous tissue and hyaline and fibrocartilage (Figure 12.36). Microscopy shows sheaves of urate crystals surrounded by foreign body giant cells and histiocytes; when viewed in polarized light they are seen to be strongly negatively birefringent. Tophi are found in the pinna of the ear, in articular cartilage with associated degenerative changes and in periarticular structures. Subchondral and subperiosteal deposition gives rise to punched-out lytic erosions in bone.

Aetiology

Hyperuricaemia is due to increased production of uric acid or to decreased urinary excretion, or both. Gout may be classified as primary or secondary.

Primary gout represents those patients who do not have another disorder causing hyperuricaemia. It is clear that there is a genetic predisposition – it has long been known that there is a familial tendency. In most cases decreased urinary excretion is responsible. Even in this group there are predisposing factors including obesity, hypertriglyceridaemia, a diet rich in purines and excessive alcohol consumption. In a few cases specific enzyme disorders have been recognized. Increased activity of 5 phosphoribosyl-1-pyrophosphate synthetase

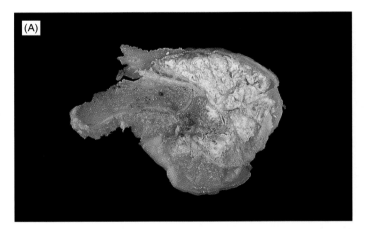

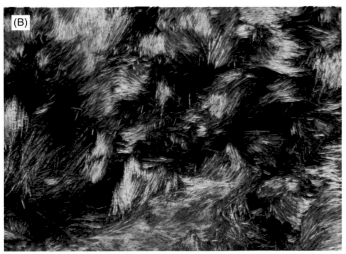

FIGURE 12.36 Gout. (A) This small toe was amputated for persistent pain. Cut section shows extensive deposition of chalky, white crystalline material within the distal phalanx and in adjacent soft tissue. On polarization microscopy (B), large sheaves of brilliantly birefringent crystals are seen.

(PRPP) and decreased hypoxanthine-guanine phosphoribosyl transferase (HGPRT) activity (Lesch–Nyhan syndrome), both result in increased urate production. Both of these extremely rare disorders are X-linked.

Secondary gout refers to those cases which develop during the course of another disease. Patients with malignancy, particularly leukaemia or myeloproliferative disorders treated by chemotherapy, without uricosuric cover commonly develop gout as a consequence of increased purine catabolism. Many drugs including thiazide diuretics interfere with renal excretion of uric acid.

Calcium Pyrophosphate Deposition Disease (Pseudogout)

Calcium pyrophosphate crystals are commonly deposited in the cartilage and juxta-articular tissues of the elderly; at least a third of those over 80 are affected. Calcium pyrophosphate deposition disease may be sporadic or familial; it may be secondary to underlying conditions including hyperparathyroidism, hypothyroidism and haemochromatosis. When the condition is recognized in younger patients a cause should be

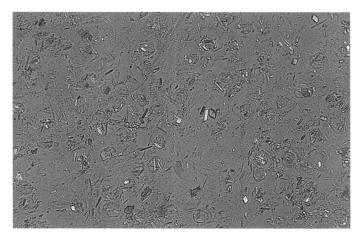

FIGURE 12.37 Pseudogout. Numerous rod-shaped crystals can be seen on polarization microscopy in fluid aspirated from the knee of an elderly man.

and give pain relief. Most prostheses are manufactured from largely inert metallic alloys and high-molecular weight polyethylene, and are anchored to the skeleton by acrylic cement or by ingrowth of bone or fibrous tissue into the prostheses. Implants made from silicone polymers are often used to replace small joints in the hands, usually in rheumatoid arthritis.

Unfortunately, in some patients the prosthesis becomes loose. This is often due to mechanical loosening in which friction between the components of the prosthesis results in fine wear products of metal or polyethylene. These, like fragments of acrylic cement, induce a reaction of macrophages and foreign body giant cells (Figure 12.38) which stimulate osteoclasts to resorb bone. As the prosthesis loosens, a vicious cycle is established. Patients may experience considerable pain and insertion of a larger prosthesis (revision arthroplasty) is often required.

sought. Mutations of the *ANKH* gene have been found in some patients with sporadic and familial disease. Calcium pyrophosphate deposition disease and osteoarthritis often coexist.

Both acute crystal synovitis and chronic deposition may occur. Acute attacks (pseudogout) lasting days to weeks may affect one or several joints, most commonly the knee. Surgery or illness may precipitate an attack. Synovial fluid contains abundant neutrophils and rhomboid and rod-shaped crystals (Figure 12.37), which show weak positive birefringence.

Chronic deposition within the menisci, articular cartilage, ligaments, tendons and joint capsule is detectable on plain radiographs as small calcified foci, an appearance known as chondrocalcinosis. The knees, hips, symphysis pubis and intervertebral discs are often affected. Although usually asymptomatic, some individuals develop subacute or chronic synovitis with morning stiffness. A white chalky precipitate is seen, while microscopy shows clusters of rod and tablet crystals.

Basic Calcium Phosphate (Calcium Apatite) Crystal Deposition Disease

Acute and chronic syndromes such as tendonitis and bursitis may occur in response to deposition of calcium apatite crystals. An erosive arthritis has also been described affecting various joints; crystals may be identified in the synovial fluid. A rapidly progressive destructive arthritis of the shoulder (so-called 'Milwaukee shoulder'), particularly affects elderly women.

Other Joint Disorders

Pathology of Joint Replacement

The management of patients with arthritis was revolutionized in the early 1960s by the development of low-friction arthroplasties (artificial joints) which can restore mobility

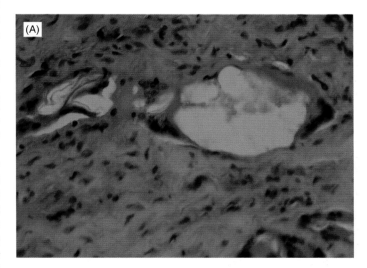

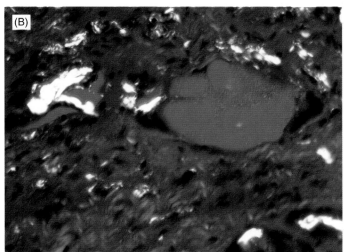

FIGURE 12.38 Reaction to a joint prosthesis. (A) Foreign body giant cells surround a pool of acrylic cement (right) and fragments of high-molecular-weight polyethylene (left). On polarization (B), the cement is not birefringent, but unsuspectedly large amounts of polyethylene are revealed.

Infection remains an important complication. It may occur in the first few months after surgery due to wound contamination, or appears insidiously years later due to haematogenous spread of organisms. Once established, deep infection is very difficult to eradicate and it may be necessary to remove the prosthesis. Coagulase positive and negative staphylococci and coliforms are often responsible, while organisms of low virulence, including anaerobes, may be cultured, sometimes with difficulty.

Rarely cancers, typically high-grade sarcomas, may arise in relation to joint prostheses, usually after several years. In view of the large numbers of operations performed, the risk to the individual is very small indeed.

Intra-articular Loose Bodies

Multiple soft loose bodies (rice or melon-seed bodies) formed from fibrin or necrotic synovium are found in tuberculous or rheumatoid arthritis. Hard loose bodies may cause repeated episodes of locking of the joint, and damage to the articular cartilage resulting in osteoarthritis. In synovial chondromatosis multiple nodules of cartilage form by metaplasia in the synovial membrane and may become ossified. Some nodules become detached and lie free in the synovial fluid. In osteochondritis dissecans (p. 341), the loose body consists of articular cartilage and underlying necrotic bone. Fracture of marginal osteophytes in osteoarthritis may occur, particularly in neuropathic joints. Rarely intra-articular fractures may result in loose bodies.

Tenosynovial Giant Cell Tumour (Pigmented Villonodular Synovitis)

This benign proliferative lesion of synovium occurs in two distinct clinical settings. Localized nodular synovitis presents as a firm, nodular swelling on the finger, often in women between 30 and 50 years. It consists of a lobulated nodule arising from tendon sheath or joint and contains giant cells and groups of histiocytes containing abundant haemosiderin and lipid, which impart a tan colour. The lesion occasionally recurs, particularly if there is diffuse involvement of the adjacent synovium, and may erode bone. Occasionally similar nodules are found in large joints alone or associated with diffuse pigmented villonodular synovitis (PVNS).

Diffuse PVNS most often involves the knee or hip joint causing pain, blood-stained effusion or locking of the joint. The synovium is thrown up into hyperplastic pigmented villi which become matted together to form solid nodular masses. The enlarged villi are covered by hyperplastic synovial cells and contain numerous macrophages containing haemosiderin and lipid. The diffuse form of PVNS is more difficult to eradicate, and tends to recur. Bone may be eroded especially in cases involving the hip joint (Figure 12.39).

In the past PVNS was thought to be an inflammatory or reactive condition, but is now more commonly regarded as a neoplasm; rare malignant forms are seen, supporting this view.

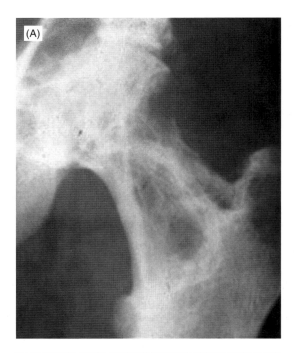

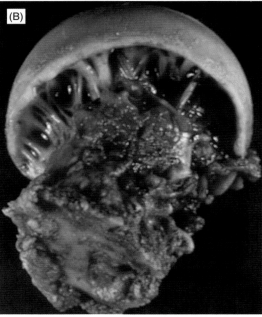

FIGURE 12.39 Tenosynovial giant cell tumour (pigmented villonodular synovitis). The radiograph of the left hip (A) and gross photograph of the resected specimen (B) show extensive erosion of the bone of the neck and inferior surface of the head of the femur. The lesional tissue is brown/tan and multinodular.

Ganglia

These common lesions occur in the soft tissue around joints or tendon sheaths, most often on the dorsum of the wrist. They develop by myxoid change in fibrous tissue with formation of thin-walled cysts containing clear glairy fluid. Sometimes there is a communication between the ganglion and an adjacent joint. Similar lesions may occur within the periosteum and sometimes within bone (intra-osseous ganglion).

Cyst of Semi-lunar Cartilage

Myxoid change may occur in the loose fibrous tissue adjacent to the lateral meniscus or in the meniscus itself resulting in a lesion histologically identical to a ganglion.

Bursitis

A bursa is a synovial lined sac, and is found chiefly over bony prominences. It may communicate with a joint and is subject to the same disorders. Repeated mild trauma may result in inflammation (as for instance in prepatellar bursitis – housemaid's knee).

Amyloidosis

Deposition of amyloid is commonly found in the synovium and degenerate articular cartilage in elderly patients who do not have systemic amyloidosis. It is of little significance; the amyloid appears to be derived from a plasma protein transthyretin. Deposition of amyloid of β_2-microglobulin origin within the synovium, articular cartilage and adjacent bone may be found in patients on long-term haemodialysis (p. 374).

SOFT TISSUE TUMOURS AND TUMOUR-LIKE LESIONS

Soft tissue tumours arise from skeletal muscle, fat and fibrous tissue and the blood vessels and nerves supplying them. They are classified on the basis of the adult tissue they resemble although they arise not from differentiated tissues but from primitive mesenchymal cells.

Most soft tissue tumours are benign, and are usually small, superficially situated lesions such as lipomas. In contrast, soft-tissue sarcomas are typically large tumours within the deep soft tissues of the limbs and retroperitoneum. Soft tissue sarcomas are a heterogeneous group of tumours of varying histological type and biological behaviour. Although uncommon they cause considerable morbidity and mortality; for this reason they are discussed at greater length than their frequency alone would warrant. Fibromatoses are a group of infiltrative and recurrent lesions which do not metastasize. A small but important group of benign reactive conditions tend to grow rapidly and may be confused histologically with sarcomas. Tumours of peripheral nerve are discussed on p. 319, those of blood vessels on p. 133, and fibrous histiocytoma and dermatofibrosarcoma protuberans on p. 504.

Benign Tumours

Lipoma

This common, slowly growing tumour is typically found in the subcutaneous tissues of the back, shoulder and neck, and the proximal parts of the limbs in patients over 40, and is usually painless. Less commonly, lipomas of deep soft tissue grow to considerable size and cause symptoms due to pressure. The pathologist must examine these tumours very carefully; some well-differentiated liposarcomas with locally aggressive behaviour closely resemble lipomas histologically. Lipomas are lobulated, encapsulated masses of mature adipose tissue. There are a number of histological variants, for example angiolipomas which contain numerous thin-walled capillaries and may be painful, especially when microthrombi form within their rich vascular network.

Leiomyoma

Benign smooth muscle tumours are much more common in the uterus (p. 409) than in soft tissue. There are three main types. Cutaneous leiomyomas arise from erector pili muscles and are usually multiple and painful. Genital leiomyomas for example arising from dartos muscle in the scrotum are usually solitary and painless, while vascular leiomyomas originate from abnormal thick-walled veins and typically form painful lumps in the legs of middle-aged patients particularly women. Leiomyomas consist of spindle-shaped cells that closely resemble normal smooth muscle cells.

Malignant Tumours

General Features

Most soft tissue sarcomas are well-circumscribed masses in deep soft tissue (Figure 12.40). Although they may appear to be encapsulated, there is microscopic invasion of the surrounding tissues; surgical 'shelling out' of the tumour is almost inevitably followed by local recurrence. The prognosis depends on several factors. The risk of local recurrence is largely related to the adequacy of surgical removal, which itself depends on the anatomical site and the skill of

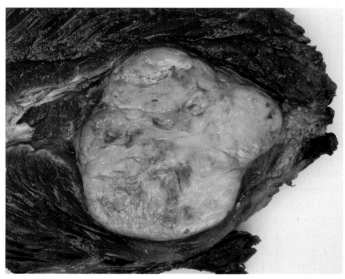

FIGURE 12.40 High-grade sarcoma. This tumour arising in the right vastus intermedialis was resected *en bloc*. The apparent degree of circumscription is deceptive as the tumour had an infiltrative pattern on histology.

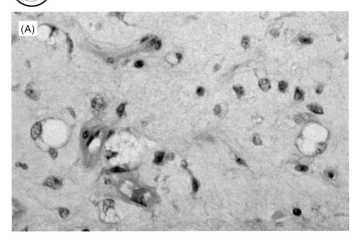

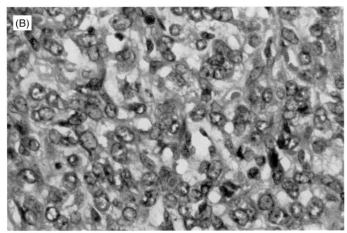

FIGURE 12.41 Myxoid/round cell liposarcoma. Myxoid liposarcoma consists of small cells in a loose myxoid background with occasional cells whose vacuolated cytoplasm contains lipid (A). Round cell liposarcoma (B) consists of closely packed and more hyperchromatic cells, some showing vacuolation. Within one tumour these two patterns may be seen as in this case. The round cell component confers a much worse prognosis.

the surgeon. Thus, a tumour confined to a single muscle compartment in the thigh may be completely removed by a 'compartmental excision' while it may be impossible to excise with a covering of normal tissue a retroperitoneal tumour or one in the popliteal fossa. Factors influencing the risk of metastases include the histological grade, extent of necrosis of tumour, size and anatomical location. There are several different histological grading systems. High-grade tumours tend to metastasize early, while low-grade lesions give problems largely from local recurrence or extension. In general the more superficial a tumour and the smaller it is, the better the prognosis.

Histological typing of sarcomas is often difficult. Even with modern techniques such as immunocytochemistry, electron microscopy and molecular and cytogenetic analysis precise histological typing is often difficult; around 5% of tumours can only be reported as 'sarcoma of uncertain histogenesis'. With few exceptions the grade of a tumour is more important than its histological type in determining prognosis. The value of cytogenetic analysis is discussed below.

Liposarcoma

Liposarcoma occurs mainly in the deep soft tissue of limbs or in the retroperitoneum in patients over 50. Several histological subtypes are described which show varying degrees of differentiation towards adipose tissue. Well-differentiated liposarcoma is a low-grade tumour which rarely metastasizes, unless it becomes associated with a high-grade non-adipose component, so-called dedifferentiated liposarcoma. Myxoid and round cell liposarcomas form a spectrum from low-grade to high-grade tumours (Figure 12.41); they share the same chromosomal translocation (p. 366). Pleomorphic liposarcomas are highly malignant tumours with early pulmonary metastases.

Rhabdomyosarcoma

While rhabdomyosarcoma is the commonest soft tissue tumour of childhood and adolescence, it is rare in older patients. Three main histological types are recognized.

Embryonal rhabdomyosarcoma occurs mainly in children, in the head and neck, genitourinary tract and retroperitoneum. Tumours occurring in the vagina or bladder project as grape-like gelatinous masses and are known as 'botryoid' (grape-like) sarcomas. They consist of spindle-shaped cells and show varying degrees of skeletal muscle differentiation. Embryonal rhabdomyosarcoma usually responds well to combined chemotherapy, radiotherapy and surgery.

Alveolar rhabdomyosarcomas occur in adolescents, particularly arising in skeletal muscle of the limbs. Tumour cells adhere to fibrous septa which divide the cells into clumps; loss of cohesion in the centre of the groups produces an alveolar pattern (Figure 12.42). The prognosis of this group of tumours remains poor. Pleomorphic rhabdomyosarcomas are very rare and occur chiefly in the skeletal muscles of older people. It is often difficult to separate this group from other pleomorphic sarcomas.

Immunohistochemical staining for muscle specific proteins, for example the intermediate filament desmin and myo-D_1, a nuclear protein expressed early in skeletal muscle differentiation, and electron microscopy to show thick and thin (myosin and actin) filaments help make a definite diagnosis.

Leiomyosarcoma

This tumour usually affects the middle aged and elderly. About half of soft tissue leiomyosarcomas arise in the retroperitoneum and have a poor prognosis; less than 30% of patients survive 5 years. Of the remainder most are found in the dermis or subcutaneous tissue. In keeping

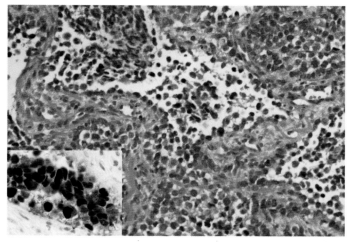

FIGURE 12.42 Alveolar rhabdomyosarcoma. The tumour is composed of sheets of round cells which show central discohesion with the formation of an alveolar or honeycomb pattern. Insert (lower left) shows that the nuclei stain with an antibody directed against myogenin, a nuclear regulatory protein involved in skeletal muscle differentiation, helping to confirm the diagnosis.

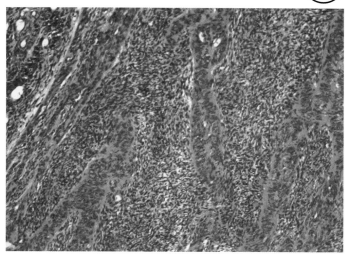

FIGURE 12.43 Biphasic synovial sarcoma. As the name suggests, there are two patterns to this tumour, namely well-differentiated glandular structures and closely packed spindle-shaped cells.

with other superficially situated sarcomas the prognosis for these tumours is better; over 90% of patients with dermal tumours and 65% with subcutaneous lesions survive 5 years. Histologically, leiomyosarcomas consist of spindle-shaped cells resembling normal smooth muscle cells which are arranged in long interlacing fascicles. Many tumours express desmin and smooth muscle actin. The principal criterion in distinguishing malignant and benign smooth muscle tumours is the number of mitotic figures. Nuclear pleomorphism without mitotic activity may be found in leiomyomas.

Malignant Fibrous Histiocytoma

This is an aggressive tumour with a high risk of recurrence and metastasis, and a poor prognosis, particularly when sited in the retroperitoneum. The distinctive histological feature is a 'storiform' pattern where cells are arranged in short bundles from a central point, likened to a cartwheel. There are several subtypes. Its histogenesis is uncertain, but it is best regarded as an undifferentiated high-grade sarcoma as is its counterpart in bone (p. 351).

Synovial Sarcoma

Despite its name this tumour is not a tumour of synovium. It is typically found adjacent to, but not in, large joints of adolescents and young adults. Sometimes the lesion has been present for many years and may have recently increased in size. Historically, the entity was defined by a biphasic pattern of a spindle-cell sarcoma with groups of epithelial cells arranged in acini and tubules (Figure 12.43). Later it was recognized that some tumours consisted of spindle cells alone; these are regarded as monophasic synovial sarcoma which contain individual cells which express epithelial antigens. A characteristic translocation, t(x;18), has been found in synovial sarcoma and this has led to a broadening of the range of histological appearances. Synovial sarcoma is an aggressive tumour, with metastases in 50–70% of patients, often many years after diagnosis.

Fibromatosis

This term includes several fibrous lesions which have a tendency to infiltrate adjacent tissues and to recur, but which do not metastasize.

Palmar fibromatosis (Dupuytren's contracture) begins as a firm nodule in the palm of middle aged and elderly patients and in time extends to form subcutaneous bands which produce flexion contractures, especially of the fourth and fifth fingers. Histologically, the palmar aponeurosis is expanded by multiple nodules of proliferating myofibroblasts. In time these nodules become heavily collagenized and poorly cellular. Similar lesions may occur in the sole of the foot, usually without contracture (plantar fibromatosis) or in the penis (Peyronie's disease).

Musculo-aponeurotic fibromatosis is seen typically in the muscles of the shoulder and pelvic girdles and in the thigh where it forms a firm mass which infiltrates widely through muscle, often further than can be identified at surgery. For this reason complete excision is difficult and repeated recurrences are common, sometimes with involvement of major structures such as the brachial plexus. Recently, it has been suggested that conservative surgery, perhaps supplemented by low-dose chemotherapy or radiotherapy, is as successful as attempts at radical surgery. Abdominal desmoids are similar lesions seen in the rectus abdominis of women during or after pregnancy but tend to be smaller, less aggressive and less likely to recur.

CHROMOSOMAL REARRANGEMENTS IN SARCOMAS

Over the past two decades, it has emerged from cytogenetic analysis of tumour specimens that many soft tissue sarcomas have characteristic chromosomal rearrangements. This finding is important for several reasons:

- Detection of a known translocation, either by cell culture and examination of chromosomes (karyotyping) or by molecular genetic techniques, may establish or confirm a precise histological diagnosis in a case where there may be diagnostic difficulty.
- More accurate staging is made possible by the identification of small numbers of occult tumour cells, for example in bone marrow biopsies or pleural fluids by molecular techniques such as reverse transcription time polymerase chain reaction (RT-PCR) which are much more sensitive than light microscopy.
- Some translocations found in a given tumour type appear to be associated with a better prognosis than examples of the tumour with a different rearrangement. For example, within synovial sarcomas, the translocation involving the *SSX1* gene correlates with a worse outcome than that with the *SSX2* gene (see Table 12.9 below).
- A more robust classification of tumours is possible. Demonstration that two histologically different tumours share the same translocation indicates that they may be part of a single biological entity. For example, the myxoid and round cell forms of liposarcoma have a very different prognosis. The demonstration of t(12;16)(q13;p11) in examples of each, together with the long-known phenomenon of round cell transformation affecting myxoid liposarcoma, indicates that the two represent the opposite ends of a spectrum. As a corollary, if two tumours thought to be closely related, for example clear cell sarcoma and malignant melanoma, do not share the same translocation, then their postulated relationship can be refuted.

- Through detection of these abnormalities much can be learned about the underlying molecular oncogenic mechanisms in these tumours.
- Finally, it is likely that through understanding these mechanisms, new targeted therapies can be designed which may have more antitumour effects than conventional cytotoxic therapies.

Table 12.9 details some of the better recognized tumours, their translocations and the underlying genetic effects. A characteristic feature is the production of hybrid genes, which encode fusion protein products. These typically act as aberrant transcriptional regulators, and promote tumour cell growth.

Ewing's Sarcoma and the *EWS* Gene

The first consistent translocation demonstrated in a sarcoma was t(11;22)(q24;q12) in Ewing's tumour (Figure 12.44). This was important because it established that a group of malignant tumours composed of small round blue cells, namely Ewing's tumour of bone and of soft tissue, so-called Askin tumour of the chest wall, and primitive neuroectodermal tumours of bone and soft tissue were all variants of the same tumour type. This kinship also established that Ewing's tumour, whose histogenesis was unknown, was a neuroectodermal tumour showing varying degrees of differentiation.

The translocation t(11;22) is found in 85% of cases of Ewing's tumour. In this rearrangement the 5′ end of the *EWS* gene on chromosome 22 fuses with the 3′ end of the *FLI1* gene on chromosome 11. *FLI1* encodes a transcription factor: the hybrid gene produces a chimeric protein which functions as an aberrant transcription factor with effects on a number of downstream genes, including some involved in apoptosis. In this way, the hybrid gene can be regarded as an oncogene. Subsequently, a number of other genes related to *FLI1* (members of the ETS group of transcription factors) have been shown to be involved in variant translocations in

TABLE 12.9 Commoner sarcomas with characteristic translocations

Tumour	Translocation	Fusion Product
Alveolar rhabdomyosarcoma	t(2;13)(q35;q14)	PAX3-FKHR
Alveolar soft part sarcoma	t(X;17)(p11;q25)	ASPL-TFE3
Clear cell sarcoma	t(12;22)(q13;q12)	ESW-ATF1
Dermatofibrosarcoma protuberans	t(17;22)(q22;q13)	COL1A1-PDGFβ
Desmoplastic small round cell tumour	t(11;22)(p13;q12)	EWS-WT1
Ewing's sarcoma	t(11;22)(q24;q12)	EWS-FLI1
Myxoid chondrosarcoma	t(9;22)(q22;q12)	EWS-CHN
Myxoid liposarcoma	t(12;16)(q13;p11)	TLS-CHOP
Synovial sarcoma	t(X;18)(p11;q11)	SYT-SSX1 or -SX2

SPECIAL STUDY TOPIC CONTINUED . . .

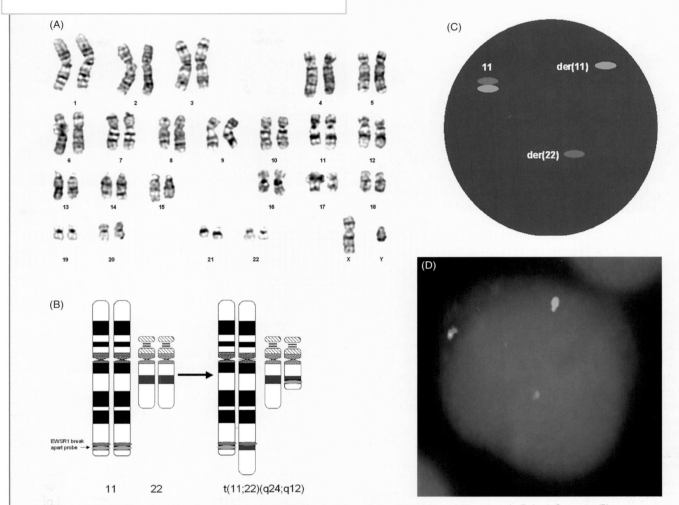

FIGURE 12.44 (A) Karyotype showing a reciprocal translocation between chromosomes 11 and 22 as seen in Ewing's Sarcoma. (B) Chromosome ideograms showing the t(11;22) translocation with chromosome 11 in black and 22 in blue. The red and green regions represent the EWSR1 break apart probe (Vysis) for the Ewing's gene. (C) Diagram showing interphase FISH pattern with the split signal indicating a translocation involving the Ewing's gene. (D) Interphase FISH image showing the pattern illustrated in C.

Ewing's tumour, for example the translocation t(11;22) (q24;q12) with an EWS-ERG fusion product.

Perhaps more interestingly, the *EWS* gene has been shown to be a partner in rearrangements with other genes in four further soft tissue tumours including extraskeletal myxoid chondrosarcoma (the *CHN* gene on chromosome 9) and some examples of myxoid liposarcoma (the *CHOP* gene on chromosome 12). The EWS gene is a member of the TET group of genes whose products have RNA binding functions. It seems likely that this gene, whose function is not yet fully understood, is important in the genesis of several forms of soft tissue sarcoma.

Much current research is directed towards fuller understanding of the functions of the genes involved in these translocations. As has already been shown in chronic myeloid leukaemia (p. 217), identification of a characteristic molecular abnormality may allow specific therapies to be devised.

Reactive Tumour-like Lesions of Soft Tissue

The clinical history in nodular fasciitis is usually of a rapidly growing tender nodule in the upper limb, especially the forearm of a young adult. Most often the lesion is subcutaneous, but sometimes muscle or deep fascia are involved. Microscopy shows loosely arranged fibroblasts randomly arranged like cells in tissue culture, with frequent mitotic figures of normal morphology (Figure 12.45). There is a prominent vascular pattern and scattered chronic inflammatory cells. This entirely benign lesion must not be misdiagnosed as a sarcoma.

Myositis ossificans occurs mainly in the muscles of the limbs of young people. Patients complain of a rapidly growing soft tissue swelling, sometimes following trauma. Many

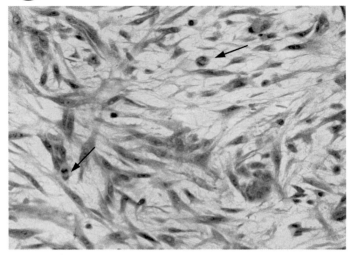

FIGURE 12.45 Nodular fasciitis. Loosely arranged fibroblasts lie randomly arranged like cells in tissue culture. While there are two mitotic figures (arrows) these are of normal appearance and although the cells vary in size the nuclei are not hyperchromatic.

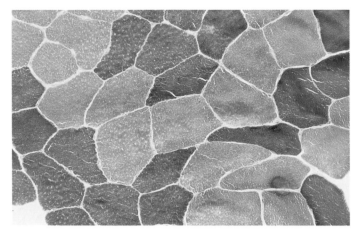

FIGURE 12.46 Normal muscle stained to show ATPase activity at pH9.4. Type 1 fibres are pale staining and type 2 are dark.

patients have low-grade fever and an elevated white blood count, suggesting infection. On microscopy there is a characteristic zoning pattern, a central zone of proliferating fibroblasts merging with areas of primitive bone formation, which may mature to form a well-defined peripheral shell of woven bone in 4–6 weeks. There is a danger that myositis ossificans is misdiagnosed as osteosarcoma particularly in the early stages, before 'zoning' has developed.

SKELETAL MUSCLE

Normal Muscle Structure

The largest tissue within the body, accounting for 40% of an average man's weight, muscle is highly organized to contract, produce movement or stability and to do work. Skeletal muscle consists of long multinucleated syncytia formed by fusion of columns of single cells. The cytoplasm contains bundles of myosin and actin filaments forming contractile myofibrils; the individual subunit is the sarcomere and these are arranged end-to-end to form muscle fibres. The parallel alignment of actin and myosin bundles gives a characteristic band-like appearance on light microscopy and alternating dark (A, anisotropic) and light (I, isotropic) bands are seen on electron microscopy. A var-iety of other proteins including α-actinin and dystrophin are found within muscle cells. The individual muscle fibre is surrounded by the endomysium; fibres are bound into fascicles by the perimysium, while the muscle itself is sheathed by the epimysium.

Muscle contracts when the relevant motor neuron is stimulated to release acetylcholine (ACh) into the cleft at the neuromuscular junction. Binding of ACh to the motor endplate results in altered permeability and an action potential is conducted over the entire surface of the membrane and into its interior through transverse tubules which dip perpendicularly into the fibre. Muscle fibres share motor nerve twigs, forming groups known as motor units based on a single anterior horn cell and the fibres it supplies. In general, the more delicate the muscle function, the fewer muscle fibres each nerve fibre innervates.

The two major proteins, actin and myosin, interact with one another in a sliding manner, akin to a rower; myosin slides past actin, binds to it, pulls back, releases and then repeats the cycle. This so called sliding filament mechanism requires continual energy provided by the breakdown of adenosine triphosphate (ATP). This reaction occurs before myosin and actin bind and the energy is stored in the cross-bridge which is cocked like a gun. A fresh molecule of ATP is required to release the linkage, explaining the phenomenon of rigor mortis, where after death muscle contraction continues until proteolysis occurs.

Fibre Types

Muscle fibres are divided into two main groups according to the type of work they are required to do. Type 1 (slow twitch; aerobic; red) fibres contain much myoglobin to provide increased oxygen uptake and are capable of continuous endurance activity, unlike type 2 (fast twitch; anaerobic; white) fibres which respond rapidly, but quickly become fatigued (Figure 12.46). Type 2 also includes some fibres with characteristics of each. The proportions vary between individuals and this may explain ability as a sprinter or marathon runner.

Diseases of Muscle

Most patients with muscle symptoms, usually undue fatigue or weakness, do not have specific muscle diseases (myopathies). Myopathies have characteristic presenting complaints which, together with laboratory investigations such as electromyography (EMG), estimation of serum levels of creatine kinase, which is released from the cytoplasm of damaged muscle cells, and muscle biopsy, allow their classification. Recently, DNA analysis and genetic assessment have changed the approach to muscle disease.

Indications for Muscle Biopsy

> **Key Points**
>
> To establish the diagnosis in:
>
> - an inflammatory myopathy before treatment
> - weakness of unknown cause
> - hereditary myopathies and dystrophies
> - to identify a treatable disorder
> - to evaluate carrier status in a female relative of a boy with Duchenne's muscular dystrophy.

Muscle biopsy is usually taken from a large proximal limb muscle, for example quadriceps, because these are most often affected. A muscle severely affected should be avoided as it may be impossible to determine the cause of the process resulting in 'endstage' muscle disease. Needle biopsies, taken under local anaesthetic, are usually adequate when specialized histochemical stains are available, especially in suspected metabolic disorders. The specimen is therefore snap frozen and stored at −70°C before cutting frozen sections as required.

The main changes seen in muscle biopsies are:

- Necrosis – usually of a segment of a muscle fibre, for example in inflammatory myopathies, but large areas of necrosis may be seen if the blood supply is affected.
- Atrophy – of either fibre type. Type 2 atrophy is seen whenever muscle is damaged in systemic disease or during steroid therapy. Neurogenic atrophy follows loss of nerve supply to a muscle fibre.
- Hypertrophy – is a compensatory response to loss of fibres in many muscle diseases especially dystrophies and in denervation.
- Regeneration – occurs if the basement membrane and endomysium remain intact. Regenerating fibres are basophilic due to increased cytoplasmic RNA.

Myopathies

Inflammatory Myopathies

This group includes polymyositis (Figure 12.47) and dermatomyositis, disorders thought to have an autoimmune aetiology. In polymyositis cytotoxic T cells attack the muscle fibre, while in dermatomyositis autoantibodies are deposited in intramuscular blood vessels. Both conditions may affect adolescents or adults and usually have a slow onset over weeks to months so that the patient often notices the weakness only when sufficiently severe that climbing stairs or lifting the arms above the head are difficult. In dermatomyositis there is a rash over the eyelids, cheekbones, sternum, elbows, knees and small joints of the hand. In severe cases, especially in adolescents, calcific deposits may affect damaged muscles.

In some patients cardiac involvement, especially of the conducting system, may cause sudden death; others develop pulmonary fibrosis. About a fifth of patients have a connective tissue disorder such as systemic lupus erythematosus, systemic sclerosis or Sjögren's syndrome. The incidence of common malignancies is slightly increased in middle-aged patients with these myopathies.

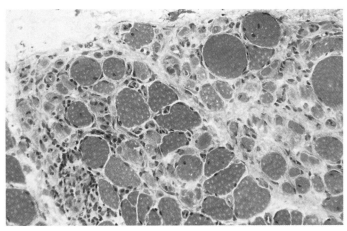

FIGURE 12.47 Polymyositis. Necrosis and regeneration of muscle fibres are accompanied by focal chronic inflammation and fibrosis.

Muscle biopsy shows necrosis of muscle fibres with subsequent phagocytosis and regeneration and focal chronic inflammation. Electromyography shows 'myopathic' changes and muscle fibre necrosis leads to an increase in serum creatine kinase.

Viral infections, notably influenza and coxsackie, may very rarely cause inflammatory myositis and the damage may be severe with rhabdomyolysis.

Metabolic Myopathies

Muscle symptoms in these disorders are related to exercise intolerance. Defects in glycogen, lipid, purine nucleotide and mitochondrial pathways can all lead to metabolic myopathies. McArdle's disease, the commonest disorder of glycogen metabolism, is an inherited recessive disorder due to lack of myophosphorylase (Figure 12.48). Exercise intolerance with stiffness is found, symptoms usually being precipitated by brief bursts of high intensity activity. Severe attacks may involve rhabdomyolysis with myoglobinuria and hence renal failure.

Mitochondrial myopathies have only relatively recently been characterized, initially by electron microscopy, but deficiencies in oxidative enzymes are now known to be responsible. They are of interest as many are due to mutations in mitochondrial rather than genomic DNA and therefore inherited through the maternal line. Many patients present with chronic progressive external ophthalmoplegia with paralysis of external ocular muscles and mild limb weakness. Cardiac conduction defects, retinopathy and seizures may also be present.

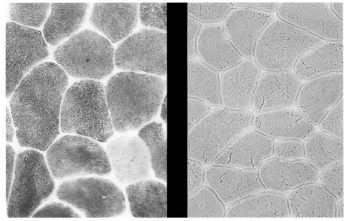

FIGURE 12.48 McArdle's disease. Muscle stained for the presence of myophosphorylase activity. Normal (left) shows abundant dark blue reaction product, which is absent in the biopsy from an affected individual (right).

Periodic Paralysis (Channelopathies)

Ion channels (see cystic fibrosis transmembrane conductance regulatory chlorine channel p. 163) are crucial components of cell membranes allowing ions to flow rapidly while maintaining extracellular and intracellular concentrations. They are selective for different ions and are controlled by specific stimuli, such as neurotransmitters. Several hereditary muscle disorders are due to mutations in ion channel proteins, frequently autosomal dominant in inheritance and usually characterized by episodic symptoms of muscle weakness and cramps, for example hyperkalaemic periodic paralysis. Malignant hyperpyrexia is a serious ion-channel disorder characterized by an abnormal response to general anaesthetics especially halothane. Intense muscle contraction starts after anaesthesia and is followed by a rapid rise in body temperature. Release of calcium from the sarcoplasmic reticulum causes massive muscle necrosis (rhabdomyolysis). The muscle relaxant, dantrolene, stops the symptoms and prevents terminal shock.

Myopathies Associated with Systemic Disease

Many systemic diseases, for example chronic heart, respiratory, liver and renal disease, cause muscle weakness. Although muscles are not primarily affected, patients may complain of muscle weakness, serum creatine kinase may be elevated and electromyography may show myopathic changes. Muscle biopsy may be normal or show mild to moderate atrophy of type 2 fibres, because these are susceptible to muscle damage of any kind. An exception is diabetes in which neurogenic atrophy is usually seen. Muscle disease usually responds to treatment of the underlying condition.

Muscular Dystrophies

Muscular dystrophies are a group of inherited conditions with an intrinsic defect of muscle and are characterized by progressive wasting and weakness.

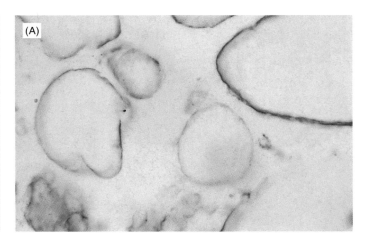

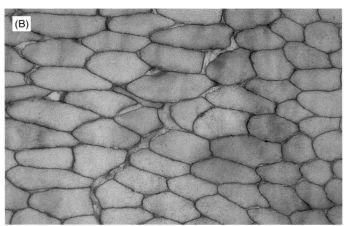

FIGURE 12.49 Becker-type muscular dystrophy. Staining for dystrophin shows patchy and variable staining (A) at the periphery of the fibres compared with the regular pattern of normal muscle (B). Staining is typically absent in Duchenne's dystrophy.

Duchenne's muscular dystrophy is the commonest dystrophy of childhood and affects 1 in 3500 male births. An X-linked recessive condition, it affects boys who present before 5 years with delayed motor function, especially a waddling gait and inability to run and, due to weakness of the pelvic girdle muscles, difficulty in rising from the floor without help of their arms. Most are confined to a wheelchair by 12 years of age and die due to cardiomyopathy or respiratory failure by the late teens or early twenties. About a third have intellectual impairment. Becker's muscular dystrophy is a clinically similar but milder form with onset in the teens and early twenties and many patients survive into middle age and beyond.

Mutations in the dystrophin gene on the short arm of chromosome X cause both disorders and its protein product, dystrophin, has been characterized. Normal dystrophin is a large molecular component of the sarcolemmal plasma membrane. When the gene is mutated, dystrophin is either absent or undetectable as in Duchenne's, or of abnormal constitution as in Becker's, the clinical phenotypes correlating well with the quantity and quality of dystrophin (Figure 12.49). In Duchenne's dystrophy two-thirds of mutations are inherited

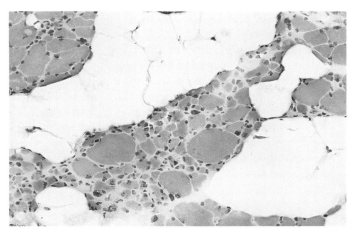

FIGURE 12.50 Duchenne's muscular dystrophy. This biopsy from advanced disease shows muscle fibres, many of which are atrophic, lying among adipose tissue.

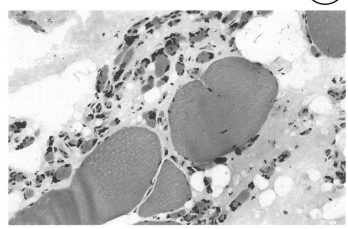

FIGURE 12.51 Neurogenic atrophy. The majority of muscle fibres are denervated and have atrophied to small fibres whose nuclei appear large. A few large hypertrophied fibres are present.

from the mother and the high figure of one-third of new mutations reflects the large size of the gene which contains several hot spots. Most patients with Duchenne's have a deletion or duplication resulting in truncation of translation and a small unstable molecule. The muscle biopsy shows a characteristic appearance with variation in muscle fibre size, some showing necrosis, and in the later stages muscle is replaced by fat and fibrous tissue (Figure 12.50).

Myotonic dystrophy, an autosomally inherited progressive neuromuscular disorder, is characterized by failure of muscle to relax after contraction (myotonia) and progressive weakness. It involves other systems, with cardiac conduction defects, cataracts, premature balding, reduced fertility and mental impairment. It is caused by an increased number of cytosine–thymidine–guanine trinucleotide repeats in an untranslated region of the dystrophica myotonia protein kinase gene. The normal gene has between 5 and 30 such repeats, while affected alleles have from 50 to several thousand. An interesting feature is the phenomenon of 'anticipation' – the clinical symptoms increase with successive generations. Electromyography and muscle biopsy show characteristic features.

A variety of other much rarer dystrophies have been described, and the mutations characterized.

Neurogenic Disorders

As muscle fibre function depends on the integrity of the whole motor unit, lesions in the motor neurone, the peripheral motor nerves and neuromuscular junction may all result in atrophy of the muscle with shrinkage of fibres. Diagnostic problems can arise because they may simulate myopathies, especially dystrophies. Among these are hereditary disorders such as spinal muscular atrophies (SMA) which fall into three broad categories: severe infantile SMA causes death from respiratory failure in infancy, milder juvenile cases with scoliosis and adults with a better prognosis. The biopsy appearances (Figure 12.51) depend on the rate and degree of denervation. Initially, atrophic fibres

are scattered at random through the fascicles, but later small clusters of tiny fibres can be identified followed by large group atrophy as more neurons fail.

Motor neuron disease (p. 310) affects upper and lower motor neurons and causes severe generalized atrophy, leading to death within 3 years or so. Similar features are seen in hereditary peripheral neuropathies, diabetes and in the post-polio syndrome.

Disorders of Neuromuscular Transmission

There are two major disorders, each with an immunological basis.

Myasthenia Gravis

This disease occurs predominantly in young women and middle-aged men, who present with abnormal fatigue of skeletal muscles with weakness on exercise and recovery after rest. The external ocular and facial muscles are usually affected causing ptosis and diplopia and there may be difficulty in swallowing, speaking and chewing. Symptoms may be restricted to the eyes but more often generalized weakness with respiratory symptoms develops, particularly in exacerbations (crises). Thymic pathology is often associated – thymic hyperplasia in young women and thymoma in older individuals.

In 90% of patients antibodies to ACh receptors occur providing a diagnostic test. The antibody titre does not correlate with the severity of the disease. In pregnant patients the antibody may cross the placenta causing transient neonatal myasthenia gravis.

Eaton–Lambert Syndrome

Unlike myasthenia gravis, in this syndrome muscle weakness improves with repeated exercise. An antibody to presynaptic structures prevents release of ACh at the nerve terminal. There is a strong association with malignancy, notably small cell carcinoma of bronchus.

SUMMARY

- Locomotor diseases, principally osteoporosis and arthritis, are a major source of morbidity, especially in middle-aged and elderly individuals, and thus of economic cost to society.
- Recent scientific studies have done much to elucidate the controlling mechanisms of bone turnover in metabolic diseases such as osteoporosis and Paget's disease and this will open avenues for new targeted therapies.
- Similar advances are being made in the biology of inflammatory joint diseases such as rheumatoid arthritis again with prospects for treatment.
- Infections of bone and joint are far less common than in past decades but awareness is important to allow early diagnosis and treatment which remain the key to preventing the tissue destruction and loss of function which characterize these in the later stages.
- Metastatic carcinomas are common in bone and cause bone destruction and major symptoms, especially in those patients in the later stages of malignancy.

- In contrast primary sarcomas of bone are rare, but those affected, throughout all ages of life, experience considerable morbidity and mortality.
- Most soft tissue tumours are benign, but those which are deeply situated, larger than 5 cm and symptomatic should be regarded as malignant till proved otherwise.
- Muscle disorders are uncommon conditions which fall into several groups including inflammatory myopathies and muscular dystrophies. For the latter, the molecular mechanisms are increasingly understood, thus offering opportunities for genetic screening and, potentially, novel therapies

FURTHER READING

Athanasou NA. *Colour Atlas of Bone, Joint and Soft Tissue Pathology*. Oxford: Oxford University Press, 1999.

Fletcher CDM, Unni KK, Mertens F. *World Health Organization Classification of Tumours: Pathology and Genetics. Tumours of Bone and Soft Tissue*. Lyon: IARC Press, 2002.

Weiss SW, Goldblum JR. *Enzinger and Weiss's Soft Tissue Tumors*, 4th edn. St. Louis: Mosby, 2001.

THE KIDNEYS AND URINARY TRACT

13

Stewart Fleming, Ian AR More and R Stuart C Rodger

CLINICAL FEATURES OF RENAL DISEASE

> **Key Points**
>
> - Renal diseases are common and account for a considerable volume of morbidity and mortality.
> - The main manifestations can be divided into several distinct types of clinical presentation.

The diseases of the kidney are complex but illustrate many of the principles of inflammatory disease, immunologically mediated disease, genetically determined disease, vascular disease and malignancy.

Heavy proteinuria in excess of 3 g/24 h (urine protein:creatinine ratio >300 mg/mmol) results in hypoalbuminaemia and generalized oedema, the three features which together constitute the nephrotic syndrome. Hyperlipidaemia is an almost invariable accompaniment and hypertension and impaired renal function may be present. The proteinuria is due to increased glomerular permeability resulting from a variety of glomerular diseases. In addition to generalized oedema there may be ascites and pleural effusions. There is increased susceptibility to infection and thrombosis including a risk of renal vein thrombosis. The acute nephritic syndrome is most frequently seen in acute proliferative glomerulonephritis. The clinical features are diffuse oedema including the facial region, hypertension and oliguria. Urinary examination reveals proteinuria, haematuria and the presence of red cell casts.

Asymptomatic proteinuria may result from the same diseases that cause the nephrotic syndrome, the main difference being that the proteinuria is of insufficient severity to cause hypoalbuminaemia and oedema. It is usually detected during a routine medical examination. Painless haematuria may result from intrinsic renal disease, diseases of the collecting system and bladder, and malignancy in the urinary tract. Microscopic examination of the urine, renal imaging and cystoscopy may be helpful in localizing the site and cause of blood loss.

Hypertension (p. 116) is usually idiopathic or essential in type but in a significant proportion of cases it is due to underlying parenchymal renal disease. The prevalence of hypertension varies among the different types of primary renal disease, and in advanced renal failure it may be as high as 80%. Hypertension is not only a consequence of renal disease but also a major cause of the progression of renal damage in a variety of different forms of intrinsic renal disease.

Renal failure, classified as either acute or chronic, has a large number of causes. In acute renal failure there is an abrupt deterioration in renal function occurring over a period of hours or days. It may be classified as:

- pre-renal – due to inadequate perfusion following circulatory collapse
- renal – due to renal parenchymal disease/damage
- post-renal – due to obstructive disorders of the urinary tract.

Chronic renal failure develops over a period of weeks, months or years. The consequences of a reduction in adequate renal function are a variety of complications due to the retention of waste products, impaired water, electrolyte and acid–base balance, loss of erythropoietin production, impaired vitamin D metabolism, activation of the renin–angiotensin system and the development of hypertension.

PROGRESSION OF RENAL DISEASE

Key Points

- Progression of renal disease is associated with a number of factors.
- Reduced renal mass may lead to hyperfiltration injury in the glomeruli.
- Tubulo-interstitial damage may be due to proteinuria and local ischaemia.
- Chronic renal failure is a gradual reduction in glomerular filtration rate.
- An international classification describes five stages of chronic kidney disease.

A number of factors may be important in the progression of renal disease from acute presentation to chronic renal disease, chronic renal impairment and end-stage renal failure. Coexisting arterial disease, hypertension, persisting activity of the original disease and some genetic factors may be important in determining the rate of progression. It has been known for some time that a reduction in nephron mass that reduces the glomerular filtration of the blood to about 30–50% of normal may result in progressive renal damage independent of continuing activity of the underlying disease. The secondary factors leading to progression are of major clinical interest because they may provide an opportunity to interrupt the cycle which leads to established renal failure. Two main histological characteristics are seen, namely focal glomerulosclerosis and tubulo-interstitial inflammation and fibrosis (Figure 13.1).

The glomerulosclerosis appears to develop as part of the response to glomerular hyperfiltration which occurs as a compensatory response to maintain renal function. The consequence of this glomerular hyperfiltration is compensatory hypertrophy and haemodynamic changes leading to endothelial and epithelial cell injury with increasing glomerular permeability to protein and increasing deposition of mesangial matrix. Many mediators of chronic inflammation and fibrosis, particularly transforming growth factor β (TGFβ), are thought to have a role in the progressive glomerular damage and loss. There is convincing evidence that a protective effect may be obtained by reducing intraglomerular pressure with angiotensin-converting enzyme inhibitors or angiotensin receptor blockade. Tubulo-interstitial damage as evidenced by tubular atrophy, interstitial inflammation and interstitial fibrosis is now recognized to be a major prognostic factor in the progression of a variety of different renal diseases. Many factors may lead to tubular injury, including urinary protein, urinary complement and immunoglobulins, cytokines liberated into the urinary filtrate or into the interstitium or local haemodynamic factors leading to relative ischaemia. The end result of expansion of the interstitial fibroblast population and in particular expansion of the interstitial extracellular matrix is a feature of the irreversible progression of renal disease.

Chronic Renal Failure

Chronic renal failure results when the functions of the kidneys have been so reduced by a chronic disease process that there is retention of nitrogenous waste products normally excreted in the urine. This reduction in glomerular filtration rate can be detected by measurement of urea and creatinine in the blood or creatinine clearance from analysis of blood and 24-hour urine samples.

Estimated glomerular filtration rate (eGFR), a laboratory calculation taking into account the serum creatinine, age, sex and race of the individual, is now the most common method of reporting renal function in adults. Using eGFR there are five recognized stages of chronic kidney disease (CKD) ranging from CKD 1 (in which eGFR is normal but there is other evidence of kidney disease such as proteinuria, chronic glomerulonephritis, calculi, scarring or polycystic kidneys) to CKD 5 (in which eGFR is <15 mL/min/1.73 m^2 or the patient is undergoing chronic dialysis or has a kidney transplant (Table 13.1). Patients with stage 5 CKD are said to have 'established renal failure', a term that has replaced 'end-stage renal failure'. Patients with stage 5 CKD who are

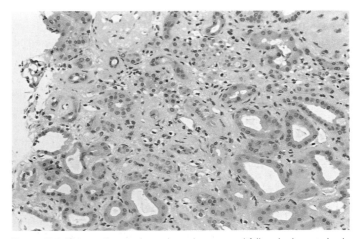

FIGURE 13.1 The renal parenchyma in end-stage renal failure is characterized by extensive glomerulosclerosis, tubular atrophy and hypertrophic and hyaline changes in the arteries and arterioles. Virtually no functioning renal parenchyma remains.

TABLE 13.1 Classification of chronic kidney disease (CKD) by eGFR

CKD Stage	eGFR(mL/min/1.73 m^2)
1 With another abnormality (e.g. proteinuria)	>90
2 With another abnormality (e.g. proteinuria)	60–89
3	30–59
4	15–29
5	<15

being treated by dialysis or who have a functioning kidney transplant are said to be on 'renal replacement therapy'.

Chronic kidney disease is common, being present in as many as 10% of the population and the incidence increases with increasing age. The commonest cause of CKD, particularly in the elderly, is ischaemic nephropathy due to hypertension or vascular disease. It is important to identify because even in its milder stages it is associated with an increased risk of cardiovascular death. As renal function deteriorates further the toxicity of nitrogenous waste products, the loss of homeostasis of fluid, electrolyte and acid–base balance and disturbances in the endocrine functions of the kidney all result in important effects. There are many diseases which may lead to chronic renal failure (Table 13.2) and their pathological characteristics are described in the appropriate sections. The biochemical, clinical and morphological changes which accompany chronic renal failure irrespective of the underlying primary renal disease are described below.

TABLE 13.2 Causes of chronic renal failure

Glomerulonephritis
Reflux nephropathy
Renal calculi
Obstructive uropathy
Diabetes
Renovascular disease/hypertension
Polycystic kidney disease
Systemic vasculitis (e.g. systemic lupus erythematosus, Henoch–Schönlein purpura)
Myeloma
Amyloidosis
Other diseases

Nitrogenous Waste Products

The clinical features of waste product retention are those of chronic poisoning and become more pronounced as renal function declines. Patients with CKD 4 and 5 complain of non-specific symptoms such as tiredness, lethargy and anorexia. Platelet function is abnormal, leading to easy bruising and bleeding from the gastrointestinal tract and disturbances of the immune system predispose to infection. In advanced renal failure fibrinous pericarditis and pneumonitis, consisting of a serofibrinous exudate in the alveolar spaces, may be present. The pulmonary changes resemble those of neonatal hyaline membrane disease but there is often partial organization of the exudate. The effects on the nervous system include peripheral neuropathy, poor concentration, sleep disturbance and ultimately coma but there are few obvious pathological changes in the brain.

Sodium and Water

In chronic renal failure the kidney's inability to control salt and water balance can lead to both overhydration and dehydration. In most cases sodium and fluid retention occur leading to hypertension and peripheral and pulmonary oedema. Less commonly but particularly where the primary renal disorder is tubular or interstitial (e.g. calculus disease) sodium and fluid depletion will occur unless a high salt and fluid intake is maintained. Loss of concentrating function due to tubular damage combined with the osmotic diuretic effect of high concentrations of nitrogenous waste products such as urea probably explain the relatively fixed output of dilute urine occurring in chronic renal failure.

Acid–Base Balance and Electrolyte Disturbance

To conserve acid–base balance the kidneys must excrete 40–60 mmol of acid (H^+) daily. In chronic renal failure total ammonia production and secretion into the tubules is reduced and there is also some loss of urinary bicarbonate, which is normally completely reabsorbed. As a result of these changes the patient with chronic renal failure is prone to develop acidosis. In renal failure, chronic acidosis may cause tissue catabolism which results in a deterioration in nutritional status and may also aggravate renal bone disease.

Excessive potassium and phosphate generated by dietary intake or protein breakdown is normally excreted by the kidney. In chronic renal failure potassium retention may occur and be exacerbated by acidosis which results in the exchange of intracellular potassium for hydrogen ions. Hyperkalaemia may cause muscle stiffness and abdominal pain but is often asymptomatic until potentially fatal cardiac arrhythmias develop. Hyperphosphataemia occurs in later renal failure resulting in calcium phosphate deposition (metastatic calcification) in the soft tissues particularly in the arterial wall, the periarticular tissues, and the conjunctivae. Pruritus is a frequent symptom in patients with advanced renal failure and calcium phosphate deposition in the skin is thought to contribute to this. These abnormalities in calcium phosphate balance are compounded by impaired activation of 25-hydroxy vitamin D in the kidney (see below) and lead to secondary hyperparathyroidism.

Endocrine Disturbances

The principal endocrine functions of the kidney concern bone metabolism, erythropoiesis and blood pressure control. Renal bone disease or renal osteodystrophy describes the various bone changes occurring in renal failure as a result of impaired activation of vitamin D, altered calcium phosphate balance and secondary hyperparathyroidism. These include osteitis fibrosis cystica, osteomalacia and osteoporosis (see Chapter 12). Anaemia is a common feature of chronic renal failure and occurs principally due to a lack of adequate production of erythropoietin from peritubular cells of the renal cortex. This secondary anaemia contributes to the symptoms of tiredness and poor exercise tolerance in renal failure and can be corrected by subcutaneous or intravenous recombinant erythropoietin treatment.

In chronic renal failure the renin – angiotensin–aldosterone system is inappropriately activated resulting in hypertension. The renal changes resulting from hypertension cause further injury to the already damaged kidneys and hence hasten the onset of renal failure. Hypertension may also contribute to left ventricular hypertrophy and vascular disease with resultant cardiac failure and the risk of cardiovascular events. Effective antihypertensive drug therapy can protect against this damage and extend the longevity of the failing kidney.

GENETICALLY DETERMINED RENAL DISEASE

The two main groups of genetically determined renal disease of note are polycystic kidney disease and genetic abnormalities of the glomerular basement membrane. Polycystic kidney disease occurs in two main forms. Autosomal dominant polycystic kidney disease is the commonest form of cystic renal disease and one of the most common genetic diseases in the community affecting approximately 1:500 to 1:1000 individuals. It accounts for about 10% of patients requiring renal replacement therapy. The disease is genetically heterogeneous and is caused by germ-line mutation in one of three separate genes. These are the polycystin 1 gene located on the short arm of chromosome 16, the polycystin 2 gene on the long arm of chromosome 4 and a third polycystic kidney disease gene, whose location is yet to be identified, which is responsible for a minority of cases. The cysts sometimes cause pain and haematuria but many of the patients with autosomal dominant polycystic kidney disease remain asymptomatic until adult life. Then there may be a progressive deterioration in renal function, usually during the third or fourth decade, leading to established renal failure particularly in those with untreated hypertension. The kidneys contain large numbers of cysts and may expand to weigh more than 1 kg (Figure 13.2). The cysts may be several centimetres in diameter and contain serous or blood-stained fluid. Cysts are present throughout the nephron (Figure 13.3). Autosomal recessive polycystic kidney disease is much less common and leads to renal failure in infancy or early childhood. There is

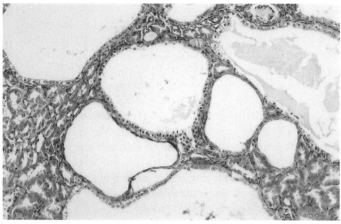

FIGURE 13.3 Histological examination of a kidney with autosomal dominant polycystic kidney disease shows cysts developing from all parts of the nephron. Intervening parenchyma is compressed and shows progressive ischaemia and hypertensive damage.

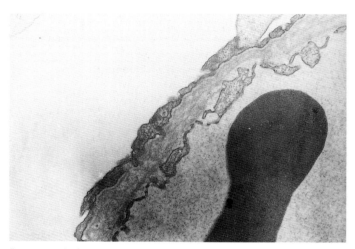

FIGURE 13.4 In Alport's syndrome there is a genetic abnormality of type IV collagen, which is an essential part of the glomerular basement membrane. As a consequence there is a failure of the basement membrane assembly with the appearance of multilayering and fragmentation.

less severe renal enlargement and the cysts are limited to dilatation of the collecting ducts. The small proportion of patients who survive infancy develop hepatic fibrosis and with age the liver complications become more significant.

The major genetically determined abnormality of the glomerular basement membrane is Alport's syndrome. This disease usually shows an X-linked pattern of inheritance and is associated with mutation in the collagen genes responsible for encoding the proteins which make up the glomerular basement membrane. Alport's syndrome may present in the first and second decade with proteinuria, haematuria and progressive renal failure but this may be delayed until later life. Males are often more severely affected than females. The disease may be diagnosed by characteristic electron microscopic appearances of the glomerular basement membrane (Figure 13.4). It is usually accompanied by high frequency nerve deafness and sometimes ocular abnormalities.

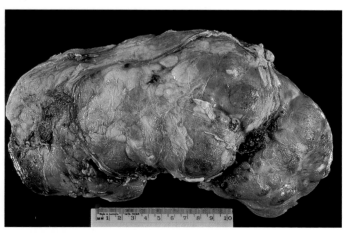

FIGURE 13.2 Autosomal dominant polycystic kidney disease. In this disease the kidney is enormously enlarged with cysts throughout the renal parenchyma. Many of these cysts will be up to several centimetres in diameter. Haemorrhage and infection within cysts is common.

13.1 SPECIAL STUDY TOPIC

GENE POLYMORPHISMS AND THE PROGRESSION OF RENAL DISEASE

There are many renal diseases in which there is variation in the risk of the disease progressing and in the rate at which it progresses. Among the features known to be important in determining progression is blood pressure control. A major determinant of blood pressure is the activity of the renin–angiotensin system. There is also evidence that the activity of this system influences glomerular filtration and the severity of proteinuria. These factors appear to contribute to chronic renal injury. These observations led to an analysis of the genes of the renin–angiotensin system in a bid to identify genetic determinants of the likelihood of progression of renal disease. Genetic polymorphisms which determined the activity of the renin–angiotensin system were identified, most prominently for the angiotensinogen, angiotensin-converting enzyme, and angiotensin receptor genes. Among these the most completely studied has been the angiotensin-converting enzyme polymorphisms.

There is a 287 base pair insertion within the *ACE* gene which correlates with the activity of the enzyme in the circulation. The insertion does not itself determine the regulation of the enzyme but is a fortuitously identified marker correlating with activity. The presence of the insertion denotes the I polymorphism and the absence of it D (for deletion). An individual can therefore be of the II, ID or DD genotype. The levels of angiotensin-converting enzyme activity in the circulation are highest for the DD genotype and lowest for the II genotype. When these genetic polymorphisms were studied in relation to renal disease it was found that they did not determine the likelihood of developing renal disease but had a strong influence on the likelihood of the disease progressing to renal failure. These studies were carried out in patients with diabetic nephropathy, IgA nephropathy and hypertensive renal disease. The same association with a poor prognosis in a DD genotype has been found for left ventricular hypertrophy, coronary artery disease and stroke. In parallel with these genetic studies has been the development of pharmacological agents which inhibit angiotensin converting enzyme, the ACE inhibitors. These act by inhibiting the conversion of angiotensin I to angiotensin II, reducing the angiotensin II in the circulation and lowering blood pressure. Combined research involving the genotypic and pharmacological approaches has now been undertaken and shown that those individuals with a D haplotype, and therefore higher levels of ACE activity, are those who are most likely to benefit from ACE inhibition. These studies have led to a better understanding of the genetic control of blood pressure and its relationship to the progression of renal disease. It is likely that in the near future the precise mechanism of regulation of the *ACE* gene and indeed of other elements of the renin–angiotensin system will be elucidated. This will give a deeper insight into the regulation of the progression of renal disease.

GLOMERULAR DISEASE

Glomerulonephritis

Key Points

- Glomerulonephritis encompasses a group of renal diseases in which the lesions are primarily glomerular, other changes in the kidney being secondary to glomerular injury.
- When the mononuclear phagocyte system is not able to remove circulating immune complexes, some will deposit in the glomerular capillaries.
- Glomerular subendothelial immune complexes damage the glomerulus in at least two ways.
- The major histological features of immune complex glomerular injury are hypercellularity, thickening of the glomerular wall and crescent formation.

Pathogenesis

Most cases of glomerulonephritis are due to injury caused by the presence of antigen–antibody complexes in the glomeruli. These immune complexes may localize within the glomeruli in the following ways:

- circulating immune complexes may be filtered out in the glomerular capillaries
- antibodies may form to constituents of the glomerular basement membrane: such antibodies become bound to the glomerular basement membrane
- circulating antibodies may react with non-basement membrane glomerular antigens, or with antigens from the plasma which have become trapped within the glomerulus to form immune complexes *in situ*
- in some instances non-antibody substances within the glomeruli may activate complement via the alternative pathway and cause glomerular damage.

Factors Influencing Deposition of Immune Complexes Within Glomeruli

The kidney receives a relatively large blood supply and the glomeruli are unusual in that their capillaries lie between two arterioles: in consequence, the glomerular capillary pressure is much greater than in most other capillary beds. In addition,

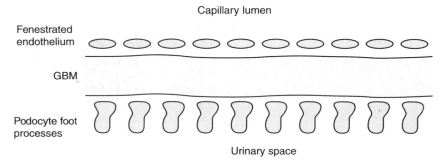

FIGURE 13.5 The glomerulus is a specialized capillary bed with close approximation of the endothelium and the epithelium (podocytes) separated only by a thin glomerular basement membrane (GBM). The endothelium is fenestrated to allow the free passage of macromolecules. The glomerular basement membrane is a product of both the endothelial and epithelial cells. The podocytes have specialist filtration structures called foot processes which align themselves on the glomerular basement membrane. This specialized capillary bed is supported by modified smooth muscle cells called mesangial cells. The latter are also phagocytic and have a major role in determining the intraglomerular pressure. Filtration occurs from the capillary lumen into the urinary filtration space.

the normal glomerular capillary wall acts as a progressive sieve: very small molecules and ions pass freely through the endothelial layer, basement membrane and epithelial slit pores to appear in the glomerular filtrate but cells and very large molecular aggregates are kept within the vascular tree by the pore size of the endothelial cells. Between these two extremes, macromolecules and antigen–antibody complexes can penetrate into the glomerular capillary wall (Figure 13.5). The depth of such penetration depends not only on molecular size, but also on their shape and charge.

The mononuclear phagocyte system removes foreign material and large protein aggregates from the blood. In normal circumstances it may remove most of the circulating immune complexes. If the system is presented with an excess of such complexes or if its activity is depressed, for example by infections, drugs or neoplasia, then it may be incapable of clearing the blood of circulating immune complexes and some will deposit in the glomerular capillaries. Other factors include the release of vasoactive agents which increase the permeability of the glomerular (and other) capillaries, and treatment with glucocorticoids which, by contrast, impedes the transfer of macromolecules across the basement membrane.

Mechanisms of Glomerular Injury by Immune Complexes

The presence of glomerular subendothelial immune complexes causes damage in at least two ways. The immune complexes activate the complement cascade, with production of the C5–9 lytic complex which damages the adjacent cells and basement membranes. Products of complement activation, notably C5a, increase capillary permeability and are chemotactic for neutrophil polymorphs and monocytes which in consequence accumulate in the lesion. These cells phagocytose immune complexes but, in doing so, secrete numerous lysosomal enzymes, some of which can degrade cell and basement membranes. There may be local activation of the coagulation cascade, either secondary to complement activation or by cell damage with the release of various enzymes and protein breakdown products. This leads to deposition of fibrin in the

lumen and walls of the glomerular capillaries. Early administration of anticoagulants in experimental immune complex nephritis has been shown to prevent some of the glomerular injury. If the injury to the glomerular capillaries is severe, components of the clotting system may escape into Bowman's space where deposition of fibrin promotes the formation of cellular aggregates or crescents which further impair glomerular function.

Glomerular Manifestations of Immune Complex Injury

The major histological features of immune complex glomerular injury can be explained by the pathogenic mechanism:

- Hypercellularity is due to an increase in the number of glomerular cells and to the arrest and emigration of neutrophil polymorphs and monocytes in response to immune complex deposition, activation of complement and endothelial injury (Figure 13.6).
- Thickening of the glomerular capillary wall as seen by light microscopy (Figure 13.7) has a variety of causes. Large subepithelial, intramembranous or subendothelial deposits of immune complexes, swelling of the damaged epithelial or endothelial cells, or prolongation of long mesangial cell processes between the endothelium and basement membrane secondary to immune complex deposition can all give rise to a thickened capillary wall. Production of the basement membrane material by endothelial and epithelial cells may also be stimulated by the presence of immune complexes.
- Crescent formation. The escape of fibrin into Bowman's space stimulates the lining epithelial cells to divide and this, together with an admixture of mononuclear phagocytes, produces a crescent-shaped mass of cells which compresses the glomerular tuft – hence the name of the lesion (Figure 13.8).

The above changes may affect the whole glomerulus (global) or part of the glomerulus (segmental).

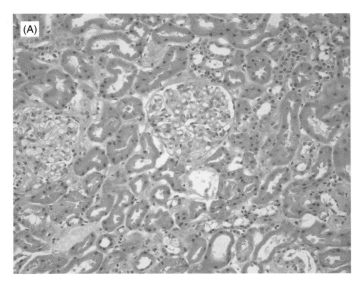

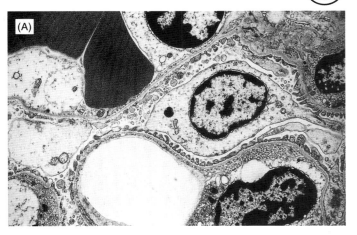

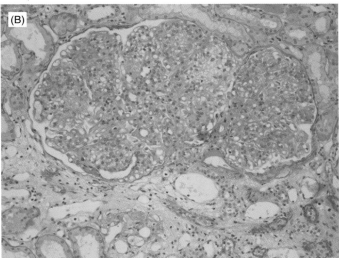

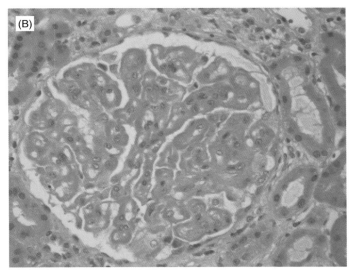

FIGURE 13.7 (A) Normal glomerular basement membrane shown by electron microscopy. (B) The glomerular basement membrane here shown by light microscopy is markedly thickened, a feature seen in a variety of diseases including membranous glomerulonephritis and diabetic nephropathy.

FIGURE 13.6 (A) Normal glomeruli. (B) These glomeruli show an increase in cellularity due to proliferation of endogenous glomerular cells, predominantly mesangial cells, and infiltration of the glomerulus by inflammatory cells.

Classification

Although the following description is not intended to be comprehensive it covers the major clinically important glomerulonephritides. Certain systemic diseases, for example systemic lupus erythematosus, diabetes mellitus and amyloidosis, can give rise to glomerular lesions resulting in clinical syndromes resembling one or other type of glomerulonephritis.

Minimal-change Nephropathy

Key Points

- Minimal-change nephropathy is the commonest cause of the nephrotic syndrome in children.
- Spontaneous remission and recurrences are common.
- Hypertension and renal impairment are usually absent.
- There are few histological changes.

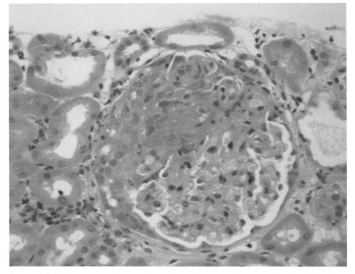

FIGURE 13.8 A crescent is a proliferation of macrophages and epithelial cells within Bowman's space but outwith the glomerular capillary bed.

General Features

Minimal-change nephropathy has a peak incidence in children between 1 and 5 years old, but occurs in children and adults of all ages. As usual in the nephrotic syndrome there is a rise in the level of blood lipids, including cholesterol, and a predisposition to infection and thromboembolism. The proteinuria is due to increased glomerular capillary permeability, and is usually highly selective, albumin being accompanied by much smaller amounts of the plasma proteins than with the less-selective proteinuria observed in most renal diseases, with or without the nephrotic syndrome. A short course of high-dose glucocorticoid therapy will usually induce remission of the nephrotic syndrome and although further relapses may occur this form of glomerulonephritis does not progress to renal failure.

Pathological Changes

Microscopically, the glomeruli look normal apart from an appearance of dilatation of the capillaries; there is no thickening of the capillary walls and no increased cellularity of the glomerular tufts. The most conspicuous glomerular change on electron microscopy is effacement of the foot processes of the epithelial cells, the basement membrane being covered externally by a layer of epithelial cell cytoplasm; the epithelial cells also show an increase in surface activity with the production of microvillous processes (Figure 13.9).

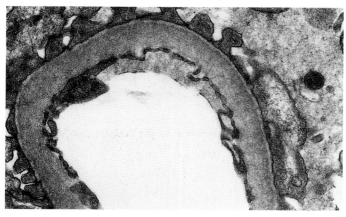

FIGURE 13.9 In minimal change nephropathy the light microscopic appearance of the glomerulus is normal. On examination by electron microscopy there is loss of the normal glomerular epithelial foot processes, known as foot process fusion, and there may be some vacuolation of the epithelium. No other abnormalities are seen in this disease.

Aetiology

The nature of this disease remains unknown. Immunofluorescence studies on the glomeruli are negative for immunoglobulins and complement. The disease is occasionally associated with routine prophylactic immunization, with hypersensitivity reactions (bee stings and asthma) and there is evidence that defects in T-cell function may be involved: this is supported by the occasional occurrence of the disease in patients with Hodgkin's disease or non-Hodgkin's lymphoma. Foot process effacement has been associated with loss of polyanion from the glomerular basement membrane,

consequent change in electrical charge and hence altered basement membrane permeability.

Focal Glomerulosclerosis

At one time thought to be a variant of minimal-change glomerulonephritis, this is now regarded as a distinct entity. The clinical features are similar to those of minimal-change glomerulonephritis, but proteinuria is *less selective* and *red cells* are more commonly present in the urine. Although most of the glomeruli appear normal, those close to the medulla show sclerosis, consisting of deposition of hyaline material with consequent obliteration of capillaries (Figure 13.10). This change is at first segmental but gradually destroys the whole glomerulus and extends peripherally to involve more glomeruli. There is associated tubular atrophy.

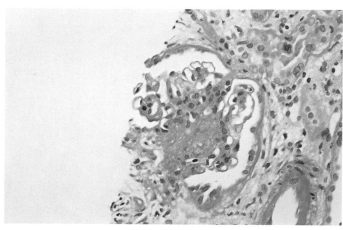

FIGURE 13.10 Focal segmental glomerulosclerosis is a disease in which there is fibrosis of part of the glomerular tuft with only a proportion of the glomeruli affected. Within the affected segment there is obliteration of the capillary spaces, extracellular matrix accumulation and sometimes the presence of foamy macrophages.

Renal biopsy is only diagnostic if it includes some of the deeper, affected glomeruli. The condition is resistant to steroid therapy although in some cases there may be an initial response. The prognosis is poor, many cases progressing to renal failure although this may take a number of years and the disease tends to recur in renal transplants. Some patients in whom a diagnosis of minimal-change glomerulonephritis is made based on a superficial renal biopsy and who eventually develop chronic renal failure are really missed cases of focal glomerulosclerosis.

Diffuse Membranous Glomerulonephritis

Key Points

- This disease is commoner in males than females.
- It usually presents as the nephrotic syndrome with non-selective proteinuria and the urine often contains small numbers of red cells.
- The main histological change is diffuse hyaline thickening of the walls of all the glomerular capillaries.

Clinical Features

This disease occurs over a wide age range, although its peak incidence is in middle age. Idiopathic membranous glomerulonephritis may remit spontaneously but a significant proportion of patients pursue an indolent course for many months or years, ending in chronic renal failure. The effects of steroids and cytotoxic drugs on the course of the disease are uncertain; because of the occurrence of spontaneous remissions, their value is difficult to assess and are still the subject of controlled trials.

Pathological Changes

The essential change is in the glomerulus, and consists of a diffuse hyaline thickening of the walls of all the glomerular capillaries. In the early stages this is minimal and hard to detect, but it becomes increasingly obvious as the disease progresses. There is no obvious swelling or proliferation of endothelial or mesangial cells, and no leucocytic infiltration. By light microscopy the capillary walls appear thickened, eosinophilic and hyaline and silver staining techniques give an appearance of spikes on the basement membrane. Immunofluorescence staining reveals immune complexes on the capillary wall. Electron microscopy shows irregular deposition of dense amorphous material in the outer subepithelial part of the glomerular basement membrane (Figure 13.11). The laying down of new basement membrane between the deposits corresponds to the spikes seen by light microscopy of silver preparations. Eventually the basement membrane spikes thicken and unite to envelop the deposits and these are gradually replaced by basement membrane, which in consequence, is considerably thickened and irregular.

In the chronic stage of the disease, the thickening of the glomerular capillary walls results in narrowing of the lumina; renal blood flow and glomerular filtration rate are seriously diminished, and uraemia and hypertension develop. Proteinuria diminishes, polyuria often develops, and the oedema tends to subside and may disappear. Microscopy of the kidneys at this stage shows gross diffuse thickening of glomerular capillary walls, some glomeruli being almost solid eosinophilic hyaline material, while others are less severely affected and still have some patent capillary lumina. Tubular atrophy secondary to ischaemia accompanies the glomerular hyalinization, and interstitial fibrosis occurs, but lipid deposits, indicative of the preceding nephrotic stage, may persist. The kidneys may be slightly shrunken, and may show the superadded changes of hypertension.

Aetiology

Examination of renal biopsies by immunofluorescence microscopy shows deposition of immunoglobulin, usually mainly IgG, along the walls of the glomerular capillaries. The deposition is diffuse throughout all the capillaries and at an early stage appears granular. As the disease progresses the deposits increase in size and number and tend to become confluent. Deposition of complement is also

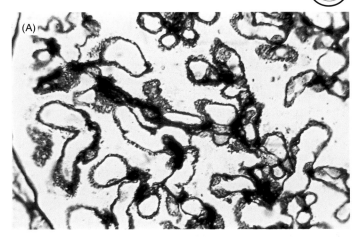

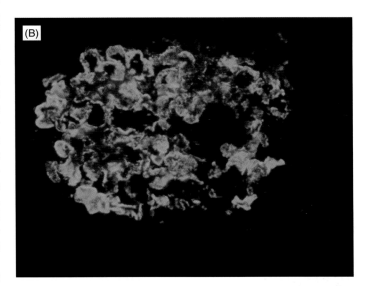

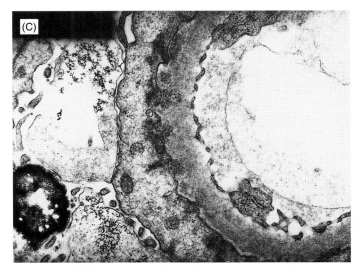

FIGURE 13.11 (A) Membranous nephropathy is characterized by thickening of the glomerular capillary walls but with normal cellularity. The thickened capillary walls exhibit a spiky appearance on silver stained preparations. (B) Immunofluorescence staining reveals the presence of immune complexes, in this case IgM, within the capillary walls as granular deposits. (C) Electron microscopic examination reveals the presence of subepithelial electron dense immune complexes.

usually demonstrable by immunofluorescence, its distribution being the same as that of the immunoglobulin(s), but it is deposited in smaller amounts and in some cases is not detectable. The low level of complement deposition may be equated with the absence of inflammatory features (cf. acute post-infectious glomerulonephritis). There is evidence to suggest *in-situ* formation of immune complexes in some types of membranous glomerulonephritis.

The nature of the antigen is unknown in most cases, but some cases are associated with infections: malaria, syphilis and hepatitis B and their corresponding (microbial) antigens have been demonstrated in the glomerular deposits in such cases. There is an association with malignant tumours and the possibility of a lymphoma or carcinoma should be borne in mind in any middle-aged or elderly patient presenting with 'idiopathic' membranous glomerulonephritis. Membranous glomerulonephritis may also occur in patients treated with certain drugs, notably penicillamine and gold salts, and is also one of the renal manifestations of systemic lupus erythematosus. In all of these associations, the glomerular deposition of Ig suggests an immune complex basis, the antigens being assumed to be derived from tumours, drugs, etc. In patients with systemic lupus erythematosus, the deposits have been shown to consist of autoantigens complexed with autoantibodies (pp. 26–27).

Mesangiocapillary (Membranoproliferative) Glomerulonephritis

This condition occurs at all ages but particularly in older children. Its presenting features may be those of the acute nephritic syndrome, the nephrotic syndrome or asymptomatic proteinuria and haematuria. Overall the prognosis is poor and many patients go on to develop chronic renal failure. The response to immunosuppression is poor, and if renal transplantation is performed the condition tends to recur in the graft.

Pathological Changes

At an early stage the glomeruli show diffuse proliferative change with increase in size and number of mesangial and endothelial cells; the mesangia in particular show increased cellularity and the lobular architecture of the glomeruli is accentuated (Figure 13.12). The capillary lumina are reduced and there is irregular thickening of the capillary walls. Silver stains may show a double basement membrane. Two main types are discernible by electron microscopy:

- In type I, discrete irregular deposits are found on the inner, subendothelial, side of the (original) basement membrane, and there is extension of the cytoplasm of mesangial cells between the endothelium and the basement membrane (mesangial interposition). A second layer of basement membrane is laid down between the endothelium and the mesangial cytoplasmic extension,

thus accounting for the double contour seen by some silver stained preparations.

- In type II, dense material is deposited within the lamina densa causing a more diffuse thickening of the basement membrane. This has sometimes led to the use of the term dense deposit disease (Figure 13.12).

A type III with both subendothelial and subepithelial deposits has also been described but is regarded as a variant of type I. The two patterns of deposition are sometimes distinguishable by light microscopy of very thin sections but are seen more readily by electron microscopy. In some cases, particularly of the type II, there is formation of small crescents in the capsule of occasional glomeruli. As the disease progresses the mesangial cells diminish in number and hyaline material accumulates, while the capillaries become progressively thickened so that glomerulosclerosis and chronic renal failure usually result.

Aetiology

The aetiology of mesangiocapillary glomerulonephritis is unknown. In type I, components of complement and immunoglobulin (IgG and/or IgM) are detectable in the capillary walls (Figure 13.12) and it is likely that the disease is of an immune complex nature. Associations with subacute bacterial endocarditis, sickle cell disease and hepatitis B, have been described. In type II there is little evidence of immune complex deposition although C3 may be found in the mesangium and around the tubules. In both types, there may be depression of C3 in the plasma and activation of the alternative pathway of complement is involved. A factor which activates C3 (the nephritic factor) has been detected in the serum in some cases. It appears to be an autoantibody to the C3bBb complex of the alternative pathway.

A familial predisposition is likely in mesangiocapillary glomerulonephritis, and, in particular, there is a syndrome linking partial lipodystrophy and the type II disease.

Focal Glomerulonephritis

This may be defined as a glomerulonephritis affecting only a proportion of the glomeruli. The lesions usually involve only part of the glomerular tuft, and may therefore be described as focal and segmental. In most patients this will be due to IgA nephropathy and the clinical features are usually microscopic or macroscopic haematuria with or without asymptomatic proteinuria. In these patients with intermittent macroscopic haematuria, episodes may be precipitated by upper respiratory tract infections, heavy exercise or certain foods/alcohol. This disease usually affects children and young adults and for many the prognosis will be good, but long-term follow-up is advised to identify the subgroup of patients who go on to develop chronic renal failure. There is no proved specific effective treatment for this form of glomerulonephritis although many studies have suggested a variety of agents might be beneficial.

Focal glomerulonephritis may also accompany a number of other systemic diseases, notably subacute bacterial

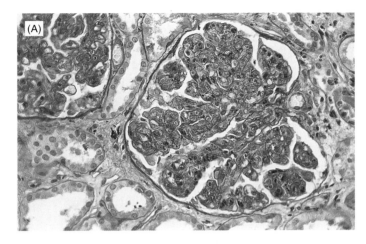

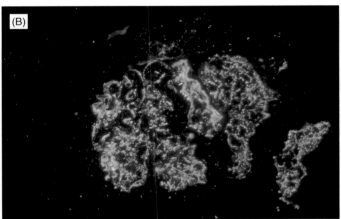

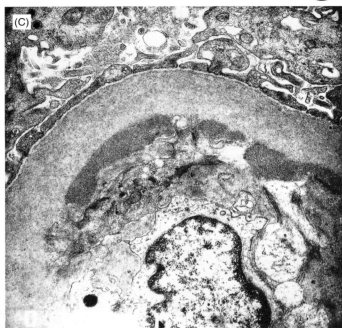

FIGURE 13.12 Mesangiocapillary glomerulonephritis, also known as membranoproliferative glomerulonephritis, is characterized by a combination of hypercellularity and capillary wall thickening. (A) At the light microscopy level the hypercellularity is seen clearly with accentuation of the glomerular) lobular architecture and a reduction in the capillary luminal space. Thickening of the glomerular capillary wall is also evident. (B) Immunofluorescence staining in cases of mesangiocapillary glomerulonephritis reveals the deposition of granules of immune complexes within capillary walls and within mesangial regions in most cases. In the example illustrated here the immunofluorescence reactivity demonstrates IgG deposition within the glomerulus. (C) Examination of cases of mesangiocapillary glomerulonephritis by electron microscopy reveals different patterns of deposition. In one form there is electron-dense thickening of the glomerular basement membrane itself. This form is known as dense deposit disease. The presence of focal electron dense deposits in the subendothelial space as shown here is the much more common form.

endocarditis (SBE), systemic lupus erythematosus (SLE), Henoch–Schönlein purpura, the microangiopathic form of polyarteritis, Wegener's granulomatosis and Goodpasture's syndrome. It must be emphasized that focal glomerulonephritis is not the only renal lesion occurring in these conditions: crescentic glomerulonephritis may develop in any of them, and is the usual lesion in Goodpasture's syndrome and the vasculitides.

Pathological Changes

The glomerular lesion consists of a cellular proliferation, probably of mesangial cells, affecting the peripheral part of one or more lobules (Figure 13.13) and in some cases accompanied by fibrinoid necrosis of capillary loops. Within the lesions, individual capillary lumina may be obliterated by eosinophilic thrombus which blends with the necrotic capillary walls. Red cells may be present in the capsular space and in the tubules, and there may also be

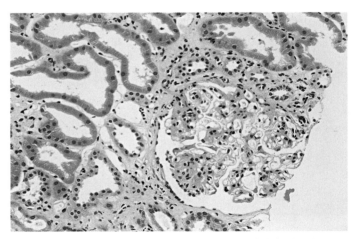

FIGURE 13.13 On occasion proliferative glomerulonephritis is focal and segmental. In these instances the hypercellularity is limited to a portion of the glomerular tuft with obliteration of capillaries and occasionally foci of necrosis.

some proliferation of the epithelial lining of Bowman's capsule, i.e. formation of small crescents. Lesions may occur in only a small proportion of glomeruli, or may involve the majority. In patients with a long history, old scarred glomerular lesions are usually seen, often adherent to the capsule. In IgA nephropathy and Henoch–Schönlein purpura nephritis there is characteristic mesangial deposition of IgA on immunofluorescence staining.

Acute Diffuse Proliferative Glomerulonephritis

Clinical Features and Course

This type of glomerulonephritis occurs at all ages, although it is more prevalent in children than in adults, but is now uncommon in developed countries. It usually follows an acute infection with Group A haemolytic streptococci – most often pharyngitis (including scarlet fever), but sometimes infections of the middle ear or skin. Glomerulonephritis develops 1–4 weeks after the onset of the streptococcal infection which usually has already resolved. Other infections, for example with *Staphylococcus aureus* and *Streptococcus*

pneumoniae have occasionally been implicated and acute glomerulonephritis may also complicate falciparum malaria, toxoplasmosis, schistosomiasis, and some acute viral infections.

The presenting features are usually those of an acute nephritic syndrome. Hypertension, moderate proteinuria and mild renal impairment are usually present and urine microscopy reveals many red cells, neutrophil polymorphs and hyaline, granular and cellular casts. During the acute phase serious complications include acute renal failure and cardiac failure due to hypertension and fluid retention. In childhood the disease has a good outcome with complete recovery in over 90% of cases but in adults the outcome is less favourable, a significant proportion developing chronic glomerulonephritis leading to chronic renal failure.

Pathological Features

Microscopically, the most conspicuous changes are diffuse enlargement and increased cellularity of the glomeruli (Figure 13.14A). The enlargement results in narrowing or obliteration of the capsular space and part of the glomerular tuft can often be seen to have herniated into the lumen

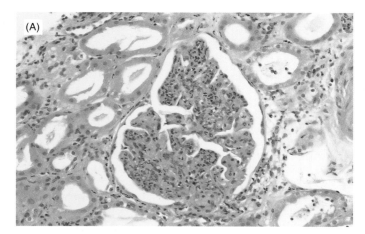

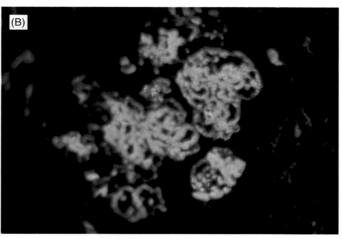

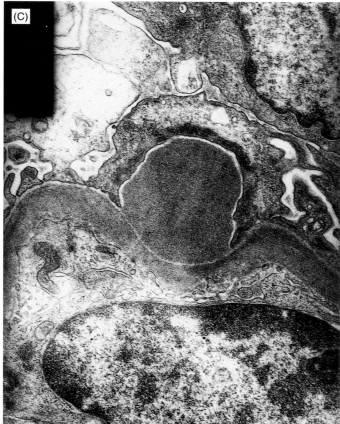

FIGURE 13.14 (A) In diffuse proliferative glomerulonephritis there is marked hypercellularity often with an influx of neutrophil polymorphs and obliteration of the capillary spaces. The glomerular capillary walls are difficult to identify within this hypercellular glomerulus. (B) Immunofluorescence in these instances reveals the granular deposition of immune complexes in the capillary walls. (C) The electron microscopic findings in diffuse proliferative glomerulonephritis are highly characteristic. In the subepithelial space there are large 'hump'-shaped electron dense deposits.

of the proximal tubule. The capillary lumina appear narrowed, and the endothelial cells are swollen. Electron microscopy shows the hypercellularity to be due to an increase of mesangial and endothelial cells; neutrophil polymorphs and macrophages are also seen but vary greatly in number from case to case.

An additional change in the glomerular tufts is an increase in the number of strands of basement-membrane-like material (mesangial matrix) demonstrable by electron microscopy in the mesangial regions. These strands are normally present between mesangial cells and are made more conspicuous by oedema. In cases which fail to resolve, the material increases in amount and contributes to the hyaline appearance of the glomeruli in the chronic stage of glomerulonephritis. Electron microscopy shows the presence of subepithelial 'humps' – deposits of electron dense material which are indicative of immune complex formation (Figure 13.14C). Smaller deposits may be seen on the endothelial surface of the basement membrane.

The epithelial cells do not show widespread effacement of foot processes, although this may occur focally. Some proteinaceous debris, and occasionally red cells, may be seen in the narrowed capsular spaces. In most cases, the epithelium of Bowman's capsule appears normal, but here and there some proliferation may be seen. Epithelial crescents are few or absent in typical cases. Changes in the rest of the kidney are secondary to the glomerular lesion: there is diffuse oedema, seen as an increase in the loose interstitial tissue between the tubules, and often accompanied by a light scattering of neutrophil polymorphs or mononuclear cells. The tubules contain protein and cellular casts, including red blood cell casts, and the epithelial cells of the proximal convoluted tubules contain hyaline droplets. Occasionally there are foci of disruption of tubular epithelial cells, possibly attributable to ischaemia secondary to the glomerular changes. Hypertension is not usually sufficiently severe or prolonged to produce changes in the heart and blood vessels.

With recovery from the disease the glomeruli return to normal, although increased numbers of cells in the mesangial zones of the glomerular lobules may persist for months, and are regarded as a retrospective diagnostic feature. Following acute diffuse glomerulonephritis, increase in the size and number of mesangial cells may persist for weeks or even months without serious sequelae. Increase in basement-membrane-like material in the mesangial areas is, however, a more serious feature; it is seen together with persistent cellular increase in those few cases which, after a latent period, develop chronic glomerulonephritis.

Pathogenesis

Immunofluorescence microscopy of renal biopsy material in cases of acute diffuse glomerulonephritis typically reveals granular deposition of immunoglobulin (usually mainly IgG) and components of complement in the glomerular capillary walls (Figure 13.14B). These findings, together with the detection by electron microscopy of dense subepithelial deposits are strongly suggestive of the deposition of immune complexes. As acute glomerulonephritis usually follows a streptococcal infection it is likely that antibodies to streptococcal products, appearing a week or so after the infection, combine with streptococcal antigens still present in the plasma, thus providing immune complexes which would, at first, be formed in the presence of antigen excess. In keeping with this there are usually low levels of serum complement components, consistent with activation of complement by an antigen–antibody reaction, and serum antistreptolysin O (ASO) titres are usually high, indicating previous streptococcal infection. It is not understood why certain types of group A streptococci, notably Griffiths types 12, 4, 1, 25 and 49 are nephritogenic, whereas other types and other microorganisms are not.

Crescentic Glomerulonephritis (Rapidly Progressive Glomerulonephritis)

This may develop without known predisposing cause, or may follow a streptococcal infection. It can supervene also in patients with the focal glomerulonephritis associated with certain diseases particularly vasculitis and Goodpasture's syndrome (see below). It can occur at any age, but is commoner in the elderly. The clinical features and urinary changes may be indistinguishable at first from those of acute diffuse glomerulonephritis but instead of regressing after a week or two, they become progressively more severe, leading to advanced renal failure after a period of days or weeks. Rarely, proteinuria may be severe enough to give rise to the nephrotic syndrome, while other cases may present in acute renal failure. Crescentic glomerulonephritis is uncommon but if diagnosed promptly immunosuppressive therapy can reverse or prevent renal failure.

Pathological Changes

Microscopy shows the most important changes to be glomerular. As in acute diffuse glomerulonephritis, there is proliferation of both endothelial and mesangial cells, with narrowing of the capillary lumina, and variable polymorph infiltration of the tuft. Although all the glomeruli are affected, some glomerular lobules may be more severely involved than others, and there may be areas of basement membrane rupture with foci of haemorrhage and fibrinoid necrosis and thrombi in some capillary lumina. Blood products may therefore escape into Bowman's space.

A characteristic histological feature is proliferation of the parietal epithelium of Bowman's capsule to form 'epithelial crescents' (see Figure 13.8) which occupy the capsular space and surround the tuft. In time, the epithelial crescents are usually replaced by fibrous tissue. Immunofluorescence studies have failed to demonstrate immunoglobulins in crescents, but deposits of fibrin are present and have been shown experimentally to stimulate crescent formation.

The tubules may be dilated and usually contain hyaline and cellular casts and red cells and proteinaceous droplets are present in the cells of the proximal convoluted tubules. There may be focal necrosis or irregular tubular atrophy and increase of intertubular connective tissue, presumably due to ischaemia resulting from the glomerular changes. In some cases hypertension is severe, and the changes of malignant hypertension become superadded. There may also be left ventricular hypertrophy and changes associated with uraemia, for example fibrinous pericarditis, anaemia and superadded infections.

A surprising feature of the disease is the rapidity with which glomerular scarring may occur: thus in cases with a history of only 2 weeks or so, biopsy may reveal sclerosis of lobules or whole glomeruli, and also fibrous adhesions between the tuft and Bowman's capsule. There is thus a combination of glomerular proliferation, necrosis, thrombosis and scarring, amounting to severe glomerular injury.

Aetiology

In the minority of cases, crescentic glomerulonephritis follows a streptococcal infection and these represent the severe end of the spectrum of acute diffuse proliferative glomerulonephritis. They show granular deposition of Ig and complement and subepithelial deposits on electron microscopy. In other cases, there is no known preceding infection, and the evidence of immune complex deposition is sometimes absent, the so-called pauci-immune group. The condition can supervene in a group of systemic conditions which may also give rise to the less serious focal glomerulonephritis. The same picture is also caused by the development of autoantibody to glomerular basement membrane in Goodpasture's syndrome.

Subacute Bacterial Endocarditis

Renal lesions are common in subacute bacterial endocarditis (SBE), but in most cases they do not lead to serious impairment of renal function and their practical importance lies mainly in the resulting haematuria, either gross or microscopic, which is of diagnostic value.

As in other organs, infarcts are common in the kidneys in subacute bacterial endocarditis and are usually nonsuppurative. Focal glomerulonephritis occurs in about 50% of cases, and tends to develop after some months. Most of the cases have been caused by *Streptococcus viridans* or *Haemophilus influenzae* but now *Staphylococcus aureus* is a recognized cause of a more acute endocarditis, particularly in intravenous drug abusers. Microscopically, a minority of the glomeruli are usually affected, and the focal lesions show capillary thrombosis, fibrinoid necrosis and proliferative changes. Blood is often seen in the capsular space and tubules, and there may be epithelial crescents. In keeping with an immune complex-mediated lesion, the serum complement levels are depressed, electron microscopy shows the presence of subendothelial and mesangial deposits and immunofluorescence studies confirm the presence of Ig. Circulating immune complexes have been demonstrated by some workers. In a minority of patients with subacute bacterial endocarditis, diffuse proliferative glomerulonephritis develops, and may progress to renal failure.

Henoch–Schönlein purpura occurs mainly in children, and gives rise to a skin rash, joint pains and colic with bloody diarrhoea due to a haemorrhagic exudate into the gut. In some cases there is a focal glomerulonephritis, with haematuria and proteinuria, and this is associated with the mesangial deposition of IgA (these histological appearances are indistinguishable from IgA nephropathy). Renal failure is either absent or mild and transient, and the kidneys usually recover completely, even after recurrent attacks. Crescentic glomerulonephritis may, however, supervene, particularly in older patients and in some other cases chronic renal failure develops after some years. Immunosuppression is of doubtful value in this form of focal nephritis except in those cases presenting with a rapidly progressive glomerulonephritis.

Goodpasture's Syndrome

In this uncommon condition, there is haematuria and proteinuria attributable to a focal glomerulonephritis. This is accompanied by haemorrhage from the alveolar capillaries which gives rise to haemoptysis and dyspnoea. The glomerular and pulmonary injuries are caused by autoantibody to basement membrane(s) causing (in the case of the kidney) a necrotizing and crescentic glomerulonephritis (Figure 13.15A) with

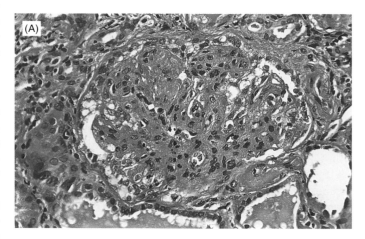

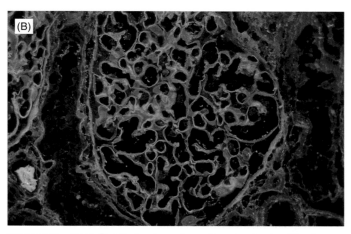

FIGURE 13.15 (A) In Goodpasture's syndrome there is a focal proliferative and necrotizing glomerulonephritis usually accompanied by crescent formation. (B) Immunofluorescence staining of renal biopsies demonstrates a linear pattern of deposition of IgG and C3 diagnostic of antiglomerular basement membrane antibodies.

GOODPASTURE'S SYNDROME

Goodpasture's syndrome is a clinical syndrome involving acute renal failure, often with pulmonary haemorrhage. It is therefore one of the so-called pulmonary–renal syndromes. The acute renal failure is usually seen in association with proteinuria and haematuria. The disease is more common in the elderly. Renal biopsy shows the syndrome to be a consequence of a proliferative necrotizing glomerulonephritis usually with a high proportion of crescents. When renal biopsy material is stained by the immunofluorescence technique to demonstrate immune complexes a linear pattern of IgG and staining for the C3 component of complement are seen on the glomerular basement membrane. Patients with Goodpasture's syndrome also have antibodies within their circulation which react with the glomerular basement membrane. These observations have led to the hypothesis that Goodpasture's syndrome is an autoimmune disease in which the patient mounts an antibody response to the constitutive components of the glomerular basement membrane. The glomerular basement membrane is an extracellular matrix comprising a number of collagens and non-collagenous glycoproteins. The autoantibodies from patients with Goodpasture's syndrome react with the type IV collagen within the basement membrane and specifically the alpha 3 domain of the type IV collagen. The autoantibodies bind to the extracellular matrix and within the glomerulus activate complement leading to a localized type III hypersensitivity reaction. The disease is therefore an example of an autoimmune disease, antibody mediated, causing type III hypersensitivity induced tissue damage.

Genetic factors play an important role in the aetiology of Goodpasture's syndrome and there is a strong association between the formation of antiglomerular basement membrane antibodies and human leucocyte antigen (HLA) DR2 alleles. During the induction of immune responses antigens are presented to immunocompetent cells on the surface of macrophages in association with the HLA molecules. The most recent research in Goodpasture's syndrome has suggested that antigenic fragments from type IV collagen presented by individuals with the appropriate DR2 alleles differ from those presented by individuals who are not susceptible to the disease. Goodpasture's syndrome is therefore a good model of antibody-mediated autoimmune disease in which there is an HLA association which determines the pattern of presentation of the autoantigen. Precisely what triggers this immune response is unclear but there is an association with hydrocarbon exposure and hydrocarbon-induced damage to the glomerular basement membrane.

linear deposition of immunoglobulin on the basement membrane (Figure 13.15B). The prognosis is poor without early treatment with plasma exchange and cytotoxic drugs.

Systemic Lupus Erythematosus

Clinically apparent renal disease occurs in upto 50% of patients with systemic lupus erythematosus (SLE) (pp. 26–27), and carries a poor prognosis. The nephrotic syndrome may develop when proteinuria is heavy, and uraemia, with or without hypertension, is an important cause of death. The essential changes are in the glomeruli, which show a great variety of lesions. These include:

- focal glomerulonephritis which is indistinguishable from the proliferative and necrotizing lesions described above, except that haematoxyphil bodies are sometimes apparent
- a focal thickening of the capillary walls with a refractile eosinophilic appearance, known as the wire-loop lesion
- hyaline thrombi in individual glomerular capillaries
- various combinations of diffuse proliferative and irregular membranous change
- diffuse membranous change resembling that seen in idiopathic membranous glomerulonephritis.

Lupus nephropathy is classified on the basis of the glomerular morphology according to well-established World Health Organization criteria (Table 13.3). The duration of these various lesions, and thus the degree of glomerular sclerosis, also vary greatly. Immunofluorescence and electron microscopy provide strong evidence that these glomerular changes represent the spectrum of immune complex injury. For example, the focal lesion is accompanied by deposition of immunoglobulin and complement in the mesangia and focally in the inner parts of the capillary walls: more extensive deposition of complexes in the inner parts of the capillary walls is seen in the combination of diffuse proliferative and patchy membranous change, while the diffuse granular pattern of deposition, much of it along the outer part of the basement membrane, is seen in the diffuse membranous lesion. Antibodies to DNA, to histones and to DNA–histone complexes have been eluted from the kidney tissue in SLE. Curious tubulo-reticular structures are sometimes seen by electron microscopy in

TABLE 13.3 WHO classification of lupus nephritis

I	No lesion by light microscopy
II	Mesangial proliferation
III	Focal (<50%) proliferation
IV	Diffuse (>50%) proliferation
V	Membranous
(VI)	Chronic renal damage

the endothelial cells. Originally thought to be viral, they are now considered to represent a response to injury by various agents, including virus infection. They are found most commonly in SLE although they have been described in other conditions, for example in human immunodeficiency virus (HIV)-associated nephropathy.

Chronic Glomerulonephritis

It is apparent from the foregoing descriptions of the various types of glomerulonephritis, that an end stage may be reached in which total glomerular function is so reduced that chronic renal failure develops. The time taken to reach this stage, and the rate of progression once it has developed, vary with the type of preceding glomerulonephritis. Hypertension, sometimes of the malignant type, usually develops and if untreated aggravates the renal tissue destruction. In cases where hypertension is absent or less severe, renal failure may progress more slowly. Chronic renal failure usually occurs because most of the nephrons have been so severely damaged by the causal disease that they are no longer functional. The remaining functioning glomeruli not only become hypertrophied but also filter off a relatively high proportion of the fluid passing through them. This hyperfunctioning state may itself cause further glomerular injury and consequently further deterioration of renal function.

In the majority of patients with chronic glomerulonephritis, there is no history to suggest preceding renal disease, and the renal lesions have progressed silently until chronic renal failure develops. In such cases, it is often not possible to decide, even by histological examination of the kidneys, what type of glomerulonephritis has led up to the chronic stage. In other cases, there is a history of previous glomerulonephritis: this may have been an acute attack of post-streptococcal glomerulonephritis years before, or the patient may have had membranous, mesangiocapillary or recurrent focal glomerulonephritis, which has progressed to the stage of chronic renal failure.

Pathological Changes and Pathogenesis

Both the kidneys are uniformly and equally reduced in size, sometimes only slightly so, but often to about one-third of normal. In those kidneys which are greatly shrunken, the capsule is often firmly adherent and the subcapsular surface uniformly and finely irregular. There is diffuse thinning of the cortex, which accounts largely for the reduction in kidney size, while the medullary pyramids are also, although less markedly shrunken. The amount of fatty tissue around the renal pelvis is increased. In contrast to chronic pyelonephritis, the calyces and renal pelvis are not distorted.

The renal arteries and their major branches show arteriosclerotic thickening, and in cases complicated by malignant hypertension the cortical mottling and haemorrhages of this condition are superimposed on the changes described above. The other organs and tissues show the changes of chronic renal failure.

Microscopically, in the small granular kidneys, it is common to find all degrees of hyalinization of glomeruli. Many are completely hyalinized and some show partial destruction. A small percentage are normal or nearly so, and may be hypertrophied. In cases in which the kidneys are not greatly shrunken the glomeruli are usually more uniformly damaged: this is seen in the chronic end stages of membranous and mesangiocapillary glomerulonephritis. The arcuate and interlobular arteries and the afferent arterioles show hypertensive changes. Where malignant hypertension has supervened the secondary glomerular changes are seen in those glomeruli not already destroyed by the glomerulonephritic process.

The tubules show extensive atrophy, many being completely lost, and there is an increase in the intertubular connective tissue and the irregular interstitial aggregation of lymphocytes and small numbers of plasma cells. In cases with some near-normal hypertrophied glomeruli, the corresponding tubules are enlarged and conspicuous, and account for the elevations which give the subcapsular surface its granular appearance. These surviving functioning tubules may show hyaline droplets in the epithelial cytoplasm and frequently contain protein casts, features which relate to the proteinuria. When malignant hypertension has supervened, there may be blood in the capsular spaces and in functioning tubules.

In cases of chronic glomerulonephritis preceded by the nephrotic syndrome, the kidneys may still be enlarged, and lipid deposits may still be visible in the cortex by the naked eye. Although the glomeruli show advanced sclerosis, their appearance may still suggest the type of glomerulonephritis responsible. All the glomeruli are affected to some extent, and the tubular atrophy is accordingly more uniform, without prominent enlarged tubules; for this reason, the surface of the kidney is often smooth and does not exhibit the granularity usually found in other forms of chronic glomerulonephritis.

Clinical Features

The clinical features and changes in other organs and tissues are those of chronic renal failure and are attributable to uraemia, and usually hypertension.

Diabetic Glomerulosclerosis

Diabetes mellitus is one of the major causes of chronic renal disease leading to chronic renal failure resulting in a requirement for renal replacement therapy. Several different abnormalities may be encountered in the kidneys of diabetic patients; these are known collectively as 'diabetic nephropathy'. Diabetic glomerulosclerosis is the most common pathology and may be associated with proteinuria, nephrotic syndrome and chronic renal failure. Although diabetic glomerulosclerosis usually develops in patients with long-standing diabetes on occasion it may present early in the clinical course and, rarely, may precede the recognition of clinical diabetes mellitus. There are three different morphological features within the diabetic glomerulus: capillary basement membrane thickening, diffuse glomerulosclerosis and nodular glomerulosclerosis. Capillary basement membrane thickening is common but requires detailed morphometric assessment to confirm its presence. Diffuse glomerulosclerosis consists of a diffuse increase in the mesangial matrix, possibly with mild proliferation of mesangial cells. This is usually also associated with thickening of the glomerular basement membrane. As the disease progresses continuing mesangial expansion and obliteration of the entire glomerulus occurs. In nodular glomerulosclerosis the glomerular lesions take the form of nodular expansions of the mesangial matrix surrounded by patent peripheral capillary loops (Figure 13.16). The expansion of the nodules with progression of the diabetic nephropathy leads to obliteration of the capillary tuft. This nodular diabetic glomerulosclerosis is pathognomonic of diabetes.

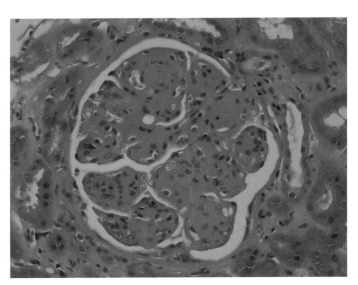

FIGURE 13.16 In diabetic nephropathy there is a nodular expansion of the mesangial matrix with thickening of the glomerular capillary walls but with no hypercellularity. Immunofluorescence staining in diabetic nephropathy is negative.

Diabetic nephropathy may also include hyaline arteriolosclerosis, increased susceptibility to pyelonephritis and papillary necrosis. Diabetic nephropathy is a progressive disease, the rate of progression being influenced by coexisting hypertension, the activity of the local renin–angiotensin system and the degree of hyperglycaemia. Recent studies have confirmed that inhibition of angiotensin generation by angiotensin-converting enzyme inhibitors or angiotensin receptor blockade has a beneficial effect on the progression of diabetic renal disease superior to that of other antihypertensive agents. Progression is less influenced by strict diabetic control.

Amyloidosis

The kidneys are one of the most frequently involved organs in amyloidosis. There is deposition of amyloid proteins around glomerular capillary basement membranes (Figure 13.17) leading to increased permeability, proteinuria and progressive renal disease. As the deposition of amyloid increases capillaries become obliterated and glomeruli extensively replaced by amyloid protein. There is secondary atrophy of tubules with interstitial fibrosis. The renal arterioles are also frequently involved in the deposition of amyloid leading to secondary ischaemic changes.

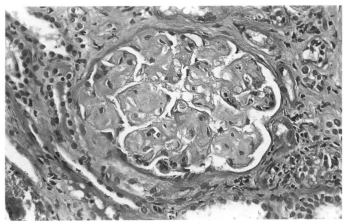

FIGURE 13.17 In amyloidosis there is marked expansion of the extracellular matrix of the glomerulus with obliteration of the capillary spaces – these features may also affect the larger blood vessels, the tubules and the interstitium of the kidney. The amyloid material stains with the Congo Red stain.

DISEASES AFFECTING TUBULES

There are two main groups of diseases affecting tubules:

● ischaemic or toxic injury leads to acute tubular necrosis
● inflammatory reactions of the tubules and interstitium are known as tubulo-interstitial nephritis.

Acute Tubular Necrosis

Key Points

- Acute tubular necrosis (ATN) is caused by ischaemic or toxic injury and regeneration of the tubular epithelium usually occurs.
- Arteriolar vasoconstriction, increased glomerular permeability, tubular obstruction and backleak of tubular fluid are all involved in the pathogenesis of ATN.
- Tubulo-interstitial nephritis may be due to an acute hypersensitivity reaction to drugs.
- Chronic tubulo-interstitial nephritis may occur with long-term use of non-steroidal anti-inflammatory drugs (NSAIDs) and excessive use of simple analgesics.

In acute tubular necrosis the kidney is injured by ischaemia (prerenal failure) or toxins or a combination of these factors resulting in cell injury and death of the tubular epithelium. The tubules are the most metabolically active part of the nephron and are therefore most vulnerable to these insults. The tubular epithelium is capable of regeneration and if the factors leading to acute tubular necrosis are corrected complete recovery of renal function can be expected. However, if the exposure is prolonged irreversible damage may occur and the outcome will be chronic renal failure or established renal failure. Examples of ischaemic and toxic causes of acute tubular necrosis are shown in Table 13.4.

TABLE 13.4 Causes of acute tubular necrosis

Ischaemic	Both	Toxic
Ruptured aortic aneurysm	Septicaemia	Drugs (e.g. aminoglycosides)
Gastroenteritis	Hepatorenal syndrome	Heavy metal poisoning
Cardiogenic shock	Pancreatitis	Rhabdomyolysis

Patients with established acute tubular necrosis are usually oliguric although in some cases urine output is maintained despite a marked reduction in glomerular filtration rate (non-oliguric acute renal failure). During this phase there is a progressive rise in urea, creatinine and other nitrogenous waste products, a failure to excrete acid and potassium and retention of sodium and water. Without dialysis these abnormalities are likely to be fatal within 2–3 days. The oliguric phase of acute tubular necrosis may last from for several hours up to several weeks and is followed by a 'diuretic phase' when urine volume increases, occasionally excessively. During this period which seldom lasts for more than a few days glomerular and tubular functions start to recover and dialysis can be stopped. Finally during the 'recovery phase' sometimes lasting many weeks, renal function returns to normal or near normal.

Pathological Changes

In fatal cases, the kidneys are usually enlarged and the cut surface bulges, due mainly to dilatation of tubules and interstitial oedema. The cortical vessels contain little blood, and the cortex appears pale, with blurring of the normal radial pattern, while the medulla is often dark and congested. Occasionally there are petechial haemorrhages in the cortex.

Microscopically, the glomerular tufts appear normal. Usually there is some granular debris in the capsular space and the parietal cells lining Bowman's capsule may be unduly prominent and cuboidal. The tubular changes are variable and depend on the severity and duration, and on the particular causal agents involved. In many cases, however, the aetiology is complex, and specific changes cannot

readily be attributed to particular causal agents. Also, it is often difficult to identify, in histological sections, which parts of the tubules have been damaged. At autopsy, the lesion is often obscured by terminal ischaemic changes and post-mortem autolysis.

In cases resulting from ischaemia, both the proximal and distal convoluted tubules are commonly dilated and the epithelial lining is flattened with basophilia of the cytoplasm and mitotic activity (Figure 13.18). These changes, which are seen as early as 3 days after the onset, appear to be sequelae to loss of tubular epithelium; the remaining cells become flattened and undergo proliferation, thus restoring epithelial continuity. In the distal tubules proliferation may be pronounced, the cells sometimes forming syncytial masses, particularly around casts. An early change seen by electron microscopy is the loss of the normal brush border from the proximal tubular cells. The time at which these cells regain their brush border correlates well with the return of renal function.

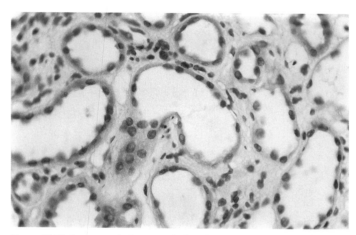

FIGURE 13.18 In a true tubular necrosis there is a flattening of the epithelial cells and many of the tubules contain cellular or acellular debris. The interstitium is oedematous but there is no significant inflammatory infiltrate.

Tubular epithelial necrosis is often not conspicuous and in many cases cannot be seen. In a minority of cases there are foci of necrosis, most numerous in the distal convoluted tubule but also occurring in the proximal tubule. This change, which is described as tubulorrhexis, may be accompanied by disruption of the tubular basement membrane and an inflammatory reaction in the adjacent interstitial tissue. This may progress to scarring and in the event of recovery lead to tubular obstruction and so loss of function of the affected nephrons.

From the ascending limb of Henle's loop onwards, the tubules contain proteinaceous and brown granular casts, and in cases associated with haemoglobinuria or myoglobinuria brown pigment casts and rounded granules of pigmented material are particularly prominent. Distension of the intertubular connective tissue by oedema fluid is conspicuous in some cases, but almost absent in others. The vasa recta of the medulla usually contain groups of nucleated cells, which appear to represent erythropoietic foci, a feature which may be analogous to that seen in the hepatic sinusoids in liver cell necrosis.

The changes described above are seen in acute renal failure resulting from shock, trauma, etc. They occur also in cases resulting from administration of the nephrotoxic poisons listed above, but in the poisoning cases there is, in addition, more extensive necrosis affecting mainly the proximal convoluted tubules of all or most of the nephrons and resulting from the direct effect of the toxic compounds or their metabolites. This nephrotoxic change is often conspicuous but, unlike tubulorrhexis, it does not involve rupture of the tubular basement membrane, and if the patient survives it is often repaired by epithelial regeneration without leaving any residual damage or scarring.

Some variation is observed in the nephrotoxic lesions brought about by different chemicals. For example, mercuric chloride tends to affect the whole of the proximal convoluted tubule, and in some instances the necrotic part of the tubule rapidly becomes calcified, resulting in permanent injury. Carbon tetrachloride causes necrosis especially of the terminal part of the proximal tubule, and also perivenular hepatic necrosis. If ethylene glycol is ingested, a small proportion of it is converted into oxalate, crystals of which form in the tubular lumens: in addition to tubular necrosis it may cause death from liver or brain injury or from acute heart failure.

Pathogenesis of Renal Failure in Acute Tubular Necrosis

Currently four factors are thought to be implicated in the renal failure of acute tubular necrosis: arteriolar vasoconstriction, increased glomerular permeability, tubular obstruction and the backleak of tubular fluid.

Arteriolar Vasoconstriction

Reduction in renal blood flow has been found in chronic renal failure, the reduced flow in acute tubular necrosis being largely confined to the renal cortex. It has been suggested that disruption in the tubular transport of sodium or chloride stimulates renin release and that the renin–angiotensin system mediates the observed vasoconstriction. This mechanism cannot, however, fully explain the facts because angiotensin promotes arteriolar vasoconstriction while the cortical ischaemia in acute tubular necrosis is due in part to constriction of the arcuate or interlobular arteries of the kidney.

Increased Glomerular Permeability

This is associated with swelling of the glomerular epithelial cells, best seen by scanning electron microscopy, in early post-ischaemic acute renal failure. This process can be mimicked by incubating glomeruli in solutions containing angiotensin, and is a second possible effect of the renin–angiotensin system. There is certainly a correlation between the extent of these glomerular epithelial cell changes and the eventual severity of post-ischaemic acute renal failure in humans.

Tubular Obstruction

Microdissection studies have shown the presence of long hyaline tubular casts, consisting largely of Tamm–Horsfall protein, which must restrict tubular flow. This is associated with raised intratubular pressure and dilated tubular lumina. The diuretic phase of acute tubular necrosis is associated with a great increase in Tamm–Horsfall protein in the urine and may indicate the flushing out of these casts. Tubular constriction also leads to afferent arteriolar vasoconstriction, which further lowers the filtration pressure gradient. Protein casts and dilated tubules are however, found in the recovery phase of acute tubular necrosis and hence tubular obstruction cannot be the whole story.

Backleak of Tubular Fluid

This can occur through the areas of basement membrane denuded of epithelial cover in acute tubular necrosis, and any rise in intratubular pressure due to obstruction by casts distal to the epithelial loss will increase the amount of such a fluid leak. Tubular obstruction also reduces glomerular filtration, but dextran-clearance studies suggest that this can explain only about 20% of the observed reduction.

It is obvious that the above-postulated mechanisms are to some extent interdependent, and it is likely that they all contribute to the observed renal failure. The more extensive necrosis of the proximal tubules, which occurs in cases attributable to various toxins, is more uniform and is explicable as a direct toxic effect on the tubular epithelium.

Tubulo-interstitial Nephritis Caused by Drugs and Toxins

In modern medical practice, drug-induced tubulo-interstitial nephritis is one of the common clinical problems facing nephrologists. Drugs may act in two main ways: first as a tubular toxin resulting in the changes of acute tubular necrosis as discussed above; and second, they may elicit an acute hypersensitivity reaction within the renal parenchyma.

Drug-induced Interstitial Nephritis

This is a well-documented form of iatrogenic disease being described in association with an increasing number of drugs, most commonly antibiotics, non-steroidal anti-inflammatory drugs and diuretics. The disease usually begins about 2 weeks after exposure to the drug and may be characterized by systemic illness such as fever and eosinophilia with or without a skin rash. In other patients acute renal impairment is the only abnormality. On histological examination of renal biopsies performed in patients with drug-induced interstitial nephritis there is pronounced oedema and infiltration of the tubules and interstitium by lymphocytes and macrophages. Eosinophils and neutrophils may be present in significant numbers. Plasma cells are found in more long-standing cases. There is a variable degree of tubular damage and regeneration is usually evident. The glomeruli are, for the most part, normal in acute tubulo-interstitial nephritis. The clinical features and morphology suggest a hypersensitivity reaction which is not dose-related but rather is idiosyncratic. It is important to recognize drug-induced interstitial nephritis because it responds satisfactorily to withdrawal of the offending drug and the patient should be made aware of the risk of recurrence on subsequent exposure to the drug.

In addition to an allergic type pathogenesis, nephropathy associated with non-steroidal anti-inflammatory drugs may involve local interstitial ischaemia because of the inhibition of the synthesis of vasodilatory prostaglandin. This is particularly important in patients who have coexisting renal disease or volume depletion. A more chronic form of drug-induced nephropathy is due to excessive long-term analgesic use. This is a disease of worldwide distribution but it appears to be more common in Australia and Scandinavia. Chronic analgesic nephropathy is characterized by a chronic tubulo-interstitial nephritis with tubular atrophy, interstitial fibrosis, chronic inflammatory cell infiltrate and, frequently, accompanying papillary necrosis. In countries with a high intake of simple analgesics it is an important cause of chronic renal failure.

Cast Nephropathy

This is a special form of toxic tubular injury. Multiple myeloma, a neoplasm of immunoglobulin-secreting plasma cells (pp. 218–220), may involve the kidney without direct invasion. The high level of circulating immunoglobulins and particularly immunoglobulin light chains predisposes the kidney to the development of cast nephropathy. The main cause of this renal pathology is related to Bence Jones proteinuria. Immunoglobulin light chains are filtered into the urinary filtrate. During the tubular reabsorption of fluid the resultant high concentrations of immunoglobulins can result in precipitation of these proteins in the tubular lumen. The protein casts thus formed damage the tubular epithelium sometimes with tubular rupture and an adjacent interstitial inflammatory cell infiltrate (Figure 13.19). In addition patients with multiple myeloma may be hypercalcaemic and hyperuricaemic resulting in nephrocalcinosis and gouty nephropathy. They may also develop renal amyloid or severe pyelonephritis. Renal insufficiency occurs in approximately half of patients with multiple myeloma.

VASCULAR DISEASES OF THE KIDNEY

The Kidney and Hypertension

Key Points

- Hyaline arteriosclerosis of the afferent glomerular arterioles is typical in hypertension whereas fibrinoid necrosis extending into the glomerular tuft is seen in the malignant phase.
- Systemic diseases causing vasculitis in the kidney are rare but important causes of renal failure.
- Thrombotic microangiopathies are characterized by thrombocytopenia, renal failure and haemolytic anaemia.
- Atheromatous renovascular disease is common in patients with peripheral and other vascular disease.

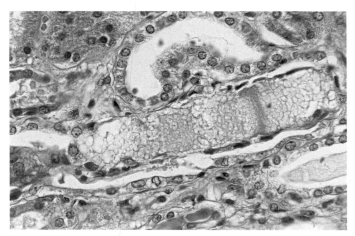

FIGURE 13.19 Patients with myeloma excrete large amounts of light chains in their urine. These light chains may precipitate as casts eliciting a tubular epithelial response and inflammation in the adjacent renal parenchyma – so-called cast nephropathy. This cast nephropathy is one of the forms of kidney involvement in multiple myeloma.

The kidney is centrally involved in blood pressure regulation through the control of salt and water balance, the production of renin and possibly other mechanisms. The kidney is also unusual in possessing a microcirculation which can to a significant degree autoregulate blood flow, thus over a range of blood pressures glomerular capillary blood flow and pressure remain constant. Disturbances in renal function are often accompanied by a rise in blood pressure and thus kidney disease is the commonest cause of secondary hypertension. Secondary hypertension in patients with renal disease is important because if untreated it accelerates the progression of renal damage which is already occurring due to the primary kidney disorder itself and this will lead to a more rapid development of renal failure.

The arterial tree of the kidney is usually affected more than other organs by hypertension and this results in varying degrees of renal damage. Chronic ('benign' or 'essential') hypertension in patients without other underlying kidney disease only occasionally causes advanced renal failure despite the development of widespread arteriosclerosis. Hyaline arteriosclerosis is usually prominent in the afferent glomerular arterioles which become tortuous, thick-walled and extremely narrowed (Figure 13.20). These arterial changes tend to cause ischaemia and because the most important lesion is the hyaline arteriosclerosis of the afferent arterioles, individual nephrons are affected. The capillary tuft of the affected glomerulus shrinks, with wrinkling of its basement membrane. The collapsed capillary tuft later becomes hyalinized and Bowman's capsule becomes filled with collagen, leading to the formation of a solid fibrous ball (Figure 13.20). The tubule atrophies and is replaced by fibrous tissue often containing some lymphocytes. This piecemeal loss of individual nephrons occurs slowly, so that in the early stages of hypertension the kidney appears normal, but with prominent arteries visible on the cut surface. As more nephrons are lost there is diffuse

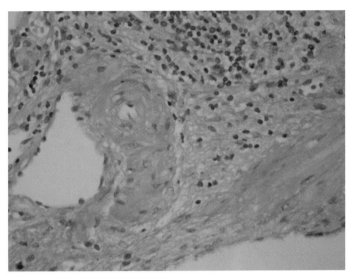

FIGURE 13.20 Hypertension affects the small arteries and arterioles of the kidney. There is a marked hyaline deposition within arteriolar walls with loss of smooth muscle cells. This leads to progressive glomerular ischaemia and glomerular fibrosis.

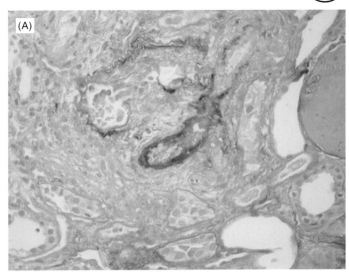

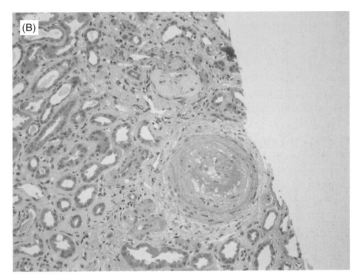

FIGURE 13.21 (A) In malignant hypertension more severe and acute vascular changes are seen in the arterioles. (B) This is characterized by fibrin deposition, platelet activation and transmural necrosis of the arteriolar wall, a constellation of features known as fibrinoid necrosis. There is little inflammatory infiltrate in fibrinoid necrosis.

thinning of the renal cortex and the kidneys become moderately reduced in size. The contraction of the small scars which replace the lost nephrons causes fine depressions on the kidney surface which becomes finely granular in appearance. If enough nephrons are lost there may be hypertrophy of the surviving nephrons which accentuates the roughening of the surface, giving rise to the so-called granular contracted kidney though the kidneys are seldom very small.

Malignant hypertension can cause acute renal failure and may arise *de novo* or supervene after a period of chronic hypertension. In contrast to benign hypertension further investigation will often reveal a cause such as glomerulonephritis. In the most acute cases the surface of the kidney is smooth and spotted with tiny petechial haemorrhages. The cut surface may show mottling due to multiple tiny infarcts. The interlobular arteries often show a proliferative myointimal thickening. Fibrinoid necrosis affects mainly the distal portions of the interlobular arteries and the afferent arterioles (Figure 13.21) but may extend into the glomerular tuft. Other glomeruli show thickening of the capillary walls with reduplication of basement membrane, congestion and capillary dilatation. There is often blood or proteinaceous fluid in Bowman's space and proliferation of the capsular epithelium may give rise to occasional crescents. Unlike glomerulonephritis, only a minority of the glomeruli are affected and the severe impairment of renal function is due to ischaemia caused by the arterial damage and superimposed thrombosis. The tubules may be atrophied or enlarged and usually contain proteinaceous or blood casts. There is hyperplasia of the renin-secreting cells of the juxtaglomerular apparatus and this morphological change correlates with the very high levels of renin and angiotensin II, which invariably occur in malignant hypertension.

Vasculitis and the Kidney

The intrarenal vessels may be involved in a variety of vasculitides particularly polyarteritis nodosa, microscopic polyarteritis and Wegener's granulomatosis. Although these are uncommon conditions they are important to recognize because of their response to immunosuppression without which they carry a poor prognosis.

Polyarteritis nodosa is a systemic vasculitis characterized by transmural necrotizing inflammation of medium-sized or small muscular arteries. The disease typically involves the kidney but may involve other vascular beds. The involvement of the renal arteries is focal and random but there is relative sparing of the glomeruli and the afferent arterioles. These may show, at most, ischaemic changes.

A 32-year-old man presented with established renal failure secondary to glomerulonephritis and hypertension. He was managed on chronic ambulatory peritoneal dialysis. He had anaemia due to defective erythropoietin production by the kidney and was given recombinant erythropoietin (EPO). His blood pressure was controlled with antihypertensive agents, including angiotensin-converting enzyme inhibitors. He underwent a rigorous medical examination but no other significant abnormalities were found. He was placed on the waiting list for renal transplantation.

Six months later a kidney became available for transplantation which showed a perfect blood group match and a good major histocompatibility complex (MHC) match. Crucially his MHC class II antigens were fully matched. He underwent renal transplantation, the new kidney being anastomosed to his iliac vessels and placed in his right iliac fossa. He was treated with conventional immunosuppressive drugs, a combination of tacrolimus, azathioprine and corticosteroids. The graft functioned well by day 5 following surgery, but at day 10 there was a reduction in his renal function. A renal biopsy was performed that showed an acute rejection episode. This was treated by increasing his dose of steroids and the graft function returned to normal. He continued well for the next 2 months until he developed a pyrexial illness with relatively normal graft function but mild liver dysfunction. He was found to have cytomegalovirus infection, a viral infection to which patients on long-term immunosuppression are more susceptible, that had been transmitted in the transplanted kidney. He was treated with ganciclovir and recovered and remains well with a functioning graft 5 years after transplantation continuing on a maintenance dose of immunosuppressive drugs.

At a later stage the acute inflammatory infiltrate disappears and there is transmural fibrous thickening of the artery wall with occasional microaneurysm formation.

Microscopic polyarteritis or polyangiitis differs from polyarteritis nodosa. This disease affects arterioles, capillaries and venules, so in the kidney there tends to be a necrotizing glomerulonephritis with frequent crescent formation (Figure 13.22). The afferent arterioles are affected but larger vessels are relatively spared. Greater than 90% of the patients have antibodies to the myeloperoxidase (MPO) component of neutrophil cytoplasmic antigen (ANCA). This disease is treated by immunosuppression and plasma exchange.

Wegener's granulomatosis is a similar necrotizing vasculitis affecting arterioles, venules and capillaries although there is a tendency also to involve medium-sized arteries. The disease characteristically includes midline lesions affecting the nose, sinuses and lung with focal necrotizing vasculitis involving the kidney. Morphologically there is a necrotizing glomerulonephritis with crescent formation and necrotizing lesions affecting the blood vessels. On renal biopsy the distinction between microscopic polyarteritis and Wegener's granulomatosis may not be possible and the categorization into these two diseases is based largely on the pattern of clinical involvement supported by the type of antineutrophil cytoplasmic antibodies detected. Greater than 90% of patients with Wegener's granulomatosis have proteinase 3 (PR3) ANCA antibodies, the titres of which correlate with disease activity.

Thrombotic Microangiopathies

In this group of disorders there is a combination of so-called malignant vascular injury, microangiopathic haemolytic anaemia and renal failure. Malignant vascular injury is a descriptive term for severe vascular lesions characterized

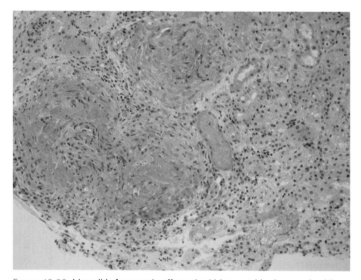

FIGURE 13.22 Vasculitis frequently affects the kidney and is characterized by a transmural inflammatory infiltrate causing localized damage with focal cellular necrosis in the blood vessel wall. Eventually this leads to ischaemia of the renal parenchyma and scarring in the blood vessel wall.

by fibrinoid necrosis and myointimal proliferation with a sparse inflammatory cell infiltrate (Figure 13.23).

Haemolytic uraemic syndrome may be of the childhood or adult type. It may be sporadic or occur in an epidemic form in which case it is particularly associated with diarrhoeal illness caused by verocytotoxin producing *Escherichia coli* (*E. coli* O157). In childhood the onset often follows an upper respiratory tract or diarrhoeal illness of ill-defined aetiology. The main features of the disease are acute renal failure, thrombocytopenia, confusion and microangiopathic haemolytic anaemia. In adults the disease may also follow an episode of diarrhoea but other causes include HIV infection, malignancy and drugs such as cyclosporin and

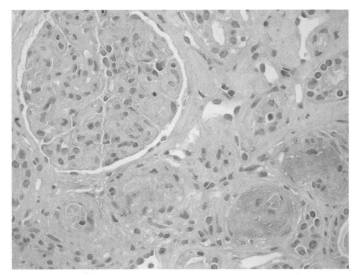

FIGURE 13.23 In the haemolytic uraemic syndrome there is fibrinoid necrosis of arterioles with fibrin and platelet deposition within glomeruli.

cisplatinum. Mutations in complement genes (e.g. factor H) have been shown to predispose to haemolytic uraemic syndrome in those cases which are familial. Haemolytic uraemic syndrome has a significant mortality in the elderly; however, most children and young and middle-aged adults survive although the recovery of renal function may be incomplete.

Thrombotic thrombocytopenic purpura (TTP) is a rarer idiopathic condition related to the haemolytic uraemic syndrome. It has many of the above features but neurological involvement is more frequent and severe and the extent of the renal failure tends to be more profound with higher mortality.

Progressive systemic sclerosis is a connective tissue disease with renal involvement. The renal manifestations include acute renal failure (scleroderma renal crisis), often irreversible, with severe hypertension. The disease occurs in a patient with the otherwise typical features of systemic sclerosis.

A syndrome resembling the haemolytic uraemic syndrome may occur in late pregnancy sometimes in association with pre-eclampsia but also seen following an uneventful pregnancy. The disease is of acute onset with renal failure, platelet consumption and a haemolytic anaemia.

The long-term outcome for renal function from all of these disorders is variable but the renal vasculature is scarred by malignant vascular injury and many patients will have residual renal impairment and hypertension.

Renal Cortical Necrosis

Bilateral diffuse cortical necrosis with sparing of the medulla is an uncommon condition but when present leads to renal failure often with incomplete recovery. It is most frequently associated with pregnancy, particularly those complicated by pre-eclampsia or placental abruption but it may occur in other disorders such haemolytic uraemic syndrome, septic shock or disseminated intravascular coagulation.

Other Vascular Diseases

Atheroma is not uncommon in the main renal arteries of patients with generalized atherosclerosis. This often occurs due to encroachment of aortic atheromatous plaque into the ostium of the renal artery, and it also occurs more distally. Renal ischaemia due to atherosclerosis of the renal arteries is an important cause of renal failure in the elderly and may also cause hypertension and cardiac failure. In some cases these features can be improved by relief of the stenosis by surgery or more often radiologically guided angioplasty.

The kidney may also be affected in the cholesterol emboli syndrome; multiple cholesterol microemboli from atheromatous plaques in the aorta become lodged in the renal vasculature, causing renal failure. Other clinical features due to cholesterol emboli occur in the skin, gastrointestinal tract and the lower limbs. In younger patients hypertension may result from fibromuscular dysplasia of the renal arteries. Senile arteriosclerosis in the kidneys of elderly normotensive people presents features similar to those of benign essential hypertension and does not seriously impair renal function.

DISEASES OF THE URINARY TRACT

Key points

- Obstruction, vesicoureteric reflux, diabetes, pregnancy, neurogenic bladder and calculi predispose to pyelonephritis.
- Urinary infection in childhood is often due to reflux nephropathy which can lead to chronic pyelonephritis if unrecognized.

Urinary Tract Obstruction

Obstruction in the urinary tract may be acute or insidious in onset and if unrelieved it will cause significant renal damage resulting in acute or chronic renal failure. It may be intermittent or complete and may be unilateral or bilateral. Urinary tract obstruction can occur at any level of the urinary tract from the urethra to the renal pelvis and may be caused by either lesions intrinsic to the urinary tract or by extrinsic lesions causing compression. The most common causes of urinary tract obstruction are summarized in Table 13.5. Urinary tract obstruction predisposes to urinary tract infection and to urinary calculus formation (see below).

Hydronephrosis

The dilatation of the renal pelvis and calyces which occurs due to obstruction of urinary outflow is termed hydronephrosis and can lead to progressive renal atrophy with fibrosis. Urinary tract obstruction with continuing

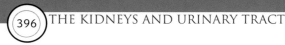

TABLE 13.5 Causes of urinary tract obstruction

Developmental anomaly
Renal stones
Renal pelvic or ureteric tumour
Retroperitoneal fibrosis
Enlarged lymph nodes
Pelvic malignancy (e.g. cervical carcinoma)

glomerular filtration leads to an increase in pressure within the renal pelvis which is transmitted back through the collecting duct into the renal parenchyma. This causes atrophy of the renal parenchyma with tubular loss occurring as an early event. The increased pressure compresses the renal vasculature altering intrarenal blood flow and further exacerbating tubular atrophy and interstitial fibrosis. Only in the later stages does the glomerular filtration rate begin to diminish. These events may be accelerated by coexisting infection or calculus formation. As the distension of the renal pelvis and calyces increases, the calyces become flattened and the underlying renal parenchyma progressively thins, ultimately forming a rim of mostly fibrous tissue surrounding the dilated pelvis and calyces. The atrophy of the renal parenchyma may be diffuse or focal so that some areas may be relatively spared while the remainder shows severe atrophy.

The clinical features of urinary tract obstruction depend to a large extent on the site and cause of the obstruction. Acute obstruction may give rise to pain due to the rapid distension of the urinary tract proximal to the obstruction. Unilateral hydroureter and hydronephrosis may be clinically silent and renal function can be adequately maintained by the other kidney. Bilateral complete obstruction will result in renal failure. Bilateral incomplete obstruction, most commonly seen in elderly men with prostatic enlargement, results initially in tubular dysfunction with an impairment of the urinary concentrating capacity. This results in polyuria, urinary frequency and nocturia. Superimposed urinary tract infection may produce additional symptoms mainly dysuria, fever and abdominal or loin pain.

Urinary Tract Infection

Urinary tract infection may involve either the bladder or the kidneys and renal pelvis, or both. The single most important criterion of urinary tract infection is the presence of bacteria in the urine, called bacteruria. In urine obtained through a bladder catheter the presence of an organism is significant while in the commonly used midstream sample there may be some contamination by urethral or perineal organisms. In these latter samples a bacterial count of or more than 10^5/mL is accepted as definitive of infection. Bacteruria in the absence of symptoms is termed 'asymptomatic bacteruria' and it is of importance under two circumstances:

- in infancy, in the presence of ureteric reflux it can lead to ascent of infection to the kidney

- in pregnancy, where it may be followed by symptomatic infection predisposing to hypertension, pre-eclampsia and prematurity.

Urinary tract infection occurring without preceding catheterization or obstruction is usually due to bacteria normally present in the faeces. The most frequently encountered organism is *E. coli* but sometimes *Klebsiella*, *Proteus* or *Pseudomonas* spp. are responsible. Infection complicating obstruction or instrumentation is commonly of a mixed bacterial type with *E. coli*, *Proteus* spp. and staphylococci being most often present. Haematogenous spread is a less frequent occurrence but may be seen arising in the course of acute pyaemia or septicaemia complicating staphylococcal infections or infective endocarditis.

By far the commonest route of infection is via the lumen of the urethra. The incidence of infection is highest in females throughout all age ranges with a male:female ratio of 20:1 in children and young adults. This sex ratio falls in old age as prostatic hypertrophy contributes to an increased incidence of urinary tract infection in elderly men. The female preponderance is due mainly to the ease with which endogenous infections can ascend the short female urethra. Precipitating factors include trauma to the perineum during sexual intercourse or childbirth. Most urinary infections in females occur in anatomically normal urinary tracts and the majority of these are confined to the bladder (cystitis). In a small percentage of females and relatively more often in males, stagnation of urine resulting from urinary tract obstruction or dysfunction is the main aetiological factor. This is caused by urethral obstruction (due to scarring or congenital urethral valves), urinary calculi, diverticula and tumours of the bladder, congenital malformations such as double ureters and neurological disorders such as paraplegia or multiple sclerosis leading to bladder dysfunction. In men prostatic enlargement secondary to hypertrophy is the commonest cause of urinary tract infection.

Cystitis is characterized by dysuria, increased frequency of micturition and sometimes haematuria. The ascent of infection to the kidneys from the bladder is usually due to vesicoureteric reflux, urinary tract obstruction or pregnancy. Vesicoureteric reflux consists of retrograde flow of bladder urine up the ureters during micturition. Reflux is normally prevented by the oblique course of the ureter through the wall of the bladder exerting a valve-like action during bladder contraction. In infancy this mechanism is less well developed and ureteric reflux more frequent. In older children and in adults reflux is less common unless associated with pregnancy or urinary tract obstruction. Vesicoureteric reflux may be demonstrated by a micturating cystogram in which dye instilled into the bladder by catheter is examined radiologically during micturition. Reflux may be seen by dye passing into the ureters or ascending to the kidney. The main importance of reflux is that it allows infected bladder urine to reach the kidneys. Bladder infection also tends to be perpetuated by reflux, as the refluxing urine returns to the bladder following micturition and there is therefore incomplete bladder emptying.

In severe reflux urine may re-enter the renal parenchyma especially at the upper and lower poles of the kidney where the papillae are compound. In such papillae the mouths of the collecting ducts are held open and refluxing urine may flow into them. These then tend to be the sites of intrarenal reflux and scarring in reflux nephropathy or chronic pyelonephritis (see below).

Pyelonephritis

Pyelonephritis is a bacterial induced inflammation of the renal pelvis, calyces and renal parenchyma. It can occur in both acute and chronic forms and may affect one or both kidneys. Most cases are due to ascending infection often associated with vesicoureteric reflux, obstructive uropathy or calculi. The predominant organisms are those which also cause cystitis.

Acute Pyelonephritis

Clinical Features

This condition is less common than acute cystitis. The symptoms of acute pyelonephritis in adults are loin pain, usually with a high fever and often rigors. There may be accompanying symptoms of cystitis. Children with acute pyelonephritis may be less unwell with fewer localizing symptoms making the condition more difficult to diagnose. In uncomplicated cases acute episodes resolve within a few days of instituting appropriate antibiotic therapy.

Pathological Changes

These comprise acute inflammation of the pelvis, calyces and renal parenchyma which, in severe cases, may progress to suppuration and abscess formation. There is purulent urine with congestion and inflammation of the pelvicalyceal mucosa. Pale linear streaks of pus may extend radially from the tip of the papilla to the surface of the cortex where adjacent lesions may fuse to produce abscesses. There may be considerable destruction of the cortex although there tends to be relative sparing of glomeruli and blood vessels. When severe there may be almost total or complete obstruction and pus may accumulate in the pelves and calyces to produce a pyonephrosis. Extension of this through the renal capsule may produce a perinephric abscess.

Chronic Pyelonephritis

Recurrent or protracted episodes of acute pyelonephritis may lead to renal parenchymal scarring. Once established this scarring causes progressive renal damage over many years even in the absence in further infection. Chronic pyelonephritis is an important cause of established kidney disease and accounts for about 15% of the European population requiring renal replacement therapy.

Clinical Features and Course

There may be a history of recurrent urinary infection, failure to thrive in early childhood or of nocturnal enuresis. In bilateral cases the condition usually presents with the features of chronic renal failure or hypertension. The diagnosis of chronic pyelonephritis is most easily confirmed radiologically with typical findings comprising asymmetrical shrinkage of the kidney, irregularity of the renal outlet due to cortical scarring and dilatation or disturbance of the calyces adjacent to the scarred areas. In some patients heavy proteinuria approaching that seen in the nephrotic syndrome may develop. These patients show secondary focal segmental glomerulosclerosis and its presence suggests the likelihood of a more rapid deterioration of renal function.

Pathological Changes

The macroscopic appearances of the kidney are important in differentiating chronic pyelonephritic scarring from other types of renal scarring. Unlike other forms of chronic tubulo-interstitial disease the pelvic and calyceal walls are thickened and distorted, their mucosa is granular or atrophic with scarring of the pyramids and usually calyceal dilatation. In contrast to chronic glomerulonephritis the renal parenchyma shows asymmetrical scarring and shrinkage, these scars being in close relationship to the deformed calyces and found mainly at the upper and lower poles of the kidney. Microscopically the pelvic and calyceal mucosa may be thickened by granulation tissue. There is often submucosal fibrosis and an intense chronic inflammatory cell infiltrate sometimes with lymphoid follicle formation. In the parenchymal scars there is tubular atrophy with thickening of the basement membranes and the interstitium is infiltrated by inflammatory cells mostly lymphocytes and plasma cells. In the late stages of the disease there is dense fibrosis with little active inflammation. The glomeruli in the scarred areas may appear normal but may show a spectrum of abnormalities with concentric periglomerular fibrosis, ischaemic injury, fibrous obliteration and hyalinization of glomerular tufts. Obliterative endarteritis affects the blood vessels. In non-scarred areas there may be compensatory hypertrophy, and vascular changes resulting from hypertension.

Rarer forms of urinary tract infection may be encountered such as tuberculosis, schistosomiasis, fungal infection or, more rarely, viral infection.

Urinary Calculi

Urinary calculi are formed by the precipitation of inorganic urinary constituents with a small amount of organic material also being incorporated. Deposition is favoured by highly concentrated urine, and hence is more frequently seen in dehydrated patients, in warm climates or at high altitude. Deposition is also increased in metabolic disorders accompanied by excretion of excess amounts of the major constituents of urinary calculi. Changes in urinary pH and the presence of urinary tract infection may also enhance calculus formation. Calculi may develop in the renal pelvis, ureter or in the bladder although some bladder calculi probably originate in the kidney and are passed down the ureter into the bladder. At this site they may enlarge by the incorporation of additional inorganic material.

The main types of urinary calculi are:

- Calcium-containing stones, the calcium salt being predominantly oxalate with lesser amounts of calcium phosphate. These comprise more than 75% of all urinary calculi and are characteristically laid down in an acid urine.
- Complex triple phosphate stones including magnesium, ammonium, carbonate and calcium components. These comprise 15% of urinary calculi and are laid down in alkaline urine. They may form an outer laminated deposit on other stones and are strongly associated with urinary tract infection.
- Uric acid and urate–uric acid stones comprise 5% of urinary calculi but affect up to 20% of patients with gout. Like calcium-containing stones they are typically laid down in an acid urine. Pure uric acid stones are radiolucent rendering their detection in a plain abdominal radiograph virtually impossible.
- Cystine stones occur in primary cystinuria, a rare but important renal disease in childhood.

The precise mechanisms of stone formation are complex and rather poorly understood. It requires both nucleation, a process whereby the stone deposition is initiated, and aggregation, whereby the stone grows in size. Some urinary constituents can promote the nucleation of others (for example urates can nucleate oxalate precipitates) and this explains why many urinary stones are mixed in composition. An increase in the urinary excretion of a particular substance is usually an important factor, typically in hypercalciuria where the increased excretion of calcium and phosphate leads to the formation of calculi. Hypercalciuria occurs in hyperparathyroidism, chronic resorptive bone disease, prolonged immobilization in bed, sarcoidosis and the milk alkali syndrome, but in most cases it is idiopathic.

Stones in the renal pelvis may be single or multiple and in some instances a single calculus may grow to occupy the entire pelvicalyceal system resulting in a so-called 'stag horn' calculus. Small calculi may pass down the ureter to the bladder giving rise to the clinical syndrome of renal colic with haematuria. They may arrest temporarily, usually at the narrower lower end of the ureter. When impaction is permanent this occurs at one of three sites, the upper end of the ureter, the level of the pelvic brim or the lower end of the ureter. This impaction and renal obstruction lead to hydronephrosis. When there is a urinary tract infection by urea-splitting bacteria such as *Proteus* spp. ammonia is produced and calculi or softer deposits composed of phosphates form within the resultant alkaline urine. These may be precipitated within the inflamed pelvicalyceal system. This combination of infection and calculus may result in pyonephrosis and ulceration. The chronic inflammation and epithelial regeneration resulting from calculi may give rise to squamous metaplasia of the lining of the renal pelvis with a subsequent increase in the risk of development of squamous carcinoma.

Stones in the bladder may be solitary or multiple and can grow to several centimetres in diameter. As with stones elsewhere in the urinary tract they increase the risk of urinary tract infection, chronic inflammation and squamous metaplasia. They characteristically give rise to symptoms such as pain and irritation with haematuria, intermittent obstruction, frequency and dysuria.

TUMOURS OF THE KIDNEY AND URINARY TRACT

Key points
- The kidney is among the 10 sites most frequently involved by malignancy accounting for 2.5% of human cancers.
- Renal cancer is associated with smoking, obesity, hypertension, exposure to petroleum vapours and possibly to a high-protein diet.
- It is more common in males than females.

Malignant Tumours

There are three main types of malignant tumour in the kidney and urinary tract. These are nephroblastoma or Wilms' tumour in children, while in adults renal cell carcinoma is the major malignancy of the renal parenchyma and urothelial carcinoma the major malignancy of the renal pelvis, ureters and bladder.

Nephroblastoma (Wilms' Tumour)

These affect about 1 in 10000 children, a figure that remains uniform across different geographical regions, and usually present between the ages of 2 and 5 years. Most cases of nephroblastoma are solitary and sporadic but up to 10% may be multifocal or bilateral at the time of diagnosis. Occasionally nephroblastoma is encountered as a feature of one of three different multisystem disorders (Table 13.6). These associations have revealed much concerning the genetics of Wilms' tumour and particularly the role of tumour suppressor genes such as *WT1*, which is located on chromosome 11p13.

TABLE 13.6 Multisystem disorders associated with Wilms' tumour

Denys Drash syndrome
WAGR (Wilms' tumour, aniridia, genital abnormalities or gonadoblastoma, mental retardation) syndrome
Beckwith–Wiedemann syndrome

Histologically these tumours are characterized by three elements (triphasic): blastema, stroma and immature tubules resembling the tissues found within the nephrogenic zone of fetal kidney (Figure 13.24). It is known that Wilms' tumour arises from oncogenic events within the

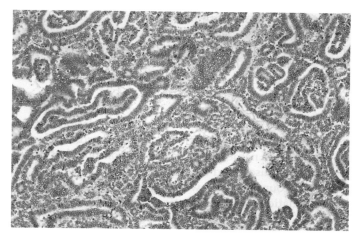

FIGURE 13.24 Wilms' tumour shows a triphasic appearance. The three histological elements comprise the undifferentiated blastema, immature epithelium and stromal connective tissue. The relative contribution of these elements varies enormously between individual cases of Wilms' tumour.

metanephric blastema of the fetal kidney and the tumour cells retain the capacity for partial differentiation into both the stromal and epithelial elements similar to the differentiation capacity of the normal metanephric blastema. The relevant amounts of these different elements within the tumour varies. In about 5% of Wilms' tumours extreme pleomorphism may be noted and this is termed 'anaplasia', which is a poor prognostic feature. Nowadays, >85% of children with Wilms' tumour are cured by the combination of surgical and non-surgical management. This compares favourably with the position 30 years ago when the cure rate was between 10% and 30%.

Renal Cell Carcinoma

Renal cell carcinomas account for more than 95% of renal malignancies in adults with a median age at presentation between 55 and 60 years. The tumours are usually sporadic but rarely familial cases may be encountered, particularly as part of the von Hippel–Lindau syndrome. This association has revealed that mutation and subsequent loss of the second or normal copy of the *VHL* gene is a key event in the development of renal carcinomas of either the sporadic or familial types. These observations also confirm the importance of the VHL gene as a tumour suppressor gene. The risk factors for the development of renal cell carcinoma are rather poorly understood; the tumour is more frequently encountered in males than females and there is a moderate association with a smoking history.

Renal cell carcinoma is usually a solitary and large tumour at the time of presentation, although the development of newer imaging techniques has led to an increase in the number of small asymptomatic renal cell carcinomas being detected and removed. The tumours are characteristically soft and yellow, frequently with areas of haemorrhage and necrosis. Invasion of the renal vein or extension beyond the renal capsule are frequent and are important measurements in defining the stage or extent of disease at the time of surgery. Bloodborne metastases to the lungs and to other tissues such as bone and brain are seen at the time of presentation in up to 20% of patients.

Histologically the commonest variant (conventional or clear cell type) is composed of uniform clear cells which are rich in glycogen and lipid (Figure 13.25). Mitoses are infrequent suggesting a slow, but nevertheless relentless, tumour growth. These tumour cells are arranged in acini, cords or sheets, and renal cell carcinomas are typically richly vascular tumours. Other histological types such as papillary (15%), chromophobe (5%) and collecting duct carcinoma (1%) may be seen. Progression to spindle cell or sarcomatoid variants may be encountered from any of these histological types and is a very bad prognostic feature. The major prognostic feature in renal cell carcinoma is the stage of tumour at the time of surgical resection. Extrarenal spread either by direct infiltration of perirenal fat or by invasion of the renal vein is strongly associated with the concurrent or subsequent development of metastatic renal cell carcinoma. The tumours often present with a triad of loin pain, haematuria and an abdominal mass but renal cell carcinoma is notorious for the frequency of paraneoplastic syndromes associated with increased production of erythropoietin (polycythemia), parathyroid hormone-related peptide (hypercalcaemia), and renin (hypertension).

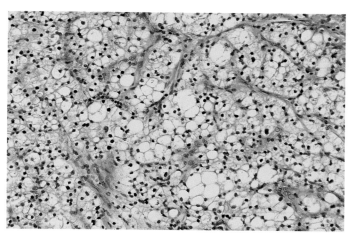

FIGURE 13.25 The most common form of renal cell carcinoma is characterized by a solid architecture composed of clear cuboidal cells supported by a rich vascular stroma. Other variants include the papillary, chromophobe and collecting duct types.

Transitional Cell Carcinoma

This, the third of the major renal and urinary tract malignancies, constitutes 90% of the tumours of the renal pelvis, ureter and bladder. They cover the full spectrum from small, relatively benign tumours to highly aggressive malignancies. They are frequently multifocal, an observation which influences the extent of surgical management of these tumours. The risk of developing urothelial carcinoma has been shown to be increased in certain industries such as dye workers and workers in the rubber industry. These tumours are also associated with cigarette smoking, analgesic

tumours may not be detectable by cervical smear until they are relatively advanced.

The main tumour types that occur in the cervix are:

- squamous cell carcinoma
- adenocarcinoma
- adenosquamous carcinoma.

The majority of cervical carcinomas are squamous in type and arise in the transformation zone, often associated with CIN. A minority of tumours are adenocarcinomas or adenosquamous carcinomas.

As at other sites, carcinomas are graded according to how closely they resemble their tissue of origin since, to some extent, this can be used to predict clinical behaviour: poorly differentiated tumours tend to behave more aggressively. The staging of tumours is more important, as stage is generally a more powerful prognostic factor. The principle is that the further a tumour has spread from its site of origin, the more likely it is to kill the patient, and the more quickly that is likely to occur. The staging of cervical carcin-oma differs from many other tumours in that 'microinvasive' carcinomas are recognized. These are diagnosed microscopically and must conform to predetermined size limits (Table 14.2). Part of the success of the cervical screening programme is that, when invasive carcinoma is identified, it is now more likely to be microinvasive – and hence curable. The more advanced stages are judged clinically, using a combination of clinical examination (often under anaesthesia) and radiological techniques. The majority of cervical carcinomas spread at least initially by direct extension into pelvic tissues. The mainstay of treatment of early (predominantly stage 1) carcinoma is therefore surgical excision either by cone biopsy or radical hysterectomy and pelvic lymphadenectomy (Wertheim's hysterectomy). More advanced stages are not surgically resectable and are treated with radiotherapy or combined chemotherapy with radiotherapy.

TABLE 14.2 Staging of cervical tumours

Stage	Definition
0	Cervical intraepithelial neoplasia (CIN)
I	Confined to the cervix
	(a) Microscopic invasion (<5 mm deep and 7 mm wide)
	(i) <3 mm deep
	(ii) ≥3 mm, <5 mm deep
	(b) Clinically visible or greater than Ia
II	Tumour invades beyond the uterus but not to pelvic wall or lower third of vagina
III	Tumour extends to pelvic side wall and/or involves lower third of vagina and/or causes hydronephrosis or non-functioning kidney
IV	Invades mucosa of bladder or rectum and/or extends beyond true pelvis (including metastasis)

Prevention and Screening

The spectrum of neoplastic cervical disease exemplifies the principle behind the role of screening in the prevention of malignant disease. If intraepithelial disease is the precursor of invasive cancer, then detection and treatment of the intraepithelial form will prevent development of the invasive form. Cervical smears are taken every 3–5 years from the age of 20 to 64 years. Cells are scraped from the surface of the cervix using a wooden spatula, and then spread onto a glass slide. The smear is stained using the Papanicolau stain, which allows the cells to be examined under the microscope for features suggestive of malignancy. These include:

- high nucleocytoplasmic ratio
- nuclear hyperchromasia
- abnormalities of nuclear chromatin pattern
- nuclear pleomorphism.

The presence of these features indicates the presence of dyskaryosis, which suggests a CIN lesion, and usually prompts referral to a colposcopy clinic for further investigation.

THE UTERINE BODY

The Endometrium

Key Points

- Dysfunctional uterine bleeding is commonly due to functional disturbance of the menstrual cycle.
- Endometrial polyps may be malignant.
- Post-menopausal bleeding is never normal.
- Endometrial carcinoma may arise from endometrial hyperplasia.
- Endometrial carcinoma tends to present early with vaginal bleeding.
- Endometrial carcinoma is curable by early surgical intervention.

Overview of the Normal Menstrual Cycle

In order to understand the abnormalities that underlie menstrual disturbances, it is important to have a basic concept of the menstrual cycle (Figure 14.8). The first (follicular) phase involves development of ovarian follicles as a result of stimulation by follicle-stimulating hormone (FSH). The fundamental features of this development are proliferation of granulosa cells, followed by formation of a space (antrum), thinning of the overlying ovarian cortex and then – as a result of a surge in luteinizing hormone (LH) secretion – ovulation. The granulosa cells secrete oestrogen which stimulates proliferation of the endometrium (proliferative phase). After ovulation, the follicle collapses and the granulosa cells transform into luteal cells (luteal phase). The structure formed from this transformation is the corpus luteum which secretes progesterone, leading to secretory transformation of the endometrium (secretory phase). This phase commences with subnuclear vacuolation of endometrial epithelial cells.

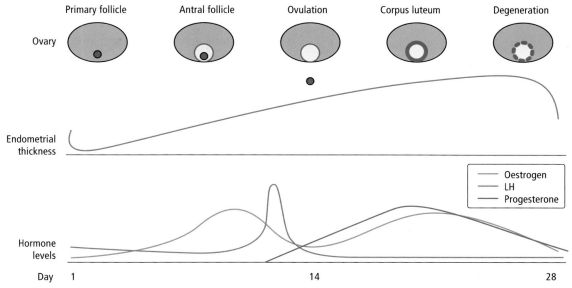

FIGURE 14.8 The major events in the menstrual cycle. The development of an ovarian follicle and its transformation into a corpus luteum is shown together with the endometrial thickness and the pattern of hormone secretion. LH = luteinizing hormone.

This is followed by supranuclear vacuolation and then the appearance of intraluminal secretion. The corpus luteum has a finite lifespan and, after approximately 14 days, begins to degenerate. Progesterone support is therefore removed from the endometrium, which undergoes apoptosis. The superficial endometrium is shed, leading to menstrual flow (menstrual phase). The basal endometrium, which does not respond to oestrogen and progesterone, remains and forms the base for the next menstrual cycle.

In the event of implantation of a conceptus into the endometrium, the corpus luteum does not degenerate but becomes a corpus luteum of pregnancy under the influence initially of LH and then human chorionic gonadotrophin (hCG) which is secreted by the placenta. Continued progestogen secretion leads to decidualization of the endometrium. It is important to appreciate that implantation does not always occur in the endometrium but may occur at other sites (ectopic pregnancy), particularly the fallopian tube. Under these circumstances, stimulation of the endometrium continues and decidualization occurs, as in normal pregnancy.

After the menopause, endocrine stimulation of the endometrium largely ceases. The endometrium therefore ceases to cycle and persists only as the basal endometrium. Many women have continued low levels of oestrogen present after the menopause (as a result of aromatization of adrenal androgens to oestrogen in peripheral fat), and hence weak proliferation may continue. This can cause post-menopausal bleeding related either to withdrawal bleeding or the formation of endometrial polyps.

Dysfunctional Uterine Bleeding (DUB)

This disorder may be defined as bleeding at an inappropriate time of the cycle in the absence of an anatomical cause. Patients present with a variety of menstrual disturbances, notably intermenstrual bleeding and menorrhagia (heavy periods). There are three main groups of functional abnormality that lead to DUB:

- anovulatory cycles
- luteal phase defects
- irregular shedding.

Anovulatory cycles typically occur at the menarche and around the menopause (perimenopausal bleeding). Failure of ovulation leads to continued endometrial proliferation. Withdrawal bleeding then occurs either when the endometrium becomes too thick to be supported by its blood supply, or as a result of fluctuation in oestrogen levels. If ovulation continually fails to occur, then endometrial proliferation may be marked, leading to simple hyperplasia of the endometrium and, in some patients, atypical hyperplasia and invasive carcinoma. This is particularly true in patients with the polycystic ovary syndrome (PCOS), one of the hallmarks of which is failure of ovulation (see p. 410). In the second group of patients, ovulation occurs but the secretory phase is abnormal. This may take the form of a coordinated delay in secretory transformation, asynchrony between glands and stroma and, perhaps most commonly, irregular ripening when only some glands develop secretory changes. A variety of physiological defects – both ovarian and endometrial – are involved in this group of abnormalities. Irregular shedding occurs when fragments of endometrium do not shed during menstruation but persist into the next cycle.

It must be remembered that a significant proportion of patients who present with menstrual abnormalities will have a physical explanation for the bleeding. The presence of fibroids (see p. 409) is a good example of this, and therefore it is important that causes other than physiological abnormalities be considered when assessing the patient.

Endometrial Polyps

Endometrial polyps are common and may present in a variety of ways, including abnormal vaginal bleeding and as an incidental abnormality identified either when a cervical smear is taken or during curettage. Endometrial polyps are most commonly benign and composed of endometrial glands and stroma with a fibrovascular core. Many are related to minor endocrine abnormalities such as anovulatory cycles. However, invasive carcinoma may present as a polyp, and it is therefore important that all endometrial polyps be submitted for histological examination.

Endometrial Hyperplasia

Endometrial hyperplasia is a spectrum of disorders ranging from simple hyperplasia (which is typically generalized) at one end to atypical hyperplasia (which is usually focal and may be associated with endometrial carcinoma) at the other end (Table 14.3). Morphologically, there are two main features of hyperplasia, namely architectural abnormality and cytological abnormality. As a general rule, those forms that show only architectural abnormality have little or no malignant potential, whereas those that show cytological abnormality are associated with either current or future risk of developing invasive endometrial carcinoma. The cause of endometrial hyperplasia is often unknown, although some cases are associated with persistent oestrogen stimulation. This may simply be the result of anovulatory cycles, such as in the perimenopausal period or in patients with polycystic ovaries, or may be due to abnormal oestrogen secretion by, for example, an ovarian tumour such as a fibrothecoma or a granulosa cell tumour (see p. 413).

TABLE 14.3 Gross and microscopic features of endometrial hyperplasia

	Simple	Complex	Atypical
Distribution	General	Focal	Focal
Component	Glands and stroma	Glands	Glands
Glands	Dilated, not crowded	Crowded	Crowded
Cytology	Normal	Normal	Atypical

Endometrial Carcinoma

Endometrial carcinoma is uncommon in women under the age of 40 years, the majority of these lesions occurring in women aged over 50. There are two main groups of patients with endometrial carcinoma. The first group includes older women in whom the tumours are unassociated with surrounding endometrial hyperplasia. The second group comprises younger women in whom the tumours tend to arise on a background of atypical endometrial hyperplasia. The latter group may have evidence of oestrogen excess such as the PCOS (particularly in women aged under 40 years) or an oestrogen-secreting tumour, for example ovarian fibrothecoma or granulosa cell tumour. Endometrial carcinoma is also associated with obesity and nulliparity. Most endometrial carcinomas present non-specifically with abnormal vaginal bleeding. In younger women, the majority of patients with such bleeding have dysfunctional uterine bleeding but, in older women – and particularly those who are post-menopausal – any bleeding should be considered suspicious and endometrial curettage performed. Hence, the adage PMB (post-menopausal bleeding) = D&C (dilatation and curettage). More recently, D&C has been replaced by pipelle endometrial biopsy.

Most endometrial carcinomas are exophytic tumours (Figure 14.9), and as they tend to grow into the endometrial cavity and cause vaginal bleeding, they present relatively early. As a result, many endometrial carcinomas are stage I at presentation (Table 14.4), and hence are curable by surgical resection. Microscopically, the majority of endometrial tumours are adenocarcinomas that morphologically resemble proliferative endometrium. These are termed type I endometrial carcinomas. A minority of tumours differentiate along other lines to resemble, for example, tubal epithelium (serous adenocarcinoma). Serous carcinomas belong to the group of type II endometrial tumours and are characterized by mutation of the *p53* gene.

TABLE 14.4 The FIGO staging system for endometrial carcinoma

Stage	Definition
I	Confined to the uterine corpus*
II	Invades the cervix, but does not extend beyond the uterus
III	Any of the following: – involves serosa – involves adnexae – tumour cells in ascites or peritoneal washing – involves vagina – pelvic or para-aortic lymph node metastasis
IV	Invades bladder and/or bowel mucosa Distant metastasis (excluding vagina, pelvic serosa or adnexa)

*Stage I is separated into three substages (IA, IB, IC), depending on the proportion of the myometrium infiltrated (confined to the endometrium, confined to the inner half of the uterine wall, and invading into the outer half of the uterine wall respectively).

Endometrial carcinoma invades directly into the underlying myometrium (see Figure 14.9), where it can gain access to myometrial and hence adnexal lymphatics. By this route, the tumour can spread to the ovaries. Surgical resection should always therefore include removal of the ovaries. Haematogenous spread may also occur. The prognosis of endometrial carcinoma depends on the grade, stage and depth of myometrial invasion. Treatment is by surgical excision and adjuvant radiotherapy if there are adverse prognostic factors.

POST-MENOPAUSAL BLEEDING

A 75-year-old woman who had her last menstrual period 20 years previously had two episodes of vaginal bleeding. Pelvic examination showed no abnormality. Endometrial curettage was performed (PMB = D&C; see p. 408), and histopathological examination of the curettings obtained showed an endometrioid endometrial carcinoma. Surgical resection was therefore performed by total abdominal hysterectomy and bilateral salpingo-oophorectomy. Pathological examination of the resected uterus showed that the endometrial cavity was filled by a polypoid tumour mass (see Figure 14.9). Histological analysis confirmed invasion of the outer myometrium and cervix, and also identified lymphatic invasion. A small tumour deposit was present in the hilum of the right ovary. These features indicated a diagnosis of Stage 3 endometrioid adenocarcinoma of the endometrium. As the tumour was of high stage, the patient was treated with postoperative radiotherapy.

This case illustrates that, although many endometrial carcinomas present at low stage, high-stage tumours may present in an identical way. This may occur as an unexpected finding, and demonstrates the need for careful pathological assessment in all cases.

Key Points

- PMB = D&C or pipelle biopsy.
- Clinical assessment may underestimate the pathological stage of endometrial tumours.

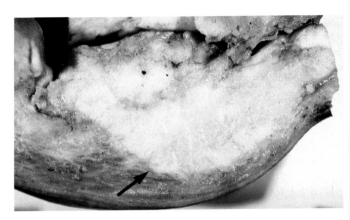

FIGURE 14.9 Macroscopic photograph of an invasive endometrial carcinoma (white). Note that the tumour is invading deeply into the myometrium (arrow).

The Myometrium

Key Points

- Painful periods that are refractory to treatment may be due to adenomyosis.
- The most common tumour of the myometrium is the fibroid (leiomyoma).
- Fibroids are benign smooth muscle tumours.
- Primary malignant tumours of the myometrium are unusual.

Adenomyosis

This disorder is sometimes referred to as 'diverticular disease' of the endometrium, by analogy with diverticular disease of the colon. The normal endometrial–myometrial junction is normally irregular but, in some women, endometrial glands and stroma extend more deeply into the myometrium and can, occasionally, be seen extending throughout the entire myometrial thickness. The degree to which these adenomyotic foci respond to hormonal stimulation is variable, and tends to be less than the lining endometrium, but this disorder is associated with both disturbances of the menstrual cycle and painful periods (dysmenorrhoea). One important point about adenomyosis is that simple endometrial curettage may not ameliorate the patient's symptoms. This disorder should therefore be considered in patients with continuing symptoms following curettage.

Leiomyomas

Tumours may arise from any of the tissue elements of the uterus, such as smooth muscle, blood vessels and nerves. By far the most common of these lesions is the leiomyoma (fibroid), which is a benign tumour arising from smooth muscle. These lesions are to some extent oestrogen-dependent and are usually multiple. They present in a variety of ways, including abnormal vaginal bleeding, a pelvic mass or pelvic pain. The latter may occur as a result of 'red degeneration' which typically occurs during pregnancy. Macroscopically, they are well circumscribed and may be submucosal (Figure 14.10), intramural or subserosal. Submucosal and subserosal fibroids are often polypoid: submucosal fibroids may present as a polyp within the

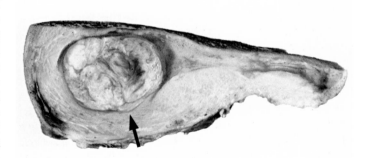

FIGURE 14.10 A submucosal uterine leiomyoma (arrow) which protrudes into the endometrial cavity. Lesions in this position may be associated with abnormal vaginal bleeding and with infertility.

endometrial cavity. Microscopically, these lesions are composed of interlacing fascicles of smooth muscle cells. There is debate regarding whether leiomyomas ever become malignant, forming a leiomyosarcoma, or whether leiomyosarcomas are malignant *ab initio*. From a practical point of view, it is important to identify leiomyosarcomas as they have metastatic capability.

A variety of uncommon and rare tumours occur in the uterus. Perhaps the most important of these is the malignant mixed Müllerian tumour, so called because of the presence of a combination of epithelial and stromal elements presumed to be derived from the Müllerian duct system. Current evidence, based on clonality analysis, suggests that these tumours are 'metaplastic' carcinomas, i.e. the stromal elements are derived from the epithelial elements by a 'metaplastic' process. These tumours are highly malignant with a poor prognosis. Finally, metastatic tumours must not be forgotten.

THE FALLOPIAN TUBE

The major disorders of the fallopian tube are salpingitis, endometriosis and ectopic pregnancy. These are dealt with elsewhere in this chapter (see pages 413–415). Primary tumours of the fallopian tube occur only rarely, and most tumours involving the fallopian tube represent direct extension from an ovarian tumour.

THE OVARY

> **Key Points**
>
> - Many ovarian cysts are not malignant.
> - Ovarian tumours may be benign, borderline or malignant.
> - Most ovarian tumours are non-functioning and tend to present late, i.e. at high stage.
> - Some ovarian tumours (thecoma, granulosa cell tumour) secrete oestrogens or androgens, and present relatively early with endometrial abnormalities or virilization.

Non-neoplastic Cysts

Non-neoplastic cysts of the ovary can be divided into three broad categories:

- functional
- inclusion
- endometriotic.

Endometriosis is discussed on pp. 414–415, and will not be considered further at this point.

Inclusion cysts are generally found within the superficial ovarian cortex, and probably arise as a result of inclusion of surface epithelium at the time of ovulation. The majority of these are of serous type, i.e. they are lined by epithelium that resembles that lining the fallopian tube.

Functional cysts are related to the cyclical development and atresia of ovarian follicles. Among functional cysts, *follicular cysts* are the most common type, and small cystic follicles are found in virtually all premenopausal ovaries. *Luteal cysts*, or cystic corpora lutea, are less common. Finally, follicular cysts may become luteinized during pregnancy to form luteinized follicular cysts.

Polycystic Ovary Syndrome (PCOS)

A specific situation in which multiple cystic follicles are present in the ovaries is the PCOS (also known as Stein–Leventhal syndrome). The clinical syndrome comprises oligomenorrhoea, infertility, hirsutism and obesity. From an endocrine point of view, there is disordered secretion of LH and FSH, leading to ovulation failure. The ovaries become enlarged and contain multiple cystic follicles. The capsule of the ovary is thickened, and there are usually no stigmata of ovulation, i.e. corpora lutea and corpora albicantes are absent. It is important to appreciate that a diagnosis of PCOS cannot be made on morphological grounds alone, and both clinical and endocrine data are also required. However, the identification of patients with this syndrome is important in view of its association with endometrial hyperplasia and carcinoma (see previously). This complication is preventable by treatment of the underlying endocrine disorder.

Ovarian Tumours

Ovarian tumours are relatively common, with the majority (approximately 80%) being benign and occurring in women of reproductive age. Malignant tumours occur in older women, most commonly aged 40–65 years, although certain uncommon tumour types do occur at a younger age. Many ovarian tumours – particularly of epithelial type – are bilateral: it is not clear whether these represent synchronous primary tumours or the spread of a single original tumour from one ovary to the other. Most ovarian tumours are non-functional and, in view of their relatively hidden anatomical location, tend to present late, usually as abdominal swelling due to the presence of a mass or associated ascites. Predisposing factors include nulliparity and gonadal dysgenesis. Recently, it has become clear that ovarian carcinoma runs in some families in association with inherited abnormalities of, for example, the *BRCA1* gene. Patients with a strong family history of breast and/or ovarian cancer can now be screened for specific molecular abnormalities.

Primary ovarian tumours arise from three distinct cell types, and are classified according to the scheme presented in Table 14.5. However, it must be remembered that, whenever a malignant ovarian tumour is encountered, the possibility that it is a metastasis should be considered, particularly if it is of an unusual histological type and is bilateral.

Epithelial Ovarian Tumours

Macroscopically, ovarian tumours may be smooth-walled cystic lesions (Figure 14.11) or contain a mixture of solid

TABLE 14.5 Classification of ovarian tumours

	Cell of origin	Type	Proportion (%)
Primary			
Epithelial	Surface coelomic epithelium	Serous Mucinous Endometrioid/clear cell Brenner Undifferentiated	65–70
Germ cell tumours	Germ cells	Teratoma Dysgerminoma Yolk sac tumour Embryonal carcinoma	15–20
Sex cord/stromal tumours	Ovarian sex cords and stroma	Granulosa cell tumours Thecoma/fibroma Sertoli–Leydig tumours	5–10
Miscellaneous	Various	Mixed Müllerian tumour	
Secondary			
Metastases	–	–	5–10

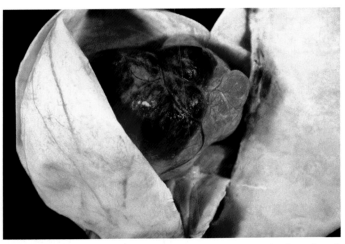

FIGURE 14.11 A benign serous cystadenoma. Note that the lesion is cystic and has smooth external and internal surfaces.

and cystic areas (Figure 14.12). Papillary tumours are also relatively frequent and tend to be of serous type (see below). It is thought that epithelial ovarian tumours arise from the coelomic epithelium that lines the surface of the ovary and that has the capacity to differentiate along a variety of paths that reflect the pluripotentiality of the Müllerian ducts. Thus, the major types of ovarian carcinoma show patterns reminiscent of tubal epithelium (serous tumours), endocervical epithelium (mucinous tumours), and endometrium (endometrioid and clear cell tumours). Other less common tumour types are also found, such as the Brenner tumour; this has a transitional morphology similar to that of the epithelium lining the urinary tract.

Each category of epithelial tumour is divided into three subcategories, based on a combination of cytological and architectural features (Table 14.6). This distinction is of fundamental importance, as the clinical behaviour of the

ABDOMINAL SWELLING

14.3 CASE HISTORY

A 54-year-old post-menopausal woman presented with a 6-month history of gradual increase in her waist size. This had been accompanied by mild constipation, but no other significant symptoms. Clinical examination of the abdomen showed 'shifting dullness', indicating the presence of ascites, while pelvic examination suggested a mass in the right adnexal region. Ultrasound examination of the abdomen and pelvis confirmed the presence of ascites and showed a 60-mm mass in the right ovary, with a possible second mass in the left ovary. The ascitic fluid was drained and a sample sent for cytological assessment. This demonstrated clusters of adenocarcinoma cells. A laparotomy was

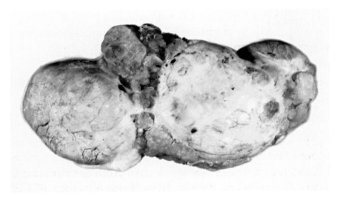

FIGURE 14.12 An invasive ovarian carcinoma. Note the presence of both solid and cystic areas. Histologically, this lesion was a serous carcinoma.

performed and total abdominal hysterectomy, bilateral salpingo-oophorectomy and omentectomy carried out. Pathological examination of the specimens showed bilateral serous carcinoma of the ovary (see Figure 14.12). The tumour in the right ovary extended through the capsule, and there were scattered tumour deposits within the omentum. A diagnosis of Stage 3 serous carcinoma of the ovary was made. The patient was treated with adjuvant cisplatin-based chemotherapy, and remained well and in remission 6 months later.

Key Points

- Ovarian carcinoma often presents late.
- Chemotherapy is an important component of the management of patients with ovarian carcinoma.

TABLE 14.6 The diagnostic criteria for epithelial ovarian tumours

Tumour	Cytological appearance	Stromal invasion
Benign	Normal	No
Borderline	Abnormal	No
Invasive	Abnormal	Yes

tumour depends almost entirely on the presence of stromal invasion. Benign tumours effectively have no malignant potential. Invasive tumours are by definition malignant. Borderline tumours are not clearly malignant but, in a small proportion of patients, may be associated with malignant features at a later date. Clinical follow-up is therefore required. The distinction between benign and borderline tumours is made microscopically. Although invasive carcinomas are often identifiable macroscopically, formal diagnosis requires histological examination. It is important to appreciate that the defining features of invasive carcinomas are stromal invasion and metastasis. Invasive tumours are staged according to the extent of spread as shown in Table 14.7.

TABLE 14.7 The FIGO staging system for ovarian carcinoma

Stage	Tumour extent
I	Limited to ovaries (a) One ovary (b) Both ovaries, no ascites (c) Malignant ascites; ruptured capsule; tumour on ovarian surface
II	Pelvic extension
III	Microscopically confirmed intraperitoneal spread or regional lymph node metastases
IV	Distant metastases

Serous tumours are the most common type, are usually cystic, and may appear papillary. A characteristic microscopic feature is the presence of psammoma bodies (Figure 14.13), which may be present in benign, borderline or malignant tumours, particularly if papillary. Mucinous tumours are more often unilateral than serous tumours. One important

complication of benign (and particularly borderline) mucinous tumours is pseudomyxoma peritonei, which occurs as a result of mucin secretion by the tumour. This mucin can spread throughout the peritoneal cavity where it may be associated with intestinal obstruction and other anatomical complications. It is now recognized that the vast majority of tumours associated with pseudomyxoma peritonei are of appendiceal origin, with secondary spread to involve the ovaries. Endometrioid and clear cell tumours are associated with ovarian endometriosis. These tumour types are important as endometrioid tumours have a relatively good prognosis, whereas clear cell tumours tend to behave aggressively.

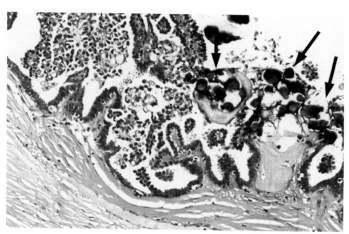

FIGURE 14.13 Microscopic appearance of a borderline serous tumour. The cells lining this cyst show cytological abnormalities, and numerous psammoma bodies are present (arrows).

Germ Cell Tumours of the Ovary

Around 95% of these are mature cystic teratomas ('dermoid cysts'). The characteristic of these tumours is that mature elements derived from all three embryonic germ layers are present. The most common elements are ectodermal (skin, hair, teeth, etc.), but endodermal (intestinal, respiratory epithelium) and mesodermal (fat, muscle) elements are also present (Figure 14.14). Rarely, malignant transformation has been described in these tumours. Immature teratomas are related to mature teratomas, but contain

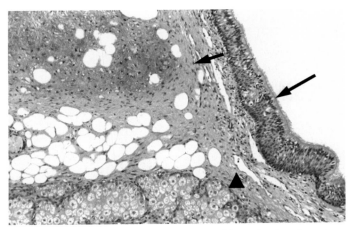

FIGURE 14.14 Microscopic appearance of a dermoid cyst showing elements from all three germ cell layers. Note the presence of cartilage (mesoderm; short arrow); respiratory epithelium (endoderm; long arrow); and sebaceous areas (ectoderm; arrow head).

immature neuroectodermal elements and behave in a malignant fashion. The importance of these is that they constitute 85% of ovarian teratomas in children.

All other types of germ cell tumour can occur in the ovary, but are uncommon. Dysgerminoma – which is the ovarian counterpart of testicular seminoma – occurs in young women and is an important diagnosis to make as the tumour is radiosensitive. Yolk sac tumours and embryonal carcinomas are rare, and highly malignant.

Ovarian Sex Cord/Stromal Tumours

These tumours differentiate along female (granulosa and theca cell tumours) or male (Sertoli/Leydig cell tumours) lines. Granulosa cell tumours are fairly common, especially in post-menopausal women; these lesions behave in a low-grade malignant fashion and may secrete oestrogens. As a result of their oestrogen secretion, the tumours are associated with endometrial hyperplasia and endometrial carcinoma (see p. 408). Ovarian fibromas and thecomas (Figure 14.15) are

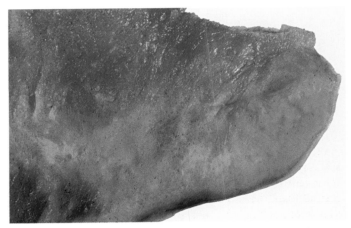

FIGURE 14.15 Macroscopic appearance of an ovarian thecoma. Note the yellow appearance, which is due to the presence of steroid hormone within the tumour cell cytoplasm.

also fairly common, but are usually benign. They too may secrete oestrogens (particularly thecomas) and may be associated with endometrial neoplasia.

Sertoli/Leydig cell tumours are uncommon and reflect the pluripotential nature of ovarian stromal cells. They may be non-functioning, but may also secrete androgens leading to virilization. Occasionally, they may secrete oestrogens.

Metastases to the Ovary

Some non-primary ovarian tumours reflect transcoelomic spread from pelvic tumours, for example from a colorectal carcinoma. Others are haematogenous or lymphatic metastases from distant sites, for example other parts of the gastrointestinal and female genital tracts. It is important to consider this possibility when assessing patients with ovarian tumours, as the identification of the primary site affects both staging and clinical management. One specific example of ovarian metastasis is the Krukenberg tumour, which is usually bilateral and associated with diffuse ovarian enlargement and the presence of signet ring tumour cells. These tumours are characteristically of gastric origin.

PELVIC INFLAMMATORY DISEASE

Key Points

- Pelvic inflammatory disease affects the whole female genital tract.
- It is associated with intrauterine contraceptive devices.
- It may be complicated by infertility and ectopic pregnancy.
- Commonly associated organisms include *Chlamydia* spp. and *Actinomycetes*.

Inflammation and consequent functional disturbance due to sexually transmitted diseases frequently affects the whole female genital tract, even when the clinical manifestations are restricted to one region. A variety of aetiological agents are important, including *Neisseria gonorrhoeae*, *Actinomyces israelii* and particularly *Chlamydia* spp. These infections have a variety of clinical consequences, including abnormal vaginal bleeding, infertility and the formation of tubo-ovarian abscesses. The clinical pattern depends upon the anatomical distribution of the inflammatory process.

Inflammation of the endometrium occurs physiologically as part of the late secretory and menstrual phases of the menstrual cycle. Endometritis is therefore defined as endometrial inflammation that is not part of the normal menstrual cycle. As with inflammation elsewhere, endometritis may be infective or non-infective; and acute or chronic.

- Acute endometritis is uncommon, and is usually bacterial. Classically, this disorder was associated with instrumentation, such as during abortion, but this is fortunately now rare.

● Chronic endometritis is more common, and is characterized by the presence of plasma cells within the endometrium. Macrophages may also be present and, when these forms aggregates (i.e. granulomata), a specific cause should be sought. Possible causes include tuberculosis, fungal infection and sarcoidosis. Granulomata are also found after transcervical resection of the endometrium, which is a procedure used relatively commonly for the treatment of dysfunctional uterine bleeding.

The most common clinical situation in which chronic endometritis is encountered is in patients with intrauterine contraceptive devices (IUCD). It is also associated with chronic pelvic inflammatory disease. In the majority of cases no organisms are identified, although it is important specifically to exclude actinomycosis and tuberculosis, if appropriate. Many cases of chronic endometritis are related to *Chlamydia* infection, which is a common cause of inflammatory damage to the fallopian tube (salpingitis) and hence infertility.

Inflammation of the fallopian tube occurs predominantly by ascending infection from the uterine cavity, and is generally accompanied by infection of other parts of the female genital tract. It may be confined to the fallopian tube (salpingitis), but often involves the adjacent ovary (salpingo-oophoritis), with adhesion of fimbriae to the ovarian surface. Such an inflammatory process can extend to the peritoneal cavity (peritonitis) and may become 'sealed off' by these adhesions, leading to formation of a tubo-ovarian abscess. Resolution of inflammation in this site usually leaves adhesions and, if these obstruct the fallopian tube, hydrosalpinx may ensue (Figure 14.16). Interference with fallopian tube function often leads to reduced fertility and predisposes to ectopic pregnancy.

ENDOMETRIOSIS

Key Points
- Definition: endometrial glands and stroma outside the uterine body.
- The pathogenesis is unknown.
- Endometriosis of the ovary frequently forms 'chocolate' cysts.

Endometriosis can be defined as the presence of endometrial glands and stroma outside the uterine body (Figure 14.17). It occurs in a wide variety of different sites (Table 14.8), but most often affects the ovaries and other sites within the

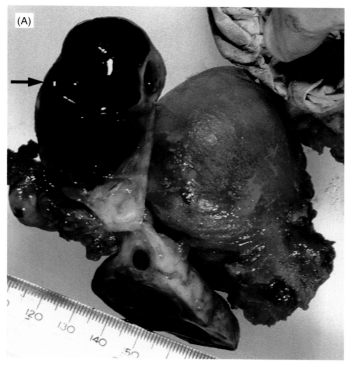

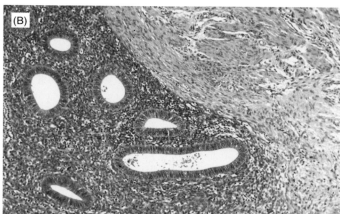

FIGURE 14.16 Resolution after adnexal inflammation has led to the formation of adhesions and a hydrosalpinx. Note that the dilated fallopian tube is 'kinked' (arrow).

FIGURE 14.17 (A) Macroscopic involvement of the ovary often takes the form of 'chocolate cysts' (arrow). (B) Microscopically, both endometrial glands and stroma are present, often with associated inflammation.

TABLE 14.8 Anatomical sites of endometriosis

Common	Uncommon	Rare
Ovary (80%)	Cervix	Lung
Uterine ligaments	Vagina	Pleura
Pouch of Douglas	Bladder	Skeletal muscle
Fallopian tube	Skin*	Small bowel

*Cutaneous involvement occurs characteristically in scars, particularly those from Caesarean sections.

pelvis, particularly the pouch of Douglas and the posterior pelvic peritoneum. Note that involvement of the serosa of the uterus is included in the definition.

The pathogenesis of endometriosis is unknown, but there are several hypothesized mechanisms, including regurgitation of menstrual endometrium (retrograde menstruation), metaplasia of surface epithelia, and vascular or lymphatic spread of normal endometrium. The former is consistent with the anatomical distribution, but it is difficult to explain the presence of endometriosis in distant sites on this basis. This is also true of the metaplasia theory.

Macroscopically, endometriosis forms multiple peritoneal nodules and, within the ovary, forms 'chocolate' cysts. The inflammation associated with the presence of endometriosis leads to the formation of adhesions which may cause secondary anatomical abnormalities, particularly of the fallopian tubes; this may lead to a reduction in fertility.

PREGNANCY

Key Points

- The placenta is formed from maternal and fetal elements.
- Abnormal vascularization of the placental bed is associated with pregnancy-associated hypertension (pre-eclampsia).
- Both maternal and fetal factors predispose to spontaneous miscarriage.
- Ectopic pregnancy may occur in any site accessible to the fertilized ovum.
- Ectopic pregnancy is an important gynaecological emergency.
- Patients with hydatidiform mole should be followed up carefully in specialist centres.

Placental Pathology

The placenta is formed from both maternal and fetal components: the decidua is formed by alteration of the maternal endometrium, and the chorionic villi and fetal membranes (including the chorion) are derived from fetal tissues. Formation of the placenta involves alteration of the maternal vascular bed within the endometrium and myometrium to support placental function and fetal demand. It is now thought that abnormality of this vascularization is the fundamental abnormality in pregnancy-associated hypertension (pre-eclampsia). Further details of placental pathology are beyond the scope of this text, but can be found in textbooks of obstetric and gynaecological pathology (see Further Reading, p. 419)

Spontaneous Miscarriage and Intrauterine Fetal Death

A significant proportion of all pregnancies end in fetal loss which occurs most frequently in the first trimester. A variety of maternal and fetal factors are involved in the maintenance of pregnancy. Therefore, pregnancy can fail as a result of a number of abnormalities: some of these are presented in Table 14.9.

TABLE 14.9 Classification of predisposing factors for spontaneous failure of pregnancy

Maternal
  Endocrine
  Physical
  Immunological
Fetal
  Chromosome abnormalities
Materno-fetal
  Infection (STORCH*; *Listeria*; parvovirus)

*STORCH = syphilis, toxoplasmosis, rubella, cytomegalovirus, herpes virus infections.

Fetal chromosome abnormalities are the most common cause of early fetal loss (Figure 14.18) that occurs up to 12 weeks of gestation. Many abnormalities have been described, including triploidy and specific trisomies. Maternal factors tend to be associated with later fetal loss. Physical abnormalities, for example uterine anomalies (e.g. uterus didelphys) and the presence of submucosal fibroids interfere with placental and fetal growth within the uterine cavity, and loss tends to occur in the second trimester. It should be remembered that these abnormalities are also associated with reduced fertility. Intrauterine death in the third trimester (stillbirth) is often of unknown cause, although evidence of ascending infection is sometimes identified. It is also associated with maternal diabetes mellitus.

Ectopic Pregnancy

Ectopic pregnancy occurs when the blastocyst implants and develops outside the endometrial cavity (Figure 14.19). This may occur in any site accessible to the fertilized ovum (i.e. pelvic peritoneum, ovary, etc.), but by far the most common site is the fallopian tube. Underlying aetiological factors that increase the chances of this happening include any fallopian tube pathology such as: current or previous salpingitis (usually as part of pelvic inflammatory disease); endometriosis; and distortion of the fallopian tube by adhesions

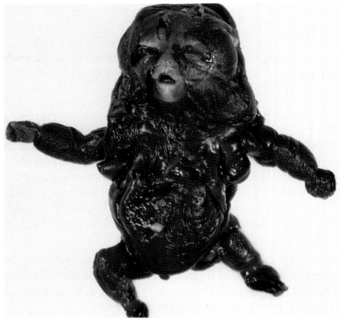

FIGURE 14.18 A spontaneously aborted fetus showing hydropic changes. Cytogenetic analysis showed a karyotype of 45,XO, indicating Turner's syndrome.

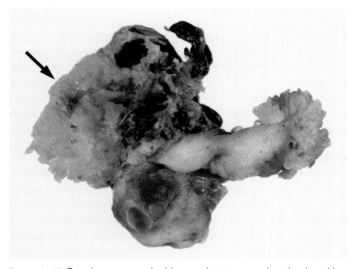

FIGURE 14.19 Ectopic pregnancy. In this case, the conceptus has developed in the lumen of the fallopian tube which has consequently ruptured. Note the presence of early placental tissue (arrow).

(e.g. those related to previous appendicectomy). The developing conceptus invades into the supporting tissues, irrespective of the anatomical site. As the fallopian tube is a thin structure with limited smooth muscle within its wall, the conceptus quickly erodes through the wall (often at around 6 weeks' gestation), with consequent intraperitoneal haemorrhage. This can be a catastrophic event as blood loss may be massive. This diagnosis should therefore be considered in any woman of child-bearing age who presents with abdominal pain or circulatory collapse. Suspicion should be even greater if there is a history of amenorrhoea. The diagnosis can

often be confirmed by carrying out a pregnancy test and examining the lower abdomen by ultrasound. Ectopic pregnancy can sometimes be treated by 'milking' the fallopian tube or by salpingotomy, but often excision of part or all of the tube (salpingectomy) is required.

Gestational Trophoblastic Disease

This is a spectrum of tumours and tumour-like conditions characterized by the proliferation of trophoblastic tissue.

Hydatidiform Mole

The most common example of this group of disorders is the hydatidiform mole, which has an incidence of approximately 1 in 2000 pregnancies in the Western world. However, it is significantly more frequent in some other parts of the world, notably Indonesia, where the incidence is as high as 1 in 80 pregnancies. Moles classically present with uterine enlargement which is 'large for dates' and may be associated with excessive vomiting (hyperemesis), related to high levels of hCG. However, the majority of patients with hydatidiform mole now do not present in this way, primarily because of the increasing use of ultrasound in the monitoring of pregnancy and the submission of most evacuated products of conception for histological examination. The classical macroscopic appearance of hydatidiform mole is a large, fleshy mass of thin-walled, translucent grape-like chorionic villi (Figure 14.20). Again, most moles do not have this appearance as the hydropic changes do not occur at early gestation. Therefore, the diagnosis is most commonly made by identifying the histological hallmark of hydatidiform moles which is trophoblastic proliferation (Figure 14.21). The fundamental cause of this is an excess of paternal chromosomes within the fertilized ovum. Hydatidiform moles are divided into two main groups: partial and complete (Table 14.10). The most likely mechanism for the occurrence of partial mole is dual fertilization of a single ovum by two separate spermatozoa. Interestingly, maternal triploidy, in which the extra set of chromosomes is of maternal origin, does not cause partial mole, although it is associated with early fetal loss. Complete

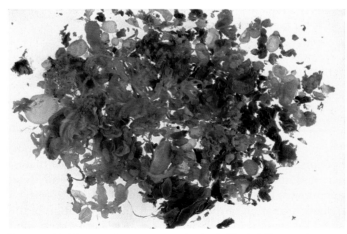

FIGURE 14.20 Macroscopic appearance of a classical hydatidiform mole.

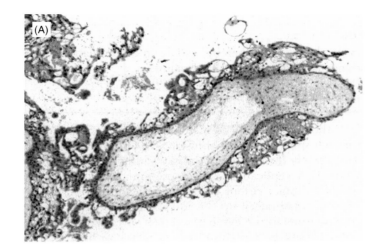

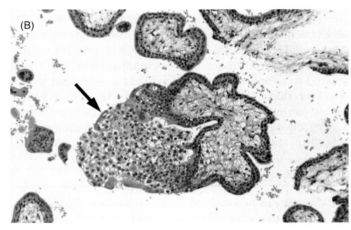

FIGURE 14.21 Microscopic appearance of (A) a hydatidiform mole showing circumferential trophoblastic proliferation. There is early stromal degeneration. This contrasts with the appearance of normal chorionic villi (B) which have polar trophoblast (arrow).

TABLE 14.10 Characteristics of complete and partial hydatidiform mole

Characteristic	Complete	Partial
Hydropic villi (if later in gestation)	All	Some
Fetus and fetal vessels	Absent	Present
Trophoblastic hyperplasia	Marked	Minimal to moderate
Ploidy	Diploid	Triploid
Sex chromosomes	85% XX, 15% XY	Most XXY

any of the three outcomes given above, but patients are generally managed as if they have choriocarcinoma as this is extremely responsive to treatment with chemotherapeutic agents, for example methotrexate.

Choriocarcinoma

Choriocarcinoma is rare in the Western world, occurring as a complication of approximately 1 in 20 000 to 30 000 pregnancies. However, as with hydatidiform mole, it is significantly more common in southeast Asia (up to 1 in 2500 pregnancies). This disorder is characterized by malignancy of trophoblastic cells. Chorionic villi are never produced. The tumour is very aggressive and frequently metastasizes, but is highly responsive to chemotherapy. Choriocarcinoma is most commonly preceded by hydatidiform mole, but may also occur following abortion, normal pregnancy and even ectopic pregnancy.

SUMMARY

The female reproductive tract is, due to its cyclical functions and ease of access of pathogens, at risk of a variety of neoplastic (often due to viral or hormonal causes) and inflammatory conditions. The role of human papilloma virus in cervical neoplasia is especially noteworthy and the prevention of this disease by cervical cytology is an indication of the potential of screening programmes. Finally, the placenta and developing fetus represent genetically different tissues which are also at risk of inflammation, developmental abnormalities and, rarely, neoplasia.

mole contains only paternal chromosomes: the precise mechanism by which this arises is not understood.

The majority of moles do not have adverse consequences. However, some recur, become invasive, or develop into choriocarcinoma. The natural history is not predictable from the histological appearance, and therefore all patients with a diagnosis of mole should be followed-up by repeated measurement of serum hCG levels. If the hCG level falls to normal, then no further treatment is required. If the level remains static or is elevated, then a diagnosis of persistent trophoblastic disease is made. This can be due to

15 THE BREASTS

Sarah E Pinder, Ian O Ellis, Andrew HS Lee and Christopher W Elston

INTRODUCTION

The female breast is in the unique position of being a gland which is non-functional except during lactation. It is, nevertheless, subject to hormonal influences, particularly throughout reproductive life, and this probably accounts for most of its pathological changes, which rarely affect the male. By far the most important disease is carcinoma, which usually presents as a palpable lump. Other lesions are mostly of significance because some of them also produce a lump or lumpiness of the breast or other symptoms which raise the suspicion of carcinoma and must therefore be investigated. The commonest of these are the fibroadenoma, which are most frequent in the third decade, and fibrocystic change, which presents particularly in the premenopausal decade. Because of the liability of the breast to injury, traumatic fat necrosis is another cause of a firm lump. Duct ectasia (dilatation of ducts) and duct papilloma may each, like carcinoma, cause a discharge from the nipple. Infection of the breast is rare except during lactation and most congenital abnormalities are of minor importance.

THE NORMAL BREAST

The breasts consist of a group of modified sweat glands, which develop from 15–25 downgrowths of the epidermis. At first solid cords, they develop a lumen and become the major (segmental) ducts, each of which opens separately at the nipple. Each segmental duct gives rise to the branching duct system of a segment of breast tissue. Before puberty the structure of male and female breast tissue is identical. In the female, under the hormonal stimulation of puberty, the duct system proliferates and lobules composed of acini and intralobular stroma bud from subsegmental ducts to form physiologically functional terminal duct lobular units (Figure 15.1). The interlobular and segmental connective tissue is less cellular and more densely collagenous and during puberty becomes infiltrated with fatty tissue; this accounts for most of the enlargement of the female breast at this time. Apart from a stratified squamous lining close to the nipple, the ducts and ductules are lined by a two-layered epithelium, an inner layer of cuboidal or columnar cells and an outer discontinuous layer of smaller, contractile myoepithelial cells. These two epithelial layers are invested in a

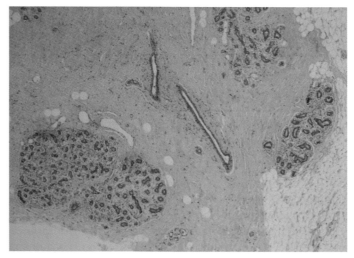

FIGURE 15.1 Normal breast. The majority of the breast is composed of stromal tissue, largely mature adipose and fibrous tissue. Within this lie the physiologically and pathologically important breast epithelial structures, from which most breast lesions are derived. The lobules of the breast form well-defined islands of small tubular structures (acini) (e.g. lower left) surrounded by intralobular stroma. The ducts are lined by a double layer of inner cuboidal or columnar epithelium over a layer of myoepithelial cells (centre).

continuous basement membrane and the duct system is ensheathed in a layer of loose connective tissue which is rich in lymphatics. There is little or no elastic tissue in the lobules, but an elastic layer surrounds the extralobular ducts.

The ductal epithelium of the mature female breast has some secretory activity, but the secretion is normally reabsorbed. During pregnancy, proliferation increases and secretory acini develop from the terminal ductular alveoli (Figure 15.2). After the menopause the breast epithelium atrophies and the lobular connective tissue changes to acellular hyaline collagen; the terminal ductules may virtually disappear, but sometimes become dilated, forming microcysts lined by flattened, attenuated epithelium. Apart from duct ectasia and duct papilloma, most lesions in the breast are believed to arise from the terminal duct lobular unit.

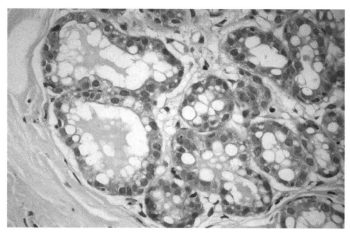

FIGURE 15.2 High-power view of lactating breast. During later pregnancy and lactation, the epithelium of the lobules becomes vacuolated with lipid-rich material, which is secreted into the lumen.

DEVELOPMENTAL ABNORMALITIES

Congenital abnormalities of the breast are rare and unimportant clinically, with the exception of polymastia (accessory breast parenchyma) and polythelia (accessory nipples). These may occur anywhere along the 'milk line' and are subject to the same disorders as normally situated breasts. Failure of development of the breast at puberty is uncommon and usually associated with ovarian agenesis, as in Turner's syndrome. Precocious development may also occur, occasionally related to the presence of an ovarian granulosa cell tumour, but usually for unexplained reasons. Adolescent or juvenile hypertrophy is the commonest developmental abnormality found. At the onset of puberty the breasts grow rapidly and out of proportion, so that they become a severe physical and psychological burden. Rarely, the hypertrophy is unilateral. The cause is unknown and the only effective treatment is surgical reduction. Microscopically, no specific abnormality is seen and the enlargement appears to be due to an overgrowth of adipose and connective tissue.

BENIGN BREAST LESIONS

The term benign breast disease is often used clinically to imply a specific pathological entity. This is clearly an over-simplification and there are a number of distinct lesions (Table 15.1) that merit discussion.

TABLE 15.1 Commonest benign breast lesions

Non-neoplastic	Fibrocystic change
	Fibroadenoma
	Hamartoma
	Sclerosing lesions including sclerosing adenosis and radial scar/complex sclerosing lesion
Benign tumours	Papilloma
	Phyllodes tumour
Infections	Acute pyogenic mastitis/abscess
Non-infectious inflammatory lesions	Duct ectasia
	Fat necrosis

Infections

> **Key Points**
>
> - Breast infections are rare.
> - They mainly occur in association with breast feeding.
> - They are caused by the introduction of staphylococci from the infant's mouth.

Acute pyogenic mastitis occurs mainly during lactation and is the result of infection via the ducts or through an abrasion of the nipple. It is most often caused by staphylococci acquired in hospital from the mouth of the suckling infant which has been colonized by the prevalent strain of *Staphylococcus aureus*. Unless effectively treated, staphylococcal mastitis may cause a loculated breast abscess; abscess formation may also occur superficial or deep to the mammary gland. Acute pyogenic mastitis may become chronic if not treated adequately, and infection with pyogenic bacteria may also start insidiously and persist, but these events are rare. Recurrent or chronic low-grade infection of the subareolar tissue occurs in some women, with scarring, distortion and sometimes fistula formation.

Tuberculosis of the breast is now rare. It may arise by haematogenous, lymphatic or direct spread, usually from the lungs or pleura. It may remain localized as a single caseating lesion, which sometimes discharges through the skin, or it may spread extensively through the breast. In view of its rarity and the occurrence of other lesions with similar histological appearances, a definite diagnosis of tuberculosis of the breast should not be made unless *Mycobacterium tuberculosis* has been detected in the lesion.

Non-infective Inflammatory Lesions

Duct Ectasia

> **Key Points**
> - Duct ectasia is of uncertain aetiology.
> - It usually presents with nipple discharge.
> - Microscopically dilatation of ducts containing foamy macrophages with a surrounding chronic inflammatory infiltrate and periductal fibrosis is seen.

Mammary duct ectasia consists of progressive dilatation of large or intermediate ducts with surrounding chronic inflammatory change. It affects one or more segments of the breast and very rarely is palpable, like a 'bag of worms'. The dilated ducts contain inspissated fatty material and their walls are thickened. Microscopically the duct epithelium appears thin, with a thickened fibrous wall that is usually infiltrated with plasma cells and lymphocytes. Foamy macrophages are often present in the lumen and in the nipple discharge.

Duct ectasia is often symptomless, but there may be a nipple discharge. Less commonly, contraction of periductal fibrous tissue may cause retraction of the nipple and raise the suspicion of carcinoma. Occasionally a dilated duct ruptures into the surrounding stroma, where its lipid contents promote a persistent inflammatory reaction with accumulation of foamy macrophages and giant cells and fibrosis; the microscopic appearances resemble those of traumatic fat necrosis and the lesion may become palpable as a firm lump. The term plasma cell mastitis is sometimes applied to duct ectasia with an unusually heavy plasma cell infiltration. The aetiology of duct ectasia is uncertain; it tends to occur most often in multipara who have not breastfed their babies, but occurs also in nullipara. There is increasing evidence that the underlying mechanism for the duct dilatation is periductal inflammation leading to destruction of the elastic network with fibrosis.

Granulomatous mastitis is a rare condition in which the terminal duct lobular unit is the site of an intense granulomatous and chronic inflammatory process with conspicuous giant cells. Terminal duct dilatation may be present, with associated foamy macrophages and, on occasion, actual abscess formation. The condition is often associated with a recent pregnancy but has also been described in nulliparous women. It should properly be termed 'idiopathic' granulomatous mastitis as the aetiology is unknown. No infectious cause has been identified, but tuberculosis should always be excluded in such a granulomatous inflammatory process. Sarcoidosis may also be associated with granulomas in the breast, but these are not confined to lobular structures.

Traumatic Fat Necrosis

> **Key Points**
> - It is caused by injury to fatty breast parenchyma.
> - It often presents as a hard ill-defined mass.
> - It may be mistaken clinically for carcinoma.
> - Microscopically a granulomatous response to lipid is seen with subsequent fibrosis.

Traumatic fat necrosis (Figure 15.3) in the fatty tissue of the breast may present as a hard lump mimicking cancer. It is caused by injury, although this may be relatively minor in the obese or pendulous breast and in many instances no history of trauma is obtained. The initial necrosis is accompanied by haemorrhage and followed by an acute inflammatory reaction. The lesion becomes heavily infiltrated by foamy macrophages containing lipid and often haemosiderin, and crystals of lipid may be deposited stimulating a foreign-body giant cell reaction. Granulation tissue forms around the lesion and gradually matures into a thick layer of fibrous tissue which, often together with calcification, accounts for the presentation as a firm or hard lump. The fibrous reaction may result in retraction of the nipple or fixation to the skin, features which increase the clinical resemblance to carcinoma.

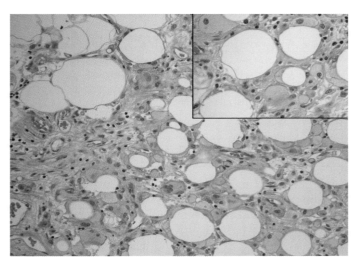

FIGURE 15.3 **Fat necrosis.** The main picture and higher power inset both show fat spaces surrounded by an inflammatory response including swollen macrophages (pale blue) which have taken up released lipid.

Reaction to Foreign Material

Leakage from silicone breast implants used for breast augmentation or as part of breast reconstruction following surgery for carcinoma is usually without harmful effect but may induce a granulomatous giant-cell reaction, causing tenderness or nodularity. This was more common in the past when silicone or paraffin would be injected directly into the breast tissues. Microscopically, fragments of the 'inert' material are seen, surrounded by macrophages and multinucleated giant cells.

Galactocele

This is a cystic swelling of a lactiferous duct which develops during lactation, apparently due to obstruction of the duct. Initially it contains creamy fluid which gradually becomes watery. Leakage of duct contents may induce a granulomatous reaction, or become infected.

Fibroadenoma

Key Points

- Fibroadenoma is one of the commonest breast lesions.
- There is localized hyperplasia rather than development of a true neoplasm.
- It presents as a well-defined mass, often in young women.
- Microscopically there is proliferation of the intralobular stroma with interspersed epithelial tubules or clefts.

Although it has previously been the convention to regard fibroadenomas as benign tumours there is considerable evidence to support the view that they are focal areas of lobular hyperplasia rather than true neoplasms. They may present at any age after puberty but are most common in the third decade, presenting as small, firm, well-defined mobile lumps, which may occasionally be multiple and bilateral. Microscopically, the dominant element is a proliferation of loose, cellular, intralobular stroma that is associated with a variable number of tubular structures (Figure 15.4). The latter appear either as elongated clefts or tubules cut in cross-section. The previous designation of 'intracanalicular' and 'pericanalicular' types, based on these patterns of stroma and epithelium, has no practical or clinical significance, and can safely be abandoned. Fibroadenomas are usually well-circumscribed lesions, but although they are easily enucleated at surgery they are not truly encapsulated. Occasionally, small foci of fibroadenomatous hyperplasia are found; these are small, microscopic lobulated areas resembling fibroadenomas, but not forming well-defined masses. Both fibroadenomatous hyperplasia and fibroadenomas may present in mammographic breast screening programmes, as associated microcalcification can form in the stroma (Figure 15.5).

Fibroadenomas are entirely benign lesions which confer no significant predisposition to subsequent carcinoma. Indeed, many surgeons avoid surgical excision once the diagnosis has been established on clinical grounds and confirmed either cytologically or histologically by needle core biopsy. Rarely, *in-situ* carcinoma, mainly of lobular type, may develop within a fibroadenoma, but this probably means that its epithelium,

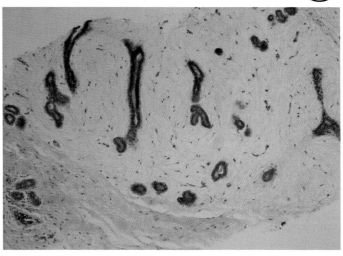

FIGURE 15.4 Fibroadenoma. A core biopsy of a fibroadenoma seen as a well-defined mass of loose myxoid connective tissue bearing ductal structures resembling tubules. A small portion of adjacent normal breast is present (bottom left).

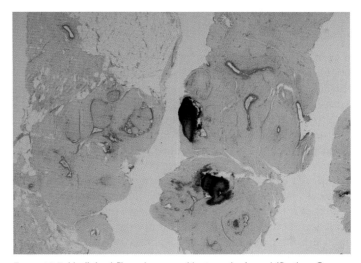

FIGURE 15.5 Hyalinized fibroadenoma with stromal microcalcification. Core biopsies from a fibroadenoma with a more hyalinized fibrous stroma than seen in Figure 15.4. Large foci of microcalcification are seen in the core on the right as irregular haematoxyphilic islands.

like that of normal breast, is not immune to carcinogenic agents.

Phyllodes Tumour

Key Points

- Phyllodes tumour usually presents in middle-aged or elderly women as a well-defined mass.
- Microscopically it is composed of cellular stroma with compressed 'leaf-like' clefts of epithelium.
- It is usually benign, although rarer borderline and malignant forms may occur.

These uncommon tumours are still referred to, entirely erroneously, as 'giant fibroadenoma' or 'cystosarcoma phyllodes'. They occur predominantly in middle-aged or elderly women and are rarely seen below the age of 40. They form large, lobulated, circumscribed masses which may grow rapidly to cause unilateral breast enlargement or even skin ulceration. Grossly, they have a whorled cut surface that resembles a compressed leaf bud (Greek phyllo = leaf) with visible clefts and cystic spaces. Microscopically, the elongated cleft-like spaces are lined by epithelial cells and the intervening stroma is cellular. The epithelial cells are regular and entirely benign, although focal hyperplasia may occasionally be present. The stromal cells are plump and may be densely packed; nuclear abnormalities are rare and mitoses variable in number. The great majority of phyllodes tumours are benign and complete excision is curative. Approximately 10% will recur locally, due to incomplete excision. It is not possible in some cases to predict behaviour and those tumours with a mitotic count above that seen in clearly benign lesions may be classified as 'borderline'. True malignant change occurs in less than 5% of cases; the stroma becomes sarcomatous and lymph node, but particularly bloodborne, metastases may develop.

Hamartoma

Hamartomas are relatively uncommon lesions which are formed from a disordered collection of lobules, stroma and fat. They may occur at any age but are predominantly seen in pre- or perimenopausal women, who present with a well-defined mass. They are, however, surprisingly often impalpable and may only be detected mammographically. Hamartomas vary in size from 1 cm to 25 cm at presentation. They have a fleshy cut surface and are composed microscopically of a mixture of morphologically normal, but disordered, fat, fibrous tissue and breast epithelial structures including lobules and few ducts. Smooth muscle may be present. Although occasionally large, these masses are entirely benign and treatment is by local excision.

Fibrocystic Change

Key Points

- Fibrocystic change is the commonest breast lesion.
- It is believed to be due to changes in hormone levels/sensitivity.
- It presents as ill-defined thickening or lumpiness in the breast in women usually aged 40–55 years.
- Microscopically, cyst formation, apocrine metaplasia, fibrosis and epithelial proliferation may be present.

A large number of terms have been used as synonyms for a group of changes which present clinically as a lump or lumpiness in the breast during the reproductive decades. They include fibroadenosis, cystic hyperplasia, cystic mastopathy, mammary dysplasia and fibrocystic disease. None is entirely satisfactory but fibrocystic change is probably the most appropriate. The condition is the commonest of all breast lesions, and produces clinical symptoms in at least 10% of women. The peak incidence is in the premenopausal decade. After the menopause there is a sharp decline in symptomatic cases. Microscopically, a range of appearances is seen and the components described below are present in variable amounts from case to case.

Cyst formation (Figures 15.6 and 15.7) results from localized dilatation of lobular and terminal ductules, and is presumably due to obstruction. Cysts are usually multiple and mostly less than 1 cm in diameter, although occasional larger ones are not unusual. They are thin walled and appear blue when seen close to the cut surface of biopsy material. The lining epithelium often becomes flattened and may be lost in larger cysts. It may also undergo apocrine

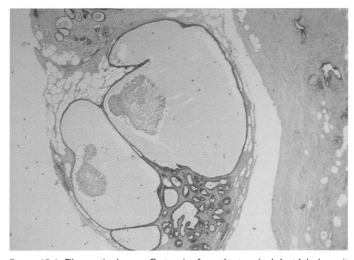

FIGURE 15.6 Fibrocystic change. Cysts arise from the terminal duct lobular unit and bear secretions. Most are less than 1 cm in diameter.

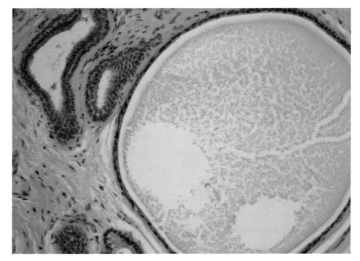

FIGURE 15.7 Microcyst in fibrocystic change. Small cysts are common in fibrocystic change. The epithelium is flattened (compare to adjacent normal epithelial lined ducts). The lumen bears flocculent secretions.

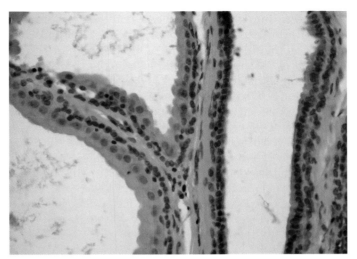

FIGURE 15.8 Apocrine metaplasia in fibrocystic change. Breast cysts in fibrocystic change are commonly lined by apocrine epithelium (seen in the left of this photomicrograph). The cells in apocrine metaplasia are larger than normal epithelium (compared to the normal epithelial cells on the right), more columnar in shape and have abundant eosinophilic cytoplasm.

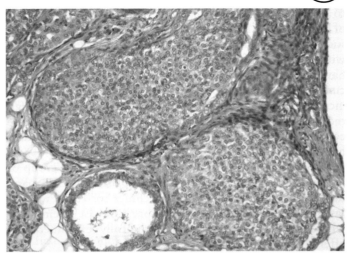

FIGURE 15.9 Epithelial hyperplasia of usual type in fibrocystic change. The duct space is no longer lined by a single layer of luminal epithelial cells but by a hyperplastic proliferation, which almost fills the ducts in this case. The cells, however, do not show significant pleomorphism or increase in size and mitoses are not prominent.

metaplasia (Figure 15.8), the cells becoming larger and columnar with a convex free margin and abundant strongly eosinophilic cytoplasm. An incomplete layer of myoepithelium can usually be detected, at least in places, under the inner apocrine epithelium of the cyst. Like the ductules from which they develop, the cysts are not ensheathed in elastic tissue. Unless haemorrhage has occurred, the cysts contain clear watery or mucinous fluid. Occasionally a cyst ruptures and causes an inflammatory reaction in the adjacent stroma, which may then become tender or painful.

Increase of fibrous stroma (fibrosis) occurs in most cases of fibrocystic change, but quantification of this process is difficult. In thin women, the normally fibrous breast stroma of young adult life persists with little change even after the menopause, but in obese women there is a progressive replacement of fibrous by fatty tissue particularly after the menopause. As age advances, the fibrous stroma becomes hyaline and relatively acellular, while the epithelial elements atrophy. It is this collagenization of pre-existing stroma without obvious fibroblastic proliferation that is responsible for fibrosis of the breast.

Epithelial hyperplasia (Figure 15.9) of significant degree occurs in approximately a quarter of cases of fibrocystic change. In the past the nomenclature has been confusing; European pathologists used the term epitheliosis whereas in the USA papillomatosis was preferred. Epithelial hyperplasia is now classified as being either of usual type or atypical. In epithelial hyperplasia of usual type several layers of epithelial cells line the ductules and the lumen may be obliterated by a solid proliferation. Nuclei are regular, and although occasional mitoses may be present they are of normal configuration.

Atypical ductal hyperplasia (ADH) is diagnosed when a small area of intraductal proliferation of epithelial cells shows features distinct from usual epithelial hyperplasia and indeed resembling low-grade ductal carcinoma *in situ* (DCIS). The degree of atypia and the overall size of the process is, however, insufficient for diagnosis of DCIS; ADH is by definition a small, microfocal lesion.

Epithelial proliferation may also take the form of lobular *in-situ* neoplasia, a term used to encompass the entities of both atypical lobular hyperplasia (ALH) and lobular carcinoma *in situ (LCIS)*. Lobular *in situ* neoplasia is usually an incidental finding in breast tissue removed for fibrocystic change. As with the intraductal proliferations (ADH vs. DCIS), the extent of this intralobular proliferation of cells is less marked in ALH than LCIS. Microscopically, small, regular, epithelial cells expand the acini of the lobules. Mitoses are few but the nuclear/cytoplasmic ratio is increased. Basement membranes remain intact. In contrast with DCIS, LCIS is often multifocal and bilateral involvement is reported to occur in up to 30% of cases.

Epithelial Proliferation and Risk of Subsequent Breast Cancer

The relationship between benign breast lesions and subsequent breast carcinoma has been the subject of great controversy. Many older studies have been seriously flawed, and it is only more recently, in studies employing careful histopathological review, that a degree of clarity has been achieved. Patients whose biopsy specimens show no epithelial hyperplasia have no increased risk; because this category accounts for approximately 70% of benign biopsies the great majority of women can be reassured, and do not require follow-up.

Hyperplasia of usual type (see above) gives an increased risk of carcinoma of about double that in women whose breasts are 'normal'. The most significant risk, up to four-fold, occurs in women whose biopsy specimens show atypical hyperplasia (either ductal or lobular), and this is doubled

Adenoma of the nipple is a rare lesion which presents as a reddened rounded nodule, sometimes mimicking Paget's disease of the nipple. It is composed of proliferating ductal type epithelium which often has a papillary structure and may indeed be a form of retroareolar benign papilloma (see above). The presence of two layers of epithelium and myoepithelium distinguishes the lesion from a carcinoma.

MALIGNANT TUMOURS OF THE BREAST

Key Points

- By far the most common malignant tumour of the breast is mammary adenocarcinoma.
- This is broadly subdivided into DCIS and invasive carcinoma.
- Other breast malignancies such as sarcoma and lymphoma are rare.

Carcinoma

With the possible exception of skin, breast cancer is the commonest of human female cancers throughout the world. During the mid-1980s mortality from cancer of the breast overtook that of every other female cancer to become the commonest cause of cancer death. However, nearly twice as many develop breast cancer as die of it. The incidence and mortality of breast cancer are high and remarkably constant in most developed countries; the incidence is increasing, especially in younger women, and this is not entirely due to an increase in the 'at-risk' population. It is more than 200 times commoner in women than in men.

Carcinoma of the breast may occur at any age, but is rare before 25 years and most common between 40 and 70 years. About 50% of invasive carcinomas occur in the upper outer quadrant of the breast (where there is the greatest proportion of breast parenchyma), the remainder being distributed equally throughout the rest of the breast. The main presenting symptom is a palpable mass and for this reason all lumps in the breast, whatever the age of the patient, must be regarded clinically as possibly malignant until proved otherwise. A cancer arising in the axillary tail may be mistaken clinically for an enlarged lymph node.

In practice, all true breast masses should be investigated and a definitive diagnosis made by fine needle aspiration cytology or, more commonly by core-cutting needle. Thus women with breast cancer can have preoperative counselling, discussions regarding appropriate treatment options can take place and surgeons can plan operations and operating time. Perioperative frozen section should be avoided (except in exceptional circumstances), particularly in small impalpable (screen-detected) lesions which may then be unavailable for full paraffin histology and assessment of prognostic factors. In the UK women aged 50–70 years are routinely invited for 3-yearly mammography as part of the UK National Health Service Breast Screening Programme (NHS BSP); in this service, lesions are most commonly detected as microcalcifications, masses, distortions or parenchymal deformities on mammography and are often impalpable.

○ 15.1 SPECIAL STUDY TOPIC

MAMMOGRAPHIC BREAST SCREENING

Although trials of the effect of tamoxifen have been reported, there is no unequivocal way at present of preventing breast cancer. Attempts to reduce the mortality from this common malignancy have therefore concentrated on early identification. Tumour size and lymph node spread of invasive breast cancer are time-dependent; small tumours (e.g. those less than 1 cm in size) are less likely to have lymph node metastases.

Although there has been some disagreement over the efficacy of breast screening programmes, randomized controlled trials (such as the HIP trial in New York and the Swedish Two-Counties studies) have indicated a reduction in mortality of approximately 20% in those invited for mammographic screening. The National Health Service Breast Screening Programme (NHS BSP) in the UK began in the late 1980s. Women aged 50–70 are now invited for 3-yearly mammography. If an abnormality is detected the woman is invited back for further assessment which includes clinical examination and further breast imaging, such as additional mammography with magnification views and ultrasound examination.

Mammographic abnormalities which may be identified include well-defined, ill-defined or spiculate masses, architectural distortions, asymmetric densities or microcalcifications. The latter is typical of DCIS (see main text). Invasive carcinoma is most often seen as a spiculate or ill-defined mass. At the time of assessment, fine needle aspiration cytology (FNAC) or, now more commonly, core biopsy samples may be taken. The aim is to obtain a preoperative diagnosis of cancer so that one-step surgery can be performed, and to be able to diagnose benign lesions. If these latter are impalpable it may be appropriate to leave them in the breast and thus to avoid unnecessary benign biopsies in well women. Features of malignancy in cytological preparations include increased nuclear size and pleomorphism and also discohesion of cells. Benign cells, conversely, are adherent to each other and are relatively small and regular. In some cases it is not, however, possible to make a definitive diagnosis on a cytological preparation.

Breast cytology samples are reported according to NHS BSP guidelines as C1–inadequate, C2 – benign, C3 – equivocal, C4 – suspicious or C5 – malignant.

Core biopsy takes a small histological sample and requires less specific expertise in histological interpretation than cytological assessment. Again, however, specific diagnosis is not invariably possible. Core biopsy samples are also reported using histological categories: B1 – normal tissue, B2 – benign lesion, B3 – lesion of uncertain malignant potential, B4 – suspicious or B5 – malignant. In the few case where definitive diagnosis is not possible on core biopsy (B3 and B4 categories) either repeated sampling, for example with a wider bore needle, or diagnostic surgical biopsy may be necessary to make a definitive diagnosis.

In general screen-detected cancers are more often lymph-node negative and smaller than symptomatic cancers. In addition they are more often of a less aggressive morphological type and of lower histological grade (see Table 15.3).

TABLE 15.3

	Proportion of screen-detected carcinomas (%)	Proportion of symptomatic carcinomas (%)
Histological type		
No special type (ductal)	28	47
Tubular and tubular mixed	49	16
Lobular	13	15
Medullary-like	2	5
Mucinous	1	1
Others	7	16
Lymph node negative	80	63
Histological grade		
Grade 1	45	19
Grade 2	40	34
Grade 3	15	47

Types of Breast Carcinoma

Carcinoma of the breast arises from the lining epithelium of the duct system. Previously it was thought that in some cases the origin was ductular and in others it was lobular, but it is now accepted that virtually all cancers are related to the terminal duct lobular unit. For a variable length of time the tumour cells remain confined within the duct system, in the form of DCIS, before breaching the basement membrane and invading the breast stroma. As elsewhere, the distinction between *in situ* and infiltrating carcinoma is extremely important and is the main pathological subdivision used.

Ductal Carcinoma In Situ

By definition the cytological changes of malignancy are present in the epithelial cells of an *in situ* carcinoma, but the basement membrane remains intact and no invasion is seen. Although carcinoma *in situ* of the breast is now known to arise from the terminal duct lobular unit, it has become conventional to recognize two types of *in-situ* carcinoma, ductal and lobular. There are significant morphological, prognostic and therefore subsequent therapeutic differences between the two, which justify subdivision into two different types. In addition, however, the name lobular carcinoma *in situ* (LCIS) is somewhat misleading, as it is now generally accepted that this is not an invariable precursor of invasive cancer. Some pathologists now use the term lobular *in-situ* neoplasia to indicate the process of either atypical lobular hyperplasia or lobular carcinoma *in situ* (see epithelial hyperplasia, above).

In symptomatic series of breast cancer the frequency of DCIS is approximately 2–5%. In the majority of these cases it presents as a palpable mass. However, DCIS is now most commonly detected in screening programmes in asymptomatic women by mammographic identification of microcalcification in the breast, and in such series the frequency is approximately 20%. Microscopically, a variable number of ducts may be involved but DCIS in general involves a single duct system within the breast.

In the past DCIS was classified according to the architectural growth pattern; thus solid, comedo, cribriform and micropapillary DCIS were described. In solid DCIS the ducts are completely filled by a disorderly proliferation of epithelial cells (Figure 15.12). There is often central comedo-type necrosis in the lumen so that lipid-rich yellow debris may be expressed from the cut surface like toothpaste from a tube. Cribriform DCIS is characterized by a geometric 'lacy' network of bridges and trabeculae. The micropapillary type consists of a proliferation of epithelial cells, which form small papillary projections into the lumen. Although this architectural classification system has some value it is clear that in many cases a mixture of one or more patterns may be present. Therefore more recent systems of categorization use the cytonuclear grade of the tumour nuclei and high-, intermediate- and low-grade DCIS are now recognized. High-grade DCIS is composed of malignant cells with abundant cytoplasm, marked nuclear pleomorphism and increased mitoses. Low-grade DCIS is formed from small, regular cells which often form cribriform or micropapillary structures, as described above. Intermediate-grade DCIS shows features less marked than those of high-grade disease and more prominent than those of low-grade DCIS.

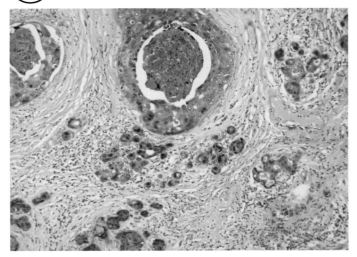

FIGURE 15.12 High-grade ductal carcinoma *in situ* (DCIS). Duct spaces are completely filled by a solid neoplastic proliferation of large, highly malignant cells. In this case the DCIS extends into the lobules as 'cancerization' of lobules; this may mimic invasion, but the process in both ducts and lobules has a surrounding myoepithelium (not shown). The DCIS within ducts bears central comedo-type necrosis.

Coarse microcalcification in the necrotic luminal debris, or fine clustered calcification in the interstices of the epithelial proliferation, form useful radiological diagnostic features for mammographic detection of DCIS. When DCIS extends along major ducts as far as the nipple, groups of carcinoma cells may enter the deeper layer of the epidermis and spread within it through the nipple and areola. The affected skin shows reactive inflammatory changes in the dermis. These changes produce a characteristic eczematous appearance named Paget's disease of the nipple (Figure 15.13) after Sir James Paget who described it in 1874. The

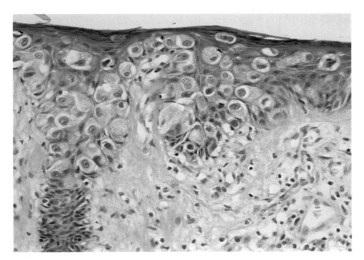

FIGURE 15.13 Paget's disease of the nipple. When DCIS extends along major ducts as far as the nipple, groups of carcinoma cells may enter the deeper layer of the epidermis and spread within it through the nipple and areola in the form of Paget's disease of the nipple. In this case, atypical malignant cells with abundant cytoplasm and large nuclei are seen in the basal layers of the nipple.

carcinoma cells usually form clusters within the epidermis and can be distinguished by their large nuclei, prominent nucleoli and abundant cytoplasm. Paget's disease is always accompanied by an underlying DCIS which may be confined to the nipple ducts or situated deep in the breast; relatively rarely nowadays there may also be invasive cancer present. At present the treatment of choice for Paget's disease of the nipple is mastectomy.

Usually DCIS is confined to one duct system in the breast, although this may overlap more than one quadrant. Because of the associated microcalcification, DCIS is now frequently identified mammographically when small and there is an increasing trend towards breast-conserving therapy (complete local excision, with or without postoperative radiotherapy) for this, as for small invasive cancers. If primary therapy is adequate the long-term prognosis of DCIS is excellent, with a 10-year survival of greater than 95%.

Invasive Carcinoma

> **Key Points**
>
> Histological types of invasive breast carcinoma:
>
> - Ductal carcinoma, now called no specific/special type (NST), is commonest (>50%).
> - Invasive lobular carcinoma (of which there are several variants) is the second commonest pattern in routine practice (approximately 15%).
> - Tubular carcinoma is much commoner in screening than symptomatic practice.
> - Medullary, mucinous and invasive cribriform carcinoma are rare.
> - Other forms such as metaplastic carcinoma are exceedingly rare.

A number of different morphological types of invasive breast carcinoma are recognized.

Infiltrating Carcinoma of No Special Type (NST) / Ductal (Figure 15.14)

Over 50% of invasive breast carcinomas fall into this category. Grossly, they form a firm, often hard, moderately defined lump usually measuring 10–40 mm in diameter. They cut like an unripe pear and it is this type which was traditionally referred to as scirrhous carcinoma. Microscopically, the tumour is composed of cords and sheets of large epithelial cells, which infiltrate in a disorganized fashion between dense bands of collagen. The cells vary in size and shape, some tubule formation may be seen and mitoses are usually present, but there are no special morphological features.

Infiltrating Lobular Carcinoma (Figure 15.15)

This accounts for approximately 10–15% of all invasive carcinomas. Although these tumours may have a scirrhous macroscopic appearance similar to ductal carcinoma, more

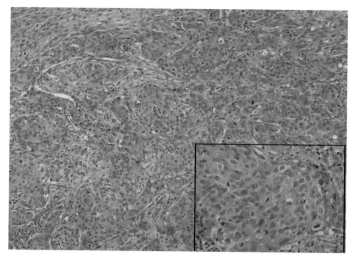

FIGURE 15.14 Invasive breast carcinoma of no special type (ductal). Invasive carcinoma is formed from irregular islands of pleomorphic malignant cells. These have no surrounding myoepithelial cells and diffusely infiltrate into the stroma. The higher power inset shows the malignant cells in more detail, with numerous mitoses.

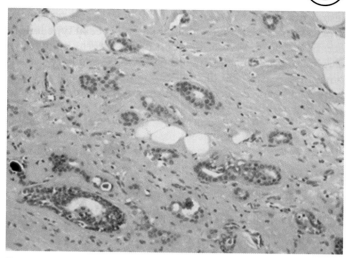

FIGURE 15.16 Tubular carcinoma. This subtype of invasive carcinoma is formed from elongated tubular structures infiltrating through a cellular fibroblastic stroma. The tubules are lined by a single layer of relatively regular cancer cells, without an associated myoepithelial layer, and with central lumina.

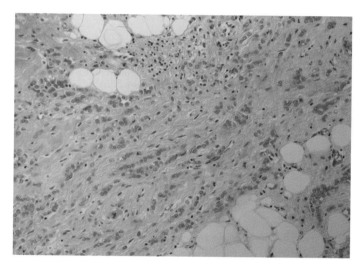

FIGURE 15.15 Infiltrating lobular carcinoma. This subtype of invasive carcinoma is composed of small, relatively regular cancer cells. Typically linear cords of carcinoma cells infiltrate diffusely as 'single files'.

frequently they are softer with an ill-defined outline. Microscopically, they are composed of small, regular epithelial cells with infrequent mitoses. Classically, linear cords of cells infiltrate diffusely as discrete or single cells within fine collagen bands giving a so-called targetoid or 'single file' pattern.

Tubular Carcinomas (Figure 15.16)

These are uncommon in symptomatic series accounting for about 2% of invasive carcinomas; this prevalence increases in screened populations to approximately 15% because these are often small impalpable lesions which are detected

mammographically as spiculate masses. Grossly these cancers may be less than 1 cm in diameter, firm and have an irregular star-shaped, stellate outline. Microscopically, there is central elastosis and elongated tubular structures radiate through a cellular fibroblastic stroma. The tubules are lined by a single layer of relatively regular epithelial cells, without an associated myoepithelial layer, and with central lumina. Mitoses are infrequent. Occasionally a mixture of tubular and cribriform structures is seen and more rarely a 'pure' invasive cribriform carcinoma is diagnosed. Although the pure tubular type is uncommon, in about 20% of invasive carcinomas a mixed pattern is seen, where a tubular structure is preserved centrally, but infiltrating ductal carcinoma is present at the periphery; some groups classify these forms as tubular mixed carcinomas or as tubular variant carcinomas.

Medullary-like Carcinomas

These account for approximately 3% of invasive carcinomas. Macroscopically, they are well-defined and soft, usually measuring between 10 mm and 40 mm in diameter. Microscopically, they are composed of syncytial masses of large epithelial cells with a conspicuous lymphoplasmacytoid infiltrate in the stoma and at the periphery, which has a pushing edge. The cells vary markedly in size and shape and mitoses are conspicuous.

Mucinous Carcinomas

These are rare (less than 1% of invasive carcinomas). Characteristically they have a well-defined gelatinous gross appearance. Histologically, the tumour is composed of clumps of small, relatively regular epithelial cells lying within lakes of mucin.

Combinations of histological patterns occur relatively commonly in the form of mixed carcinomas, for example a

grade 1. Low-grade cribriform DCIS was also present. Excision was widely complete by more than the required distance of 5 mm. Despite the low histological grade, one of the five axillary nodes removed contained metastatic carcinoma and the tumour was thus of lymph node stage 2 (fewer than four lymph nodes involved). The tumour was also examined by immunohistochemistry to determine whether oestrogen-receptor expression and HER2 protein were present; strong, extensive staining for oestrogen receptor was seen (100% of nuclei were positive) indicating that the tumour would respond to hormone therapy such as tamoxifen, if this was felt appropriate. No membrane immunoreactivity for HER2 protein was present and the tumour was therefore regarded as HER2 negative.

Despite the node metastasis, the patient's Nottingham Prognostic Index Score was 3.28 and her prognosis predicted to be good (Figure 15.20). More than 83% of patients in this good prognostic group are alive at 10 years' follow-up.

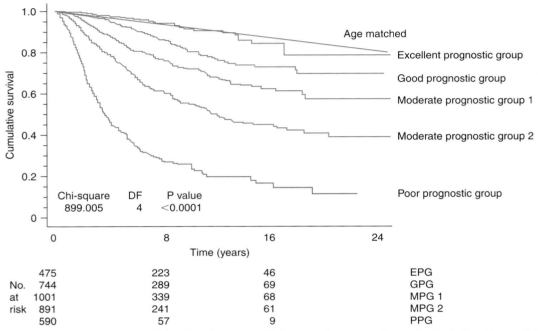

FIGURE 15.20 Overall survival curves for patients with invasive primary operable breast carcinoma according to the Nottingham Prognostic Index (NPI) groups from data from the Nottingham Tenovus Primary Operable Breast Cancer Series. Each of the five lines shows survival for women within that range of NPI scores, namely excellent, good, moderate 1, moderate 2 and poor prognostic groups.

Aetiology of Breast Carcinoma

No single causal agent has been found, but a number of predisposing factors have been identified. The incidence of breast cancer, like carcinomas in general, increases with age, but the increase occurs earlier than for most cancers, being most rapid between the ages of 30 and 50 years, after which it rises more slowly to a maximum in old age. The strongest aetiological factor is a positive family history; there is a definite increased risk if a female relative, i.e. mother, maternal grandmother or sister, has had breast cancer. Occasional families exist in which there is a very high incidence of breast cancer, and these patients may have a genetic predisposition (see Special Study Topic 15.2).

Although differences in racial susceptibility have been established (the incidence is lower in China and Japan) this is almost certainly due to environmental factors, since the incidence rises in 'Westernized' Japanese women. There is good evidence that exposure to female sex hormones, and oestrogen in particular, is an important factor in the development of breast cancer, but it is not certain whether there is a systemic effect or an increase in target organ sensitivity. Some risk factors have been identified; apart from the obvious difference in the incidence in men and women, the risk in women is increased by early menarche and late menopause, whereas early first pregnancy and oophorectomy before the age of 35 years have a protective effect. There is still no complete agreement concerning the role of oral contraceptive therapy or hormone replacement therapy in the aetiology of breast cancer and the degree of risk they may confer. The balance of epidemiological evidence is that long-term users of the contraceptive pill are at an increased risk. The higher doses of sex hormones used in older formulations of hormone replacement therapy also increase risk. These data, however, are difficult to interpret because of the large number of variable factors involved and the combinations of hormones and changes of formulation and dose.

Predictive Markers in Invasive Breast Carcinoma

Oestrogen Receptor

In many women with breast cancer the course of the disease may be influenced by alterations in the hormonal background of the patient. This was first demonstrated by Beatson in Glasgow in 1896 when he carried out bilateral oophorectomy in women with advanced breast cancer. The oestrogen receptor (ER) competitor tamoxifen or, more recently the aromatase inhibitors, have been used successfully in the treatment of hormone receptor positive metastatic disease. Measurement of oestrogen receptor protein in tumour samples provides a good prediction of likely response to endocrine therapy; a favourable response is unlikely if oestrogen receptor cannot be detected. Oestrogen receptor status is now routinely examined in tissue sections from invasive breast cancers using immunochemistry (Figure 15.21). Thus the likelihood of response to hormone therapy can be predicted and the most appropriate therapy selected.

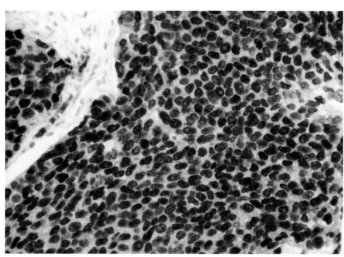

FIGURE 15.21 Oestrogen receptor immunohistochemistry in invasive breast carcinoma. Sheets of invasive breast carcinoma cells stained immunohistochemically with antibody against oestrogen receptor. The nuclei of this cancer all show strong reactivity (as intense brown staining) and this tumour is strongly oestrogen-receptor-positive, indicating a good chance of response to hormone therapy.

HER2

HER2 is a member of the human epidermal growth factor receptor family and encodes a transmembrane tyrosine kinase receptor. It is expressed in approximately 25% of invasive breast cancers and is associated with a poorer patient outcome in several studies, although it is also more commonly present in tumours with a poor profile in general (e.g. worse histological grade). More recently, however, drug therapy using humanized monoclonal antibodies against the HER2 protein has been developed and proven valuable in the treatment of that subgroup of women who have cancers which overexpress the protein on the surface of the tumour cells or have amplification of the gene. Herceptin (trastuzumab) has proved efficacious in both women with metastatic and early breast cancer (without metastasis) and it is now recommended that all invasive breast cancers are tested for the presence of excess protein on the cell surface by immunohistochemistry (Figure 15.22) or for amplification of the gene by fluorescent *in-situ* hybridization (Figure 15.23).

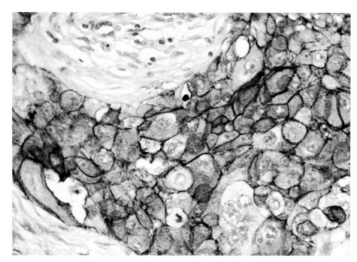

FIGURE 15.22 HER2-positive breast cancer. Invasive breast cancer with strong positive staining of HER2 protein on the surface of the cell membranes (3+ staining).

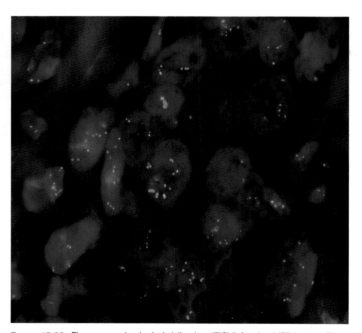

FIGURE 15.23 Fluorescent *in-situ* hybridization (FISH) for the *HER2* gene. The number of copies of the *HER2* gene in the tumour cell nucleus is assessed with fluorescence microscopy and the number of signals (red dots) is counted per cell and compared with the number of signals for chromosome 17 (green dots). A ratio of *HER2* gene to chromosome 17 of more than 2 is considered positive, as here.

GENETICS OF BREAST CANCER

The development of malignancy is related to abnormalities in structure and/or function of tumour suppressor genes and oncogenes. A great many genes have been found to show aberrations in invasive breast carcinoma including members of the tyrosine kinase family of growth factors such as epidermal growth factor and *HER2*, c-*myc*, the tumour suppressor gene *p53* and members of the ras family. Many of these abnormalities are seen in sporadic cases of breast cancer. Although inherited cases account for only 5–10% of breast cancer, it is clear that some families have a significantly greater risk than the general population for the development of breast cancer. In particular it is likely that a true hereditary factor is implicated if the disease is diagnosed at a young age, is bilateral or if many family members are affected. In some families with breast cancer, ovarian carcinoma may also be seen and in others both males and females may be affected.

It is clear that there is not a single gene which is mutated in all cases of familial breast cancer. One of the first abnormalities to be identified was a mutation in the tumour suppressor gene *p53* (also seen in sporadic breast cancer) on the short arm of chromosome 17. Li–Fraumeni syndrome is a cancer family syndrome with a germ-line mutation in *p53* causing breast cancer but also sarcomas, various childhood malignancies and gliomas. This autosomal dominant inherited condition is, however, associated with less than 5% of familial breast cancers. However, breast cancer associated gene 1 (*BRCA1*) and subsequently gene 2 (*BRCA2*) have been cloned. These are also of autosomal dominant inheritance. It remains uncertain precisely what function these genes products play in normal tissue. It is nevertheless clear that mutations in these genes are associated with differing risk of breast and ovarian cancer. *BRCA1* is associated with an overall lifetime risk of 85% of developing breast cancer but the site of the mutation appears to be important with relation to the differing risks of breast and ovarian cancer.

BRCA1 appears to be implicated in approximately 45% of familial breast cancers and *BRCA2* in another 40%. *BRCA2* mutations are found in those families where male breast cancer is also seen. Other genetic syndromes account for only approximately another 5% of hereditary breast cancers; thus it seems likely therefore that other breast cancer associated genes have yet to be discovered, probably low penetrance genes in combinations.

A woman may have several close relatives who have developed breast cancer, and as described above, the likelihood of a genetic aetiology is increased if they did so at a young age. Her statistical risk of developing breast carcinoma can be ascertained by comparison with large epidemiological series. Risks are often quoted in terms of 'relative risk' in comparison to the general population, but for an individual patient this may be difficult to understand and thus unhelpful. For example a relative risk of 10 times the population does not mean that the patient is at 10 times the risk of 1 in 12 for the population lifetime risk. In particular, the relative risk differs according to the woman's age. Thus a cumulative risk for an individual is more helpful and can give an estimated risk of developing cancer over a lifetime.

The risk of any individual in a breast cancer family of developing carcinoma, however, depends on whether they have inherited the genetic mutation present. If the specific abnormalities can be identified in the affected family member's tissue/blood it can be sought in the patient. If a *BRCA1* mutation has indeed been inherited, the risk for the individual approaches 100% over their lifetime. These women may choose to have bilateral preventative/prophylactic mastectomy or to attend high-risk clinics with regular clinical examination and breast imaging. If a mutation cannot be identified in the family members or tissue is not available, the absence of an abnormality in the patient does not preclude the presence of an abnormal gene, because present screening techniques will not identify 100% of mutations. In these latter women risk must be estimated from the epidemiological data.

Other Malignant Tumours of the Breast

Sarcomas

Most types of malignant connective tissue tumour have been described in the breast, but all are very rare. The prognosis of angiosarcoma, once thought to be invariably fatal, is now known to depend on the degree of differentiation of the vascular endothelium. These malignant vascular tumours have an association with radiotherapy and have been described after irradiation following wide local excision for breast cancer in the overlying subcutis. Other sarcomas are exceedingly rare and their clinical behaviour is thus not clear from the published literature; liposarcomas, leiomyosarcomas and fibrosarcomas appear to behave in an essentially similar fashion to those in other sites in the body.

Lymphomas

The breast is an unusual primary site of lymphomas, diffuse large B-cell lymphoma being the least rare. Its distinction from carcinoma preoperatively is important in order to avoid unnecessary mutilation. Involvement of the breast in disseminated lymphomas and in granulocytic leukaemia is commoner. For example, young girls with Burkitt's lymphoma may develop bilateral breast involvement. Disseminated lymphoma, granulocytic sarcoma (CML) and myeloma may rarely present with breast masses before disease elsewhere becomes evident.

THE MALE BREAST

Hypertrophy (Gynaecomastia)

Key Points

- Hypertrophy of the male breast is due to changes in sex hormone levels.
- It is commonest in older men (chronic liver disease, prostatic cancer treatment, some other medication) but may occur at puberty.
- Microscopically an increase in the stroma is seen with duct enlargement and sometimes epithelial hyperplasia.

The male and female breasts are essentially similar until the onset of the secondary sex characters at puberty; in some adolescent males one or both breasts may then enlarge. This is known as pubertal hypertrophy and is rarely marked, but may cause pain, discomfort or embarrassment. It is due mainly to increase of stroma and enlargement of ducts, but without lobule formation. The hyperplastic duct epithelium may be surrounded by a zone of oedematous, fibrillary stroma. It tends to regress and operative removal is rarely necessary. Similar changes may occur in old age. Both pubertal and senile hypertrophy are due to changes in levels of sex hormones. Gynaecomastia occurs in response to high oestrogen levels, for example in chronic liver disease, in prolonged hormonal therapy for prostatic cancer, and reportedly in workers involved in the manufacture of oestrogens. Less commonly, it is induced by digitalis or some other drug. Very rarely hypertrophy results from an underlying endocrine disease such as feminizing tumour of the adrenal cortex. Testicular injury is an extremely rare cause. In chromatin-positive Klinefelter's syndrome the enlarged breasts show lobules histologically, comparable to those of the normal female breast.

Tumours

Tumours in the male breast are rare. Carcinomas are morphologically the same as those in the female organ and

similarly the prognosis is poor if spread has occurred to the lymph nodes (and to the chest wall). Paget's disease of the male breast is exceedingly rare. Metastatic tumour, for example from a bronchial or prostatic carcinoma occasionally occurs in the male breast, as metastases from other malignancies may be seen in the female breast. Thus, as in the female, the male breast may be involved in generalized lymphoid neoplasms and leukaemias.

SUMMARY

- Benign lesions of the female breast are frequently seen in clinical practice; the most common lesions are fibrocystic change and fibroadenomas.
- The importance of benign lesions lies chiefly in exclusion of malignancy; particular mimics of carcinoma are fat necrosis, radial scars and sclerosing adenosis.
- Risk factors for breast cancer are female sex, increasing age, northern European or American descent, previous personal or family history of breast cancer, uninterrupted menses and atypical epithelial proliferative disease.
- Ductal carcinoma *in situ* is believed to be a true precursor of invasive tumour and is often identified mammographically as microcalcifications.
- Invasive breast cancer is of heterogeneous microscopic appearance and variable prognosis.
- The most important features in predicting prognosis are lymph node stage, histological grade and tumour size.
- Diseases of the male breast are rare; the most common abnormality is gynaecomastia (hypertrophy) due to changes in sex hormone levels.

FURTHER READING

NHS Cancer Screening Programmes. *Guidelines for Non-operative Diagnostic Procedures and Reporting in Breast Cancer Screening*. London: NHS BSP, Publication No. 50, 2001.

Rosen PP. *Rosen's Breast Pathology*, 2nd edn. Philadelphia: Lippincott Williams & Wilkins, 2001.

Royal College of Pathologists/NHS Cancer Screening Programmes. *Pathology Reporting of Breast Disease*. London NHS Breast Screening Programme (NHS BSP) Publication No. 58, 2005.

Tavassoli FA, Devilee P. *World Health Organization Classification of Tumours. Pathology and Genetics. Tumours of the Breast and Female Genital Organs*. Lyon: IARC Press, 2003.

16

David Ansell and Robin Reid

OUTLINE OF THE MALE REPRODUCTIVE SYSTEM

The male reproductive system comprises the following structures:

- The testes, in which the testicular tubules produce spermatozoa, and the interstitial (Leydig) cells the male hormone testosterone. Spermatozoa pass from the testis through the epididymis, vas deferens and seminal vesicles to the urethra, and thence to the exterior via the penis at ejaculation.
- The prostate gland, which lies at the base of the bladder and surrounds the prostatic urethra. In the normal male this gland is about the size of a sweet chestnut and adds secretions to semen necessary for sperm viability. It must be stressed that the seminal vesicles are NOT a place of storage for sperm.

Tumours of the testis and prostate are increasing in incidence in the Western World. Testicular tumours are the most common malignant solid tumour in young men aged between 20 and 35 years. Some 30 years ago, these teratomatous tumours had a very poor prognosis, and more than 50% of patients with such lesions died within 2 years. With modern platinum-based chemotherapeutic regimes however, 90% or more of patients can be cured, even if they have metastatic disease. Prostate cancer is now the second most common malignant cause of death in older men in England and Wales, having recently overtaken colorectal cancer, though bronchial carcinoma remains the major killer.

THE TESTIS

Congenital Abnormalities

Cryptorchidism

Cryptorchidism, or maldescent, is the most common congenital abnormality. The testis develops embryologically from the genital ridge adjacent to the mesonephros. During intrauterine development it descends into the scrotum under the influence of the gubernaculum. This process may be halted at any level to produce this condition. Spermatogenesis will only proceed satisfactorily in the lower temperature of the scrotum, and cryptorchidism is a significant cause of male infertility. Maldescent is also an important cause of testicular tumours, both within the undescended testis and in the contralateral organ. It is therefore important to investigate the position of any undescended testis in male infants and, if possible, to bring it down into the scrotum (orchidopexy). Laparoscopy now enables the urologist to locate the intra-abdominal testis in a non-invasive manner and to remove it if it cannot be brought down into the scrotum surgically. This investigation will also reveal the rare cases of anorchia (congenital absence of testis) and those of the vanishing testis, where only epididymal remnants are identified at the site of the testis with no remaining testicular tubules present. Most of these cases are thought to be due to previous intra-abdominal torsion.

Torsion

Torsion of the testis after infancy is usually ascribed to an unusually long mesorchium, the 'mesentery' that unites the body of the testis with the epididymis. Young men with this condition present with an acute onset of unilateral pain in the scrotum due to rotation of the testis around the mesorchium, with resultant obstruction of the venous return from the testis, which rapidly becomes engorged with blood. Early diagnosis is essential as prompt reversal of the rotation and fixation of the organ results in complete resolution, whilst delay leads to infarction and death of the testis.

Inflammatory Conditions

Inflammation of the testis (orchitis) may be due to many infective agents. The most common viral cause is mumps, and orchitis is common in men suffering from this infection. The viraemia in mumps also causes inflammation of other organs besides the salivary glands and the testes (e.g. the pancreas and ovary), although clinical symptoms from these organs are uncommon. Previous mumps orchitis may lead to infertility.

16.1 CASE HISTORY

TESTICULAR TUMOUR

A 21-year-old man noticed a painful lump in his testis and went to his general practitioner, who provisionally diagnosed epididymo-orchitis and prescribed a course of antibiotics. The swelling and pain continued despite treatment, and the patient was referred to a urologist. On questioning, he admitted to mastodynia and was referred for an ultrasound examination of the testis, which revealed a tumour (Figure 16.1). Blood taken for tumour markers at this time showed a raised human chorionic gonadotrophin (hCG) level (the cause of his mastodynia).

Radical orchidectomy was performed. The excised tumour had a very haemorrhagic cut surface (Figure 16.2) typical of choriocarcinoma (malignant teratoma trophoblastic; MTT). This was confirmed at histology, which showed multinucleate syncytiotrophoblast cells in association with cytotrophoblast (Figure 16.3). Postoperatively the patient's tumour markers returned to normal, and computed tomography scanning showed no evidence of any metastases (Stage 1 tumour). Vascular invasion was noted histologically, and so the patient was given limited chemotherapy. Currently he is alive and well 5 years later.

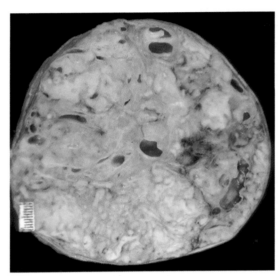

FIGURE 16.2 Orchidectomy specimen with most of the testis replaced by a solid tumour which is partly necrotic and haemorrhagic. Choriocarcinomas (malignant teratoma trophoblastic, MTT) are typically haemorrhagic.

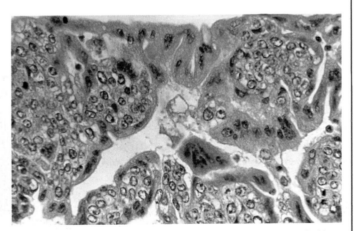

FIGURE 16.3 Choriocarcinoma (MTT) with multinuclear syncytiotrophoblast and cytotrophoblast cells. These cells can be shown to contain human chorionic gonadotrophin (hCG) by immunohistochemistry.

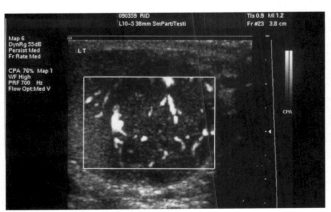

FIGURE 16.1 Testis ultrasound with power Doppler angiogram showing a well-defined low echo mass with increased blood flow, suggesting a well-vascularized tumour.

The vasa and seminal vesicles drain into the urinary tract, and so it is not surprising that retrograde spread of urinary tract organisms along the genital tract may lead to acute inflammation. Infections of the testis from this source affect both testis and epididymis, referred to as acute epididymo-orchitis. Patients with this condition present with testicular pain and swelling and systemic symptoms such as fever (distinction from torsion is important, as this needs urgent surgery); antibiotic treatment is usually curative in these cases. Young patients with painless testicular swelling should not be diagnosed as epididymo-orchitis, as most will have a testicular tumour requiring urgent investigation and treatment. Tuberculosis of the urinary tract may lead to tuberculous epididymo-orchitis; this affects the epididymis before spreading to the testis, and ultimately may lead to sinuses draining from the area of infection onto the scrotal skin.

Infertility

In a significant proportion of couples presenting with infertility it is the male who is responsible. The role of testicular biopsy in the investigation of men with low sperm counts or azoospermia is contentious, as there is considerable doubt as to whether there is any effective treatment, apart from in those patients with obstruction. Surgical attempts to relieve the obstruction should only be performed when a previous testicular biopsy has shown effective spermatogenesis. However, now that intracytoplasmic sperm injection (ICSI) of ova *in vitro* is possible, biopsy is increasingly performed to confirm that sperm are present in the testis, which can be recovered surgically to be used in this technique.

A number of patients who have had a vasectomy for contraceptive purposes are subsequently found to have spermatozoa in their ejaculate, having previously been azoospermic. This is the result of vasitis nodosa, when spermatozoa released into the tissues at the site of section of the vas deferens elicit a granulomatous inflammatory response within which epithelial cells from the vas deferens ramify and connect with those of the other portion of transected vas deferens such that continuity is re-established.

For endocrine causes of male infertility see Chapter 17.

Tumours

The vast majority of testicular tumours (>95%) are derived from the germ cells of the testis. The other 5% comprise a heterogeneous group which are rarely encountered clinically and are derived from a variety of tissues (Table 16.1).

Aetiology

The association of germ cell tumours and cryptorchidism has been known for many years, although the stated increased risk associated with this abnormality varies considerably in different publications, from a four-fold increase in patients with this condition in some reports, to a forty-fold increase in

TABLE 16.1 Non-germ cell tumours of the testis

Tumour group	Example
Sex cord/gonadal stromal	Leydig cell tumours, Sertoli cell tumours
Mesenchymal	Embryonal rhabdomyosarcoma, leiomyosarcoma
Haemopoietic	Malignant lymphoma, leukaemic infiltrates
Metastatic	

others. It is probable that the increased incidence in these patients is in part genetic, since cryptorchidism is often associated with other congenital abnormalities of the urogenital tract, and unilateral cryptorchidism is also associated with an increased incidence of tumours in the contralateral testis. There is also a small familial incidence of testicular tumours, and these are associated with abnormalities of chromosome 12p.

The incidence of testicular tumours in Western countries has increased considerably over the past few decades, and this has been attributed to an increase in oestrogenic substances in the environment. These may come from a variety of sources, from the administration of oestrogens to mothers at risk of miscarriage to metabolic byproducts of chemicals used extensively in packaging. Support for this proposition is provided by the reported decrease in sperm counts of the typical Western male over the past 15 years, which can also be attributed to environmental oestrogenic substances.

Intratubular Germ Cell Neoplasia

The precursor lesion of testicular germ cell tumours is thought to be intratubular germ cell neoplasia (ITGCN). This may be regarded as a variety of carcinoma *in situ* occurring within the testicular tubules. These cells are recognizable histologically, being larger and more pleomorphic than normal spermatogonia (the cells from which spermatozoa develop). ITGCN is seen in tubules adjacent to the majority of testicular germ cell tumours, and it has also been seen in biopsies taken from cryptorchid testes of patients who have subsequently developed a tumour in the same testis.

Terminology

Testicular germ cell tumours are confusing in that different classifications and terms are employed on the two sides of the Atlantic. The tumours can be subdivided primarily into two main groups. The first group – seminomas – are thought to be derived from normal sperm-producing cells, and their terminology does not elicit any controversy. The other group of tumours is considered to be derived from totipotent germ cells within the gonad which have the capacity to differentiate into all varieties of benign and malignant tissues, thus potentially producing a bewildering spectrum of histological appearances. This is where the confusion and contention arises. The American and World Health Organization (WHO) classifications describe and list the tissues present in these tumours, thereby producing a long and complicated list of possible diagnostic terms. The British classification attempts to simplify this by calling all these tumours teratomas on the assumption that they have the potential to produce tissues from all three germ cell layers, although these may not be seen in the tumour under consideration. However, as the more malignant non-seminomatous germ cell tumours do not contain differentiated tissue from a variety of cell layers, the Americans will not accept the general term 'teratoma', reserving it only for those tumours in which such differentiated tissues foreign to the testis are found. In an attempt to resolve this dispute there is increasing use of the term 'non-seminomatous germ cell tumour' (NSGCT) as an umbrella name for all these tumours.

It is very important clinically to differentiate seminomas from NSGCTs, as they are managed clinically in completely different ways. Approximately 40% of testes containing a germ cell tumour actually have both seminoma and non-seminoma present, and these combined tumours are managed clinically as NSGCTs.

Seminoma

Key Points

- Occurs at age 30–50 years.
- Spreads predominantly via the lymphatic system.
- Is very radiosensitive.
- Most do not produce serum tumour markers.

These tumours occur in middle-aged men (aged 30–50 years) and usually present as an enlarged, painless testis. Most patients will not have raised tumour markers, but a small number have a raised serum hCG level. These tumours have a characteristically uniform, slightly lobulated cut surface (Figure 16.4), and histologically are composed of large cells with clear cytoplasm and vesicular nuclei with a significant associated lymphocytic infiltrate (Figure 16.5). Those cases with a raised serum hCG level also contain multinucleate giant cells (syncytiotrophoblast); despite this, they have the same prognosis as those tumours not containing giant cells.

These tumours spread via the lymphatic system, and enlarged para-aortic abdominal lymph nodes are the first sign of metastatic spread. Occasionally, lymphadenopathy is the presenting symptom – these patients almost always have an unrecognized primary tumour in the testis. On rare occasions no primary testicular tumour is found, and these tumours are thought to have arisen from germ cells in the genital ridge that have not migrated down into the scrotum within the testis, and which have developed into a tumour in this ectopic site.

Seminomas are extremely radiosensitive, and most patients will be cured by this treatment, if administered correctly.

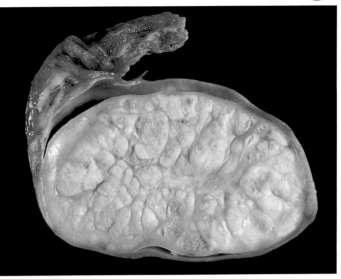

FIGURE 16.4 Seminoma of the testis. Lobulated, creamy white tumour replaces most of the body of the testis, but there is no necrosis.

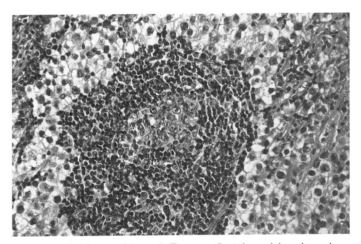

FIGURE 16.5 Seminoma of the testis. Tumour cells at the periphery have clear cytoplasm and well-demarcated cell borders. Centrally, there is a lymphoid follicle; this is a common occurrence in these tumours.

Non-seminomatous Germ Cell Tumour (NSGCT)

Key Points

- Occurs in the 20- to 30-year-old age group.
- Spreads via blood vessels.
- Is not radiosensitive, but responds to appropriate chemotherapy.
- Majority of cases secrete AFP and/or hCG into the serum.

As noted above, these tumours have the potential to differentiate into the whole spectrum of embryonic and extra-embryonic tissues. Extraembryonic tissue comprises trophoblast, as seen in the placenta and yolk sac tissue from the organ of that name. These two tissues secrete human chorionic gonadotrophin (hCG) and α-fetoprotein (AFP) respectively, and patients with tumours containing these histological elements have raised levels of these substances in their serum (so-called tumour markers). In practice, 80% or more of NSGCTs will have raised levels of one of these tumour markers in the serum. Elevation of serum tumour markers is rarely of diagnostic importance, since the common presentation of testicular tumour is an enlarged, painless testis. However, these markers may aid diagnosis in those patients who present with symptoms arising from a metastasis. Their value lies in the post-operative management, for if previously elevated values do not return to normal after surgery, the presence of metastases is indicated. The markers are also used to monitor patients during follow-up, as rising values indicate the recurrence of tumour.

Histology

The most common malignant element seen is sheets of anaplastic cells of epithelial appearance (embryonal carcinoma to the Americans; malignant teratoma undifferentiated or MTU to the British) (Table 16.2; Figures 16.6 and 16.7). When this is accompanied by differentiated elements such as cartilage, skin, glandular tissue and muscle, the British classification refers to the tumour as 'malignant teratoma intermediate' (MTI), and the American classification as 'teratoma with malignant component'.

Very occasionally only mature, benign-looking tissue is seen in a tumour; these the American classification is happy to call teratoma, and the British teratoma differentiated (TD). Although malignant tissue may not be demonstrable, these tumours should be followed up clinically in an identical manner to other NSGCTs as a significant number develop metastases later and require chemotherapy. This apparently contradictory behaviour is presumed to be due to malignant tissue not detected by pathological sampling. Such behaviour is in marked contrast to the common teratoma of the ovary (dermoid cyst), which almost always behaves in a benign fashion.

Many tumours contain small quantities of yolk sac or trophoblastic tissue, as mentioned earlier. The most common NSGCT in prepubescent boys consists almost entirely of yolk sac tissue. Tumours containing significant quantities of trophoblastic tissue with both cytotrophoblastic and syncytiotrophoblast are particularly aggressive – they have identical histological features to choriocarcinoma of the placenta, and are given this name by the Americans, whilst the British use the term malignant teratoma trophoblastic (MTT).

Macroscopically, non-seminomatous tumours have a more variable appearance than seminoma. The malignant areas are soft, brownish and often haemorrhagic, whilst the differentiated areas are white and frequently cystic (Figure 16.6). Metastatic spread is via the bloodstream, the lungs being the most common site of secondary lesions. Those tumours associated with very high serum levels of hCG often present with grossly haemorrhagic metastases in liver, lungs or brain, and have a much worse prognosis than other NSGCTs.

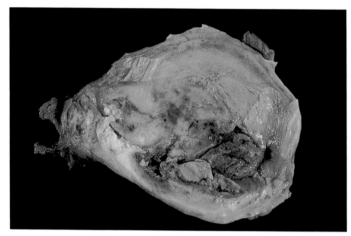

FIGURE 16.6 Malignant teratoma of testis with extensive haemorrhagic necrosis.

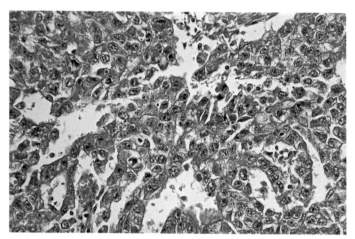

FIGURE 16.7 Embryonal carcinoma – the most common malignant element seen in malignant teratomas. The tumour cells have an epithelial (carcinomatous) appearance.

TABLE 16.2 Comparison of classifications of non-seminomatous germ cell tumours

Histology	British	American/WHO
Benign differentiated tissue only	Teratoma differentiated (TD)	Mature teratoma
Malignant tumour with differentiated tissue present	Malignant teratoma intermediate (MTI)	Teratoma with malignant areas
Undifferentiated malignant epithelial tumour only	Malignant teratoma undifferentiated (MTU)	Embryonal carcinoma
Malignant trophoblast	Malignant teratoma trophoblastic (MTT)	Choriocarcinoma

INCIDENCE OF TESTICULAR TUMOURS

The cause or causes of the increasing incidence of testicular tumours in young men is far from clear. The role of testicular maldescent has been known for many years, but this accounts for only a small percentage of tumours. However, the fact that the tumours in men with cryptorchidism may occur in the contralateral testis, the established increased risk of tumour in the other testis in patients who have had one tumour, and the occasional cases of familial tumours all point to a genetic cause in some patients.

Much interest and study has also been applied to the possible carcinogenic effects of increased quantity of oestrogens, or substances with oestrogenic properties, in the environment today. The rise in number of testicular tumours in Western countries has been associated with a reported fall in the sperm count of males in those countries where this rise has been noted. Similarly, reports of male fish with ambiguous genitalia occurring in water which has been contaminated by chemicals indicates the occurrence of oestrogenic material in the environment.

Further Reading

Anonymous. Studies highlight chemical threats to reproduction. *Br Med J* 1995; **311**: 1.

Skakkebaek NE, Sharpe RM. Are oestrogens involved in falling sperm counts and disorders of the male reproductive tract? *Lancet* 1993; **341**: 1392–1395.

THE PROSTATE

The prostate gland sits at the base of the bladder, and surrounds the proximal urethra. The seminal vesicles, which lie posterosuperiorly, receive the vas deferens from the testis, and drain into the posterior prostatic urethra adjacent to a small promontory, the verumontanum, which is easily seen at cystoscopy. The seminal vesicles do not store the spermatozoa but, like the prostate gland, produce secretions necessary for the nurture of spermatozoa. The prostate is composed of numerous glandular acini which drain via ducts into the urethra. One of the secretions of these glands is prostate-specific antigen (PSA) which may be detected in blood; elevated levels are found in patients with carcinoma of prostate, but levels are also raised when the gland is either large or inflamed.

In older men (aged 50 years and above), there is a gradual enlargement of the prostate, a condition known as 'benign nodular hyperplasia'. This may produce severe urinary symptoms such as urgency, frequency and dysuria and, in extreme cases, acute urinary retention. In this same age group, adenocarcinoma arises in this organ, and is an important cause of death with the ever-increasing longevity of the Western male. A detailed description of the lobular anatomy of the prostate would be inappropriate, but it is important to note that benign nodular hyperplasia occurs in the central portion of the gland (often called the middle lobe), whereas the majority of carcinomas occur in the periphery. Operations to treat benign nodular hyperplasia (transurethral resection [TURP] and retropubic prostatectomy) remove the central part of the gland only, and do not necessarily remove or even detect coexisting carcinomas. Such surgery is therefore not effective treatment for this tumour.

Congenital abnormalities of the prostate and seminal vesicle also occur, but are uncommon and rarely of any clinical significance.

Inflammatory Conditions

Histological examination of prostatic tissue removed for obstructive symptoms will often show a small number of both acute and chronic inflammatory cells associated with prostatic acini, although these are rarely associated with clinical symptoms. Clinically significant, more extensive acute or chronic inflammation of the prostate is less common:

● Acute prostatitis, with microabscess formation, may complicate conditions in which there is some degree of immune paresis, and is particularly common in diabetics.

● Chronic prostatitis is a recognized clinical entity in which patients present with pelvic pain and in whom pus cells can be seen in the urine after massaging the prostate per rectum. This condition usually responds to appropriate antibiotic therapy.

● A number of patients present with pain in the prostate, but do not have inflammatory cells in their urine. In these cases there is probably a significant psychological component, and this condition is labelled prostatodynia.

In some cases of severe chronic inflammation within the prostate there is a significant granulomatous element with multinucleate giant cells and numerous histiocytes. This is a non-specific inflammatory response to prostatic secretions within the stroma following rupture of ducts. This non-specific granulomatous prostatitis is important clinically as the inflammation produces a firm gland which may be mistaken for carcinoma at rectal examination, and may also give a raised level of serum PSA, thus adding to diagnostic confusion. An important differential diagnosis of granulomatous prostatitis is tuberculous prostatitis, as patients with genitourinary tuberculosis (TB) may have infection in the prostate. The granulomata in this condition often have true caseation necrosis, and acid-fast (tubercle) bacilli may be demonstrable in Ziehl–Neelsen-stained sections. Patients with granulomatous prostatitis suspicious of TB should have an early morning urine sample examined microbiologically for tubercle bacilli.

Benign Nodular Hyperplasia

Key Points

- Arises from excessive growth of the central group of glands.
- Produces frequency and dysuria, and occasionally urinary retention.
- Significant cause of renal failure in older men, causing obstructive uropathy.
- May give a significantly raised serum level of PSA.

This common condition in middle-aged and elderly males is almost certainly due to some disturbance in the balance of male hormone production, as it does not occur in castrates. The condition is caused by an overgrowth of the various stromal elements of the prostate, glands, smooth muscle and fibrous tissue, thereby producing glandular and stromal nodules which distort the prostatic urethra. The condition affects only the central and superior portions of the gland, and when excessive may produce a rounded nodule of prostate at the base of the bladder between the ureteric orifices (Figure 16.8). This acts like a ballcock, obstructing the urethral orifice when bladder pressure rises at micturition. The bladder wall of these patients is thickened and trabeculated. In severe cases acute or chronic renal failure may occur due to ureteric blockage; this is referred to as obstructive uropathy.

Carcinoma

Key Points

- Usually arises in the periphery, and not always sampled in TURP specimens.
- Is preceded by prostatic intraepithelial neoplasia (PIN).
- Second most common cause of cancer deaths in males in the UK.
- Very variable natural history.
- Boney metastases often osteoblastic.

The majority of tumours of the prostate are adenocarcinomas (benign tumours are extremely rare) (Figure 16.9). Prostatic carcinomas vary considerably in their degree of differentiation, and this in part determines the natural history of the disease, although not entirely (see below). Like many other epithelial neoplasms, invasive prostatic carcinoma is preceded by in-situ tumour (PIN). Carcinoma of the prostate is now the second most common malignant cause of death in Western males, though whether this is a true increase in incidence or is due to men living longer and not dying of other diseases (e.g. ischaemic heart disease, lung cancer) is uncertain and debatable.

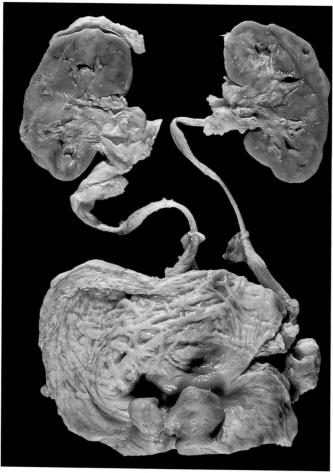

FIGURE 16.8 Benign nodular hyperplasia of the prostate. Hypertrophy of the central portion of the gland (middle lobe) projects into the base of the bladder. Obstruction of urinary flow has produced hypertrophy of muscle of bladder wall, giving this trabeculated appearance and also a degree of ureteric dilatation and hydronephrosis.

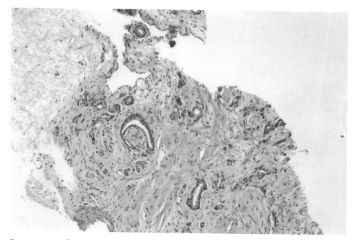

FIGURE 16.9 Carcinoma of prostate gland, seen in a needle biopsy. The tumour can be seen encircling a nerve in the centre.

Aetiology and Epidemiology

Growth of prostatic glandular cells – both benign and malignant – requires testosterone and dihydrosterone, and this was the first tumour in which hormone dependency was demonstrated. In the early 1940s, Huggins showed that castration was an effective treatment for some cases of metastatic prostate cancer, and this formed the basis of antiandrogen therapy which is still employed widely today. In a minority of cases there is a familial component; there is also a wide ethnic variability, the tumour being more common in African blacks and less frequent in Hispanics and Orientals. Although the tumour occurs in the same age group as benign nodular hyperplasia, the two conditions are not thought to be causally related.

Studies of the natural history of this tumour are problematical due to its variable biological behaviour. Post-mortem studies conducted in the past revealed that many older men who had died of unrelated causes had histological carcinomas in their prostate (latent carcinoma), and that the incidence of these increased with age. Similarly, histological examination of prostatic tissue removed for benign hyperplasia often reveals adenocarcinoma, although this was not suspected and the patient shows no evidence of metastatic disease (incidental carcinoma). Many incidental carcinomas do not develop metastatic disease, and in the past such patients were not treated. However, recent long-term follow-up of such cases has shown that a significant number develop metastases many years later, which suggests that younger patients found to have such tumours might benefit from treatment.

The only effective treatment for prostatic carcinoma is radical prostatectomy in which the entire gland is removed (including the peripheral portion not excised at TURP, or retropubic prostatectomy) (Figure 16.10). This operation was often followed by impotence and incontinence, but during the 1980s nerve-sparing techniques were developed which preserved potency. Indeed, this approach has now become an acceptable treatment for gland-restricted prostatic carcinoma. At about the same time that this operation was developed, screening for prostate cancer by

measurement of serum PSA levels became available. By using this technique patients with small, operable tumours could be identified and considered for surgery.

Serum PSA levels may be elevated in a number of conditions, and therefore needle biopsies of the prostate are taken to confirm malignancy. These are often taken under the guidance of transrectal ultrasound (TRUS), which may identify localized abnormalities. Biopsies are frequently taken from different parts of the gland; these are referred to as sextant biopsies.

The usual criteria used to identify patients with small tumours likely to benefit from radical surgery are:

- serum PSA level
- size of the tumour (from TRUS examination or evaluation of the amount of tumour in the needle biopsies)
- the grade of tumour.

Prostatic cancer is graded using the Gleason system, which grades tumours by the degree of glandular differentiation only, and ignores cytological detail. Tumours are graded from 1 (very well differentiated) to 5 (anaplastic). As many tumours have a variable degree of differentiation, this system attributes primary and secondary grades for those lesions with two patterns. Tumours are thus given two Gleason grades – for example 3:4 – and these are summated to give a Gleason score (in this example of 7). If the tumour is uniform, the grade is repeated, i.e. 3:3.

Needle biopsies of the prostate gland taken to detect carcinoma are not always easy to diagnose. The malignant cells have the usual criteria of malignancy, but the small tumours detected by screening programmes are often well-differentiated. Normal prostatic acini are surrounded by a thin layer of basal cells which are not present around malignant glands, and their absence can be detected by immunostaining with high molecular-weight cytokeratins that stain basal cells, but not acinar cells. Prostate cancer cells also have a predilection for infiltrating lymphatics and the spaces around nerves. The presence of perineural infiltration is also an indicator of malignancy.

Examination of radical prostatectomy specimens is performed to confirm the presence of malignancy, and to compare the Gleason score with that seen in previous biopsies. The resection margins are examined carefully to assess whether the tumour has been adequately excised, although it is not common practice to treat patients with positive margins. In fact, many patients with positive margins are apparently free of clinically significant disease at 5 or more years later. Active treatment is usually only considered if and when the serum PSA levels start to rise.

Tumour Spread

Local spread into the base of the bladder is common, and such tumours may be difficult to differentiate from primary bladder cancer. Immunocytochemistry is useful in this situation, as prostatic cancer cells invariably contain PSA and prostatic acid phosphatase (PSAP). Extension posteriorly into the rectum is uncommon, as there is a dense layer of fascia between the two organs.

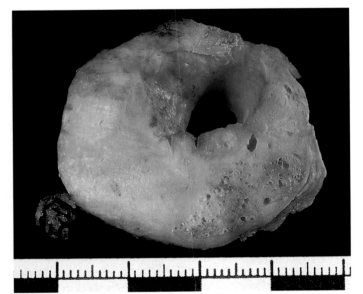

FIGURE 16.10 Carcinoma of prostate gland in radical prostatectomy specimen. The tumour occupies most of gland on the left of the picture.

Prostate cancer metastasizes primarily via the lymphatics, initially to the pelvic and para-aortic lymph nodes. Some surgeons will sample pelvic lymph nodes by frozen section at the time of radical prostatectomy and cancel the operation if metastasis to local nodes is found. Spread to bones is also common; these metastases are frequently osteosclerotic (osteoblastic), and radiologically may be mistaken for Paget's disease. Alkaline phosphatase levels will be elevated in both conditions, but PSA only with secondaries from prostatic cancer. Bone metastases are commonly seen in the lumbar vertebrae and pelvis (Figure 16.11). This has been attributed to the extensive venous plexus connecting the prostate and this portion of the skeleton, but it is more probable that this is the part of skeleton most commonly seen by urologists in intravenous urography (IVU), and plane X-radiography of the bladder as whole body imaging reveals secondaries throughout the skeleton in most of these patients.

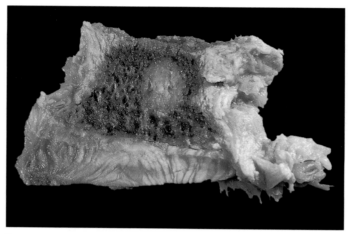

FIGURE 16.11 Osteosclerotic (osteoblastic) metastasis of carcinoma of prostate gland in a vertebral body.

16.2 CASE HISTORY

PROSTATIC ADENOCARCINOMA

A 53-year-old man went to his general practitioner complaining of backache. An X-radiograph of his lumbar spine showed sclerotic areas in lumbar vertebrae which were considered to be most probably metastatic prostatic carcinoma rather than Paget's disease of bone (Figure 16.12). This was supported by finding a firm, irregular prostate gland on digital rectal examination (DRE), and a raised serum level of PSA.

In view of the side effects of oestrogen-like drugs (impotence, venous thrombosis) in a relatively young man, it was considered mandatory to establish a tissue diagnosis. A transrectal needle biopsy of prostate was taken, and this confirmed the diagnosis of a well-differentiated adenocarcinoma (Figure 16.13).

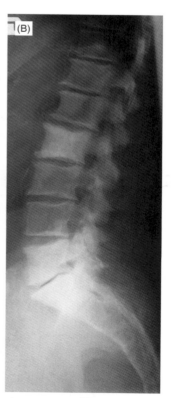

FIGURE 16.12 Anteroposterior (A) and lateral (B) radiographs of the lumbar spine of the patient. The bodies and posterior elements of L2, L5 and S1 vertebrae are sclerotic. There are also areas of patchy sclerosis in other vertebral bodies and in the right iliac bone. This is the typical appearance of skeletal metastases from prostate cancer.

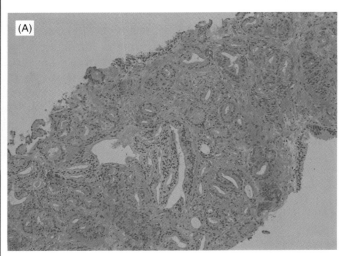

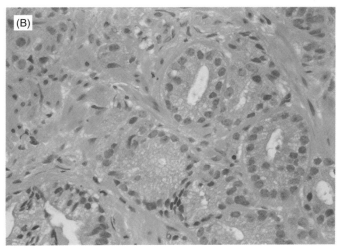

FIGURE 16.13 Needle core biopsy of prostate: (A) low power; (B) high power This is a well-differentiated adenocarcinoma, which is subtly different from normal in its diffuse non-lobular pattern of growth, and glands lined by single layers of cells with prominent nucleoli.

THE PENIS AND SCROTUM

Congenital Abnormalities

Cryptorchidism has been discussed previously (see p. 438). Important congenital abnormalities of the penis include:

- hypospadias, in which the urethra opens onto the ventral aspect of the penile shaft, following incomplete fusion of the urethral folds during embryological development
- epispadias, when the urethra opens onto the dorsal aspect of the shaft; this is frequently associated with bladder exstrophy due to abnormal differentiation of the cloacal membrane.

Inflammatory Conditions

The penis is involved in many sexually transmitted diseases, but discussion of these will be found in texts relating to dermatology and microbiology. Viral warts of the penis, condylomata acuminata, are not uncommon and have the same histological appearance and natural history as those seen in the female genitalia and around the anus. The prepuce – especially in patients with recurrent infections of the underlying glans (balanitis) – may be discoloured and white. This has similarities to 'leucoplakia' of the vulva. Histological examination of some of these show the features of lichen sclerosus; in preputial skin this condition goes under the exotic name of balanitis xerotica obliterans.

Tumours (Carcinoma)

Key Points

- Uncommon in UK, but very common in Third-World countries.
- Never occurs in men circumcised soon after birth.
- May be related to human papilloma virus (HPV) infection.
- Spreads to inguinal lymph nodes, but these may be enlarged due to inflammation beneath prepuce rather than to metastases.

Worldwide, squamous cell carcinoma of the penis is a common tumour, although it is relatively rare in Western communities. The tumour usually arises on the internal aspect of the prepuce, or on the glans (Figure 16.14). It may thus not be readily seen and there may be delay in presentation. The tumour is not seen in men who are circumcised at birth, and it is generally accepted that poor hygiene is an important aetiological agent. The role of human papilloma virus (HPV) virus is uncertain, although there are reports of penile carcinoma in the partners of women with carcinoma of the cervix. The tumour spreads by lymphatics to the inguinal lymph nodes which are almost invariably enlarged, although often this is due to a reaction to the concurrent infection rather than to metastatic spread.

Squamous cell carcinoma of the scrotum is rare, but is of historical interest in its occurrence in men who had swept chimneys by crawling through them as children. This finding

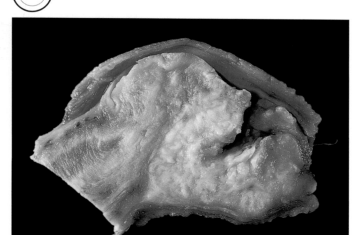

FIGURE 16.14 Carcinoma of the penis, arising beneath the prepuce and destroying much of the glans.

was originally reported by Percival Pott in the eighteenth century, and was the first description of a tumour being caused by a chemical agent. In the nineteenth century, tumours of the same site were described following excessive exposure to machine oil in factory workers; this was known as mule-spinner's carcinoma.

SUMMARY

Testicular cancer is a relatively uncommon tumour, which occurs in young men and is increasing in incidence in the UK. Modern chemotherapeutic regimes cure 95% or more of patients, including those with metastatic disease.

Prostate cancer is a common tumour in older men, and its incidence is also increasing. In theory men can be screened for this tumour by measurement of PSA levels in the blood, but there is considerable debate as to the correct way to manage patients with non-metastatic disease. Although some tumours respond to hormone manipulation there is increasing use of radical surgery and radiotherapy, although the effectiveness of these treatments is not satisfactorily established.

FURTHER READING

Al-Nafussi A. *Tumour Diagnosis. Practical Approach and Pattern Analysis*, 2nd edn. Chapter 11. London: Hodder Arnold, 2005.

Eble JN, Santer G, Epstein JI, Sesterhenn IA. *World Health Organization Classification of Tumours. Pathology and Genetics. Tumours of the Urinary System and Male Genital Organs*. Lyon: IARC Press, 2004.

THE ENDOCRINE SYSTEM

Anne Marie McNicol and Alan K Foulis

INTRODUCTION

The endocrine system is very important in maintaining normal homeostasis, by interacting with the central and peripheral nervous systems and the immune system. The system can be considered as comprising two main parts:

● The classical endocrine system, consisting of the pituitary, thyroid, adrenal and parathyroid glands, the islets of Langerhans in the pancreas, and the endocrine cells of the testis and ovary. These secrete hormones into the bloodstream, and these interact with cells at distant sites.
● The diffuse endocrine system, which comprises cells scattered singly or in small groups within other tissues, such as the gut, lung and skin. These release chemicals that affect the function of other cells in the local environment – termed paracrine signalling. The physiological roles of these cells are poorly understood and, consequently, little is known of the diseases that affect them. Hence, this chapter will deal only with abnormalities of the classical endocrine glands.

Endocrine diseases present in two main ways. First, the gland secretes too much or too little hormone, resulting in a specific clinical syndrome. Second, there is an increase in size due to hyperplasia or tumour. A mass may be noticed by the patient, or it may cause symptoms due to pressure on local structures. If a malignant tumour develops, the symptoms or signs may be related to invasion or metastases. Sometimes there is a combination of hormonal and mass effects.

Some endocrine diseases are familial. These include the autoimmune diseases where the patterns of inheritance are still to be fully defined. There are also a number of syndromes in which specific types of endocrine tumours occur in a familial setting, the most common being multiple endocrine neoplasia, type 1 and type 2 (MEN1, MEN2). These are discussed in more detail on pages 472–473. The unravelling of their molecular genetic background raises the practical and ethical problems of genetic screening and counselling.

Very few of the diseases discussed in this chapter are common. However, it is important to recognize them, as they may cause significant morbidity if untreated, and, in most instances, they can be treated with good effect.

The final diagnosis in endocrine pathology must in general be based on a combination of clinical, biochemical and pathological findings. Some recent technical advances have permitted pathology to contribute more specific information.

Techniques in Endocrine Pathology

These include:

● conventional histopathology
● immunohistochemistry
● electron microscopy
● *in-situ* hybridization
● cytogenetics and molecular genetics.

In the past, it was difficult to understand the functional aspects of endocrine tissues by histological examination. Immunohistochemistry, *in-situ* hybridization and ultrastructural analysis have made significant advances in our understanding of normal function, and of the changes that occur in disease. In many instances, these techniques now also contribute to diagnosis.

Immunohistochemistry

Antibodies to specific hormones or other cellular proteins are applied to tissue sections, and the sites of binding are visualized by histochemical techniques which generate

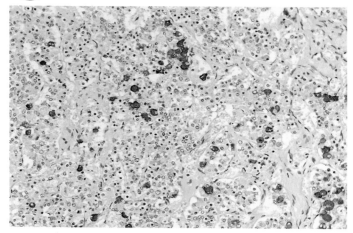

FIGURE 17.1 Section of anterior pituitary gland stained by the immunoperoxidase technique with an antibody to ACTH. Corticotrophs (ACTH-producing cells) are scattered among immunonegative cells, producing other hormones.

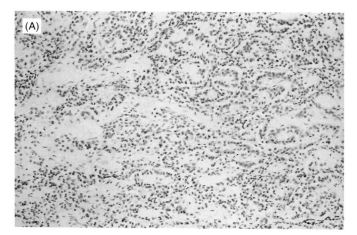

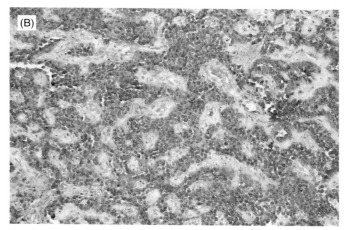

FIGURE 17.2 Sections from a pituitary tumour in a patient with hyperprolactinaemia. (A) Immunostaining for prolactin is negative, because the tumour cells are not storing the hormone. (B) *In-situ* hybridization for prolactin mRNA gives a positive signal, confirming that the tumour is producing the hormone.

a coloured signal where the protein is localized (Figure 17.1). We now know that some tumours produce hormones but do not secrete them, and that others synthesize more than one hormone. We can also show that a tumour is of neuroendocrine origin, even when it is not synthesizing known hormones, because it is possible to localize other proteins produced by this type of cell (e.g. neurone-specific enolase, PGP9.5, chromogranins, CD56 [NCAM, neural cell adhesion molecule]).

In-situ *Hybridization*

This technique allows the presence of messenger RNAs (mRNAs) to be demonstrated, and can therefore confirm that a tumour is the source of increased circulating hormone, even if it does not store sufficient to be detected by immunohistochemistry (Figure 17.2). The method is based on the natural complementary base pairing of nucleotides. A nucleotide probe (DNA or RNA) complementary to a sequence within the specific RNA binds to it on the tissue section. This probe is labelled so that sites of binding can be detected by immunohistochemistry or autoradiography.

Electron Microscopy

This has been a powerful tool in endocrine pathology, particularly when coupled with immunocytochemistry. Very precise classification of cell types is possible, based on the morphology of neurosecretory granules and the distribution of organelles. However, it is now possible to gain much of this information by using immunohistochemistry.

PITUITARY GLAND

The pituitary gland consists of two lobes. The anterior (adenohypophysis) arises from the oral cavity and accounts for about 75% of the gland's weight; the posterior (neurohypophysis) grows down from the brain and remains connected to the hypothalamus by the pituitary stalk. The gland sits in a bony

cavity, the sella turcica, covered by a layer of dura perforated by the pituitary stalk. It lies below the optic chiasma, and the cavernous sinuses lie laterally. Any significant enlargement can result in pressure on these structures.

Anterior Pituitary

The anterior lobe secretes six classical hormones: growth hormone (GH); prolactin (PRL); adrenocorticotrophic hormone (ACTH); thyroid-stimulating hormone (TSH); and the gonadotrophins, follicle-stimulating hormone (FSH) and luteinizing hormone (LH). These are released into the circulation and regulate target organs at distant sites. Other peptides, growth factors and cytokines are also produced, which may have paracrine actions. The secretion of anterior pituitary hormones is mainly under the control of hypothalamic releasing and inhibiting factors, carried directly in the hypothalamic–pituitary portal system. The primary capillary plexus lies in the median eminence of the hypothalamus, where these factors are secreted. Blood passes down venous channels in the pituitary stalk to the secondary capillary plexus in the anterior lobe. There is negative feedback by hormones from the target organs at both pituitary and hypothalamic levels, and also by pituitary hormones on the hypothalamus. Basal levels of many anterior pituitary hormones show a circadian rhythm, and may be altered by external stimuli.

Growth Hormone

The secretion of GH by somatotrophs is regulated by two hypothalamic factors: growth hormone-releasing hormone (GHRH) stimulates, while somatostatin (SMS) inhibits release. GH has direct effects, including the stimulation of protein synthesis in liver and muscle and lipolysis of fat stores. Indirect effects include skeletal growth mediated by insulin-like growth factor I (IGF-I), which also exerts negative feedback on GH release from the pituitary.

Adrenocorticotrophic Hormone

This is produced in corticotrophs from a large precursor molecule, proopiomelanocortin (POMC). Its release is stimulated by corticotrophin-releasing factor (CRF) and vasopressin (VP). It regulates the secretion of glucocorticoids by the adrenal cortex: these exert negative feedback on both CRF and ACTH secretion.

Glycoprotein Hormones

FSH, LH and TSH are glycoproteins consisting of two subunits. The α-subunit is common to all three, but each has a specific β-subunit. FSH and LH are produced in the same cells (gonadotrophs). In men, FSH stimulates spermatogenesis and LH regulates Leydig cell function, whereas in women, FSH is involved in the regulation of follicle growth, while LH is related to ovulation and development of the corpus luteum. The absolute and relative levels of the two hormones vary with the menstrual cycle. The hypothalamic peptide, gonadotrophin-releasing hormone (GnRH) is important in the stimulation of both FSH and LH secretion, while androgens and oestrogens exert negative feedback.

TSH, secreted by thyrotrophs, stimulates the thyroid follicular cells. Its secretion is stimulated by thyrotrophin-releasing hormone (TRH), with negative feedback from thyroid hormones.

Prolactin

This stimulates the breast during lactation. Circulating basal levels are similar in men and women, but no specific function has yet been identified in the male. In contrast to the other pituitary hormones, the dominant regulatory influence of the hypothalamus is inhibitory, effected mainly by dopamine.

Anterior Pituitary Hyperfunction

> **Key Points**
>
> Anterior pituitary hyperfunction is associated with:
>
> - acromegaly
> - Cushing's disease
> - hyperprolactinaemia
> - rarely, hypersecretion of other hormones.

Hyperactivity of the anterior pituitary is usually associated with excess hormone secretion from a pituitary adenoma. Less commonly, excessive release of hypothalamic stimulating factors causes hyperstimulation of the pituitary. Rarely, ectopic release of these peptides from a neuroendocrine tumour at another site (e.g. endocrine tumour of the pancreas) results in the hypersecretion of pituitary hormones.

Acromegaly

Acromegaly is caused by excess GH secretion in adult life, usually from a pituitary adenoma. There is overgrowth of soft tissues and bone with enlargement of the feet and hands, and a characteristic facial appearance with prognathism and widening of the nose. Osteoarthritis often results from the irregular bone growth. Nerve entrapment can cause pain and paraesthesia. Internal organs also enlarge, with cardiomegaly and hypertension. There is a two-fold increase in mortality if the disease is untreated, mainly from cardiovascular complications. Effects on general metabolism cause abnormal glucose tolerance and sometimes diabetes mellitus (see Case History 17.1). *Gigantism* occurs when GH excess occurs before the epiphyses have closed.

Cushing's Disease

Cushing's syndrome (see below) is the result of excessive circulating free glucocorticoids. About 70% of cases are due to hypersecretion of ACTH from the pituitary gland, known as Cushing's disease. Almost all patients have an ACTH-secreting adenoma. Corticotroph hyperplasia is present in a minority of cases, possibly caused by excessive secretion of CRF and/or VP by the hypothalamus.

Hyperprolactinaemia

If PRL is secreted in excess in a premenopausal woman, the menstrual cycle is abnormal, and the patient presents with amenorrhoea, infertility and occasionally galactorrhoea. In men, hyperprolactinaemia may cause loss of libido or infertility, but is usually asymptomatic, as it is in post-menopausal women. Thus, while PRL-secreting adenomas are often diagnosed in young women even when small, they do not usually manifest themselves in other patients unless large enough to cause pressure effects.

In contrast to the other hormones, hypersecretion of PRL has a number of causes other than tumour. Anything that interferes with normal transport of dopamine to the anterior lobe or with its turnover or metabolism may result in hyperprolactinaemia (Table 17.1). The physiological rise of PRL in pregnancy and lactation must never be forgotten in a differential diagnosis.

Hypersecretion of Other Hormones

TSH-secreting tumours are a rare cause of hyperthyroidism. Gonadotrophin excess is usually asymptomatic.

ACROMEGALY

Clinical History

A 52-year-old man was referred to an oral surgeon because of marked prognathism and distortion of his bite, and was subsequently referred to an endocrinologist. The patient gave a history evolving over 5 years, during which time he had noticed two increases in shoe size. His hands had also increased to the extent where he could no longer wear his ring. He complained of intermittent paraesthesia of his hands in a distribution consistent with carpal tunnel syndrome. He had been aware, for several years, of excessive sweating and recurrent occipital headaches. He had also been troubled by pain in his hands, knees and hips, consistent with osteoarthritis. The evolution of the facial changes is shown in Figures 17.3 and 17.4.

Biochemistry

Initial investigations showed raised growth hormone (GH) levels of between 12 and 50 mU/L, with an average of 32 mU/L (normal range up to 10 mU/L). Insulin-like growth factor I (IGF-I) levels were also raised. At a GH level of 18.7 mU/L, the IGF-I level was 701 µg/L (normal 80–360 µg/L). During a glucose tolerance test, the patient exhibited a normal glucose profile, but his GH level failed to suppress. These findings were all consistent with a diagnosis of acromegaly.

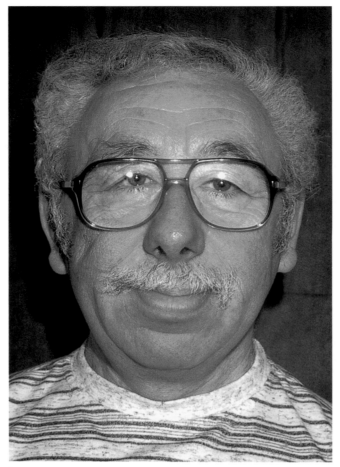

FIGURE 17.4 The patient's appearance at the time of presentation in 1997.

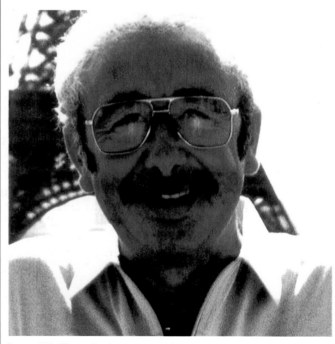

FIGURE 17.3 The patient's appearance in 1990.

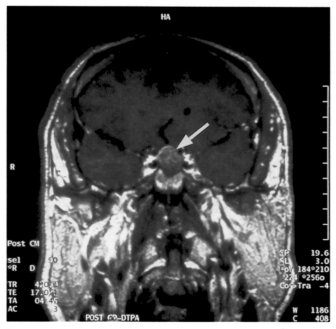

FIGURE 17.5 Enhanced MRI scan showing the pituitary tumour (arrow).

Magnetic resonance image (MRI) scanning (Figure 17.5) showed a 2-cm pituitary adenoma with no invasion of the cavernous sinus, but minor displacement of the optic chiasma. The patient's visual fields were normal, and he was treated with octreotide subcutaneously prior to surgery, the aim of which was both to reduce GH levels and to shrink the tumour. The pituitary adenoma was removed at transsphenoidal surgery, and was confirmed as a GH-producing tumour by immunocytochemistry (Figure 17.6).

Postoperatively, the GH levels fell to 1.1 mU/L and IGF-I levels to 142 µg/L. Currently, the patient feels well although, as is usual, the bony and soft tissue changes have not fully regressed.

(Case history produced with the help of Dr AR McLellan and Professor GM Teasdale.)

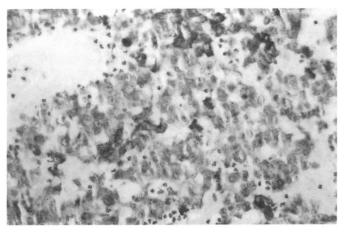

FIGURE 17.6 Section of pituitary adenoma immunostained for growth hormone, confirming it as the source of secretion.

TABLE 17.1 Causes of hyperprolactinaemia

- Prolactin-secreting adenoma of pituitary gland
- Pituitary stalk pressure, e.g. by another type of tumour
- Hypothalamic destruction by tumour or inflammation
- Drug therapy
   dopamine receptor antagonists (phenothiazines, metoclopramide)
   drugs affecting dopamine turnover (methyldopa, reserpine)
- Primary hypothyroidism
- Idiopathic
- Physiological (pregnancy)

Hypopituitarism

Key Points

Hypopituitarism is associated with:

- pressure from a pituitary tumour
- iatrogenic complications following pituitary surgery or irradiation
- Sheehan's syndrome.

Deficiency of several hormones is usually caused by destruction of the pituitary gland, the stalk or the hypothalamus. In developed countries, the most common cause is now pressure from an expanding pituitary tumour or damage following pituitary surgery. Sheehan's syndrome (pituitary necrosis secondary to post-partum haemorrhage) is still the leading cause where obstetric services are poorly developed. Irradiation of the pituitary or adjacent structures may also result in hypopituitarism as a late complication. Occasional cases are the result of trauma, inflammation (including autoimmune hypophysitis), or intrasellar tumours other than pituitary adenomas. Langerhans' cell histiocytosis or granulomatous diseases may affect the production of hypothalamic releasing hormones. Suprasellar tumours (e.g. craniopharyngioma) can destroy the hypothalamus or stalk.

The clinical manifestations are variable. Gonadotrophin deficiency usually presents first with amenorrhoea in women, impotence in men, and loss of secondary sex characteristics and libido. Low circulating GH levels are usually asymptomatic. Lack of TSH and ACTH cause hypothyroidism and hypoadrenalism, presenting as nausea, vomiting, hypotension and occasionally fatal collapse.

Isolated hormone deficiencies are usually the result of genetic abnormalities in the expression of specific hormones. GH deficiency is a cause of growth retardation, and there is occasional lack of ACTH or gonadotrophins.

Pituitary Adenomas

These are the most common lesions of the anterior pituitary gland, comprising about 10% of intracranial neoplasms in neurosurgical practice. They are found more commonly at autopsy, indicating that the majority cause no clinical symptoms because they do not secrete excess hormone. Most of these lesions are sporadic, but they may occur as part of the multiple endocrine neoplasia type 1 (MEN1) syndrome (p. 472). They are classified as microadenomas (<10 mm diameter) and macroadenomas (>10 mm). Small tumours are usually recognized only if they secrete excess hormone. Larger tumours usually present even if they are non-functional because of local pressure effects (Figure 17.7). If they compress the optic chiasma or nerves, visual disturbances may occur (classically homonymous hemianopia). Headache is not uncommon. Pressure on the para-adenomatous gland may cause atrophy and hypopituitarism.

A minority of these tumours show aggressive behaviour, with spread into the hypothalamus and brain that eventually

are shown in Table 17.4. There is weight gain and general lethargy with cold intolerance. Skin and hair are dry and accumulation of mucopolysaccharides in connective tissue result in a thickening of the skin, hoarseness, and pain and paraesthesia when nerves are trapped. There is intellectual impairment. Change of mood may progress to psychosis. In severe deficiency, hypothermia and coma can develop. Raised blood cholesterol levels increase the risk of cardiovascular disease.

TABLE 17.4 **Causes of hypothyroidism**

- Autoimmune thyroid disease
  Hashimoto's thyroiditis
  primary myxoedema
- Severe iodine deficiency
- Dyshormonogenesis
- Following thyroid surgery or radio-iodine therapy
- Ingestion of goitrogens
- Hypopituitarism

Cretinism is due to severe hypothyroidism in infancy. Thyroid hormones are critical for normal brain development, and these children show signs of mental retardation, neuromuscular abnormalities, deaf-mutism and retarded growth. There is a goitre when it is caused by severe iodine deficiency, or by inherited defects of the enzymes involved in thyroid hormone synthesis. Rarely, thyroid agenesis or hypoplasia occurs, and in these cases goitre is absent. It is extremely important to make an early diagnosis because hormone replacement permits normal development.

Functional Disorders

Non-toxic Nodular Goitre

Key Points

- Non-toxic nodular goitre is the most common thyroid disease.
- It is either endemic or sporadic.
- There is nodular enlargement of the thyroid gland.
- Affected individuals may be either euthyroid or hypothyroid.

Non-toxic nodular goitre is the most common lesion in thyroid pathology. When there is absolute or relative iodine deficiency, reduced levels of thyroid hormones result in increased TSH secretion by the pituitary. This induces hyperplasia in an attempt to increase thyroid hormone output. The demands are usually intermittent, and the gland undergoes cycles of growth and involution, resulting in the well-recognized picture of multinodular goitre, with nodules consisting of follicles of varying size, fibrosis, haemorrhage and focal inflammation. Enlargement is usually asymmetrical, and the gland may weigh up to several hundred grams

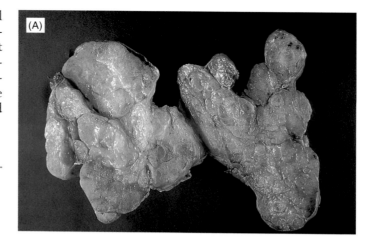

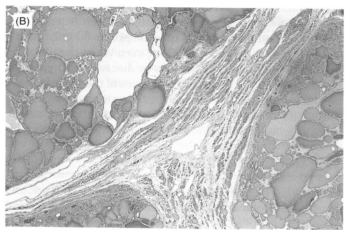

FIGURE 17.9 **(A)** A cut section through a multinodular goitre showing gross asymmetrical enlargement. **(B)** Nodularity is clear on histological assessment.

(Figure 17.9). Occasionally, simple goitre may produce signs or symptoms suggestive of tumour. When one nodule is larger than the others (dominant nodule), fine needle aspiration cytology or even partial thyroidectomy is required to distinguish the two. Occasionally, there may be compression of trachea, oesophagus or recurrent laryngeal nerve.

On an epidemiological basis, two forms are defined:

- Endemic goitre affects more than 10% of the population, occurring in areas with absolute deficiency of iodine, usually far from the sea, reflecting seafood as the major source of iodine. These areas include the Andes, Himalayas and Alps. The introduction of iodized salt has reduced the incidence. Goitre usually develops in childhood, and the sexes are equally affected.
- Sporadic goitre is due to a relative lack of iodine in individuals. It reflects inadequate intake; inherited abnormalities in thyroid hormone production; and ingestion of goitrogens, i.e. substances that interfere with hormone synthesis. These include vegetables of the *Brassica* family, excessive fluoride, or drugs such as *p*-aminosalicylic acid and sulphonylureas. Some people also suggest that autoimmune mechanisms may be involved.

TABLE 17.5 Autoantibodies in thyroid autoimmune disease

Antithyroperoxidase	Present in >80% of patients with chronic thyroiditis: also found in 10% of normal adults
Antithyroglobulin	–
Anti-TSH receptor	–
thyroid-stimulating immunoglobulins (TSI)	Stimulate activity
thyroid growth-stimulating immunoglobulins (TGI)	Stimulate growth
receptor-blocking antibodies	? Contribute to hypothyroidism

Autoimmune Thyroid Disease

Key Points

- Autoimmune thyroid disease is associated with antibodies to thyroid antigens.
- The clinical picture varies according to the antibodies produced.
- Women are more commonly affected than men.

This group of diseases – Graves' disease, Hashimoto's thyroiditis, and primary myxoedema – are characterized by lymphoid infiltration of the gland and by the presence of circulating antibodies to various components of thyroid follicular cells (Table 17.5), some of which are thought to play an active role in pathogenesis. Thyroid-stimulating immunoglobulins (TSI) bind to and activate the TSH receptor, causing the increased secretion of thyroid hormones usually seen in Graves' disease. Other antibodies are thought to stimulate growth, and may be important in goitrogenesis in Hashimoto's thyroiditis. Receptor-blocking antibodies may contribute to hypothyroidism and to thyroid atrophy in primary myxoedema. These diseases may be familial, and are associated with other organ-specific autoimmune diseases (Table 17.6).

TABLE 17.6 Familial associations of thyroid autoimmune disease

- Addison's disease
- Pernicious anaemia
- Type 1 diabetes mellitus

Graves' Disease

This is characterized by a diffuse goitre and hyperthyroidism. It mainly affects women aged 20 to 40 years. The gland is diffusely hyperplastic and hyperaemic, clinically resulting in a bruit on auscultation. In the untreated case, the thyroid epithelium is hyperplastic and there is little colloid storage. Lymphocytic infiltration is usually less marked than in Hashimoto's thyroiditis.

It is unusual now to see the classical histological features of the disease because of effective drug therapy. A minority of patients relapse and come to surgery, but are usually euthyroid at the time of operation because of treatment with antithyroid drugs, with or without the addition of iodine. Their thyroids show complex histological features, antithyroid drugs inducing more marked follicular hyperplasia, while iodine reduces vascularity and increases colloid storage. This emphasizes the importance of a full clinical history in the interpretation of the histological appearances in endocrine disease.

Hashimoto's Thyroiditis

This is a disease of middle-aged women, in whom it occurs 20 times more commonly than in men. There is a diffuse, firm, painless goitre (Figure 17.10). Initially, the patient is usually euthyroid, but 80% become hypothyroid. The occasional patient is hyperthyroid at presentation, presumably due to the presence of TSI. High-titre antiperoxidase antibody is usually present. The gland is widely infiltrated and replaced by lymphocytes, plasma cells and macrophages, often with germinal centre formation (Figure 17.11). The thyroid follicular cells are enlarged with eosinophilic granular cytoplasm due to accumulation of mitochondria (Askanazy or Hürthle cell change).

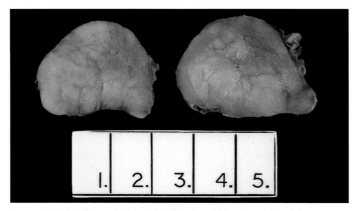

FIGURE 17.10 Hashimoto's thyroiditis. The thyroid is enlarged, and the cut surface is pale in contrast to the normal brown appearance.

Primary Myxoedema

This disease affects mainly elderly women. The thyroid is atrophic, largely replaced by fibrous tissue with a lymphoid infiltrate. The patients are severely hypothyroid and are the most likely to present with hypothermia and coma.

Focal chronic thyroiditis is seen in 15–20% of autopsies from patients with no clinical evidence of thyroid disease. This may represent subclinical autoimmune disease, as

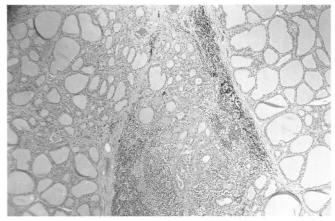

FIGURE 17.11 Hashimoto's thyroiditis showing the diffuse lymphoid infiltrate with destruction of the thyroid epithelium.

the incidence is similar to that of thyroid autoantibodies in the general population.

Lymphocytic thyroiditis occurs in children and young adults who present with goitre and sometimes hyperthyroidism. It may be a precursor of Hashimoto's disease.

Other Forms of Thyroiditis

- Acute thyroiditis may occasionally develop in bacteraemia or by local extension of inflammation.
- Giant cell (de Quervain's) thyroiditis, also known as *subacute thyroiditis*, presents as a painful goitre. It is probably viral in origin, and there are often preceding general or upper respiratory signs and symptoms. Women are affected three times as often as men. Hyperthyroidism and the presence of thyroid antibodies are usually transient. Although there is an initial acute inflammation, followed by a granulomatous response, the whole process may resolve. Even if some fibrosis persists, there are no long-term functional effects.
- Riedel's thyroiditis. In this very rare disease the thyroid is replaced by dense fibrous tissue, which often extends into perithyroidal tissues, mimicking invasive carcinoma. It may present as a goitre or with symptoms related to involvement of trachea or recurrent laryngeal nerve. The aetiology is unknown, but some patients also have retroperitoneal or mediastinal fibrosis.

Thyroid Tumours

Key Points

Thyroid tumours include:

- follicular adenoma
- follicular carcinoma
- papillary carcinoma
- medullary carcinoma
- anaplastic carcinoma
- lymphoma.

Thyroid tumours usually present as solitary nodules, and most are 'cold' on scanning, as they concentrate radioactive iodine less actively than the surrounding gland. Some 70% of clinically apparent solitary nodules are, however, dominant nodules in a multinodular goitre; the rest are tumours (mostly benign). Thyroid cancer is rare, and accounts for less than 1% of all cancers and less than 0.5% of deaths from cancer. Cold nodules in men and in younger women should be regarded as more suspicious than those in middle-aged women. Most tumours arise from follicular cells, the majority being follicular adenomas. There are two types of carcinomas – follicular and papillary – which develop and behave differently. The C cells give rise to medullary carcinoma.

Follicular Adenoma

These are the most common thyroid neoplasms, presenting most frequently in women aged over 30 years. They are usually non-functional, but may occasionally secrete excess thyroid hormones. They are generally encapsulated and compress the surrounding gland. Haemorrhage, degeneration and fibrosis may occur. The lesions show a variety of histological appearances, but these have no clinical importance. It can sometimes be difficult for a pathologist to distinguish between an adenoma and a hyperplastic (adenomatoid) nodule in a non-toxic goitre, but again this has no clinical significance.

Follicular Carcinoma

These comprise 15–20% of all thyroid cancers, but they are more common in areas of iodine deficiency. Their peak incidence is in the fifth decade of life, with one-third of cases occurring over the age of 50 years. These lesions are also more common in women. They metastasize by the vascular route, particularly to bone and lung. The overall survival is reported at about 50%. Two variants are recognized: encapsulated, so-called 'minimally invasive' carcinoma, where vascular and capsular invasion is seen only on microscopic examination (Figure 17.12); and 'widely invasive'

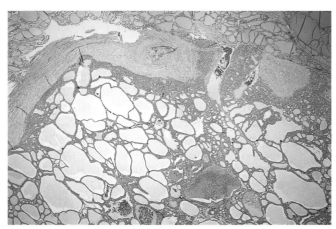

FIGURE 17.12 Follicular carcinoma. Tongues of tumour are seen breaching the capsule and invading the surrounding gland in this minimally invasive follicular carcinoma of the thyroid.

tumours, where obvious spread is seen throughout the gland or beyond (Figure 17.13). The latter have a poorer prognosis than the former.

Papillary Carcinoma

All papillary tumours of the thyroid are regarded as malignant. They account for 60–70% of all thyroid cancers, occur in young adults (aged 30–40 years), and are three times more common in women than in men. They have good prognosis overall, with a 5-year survival approaching 90%. They are not usually encapsulated, and may be multifocal. For this reason, some surgeons perform total thyroidectomy. Some 40% of patients have metastases in local lymph nodes at presentation, but this does not seem to alter the prognosis. The patient may first present with an enlarged lymph node if the thyroid primary is very small. In the small minority where the tumour has spread through the thyroid capsule or there are distant metastases, the prognosis is worse.

These lesions almost all show papillary structures (see Figure 17.18). Some have fibrosis, and psammoma bodies are present in about half. There are characteristic cytological features, with clear or grooved nuclei. Some tumours with these nuclear features have mixed papillary and follicular, or only follicular, architecture (the follicular variant of papillary carcinoma). These behave in the same way as the classical papillary tumours. Some less common variants (e.g. tall cell variant) exhibit more aggressive behaviour.

Medullary Carcinoma

These account for 5–10% of thyroid cancers. Between 10% and 20% are familial, forming part of the MEN2 syndrome

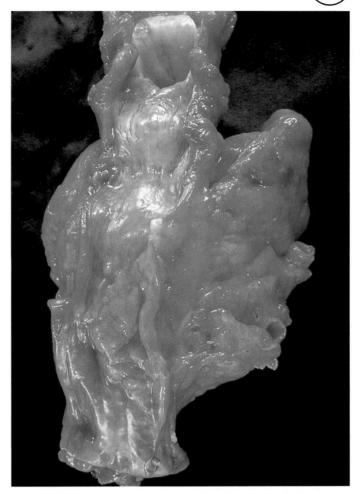

FIGURE 17.13 This autopsy specimen shows invasion of the trachea and oesophagus by a follicular carcinoma of thyroid.

17.2 CASE HISTORY

INVESTIGATION OF A THYROID LUMP

A 32-year-old woman presented with a lump in the right side of her neck (Figure 17.14). She had no other symptoms, but on examination the lump was clearly related to the thyroid. A radio-iodine scan showed a cold nodule (Figure 17.14). The thyroid function tests were normal.

Fine needle aspiration cytology showed the cellular appearances of a follicular lesion (Figure 17.15). In such cases, surgical removal is necessary to distinguish between follicular adenoma and follicular carcinoma. The pathologist must sample widely the interface of the lesion and normal gland and look for penetration of the capsule, or of invasion into vessels within the capsule or in the normal gland. At operation, there was a 3-cm diameter nodule in the right lobe of the thyroid, and a lobectomy was performed. Histological examination demonstrated both capsular (Figure 17.16) and vascular (Figure 17.17) invasion,

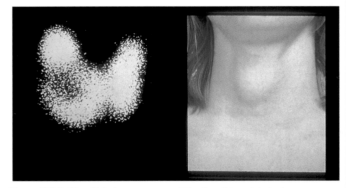

FIGURE 17.14 The clinical appearance of the thyroid nodule is shown on the right, with the radio-iodine scan on the left.

the diagnosis being minimally invasive follicular carcinoma. The patient went on to have a completion thyroidectomy.

(Case history produced with the help of Drs HW Gray and CJR Stewart.)

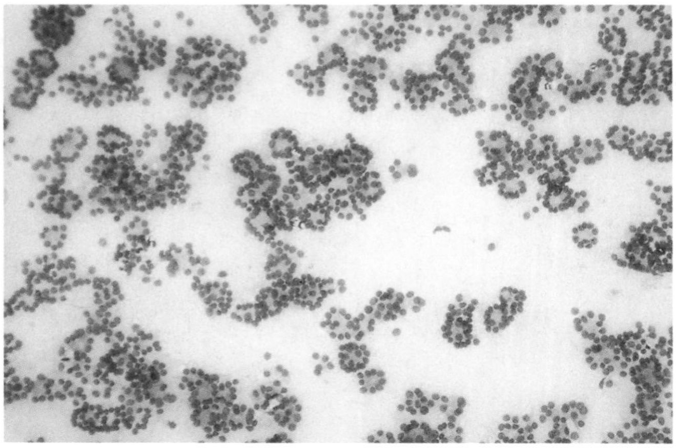

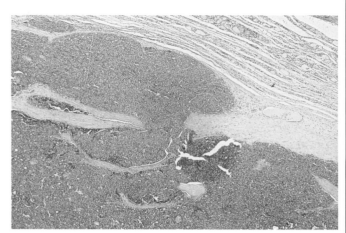

FIGURE 17.15 The fine needle aspiration cytology specimen showed a microfollicular pattern, consistent with a follicular neoplasm. (Leishman).

FIGURE 17.16 The follicular carcinoma shows capsular invasion.

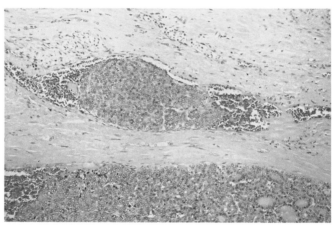

FIGURE 17.17 Vascular invasion is also seen.

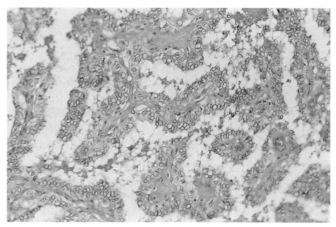

FIGURE 17.18 Papillary carcinoma of thyroid showing papillae with fibrovascular cores and classical optically clear nuclei.

(see p. 473). These lesions are slightly more common in women. Sporadic tumours are usually unilateral, and the majority present between the ages of 40 and 60 years. In contrast, familial cases are usually bilateral and multifocal, arising from C-cell hyperplasia, and often present before the age of 25 years. Histologically, medullary carcinomas differ from the other tumours. They consist of cells with an alveolar or trabecular arrangement, and they are immunopositive for calcitonin (Figure 17.19). Amyloid, formed from the calcitonin precursor, is seen in about 50% of cases. The tumours may secrete other hormones such as ACTH or serotonin, and this may occasionally result in ectopic hormone syndromes. These tumours show both lymphatic and vascular spread. The overall 10-year survival is around 50%.

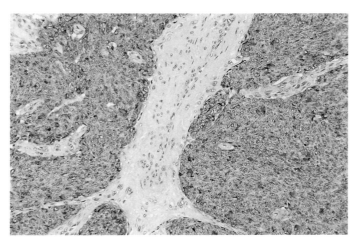

FIGURE 17.19 Medullary carcinoma of thyroid showing immunopositivity for calcitonin (brown).

Other Tumours

Occasionally in older women, a rapidly growing anaplastic carcinoma occurs. These are highly malignant and usually present as a rapidly growing mass. They probably represent progression of a pre-existing follicular or papillary tumour.

Benign and malignant tumours may rarely arise from the connective tissue or vascular components (e.g. haemangiomas). Occasional metastases are seen, usually from the lung, breast or gastrointestinal tract.

In 1–2% of patients with Hashimoto's thyroiditis, B-cell lymphoma develops. This may also present as a rapidly expanding mass. Differentiation from anaplastic carcinoma can be made using fine needle aspiration cytology.

Aetiology

The molecular genetic pathways involved differ in follicular and papillary tumours. Mutations in *ras* oncogenes play

◯ 17.1 SPECIAL STUDY TOPIC

RADIATION AND THYROID CANCER

The general carcinogenic effects of radiation are well known. Exposure to particulate radiation produces double-stranded breaks in DNA, and can therefore result in a number of changes, including deletions and chromosomal inversions or translocations. Increased numbers of thyroid cancers among survivors of the Hiroshima and Nagasaki atomic bombs, and also following therapeutic irradiation of the head and neck, first raised the possibility that radiation might be involved in the pathogenesis of the disease. The thyroid may be exposed to radiation in two ways: first by external irradiation; and second by exposure to radioactive iodine. These are discussed separately below.

The thyroid appears to be much more susceptible to radiation-induced tumorigenesis in children than in adults. This may reflect a requirement for hormonal or growth factor stimulation in the pathogenesis, but this aspect remains to be elucidated.

External Radiation

In the early days of therapeutic irradiation its long-term effects were not appreciated, and it was used in the treatment of minor conditions in children, including tinea capitis and tonsillar hyperplasia or thymic enlargement. Around 1950, an increased incidence of thyroid cancer in people who had undergone such irradiation in childhood was first reported, and this has been extensively confirmed. Pooling of data from a number of series indicates an average excess relative risk of 7.7 per Gy. In children, it appears that the thyroid has one of the highest risk coefficients observed for any organ, with increased risk at levels as low as 0.1 Gy. The effects of the atomic bombs in Japan were also related to external radiation because the explosions occurred at high altitude and there was little radio-iodine fallout.

Radio-iodine Exposure

^{131}I is given both as a diagnostic tool in thyroid disease and, at higher doses, as a therapeutic agent in hyperthyroidism. There is no evidence to suggest that this results in an increased risk of thyroid cancer. Studies on fallout-induced thyroid cancer following atomic bomb testing support this, and suggest that the increased risk is due to short-lived radioiodines, ^{132}I and ^{133}I. However, these studies have been unable to produce a risk coefficient for exposure.

On April 26, 1986, the nuclear reactor in Chernobyl exploded, releasing 10^{19} becquerels (Bq) of radioactive substances into the atmosphere, including about 1.8×10^{18} Bq of ^{131}I, and 3.6×10^{18} Bq of short-lived radio-iodines (^{133}I and the precursor of ^{132}I, tellurium). The southern part of Belarus was most affected. Larger doses of radioactive iodine were inhaled and ingested on food, giving high doses to the thyroid. Milk is the main source of ingestion of radio-iodine, meaning that children would have a higher intake than adults. This is an iodine-deficient area, with incomplete iodine supplementation, and this probably raised the thyroid dose. An increase in thyroid cancer in children was noted as early as 1990. The annual incidence rose to more than 20 per 100 000 children – an increased morbidity rate of 55.7 compared to the 10 years before the accident – and about 2000 cases have now been documented. The average excess absolute risk per unit thyroid dose for children has been estimated as 2.1 per 10^4 children/year/Gy. A two- to four-fold increase has been reported in adults, but it is not known whether this is real, or is the result of increased detection. If potassium iodide had been administered at the time as a competitive blocker of radio-iodine uptake it would most probably have reduced the incidence in susceptible groups.

Tumour Type and Molecular Genetics

Almost all radiation-induced thyroid tumours are papillary carcinomas. From studies of the post-Chernobyl tumours, it appears that those that developed after a short latent period are less well differentiated and more invasive than those that developed after a longer latent period.

The molecular genetic changes in papillary carcinoma are not fully elucidated. In about 35% of sporadic adult cases, there is oncogenic rearrangement of the *RET* proto-oncogene on chromosome 10q11.2, which encodes a receptor tyrosine kinase. A number of rearrangements have been identified, the most common known as *RET/PTC1* and *RET/PTC3*. In all of these the gene loses the ligand binding and transmembrane domains and fuses to another gene at its 5′ end, coming under regulation of the fused gene. In *RET/PTC1*, there is a chromosomal inversion and fusion with the *H4* gene and in *RET/PTC3* with the *ELE1* gene. There is emerging evidence that the *RET/PTC3* rearrangement is associated with the less well-differentiated tumours of short latency, with *RET/PTC1* more common in those tumours with a longer latent period.

Less frequent rearrangements of the gene encoding the receptor tyrosine kinase for nerve growth factor (*NTRK1*) are also found in both sporadic and radiation-induced tumours. Point mutations in the *BRAF* proto-oncogene, which are found in about one-third of sporadic papillary carcinomas, are rare in radiation-associated tumours.

These rearrangements of *RET* and *NTRK1* result in ubiquitous expression of the fused proteins; the ability to dimerize and thus become active in the absence of ligand; and translocation to the cytoplasm where they may interact with unusual substances. All of these processes are probably important in the neoplastic process.

TABLE 17.7 Comparisons of *RET* proto-oncogene rearragements in sporadic papillary carcinoma of thyroid and in radiation-induced papillary carcinoma in Belarus

	Sporadic	Radiation
Total *RET*	c. 16%	c. 61%
RET/PTC1	16%	13.6%
RET/PTC2	Rare	Not identified
RET/PTC3	Rare	39%
RET/other	Not identified	8.4%
None	c. 84%	39%

Mutations in the *ras* and $G_s\alpha$ (GTP-binding α subunit of the adenylate cyclase stimulatory protein), which have been identified in sporadic adult follicular tumours, have not been identified, nor have mutations in *p53*, which are seen in anaplastic thyroid tumours.

Further Reading

Furmanchuk AW, Averkin JI, Egloff B, Ruchti C, Abelin T, Schappi W, Korotkevich EA. Pathomorphological findings in thyroid cancers of children from the Republic of Belarus – a study of 86 cases occurring between 1986 (post-Chernobyl) and 1991. *Histopathology* 1992; **21**: 401–408.

Rabes HM, Klugbauer S. Molecular genetics of childhood papillary thyroid carcinomas after irradiation: high prevalence of RET rearrangements. *Recent Results Cancer Res* 1998; **154**: 248–264.

Robbins J. Lessons from Chernobyl: the event, the aftermath, the fallout: radioactive, political, social. *Thyroid* 1997; **7**: 189–192.

a role in some follicular tumours, and are said to be associated with metastases. Iodine deficiency seems to favour *ras* mutation. In contrast, intrachromosomal inversions involving the *RET* proto-oncogene on chromosome 10 or *NTRK1* on chromosome 1 and mutations in *BRAF* are involved in papillary carcinoma. Mutations in the *p53* tumour suppressor gene have been identified only in undifferentiated tumours. The role of radiation is reviewed in Special Study Topic 17.1.

Activating mutations in the *RET* gene are involved in medullary carcinoma arising as part of the MEN2 syndrome. This does not play a significant role in sporadic tumours.

Miscellaneous Disorders

Occasional abnormalities of thyroid descent occur, most commonly lingual thyroid. Thyroglossal duct cysts are situated in the midline and develop from persistence of the lower

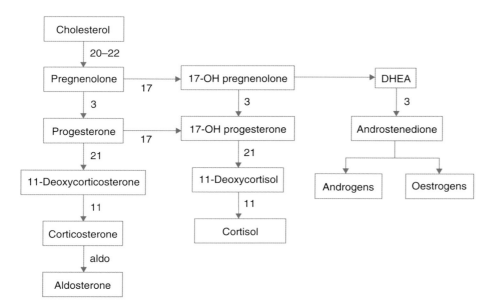

FIGURE 17.20 Pathways of adrenal steroidogenesis. The enzymes involved are: 20–22 = 20,22 desmolase (CYP 11A); 3 = 3β-hydroxysteroid dehydrogenase; 21 = 21 hydroxylase (CYP 21); 11 = 11β-hydroxylase (CYP 11B1); aldo = aldosterone synthase (CYB 11B2). DHEA = dehydroepiandrosterone.

part of the tubal downgrowth that gives rise to the gland. Amyloid may be seen, either as part of systemic amyloidosis or as an isolated finding.

ADRENAL GLANDS

The adrenal glands lie above the kidneys and comprise the outer cortex of mesodermal origin and the inner medulla, derived from neuroectoderm. In the adult, the glands weigh about 4 g in cases of sudden accidental death. However, stimulation by ACTH causes them to increase in size, and the stress of terminal illness results in an average weight of 6 g at hospital autopsy. The cortex and medulla will be dealt with separately.

Adrenal Cortex

The adrenal cortex consists of three zones: the zona glomerulosa, the zona fasciculata and the zona reticularis, which synthesize a range of steroid hormones (Figure 17.20). The zona glomerulosa, which is dispersed focally below the capsule, secretes the mineralocorticoid aldosterone, and is regulated by the renin–angiotensin system. Aldosterone plays a major role in the regulation of plasma volume and of potassium balance, mainly by effects on the kidney. The zona fasciculata and zona reticularis produce glucocorticoids, mainly cortisol. Glucocorticoids have wide-ranging effects on general metabolism, promoting gluconeogenesis, and inhibiting protein synthesis. They have anti-inflammatory and immunosuppressive effects, particularly affecting T cells. Actions on bone metabolism favour the development of osteoporosis. The gland also secretes sex steroids, probably from the zona reticularis. These are mainly androgens, but may undergo peripheral conversion to oestrogens.

Adrenocortical Hyperfunction

> **Key Points**
> - Cushing's syndrome.
> - Conn's syndrome (hyperaldosteronism).
> - Adrenogenital syndrome.
> - Adrenocortical tumours.

There are three main syndromes within this spectrum, relating to the hypersecretion of glucocorticoids, aldosterone or sex steroids.

Cushing's Syndrome

This is the result of the excessive secretion of cortisol, although some of the features may be caused by the secretion of cortisol precursors with mineralocorticoid effects. If undiagnosed, or untreated, there is a high morbidity and mortality. Cushing's syndrome occurs most commonly in women, but may also present in men, and, rarely in children. The administration of excessive doses of therapeutic steroids may induce an iatrogenic form of the disease.

The clinical picture is characteristic (Figure 17.21). Increased protein breakdown leads to a loss of muscle bulk, particularly on the limbs; centripetal deposition of fat results in a moon face, buffalo hump and truncal obesity; inhibition of protein synthesis and abnormal collagen maturation cause abdominal striae. There is hypertension. Osteoporosis may lead to vertebral collapse. Proximal myopathy is common. Diminished glucose tolerance is present, with hyperglycaemia and glycosuria in up to 20% of cases. Wound healing may be delayed. Mental symptoms are common, with depression and sometimes psychosis. In some cases, there is also excess secretion of androgens, with hirsutism, amenorrhoea and virilization.

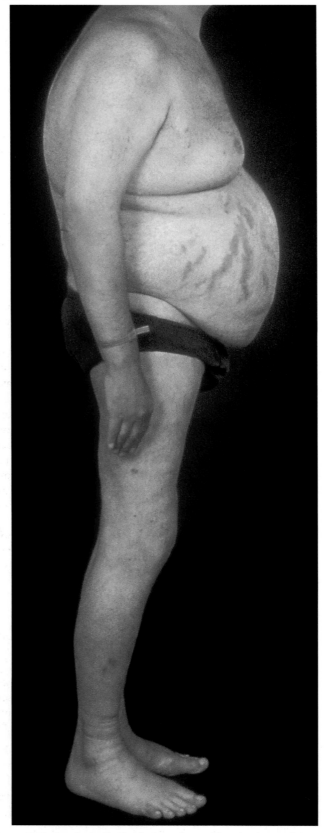

FIGURE 17.21 A patient with Cushing's syndrome. Note the characteristic obesity of the neck and trunk and the relative wasting of the limbs. (Figure courtesy of Professor JMC Connell, University of Glasgow.)

TABLE 17.8 Proportions of causes of Cushing's syndrome

Pituitary adenoma	67%
Adrenal tumour	15%
adenoma	
carcinoma	
Ectopic ACTH syndrome	17%
Ingestion of glucocorticoids	

The main causes of Cushing's syndrome are shown in Table 17.8, and are outlined below.

Cushing's disease (pituitary-dependent Cushing's syndrome)

This accounts for about 70% of Cushing's syndrome cases. There is excess ACTH secretion from the pituitary, usually from a tumour (pp. 453–454). This causes hyperstimulation of the adrenals and bilateral cortical hyperplasia, which may be either diffuse or nodular. In diffuse hyperplasia, the gland is increased in weight to between 6 and 12 g, and the cortex is broadened. In the less common nodular hyperplasia, obvious nodules visible to the naked eye are present and the glands may be markedly enlarged. Why these nodules develop is unknown, but they are more common in longstanding disease. The raised plasma glucocorticoids can be suppressed by high doses of dexamethasone. ACTH levels are usually just above normal, with loss of the circadian rhythm.

Adrenocortical tumours with autonomous secretion of cortisol

These cause about 20% of cases in adults, with 80% occurring in women. Approximately half are malignant. In children, adrenocortical tumours cause 50% of cases, and carcinoma is more common. Particularly with malignant tumours, the production of sex steroids also causes virilization (so-called 'mixed' Cushing's syndrome). The excess glucocorticoids suppress ACTH secretion by the pituitary, which results in atrophy of the contralateral adrenal and of the adrenal remnant adjacent to the tumour. If the tumour is removed surgically, the patient must receive glucocorticoids until ACTH secretion is re-established and the remaining adrenal regenerates. The raised cortisol levels in these patients cannot be suppressed by dexamethasone. Plasma ACTH levels are low or undetectable.

Ectopic ACTH syndrome

In the remaining cases, there is secretion of ACTH by a non-pituitary tumour. These include small cell carcinoma of lung, thymic carcinoids and endocrine tumours of the pancreas. Patients with lung cancer may not develop full-blown clinical features because of the other effects of a rapidly progressing tumour. There is bilateral diffuse adrenal hyperplasia, and the glands are usually heavier than in Cushing's disease, weighing up to 20 g each. The high glucocorticoid levels are not suppressed by dexamethasone. ACTH levels and those of ACTH precursors are raised, usually to higher levels than in Cushing's disease.

Conn's Syndrome (Primary Hyperaldosteronism)

This is characterized by hypertension, periodic muscle weakness or paralysis, muscle cramps and tetany, nocturia and polyuria. There is hypokalaemia, metabolic alkalosis (high serum bicarbonate), high plasma aldosterone and low renin, indicating autonomous secretion of aldosterone. Some 80% of patients have an adrenal adenoma (Figure 17.22), with three-quarters of these occurring in women. Carcinomas are rare. In the remaining cases, there is bilateral hyperplasia of the zona glomerulosa of unknown cause. The surgical removal of an adenoma can be curative if performed before the vascular changes of hypertension become established.

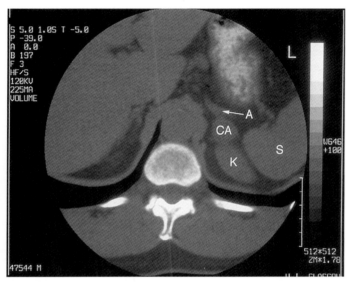

FIGURE 17.22 Computed tomography scan of the abdomen in a patient with Conn's syndrome. An adenoma (CA) is seen in the left adrenal, continuous with normal adrenal tissue (A). The kidney (K) and spleen (S) are also shown. (Figure courtesy of Professor JMC Connell, University of Glasgow.)

Secondary hyperaldosteronism

Increased activity of the renin–angiotensin system will stimulate aldosterone secretion. This can occur in kidney disease where there is renal ischaemia (p. 119), in oedema and occasionally with a renin-secreting tumour. Plasma levels of both aldosterone and renin are high.

Adrenogenital Syndrome

Adrenal tumours

These may secrete sex steroids, more usually androgens. This is more common in carcinomas than in adenomas, and in women it results in virilization (clitoromegaly and hirsutism). Occasionally, secretion of oestrogens may cause gynaecomastia and penile and testicular atrophy in men.

Congenital adrenal hyperplasia

This is associated with a group of diseases which are the result of inherited mutations in the genes encoding the enzymes and other proteins involved in steroidogenesis. Reduction in cortisol secretion causes reduced negative feedback and ACTH secretion is increased in an attempt to produce normal levels of cortisol. This usually also results in an increase in androgen secretion. Intermediate steroids with mineralocorticoid effects may also be secreted in excess. The clinical picture depends on the combination of steroids secreted. The increased stimulation leads to massive adrenocortical hyperplasia. The most common form is the 21-hydroxylase deficiency, with a mean incidence of 1 in 14 000. Female infants have clitoromegaly and various degrees of labial fusion. The internal reproductive tract is normal. Males present with precocious puberty. In two-thirds of cases, aldosterone synthesis is also impaired, and these infants have features of salt loss with dehydration, vomiting and hypotensive collapse. Deficiency of 11β-hydroxylase is one-fifth as common. Deoxycorticosterone accumulates along with androgens, causing hypertension in addition to virilism.

Adrenocortical Tumours

It is unclear how common adrenal adenomas are as they are usually diagnosed in life only when they secrete excess hormone. At autopsy, nodules can be found in about 5% of adrenals, and the results of clonality studies have suggested that the larger lesions are neoplastic. More of these are now being identified in live patients, mainly because people have their abdomens scanned during the investigation of other diseases. This raises the problem of what to do with the lesion, if found. At present, if there is no evidence of significant hormone secretion and the lesion is less than 3 cm in diameter, and does not grow on sequential scanning, most surgeons would not remove it. This approach is based on the low probability of malignant potential, and the fact that carcinomas tend to be larger tumours. However, carcinomas can be small, so there is a risk of missing one using this strategy.

Functional adenomas may secrete cortisol, aldosterone or sex steroids. They resemble normal adrenal cortex histologically, and tend to have a preponderance of lipid-laden, fasciculata-like cells.

Adrenocortical carcinoma

This has an incidence of only 1–2 per million of the population. Most of the lesions are clearly malignant at presentation, with local spread and/or metastases (Figure 17.23). The prognosis is poor. The histological distinction between benign and malignant tumours can be difficult, and is based on analysis of a number of factors. Tumours secreting androgens, oestrogens or precursor steroids are more likely to be malignant.

Aetiology

Adrenal carcinomas show widespread cytogenetic changes, but the critical molecular genetic events involved in their pathogenesis are still under investigation. The *MEN1* gene does not appear to be involved in sporadic tumours. Abnormalities in *p53* may play a role in tumour progression. The *ras* oncogenes are not mutated. Overexpression of

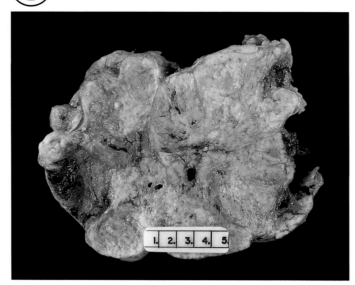

FIGURE 17.23 Adrenocortical carcinoma, showing necrosis and haemorrhage. This tumour was causing Cushing's syndrome.

insulin-like growth factor II (IGF-II) has been shown in carcinoma, and IGF-I and members of the epidermal growth factor and transforming growth factor β families may also play a role in regulating growth.

Adrenocortical Hypofunction

> **Key Points**
>
> - Acute adrenocortical hypofunction may result from meningococcal septicaemia and other infections.
> - Chronic adrenocortical hypofunction may result from autoimmune adrenalitis or tuberculosis.

In both acute and chronic hypofunction, about 90% of the cortex must be destroyed before clinical symptoms are present. Adrenocortical failure may be the result of primary disease of the adrenal gland, or may be secondary to lack of ACTH release from the pituitary, most commonly as one aspect of panhypopituitarism.

Acute Adrenocortical Insufficiency

This is a rare complication of septicaemia, particularly due to meningococcal infection, and is known as Waterhouse–Friderichsen syndrome. It is seen less frequently with other bacteraemic infections, including *Pneumococcus* sp., *Staphylococcus* sp. or *Haemophilus influenzae*. The condition presents with vomiting, salt loss with hyponatraemia, hyperkalaemia, hypoglycaemia and dehydration, causing collapse, hypotension and sometimes death. Patients often have high fever and a purpuric rash. There is haemorrhage into the adrenal glands, with extensive cortical necrosis. In the past, it was thought that the adrenocortical failure played a major role in the vascular collapse, but it is now realized that it is probably a minor component, the major factors being the massive bacteraemia and endotoxaemia which result in disseminated intravascular coagulation and shock.

Acute adrenocortical failure superimposed on chronic failure (Addisonian crisis) may occur when increased demands are made on a chronically failing adrenal cortex by, for example, infection or trauma. In addition, a lack of corticosteroid cover in adrenalectomized patients may precipitate adrenal failure, as may the sudden withdrawal of glucocorticoids from patients on long-term treatment. It is critically important therefore that patients receiving glucocorticoids should be made fully aware of the risk of discontinuing these drugs. Acute adrenocortical failure may also be part of the acute presentation of congenital adrenal hyperplasia.

Chronic Adrenocortical Insufficiency (Addison's Disease)

In chronic adrenal insufficiency, there is general lethargy, muscle weakness, hypotension, anorexia and pigmentation of skin and mucous membranes. The most common cause of chronic insufficiency is now autoimmune adrenalitis, which accounts for 75% of cases. The adrenals are atrophic, with an infiltrate of lymphocytes and plasma cells. The medulla is not affected. There is an association with other organ-specific autoimmune diseases, such as autoimmune thyroid disease, pernicious anaemia (p. 236), vitiligo and insulin-dependent diabetes mellitus (p. 468).

The second most common cause is tuberculosis, in which the medulla is also destroyed. The adrenals are enlarged and consist of masses of caseous material often with calcification that may be seen on X-radiography. Occasionally amyloidosis, fungal infection or secondary tumour may result in adrenal failure.

Chronic adrenal insufficiency results in corticotroph hyperplasia with increased ACTH secretion by the pituitary. Occasionally, a pituitary adenoma may form.

Adrenal medulla

The main component of the medulla is the phaeochromocytes or chromaffin cells which secrete the catecholamines, adrenaline and noradrenaline. Nerves and ganglion cells are also found. Tumours are the only important pathology.

Phaeochromocytoma

Phaeochromocytomas arise from the chromaffin cells (Figure 17.24), and produce symptoms related to catecholamine excess, which may at first be intermittent. These include hypertension, palpitation, sweating and sometimes collapse. There is hyperglycaemia and glycosuria. They occur in both sexes across a wide age range, but are rare in children. Historically, about 10% of cases were thought to be familial, most often as part of the MEN2 syndrome (p. 473). However, the recent identification of familial cases associated with mutations in the succinate dehydrogenase genes suggests that about 20% are familial. In MEN2, about half of the individuals have bilateral phaeochromocytomas. Bilateral tumours may also occur sporadically. Less than

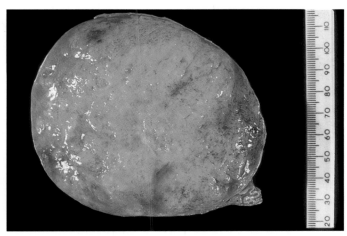

FIGURE 17.24 Phaeochromocytoma removed from a patient with hypertension. The normal adrenal can be seen to the bottom right.

The parathyroid glands secrete parathyroid hormone, which regulates serum calcium levels by effects on bone, kidneys and gut. Secretion is controlled by circulating calcium, via the calcium sensing receptor.

Hyperparathyroidism

Hyperparathyroidism is classified as:

- primary, when excessive secretion of parathyroid hormone is autonomous
- secondary, when the glands hypersecrete parathyroid hormone in response to increased physiological stimulation, most often in chronic renal failure
- tertiary, when autonomous hypersecretion of hormone develops on a background of secondary hyperparathyroidism.

Primary Hyperparathyroidism

This is a disease of middle age, and is slightly more common in women than in men. Patients may present with general tiredness and muscle weakness, and are often now diagnosed at this stage before significant pathology develops. In the past, more people presented with renal calculi and some developed severe bone disease with osteitis fibrosa cystica. Other complications include duodenal ulceration and acute pancreatitis. Metastatic calcification may cause nephrocalcinosis and renal failure, and may affect the soft tissues, heart and other organs.

In 80% of patients, there is a single parathyroid adenoma, and removal of this results in cure. In 15–20% of cases, there is enlargement of more than one gland, termed primary hyperplasia. Parathyroid carcinoma accounts for only 2–3% of cases. At the time of surgery it is often clear that a carcinoma is infiltrating the surrounding tissues, and hence the surgeon may have difficulty in removing it. As with other endocrine tumours, it can be difficult for the pathologist to predict malignant behaviour if the tumour is not obviously invasive or metastatic.

Primary hyperparathyroidism may occur as part of the MEN1 and MEN2 syndromes. Hyperplasia (Figure 17.25) may be found in these cases.

Secondary Hyperparathyroidism

Persistent low serum levels of ionized calcium will result in increased stimulation of parathyroid hormone release, and result in hyperplasia. This occurs most commonly in chronic renal failure, but it may also be seen in malabsorption syndromes and with vitamin D deficiency.

Occasionally, a patient with secondary hyperparathyroidism becomes hypercalcaemic; this is referred to as tertiary hyperparathyroidism. It is thought that some cells in a parathyroid gland become autonomous, i.e. insensitive to the controlling effect of Ca^{2+}, and an inappropriately high level of hormone results. In some cases an adenomatous nodule may develop.

10% of all tumours are malignant. The lesions usually consist of cells arranged in an alveolar or trabecular pattern. It is difficult to predict tumour behaviour on histological grounds. They may occasionally produce ectopic hormone syndromes, secreting ACTH or VIP, that causes the WDHA (watery diarrhoea, hypokalaemia and achlorhydria) syndrome.

Similar tumours may arise in extra-adrenal paraganglia, most commonly in the organs of Zuckerkandl. These are more often malignant than intra-adrenal tumours.

Other Tumours

Neuroblastoma is a tumour arising in children from the primitive cells of the medulla. Benign tumours may arise from the other components of the medulla and include neurofibroma and ganglioneuroma, fibroma and angioma.

Occasionally pseudocysts may develop, due to haemorrhage into adrenal tumours. Haemopoietic tissue is frequently seen in the adrenal cortex at autopsy. This may coexist with adipose tissue, the so-called myelolipoma. Metastases are common, particularly from bronchial carcinoma.

PARATHYROID GLANDS

There are usually four parathyroid glands, lying posterior to the thyroid gland – two at the upper and two at the lower poles. However, one or more glands may be intrathyroidal, or lie in the lower neck or upper mediastinum close to the thymus. The total weight is 120 mg in adult males and 140 mg in females, the upper limit of normal for an individual gland being 50 mg. The glands contain two main cell types: (i) chief cells, which form the main functional group, are usually eosinophilic, but may also appear clear, depending on the intracellular glycogen content; and (ii) oxyphil cells, which are slightly larger, with a strongly eosinophilic rather granular cytoplasm, due to the presence of large numbers of mitochondria. The number of oxyphil cells increases with age. Stromal fat is seen after puberty, and constitutes up to 30% of the normal adult gland.

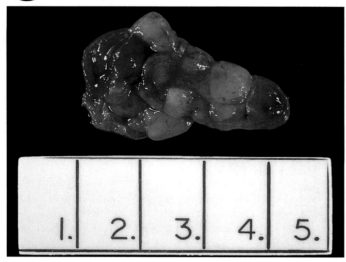

FIGURE 17.25 Nodular parathyroid removed from a patient with multiple endocrine neoplasia, type I (MEN1) who had hypercalcaemia. The other glands were also nodular, but much smaller.

Hypoparathyroidism

Deficiency of parathyroid hormone causes hypocalcaemia and hyperphosphataemia. The low calcium level causes increased muscular tone and, if severe, tetany. Patients often develop cataracts, and may have psychological changes and convulsions. The most common cause is surgical removal of the glands, sometimes inadvertently during thyroidectomy or head and neck surgery. This condition forms part of the Di George syndrome (p. 28), coupled with immunological deficiencies. This is due to hypoplasia or aplasia of both parathyroids and thymus, caused by abnormal development of the third and fourth branchial arches. Very rarely, auto-immune parathyroiditis is the cause, sometimes associated with other autoimmune organ-specific diseases.

DIABETES MELLITUS

Key Points

Diabetes mellitus is:

- an extremely common metabolic disorder, which is rising in prevalence
- known as 'syndrome of inadequate insulin action'
- the type 1 condition is insulin-dependent diabetes mellitus (IDDM)
- the type 2 condition is non-insulin-dependent diabetes mellitus (NIDDM)
- eye, renal, vascular and neurological complications are commonplace.

Diabetes is not a single disease, but is rather the pathological and metabolic state caused by inadequate insulin action. A feature common to all types is glucose intolerance. Diabetes is defined clinically as either a fasting plasma glucose level greater than 7.8 mmol/L (140 mg/dL) or a 2-hour post-prandial plasma glucose greater than 11 mmol/L (200 mg/dL).

Insulin is a major anabolic hormone which promotes the uptake of glucose by cells and the formation of intracellular glycogen from glucose. It also stimulates cells to utilize amino acids for protein synthesis rather than for gluconeogenesis, and it promotes the uptake of free fatty acids by adipose tissue. A lack of insulin, therefore, results in a general catabolic state with loss of weight, hyperglycaemia, diminished protein synthesis, increased gluconeogenesis, and hyperlipidaemia due to lipolysis in adipose tissue. Although the renal threshold is usually raised, there is heavy glycosuria which results in an osmotic diuresis, causing dehydration and thirst. In the liver, excess free fatty acids are converted via acetyl-CoA into ketone bodies which, in the absence of available glucose, are metabolized for cellular energy. The ketone bodies (acetoacetic acid, β-hydroxybutyric acid and acetone) dissociate to produce hydrogen ions, with a resulting metabolic acidosis (ketoacidosis). This complex of metabolic disturbances produces hyperosmolarity, hypovolaemia, acidosis and electrolyte imbalance, which have serious effects on the functions of neurones and result in one form of diabetic coma – ketoacidotic coma. The other major form – hyperosmolar non-ketotic coma – results from massive dehydration and profound hyperglycaemia in the absence of ketoacidosis. Relative or absolute overdosage with insulin causes hypoglycaemic effects, including coma which, unless treated, may be fatal.

Classification of Diabetes

Over 99% of cases of diabetes are caused by two diseases: type 1 diabetes (insulin-dependent diabetes mellitus; IDDM); or type 2 diabetes (non-insulin-dependent diabetes mellitus; NIDDM). Type 2 diabetes is 10 times more common than type 1. The principal differences between the two are detailed in Table 17.9. Specific diseases in which diabetes occurs as a secondary event include chronic pancreatitis, haemochromatosis, cystic fibrosis, acromegaly, Cushing's syndrome and glucagon-secreting islet cell tumours. In haemochromatosis, excess iron is taken up by B cells, but not by other islet endocrine cells, resulting in inhibition of insulin synthesis.

Complications of Diabetes

- Atheroma.
- Hypertension.
- Diabetic nephropathy.
- Diabetic retinopathy.
- Bacterial infection.
- Peripheral neuropathy.

Coma due to lack of diabetic control is now a relatively rare cause of death, and the mortality and morbidity of diabetes are due to the above complications.

TABLE 17.9 The two main diseases which result in diabetes

Type 1 diabetes	Type 2 diabetes
Onset under age 40 years	Onset over age 40 years
Thin patient	Obese patient
Affects 1 in 400 of population in UK	Affects at least 1 in 40 of population in UK
Liable to ketoacidotic coma	Liable to hyperosmolar non-ketotic coma
Always requires insulin for therapy	Does not always require insulin for therapy
Concordance rate for monozygotic twins 40%	Concordance rate for monozygotic twins 100%
Genetic link with class II MHC antigens	No genetic link with class II MHC antigens
Islet cell antibody present	Islet cell antibody absent
Insulitis present	Insulitis absent
B cells destroyed in pancreas	B cells not destroyed in pancreas
Islet amyloid absent	Islet amyloid present

 17.2   SPECIAL STUDY TOPIC

TYPES OF DIABETES MELLITUS

Type 1 Diabetes

Aetiology and Pathogenesis

In this disease, insulin-secreting B cells are selectively destroyed in the pancreatic islets, but A, D and PP cells are preserved. The process of B-cell destruction appears to take many years, and the patient presents clinically with diabetes when about 80% of the B cells are lost. Islets in which there is active B-cell destruction are inflamed; this is termed insulitis (Figure 17.26). The infiltrate consists mainly of lymphocytes with a few macrophages.

Autoimmunity

Type 1 diabetes is an organ-specific autoimmune disease (Atkinson and Maclaren, 1994) in which both humoral (islet cell antibodies) and cell-mediated immunity are directed towards the B cells. At clinical presentation at least 80% of patients have circulating cytoplasmic islet cell antibodies. Some 15% of patients develop other organ-specific autoimmune diseases such as thyroiditis, pernicious anaemia or autoimmune Addison's disease.

Genetic Factors

There is a significant link between type 1 diabetes and the class II major histocompatibility complex (MHC) genes – *DP*, *DQ* and *DR* in man. Persons carrying the DR3 allele have a relative five-fold risk of developing type 1 diabetes. The risk for *DR4* is seven-fold, and that for *DR3/DR4* heterozygotes is 14-fold. There is an even stronger association with the *DQ* gene. However, the concordance rate between identical twins is only 40%, indicating the involvement of non-genetic factors in the pathogenesis of the disease.

Environmental Factors

If diabetes is an autoimmune disease occurring in a genetically susceptible population, what are the environmental triggers that might precipitate the development of autoimmunity? Two theories exist. First, the process may be initiated by a viral infection. Up to 30% of patients presenting with type 1 diabetes have serological evidence of a recent or continuing enteroviral infection (usually Coxsackie B virus). This virus is capable of specifically infecting islet B cells. Other viruses that have been implicated are mumps and rubella viruses. Second, the type of infant diet may influence the development of the disease (Ellis and Atkinson, 1996). Epidemiological studies have suggested that exposure to cows' milk antigens before 6 months of age may also play a part. It is conceivable that

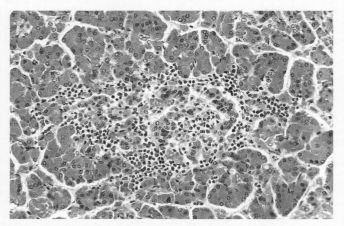

FIGURE 17.26 Insulitis. Lymphocytes infiltrating and destroying an islet.

an immune response to a bovine antigen in food may precipitate autoimmunity by crossreacting with an antigen on the B cell.

The Pancreas in Type 1 Diabetes (Figure 17.27)

At clinical presentation of diabetes, two distinctive abnormalities can be seen in the islets in the pancreas (Foulis, 1989). First, many of the B cells that remain express interferon-α – a cytokine which is secreted by a cell in response to viral infection. Second, occasional B cells express class II MHC molecules (HLA-DR).

Interferon-α expression appears to be the earlier of these two events in the disease process, and raises the question as to whether the B cells are infected by a virus at this stage, although no convincing evidence of this has yet been found. Islet inflammation secondary to the secretion of interferon-α by B cells may release certain other cytokines which might cause already damaged B cells to express class II MHC. Such class II MHC molecules are necessary for antigen presentation to helper T lymphocytes, the cells which initiate the immune response. Thus, the islet B cells in type 1 diabetes may become antigen-presenting cells, presenting cell-specific antigens to which there is no tolerance. This may stimulate autoimmunity directed against their own antigens, and lead to their destruction.

Type 2 Diabetes

The pancreas at clinical presentation of this disease does not show the same dramatic loss of B cells as that seen in type 1 diabetes. However, in about 70% of cases amyloid is present within islets (Figure 17.28). The chemical nature of the amyloid protein has now been determined. It consists of a 37-amino-acid peptide known variously as islet amyloid polypeptide or amylin. This protein is produced by B cells in both normal and diabetic subjects.

Patients with type 2 diabetes, obese people, and 25% of the normal population show resistance to the action of insulin. These people thus have to hypersecrete insulin in order to achieve metabolic homeostasis. Whilst in many normal people this, possibly genetic, disorder may cause no illness, it is proposed that in a minority there is eventual B-cell exhaustion with falling insulin secretion and hence the development of type 2 diabetes. Thus, there may be both a qualitative and quantitative insulin insufficiency. The concordance rate for type 2 diabetes among monozygotic twins is 100%, suggesting that the failure of B cells to cope with prolonged insulin resistance may also be genetic. By the time the patient presents with type 2 diabetes there is a marked reduction in insulin response to a glucose load. The accumulation of amyloid in the islets may reflect long-standing B-cell hyperfunction where the islet amyloid polypeptide has been hypersecreted in parallel with insulin. It is interesting in this regard that amyloid of the same composition is also found in some insulinomas.

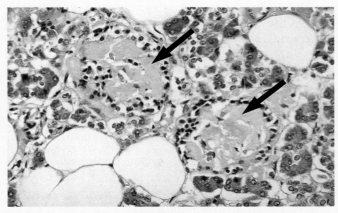

FIGURE 17.28 Amyloid (pink indicated by arrows) largely replacing two islets.

References

Atkinson MA, Maclaren NK. The pathogenesis of insulin-dependent diabetes mellitus. *N Engl J Med* 1994; **331**: 1428–1436.

Ellis TM, Atkinson MA. Early infant diet and insulin-dependent diabetes. *Lancet* 1996; **347**: 1464–1465.

Foulis AK. In Type 1 diabetes, does a non-cytopathic viral infection of insulin- secreting B-cells initiate the disease process leading to their autoimmune destruction? *Diabetic Med* 1989; **6**: 666–674.

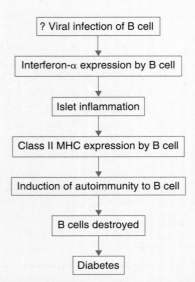

? Viral infection of B cell

↓

Interferon-α expression by B cell

↓

Islet inflammation

↓

Class II MHC expression by B cell

↓

Induction of autoimmunity to B cell

↓

B cells destroyed

↓

Diabetes

FIGURE 17.27 Immune events in the pancreas in type 1 diabetes.

Cardiovascular Complications

It is customary to speak of diabetic macroangiopathy, most commonly affecting large muscular arteries, and diabetic microangiopathy, affecting arterioles and capillaries. The former is simply atheroma, which tends to develop early and become severe in diabetics of either sex. This – plus the fact that 50% of patients with type 2 diabetes have hypertension – results in 80% of adult diabetic deaths being due to cardiovascular, cerebrovascular or peripheral vascular diseases. In diabetic patients with peripheral vascular disease, the small muscular arteries of the lower leg and foot are commonly affected. Thus, a toe may be gangrenous in the presence of normal femoral and popliteal pulses due to the fact that relatively small vessels are narrowed by atheroma.

In diabetic microangiopathy, two types of lesion have been described: first, a thickening of the basement membrane or an accumulation of basement membrane-like material in capillaries; and second, endothelial cell proliferation together with basement membrane thickening. The cause of the microangiopathy is uncertain, but it affects diabetics of all types, appears to be related to the duration of the disease, and is aggravated by poor diabetic control. It is responsible for diabetic retinopathy (p. 325) and diabetic nephropathy (pp. 388–389). Diabetic retinopathy is the most common cause of blindness under the age of 65 years in developed countries.

Infections

There is an increased susceptibility to bacterial and fungal infections in diabetes. Boils, carbuncles and urinary tract infections – sometimes complicated by pyelonephritis and renal papillary necrosis – are of frequent occurrence, and may precipitate diabetic coma. Diabetics have an increased risk of tuberculosis, especially of the lungs, and unless treated the disease tends to progress rapidly.

Other Pathological Effects

Trophic disturbances – such as ulceration of the fingers or toes and neuropathic arthropathy – may develop as complications of diabetic peripheral neuropathy. It is noteworthy that atheroma, diabetic microangiopathy, peripheral neuropathy and susceptibility to infections all tend to promote gangrene of the extremities in diabetes.

Recent large studies have shown that the incidence of diabetic complications in both type 1 diabetes and type 2 diabetes can be reduced by treating hypertension vigorously and ensuring strict control of blood sugar levels.

GONADS

Testis

The adult testes are paired ovoid organs within the scrotum, and weigh 15–20 g each (see also Chapter 16). They comprise mainly the seminiferous tubules, which contain Sertoli cells and germ cells in the various stages of maturation from spermatogonia to spermatozoa. The Sertoli cells secrete growth and inhibitory factors that play important roles in the maturation of the germ cells, and an androgen-binding protein which binds testosterone. Spermatogenesis is mainly under the control of FSH from the pituitary and testosterone, secreted by Leydig cells.

Male Pseudohermaphroditism

Male pseudohermaphroditism is a rare condition in which the karyotype is 46,XY, and the individual has bilateral testes, but has ambiguous or female internal and external genitalia. The condition is usually due to inherited mutations in one of the genes encoding the enzymes involved in androgen synthesis or in the androgen receptor gene.

Disorders of Puberty

These comprise two broad groups of precocious puberty and delayed puberty.

Precocious puberty may be due to premature activation of the hypothalamic-pituitary-gonadal axis (HPG). It may be induced by testosterone secretion from a Leydig cell tumour, or by chorionic gonadotrophin secretion from a tumour. It is also seen in some variants of congenital adrenal hyperplasia (p. 465) where the adrenal glands are secreting large amounts of androgens.

The most common congenital form of delayed puberty is Kallmann's syndrome, which is associated with absent or reduced secretion of GnRH from the hypothalamus, and thus of gonadotrophins from the pituitary. It is usually associated with anosmia or hyposomia. This presumably reflects abnormalities in hypothalamic development. It is an X-linked condition, but the gene involved has not yet been identified. Hypopituitarism can also result in delayed puberty, but there will probably also be deficiencies in other hormones.

Hypergonadotrophic hypogonadism is usually the result of impaired production of testosterone. It is found in Klinefelter's syndrome (XXY genotype) and in Sertoli cell-only syndrome, where spermatogenesis does not occur and only Sertoli cells are seen in the tubules.

Infertility

There are numerous causes of infertility. Some are related to chromosomal defects, or to primary hypofunction of the HPG axis. However, secondary changes in the HPG axis may also be seen in diseases of other endocrine organs, and in chronic diseases of other organs such as the kidneys and liver. Infertility may also follow on chemotherapy or exposure to toxic substances.

Hormonal Aspects of Testicular Tumours

Human chorionic gonadotrophin is secreted when choriocarcinoma forms part of a mixed germ cell tumour. Leydig cell tumours can secrete a variety of androgens and other steroids, and in children this may result in precocious puberty.

Ovary

The ovaries are paired intra-abdominal organs with complex anatomy, physiology and biochemistry, and are dealt

with elsewhere in some detail (see Chapter 14). Their main function is the production and release of the mature oocyte. This requires multiple interactions between the follicles and the stroma, with the production of steroids, peptide hormones and growth and inhibitory factors.

Pseudohermaphroditism

In the female, this is usually caused by the excessive androgen secretion of congenital adrenal hyperplasia (p. 465); the ovaries are normal in these patients.

Infertility

Because of the complexities of the menstrual cycle, there are a wide range of causes of female infertility, and these are discussed in detail in many textbooks of gynaecology. The causes of infertility include primary ovarian disease and abnormalities of the HPG axis. In this context, hyperprolactinaemia (see Table 17.1) should be considered. As with the male, diseases of other endocrine glands and chronic diseases of other organs may also result in infertility.

Hormonal Aspects of Ovarian Tumours

It is now recognized that most ovarian tumours have the potential to secrete hormones, although this may not result in the production of clinical symptoms. Sex cord/stromal tumours (p. 413) are often associated with hormone production. Excessive oestrogen production from a granulosa cell tumour may result in menstrual disturbances, in postmenopausal bleeding, or in sexual precocity. Androgen secretion from other variants may result in virilization and hirsutism. In epithelial tumours, hormone production is usually by the stroma, and is most often of oestrogens, androgens and progesterone. Occasional cases of ectopic hormone secretion are found.

Hormonal Aspects of Non-neoplastic Ovarian Disease

Patients with polycystic ovary syndrome present with obesity, oligomenorrhoea or amenorrhoea, hirsutism and infertility. There is also evidence of excess oestrogen secretion, with endometrial hyperplasia and sometimes even endometrial carcinoma. The ovaries are enlarged and contain multiple cysts. The basic defect is unknown, but there are multiple abnormalities within the HPG axis with raised and fluctuating levels of LH, low levels of FSH, and enhanced sensitivity of gonadotrophs in the pituitary to GnRH.

In older women, stromal hyperplasia may occur, and this is associated with obesity, hypertension, abnormal glucose tolerance and virilization.

 17.3 SPECIAL STUDY TOPIC

MULTIPLE ENDOCRINE NEOPLASIA (MEN) SYNDROMES

It has been appreciated for some time that particular tumours of the endocrine glands show familial associations. In these syndromes, tumours occur in more than one endocrine gland in the same individual, or in a number of members of the family. The two main types are the multiple endocrine neoplasia (MEN) syndrome type 1 and type 2. Both are inherited in an autosomal dominant manner, but the pattern of tumours differs. Familial predisposition to neoplasia is usually associated with the inheritance of a germline mutation in a specific gene. The acquisition of genetic change in the other allele results in the development of the tumour. The tumours are preceded by hyperplasia and present at an earlier age than in sporadic cases. Advances in molecular genetic techniques now permit the screening of people at risk once the gene of interest has been identified. This process is easier if a few hotspots for mutation are defined. The genes involved in the MEN syndromes have both now been recently characterized, and screening programmes established for MEN2, but not routinely for MEN1.

Multiple Endocrine Neoplasia Type 1 (MEN1)

This syndrome is characterized by tumours of the parathyroid, pancreas and other gastrointestinal neuroendocrine tissues and anterior pituitary. In some cases, adrenocortical tumours occur, and also tumours of the skin, including lipomas, collagenomas and angiofibromas. Parathyroid tumours arise in about 95% of affected individuals, and are usually the first to present clinically, resulting in hypercalcaemia. Endocrine tumours of the pancreas are seen in about 40% of cases. Insulinomas will often be identified in patients under the age of 40 years, whereas gastrinomas tend to occur later in life. Pituitary tumours usually present over the age of 40 years. The age-related penetrance has been calculated as 7% at 10 years of age, 52% at 20 years, rising to 98% at 40 and 100% at 60 years.

The gene involved was mapped to chromosome 11q13 in 1988, but was not characterized until 1997. The MEN1 tumor suppressor gene consists of 10 exons spanning more than 9 kb of genomic DNA. It encodes a 610 amino acid protein, named menin. This is primarily a nuclear protein that is ubiquitously expressed, but its function has not yet been elucidated. Mutations have been identified in the coding region in MEN1 families. Most are predicted to give rise to a truncated menin protein, presumably with

loss of function. There is no link between particular mutations and the phenotype. In addition, the mutations are scattered throughout the whole of the coding region, with no obvious hotspots. This means that it is difficult to set up routine analyses to screen individuals at risk. There is currently great interest in defining the function of the menin protein, and in determining why these particular organs are the sites of tumorigenesis.

Multiple Endocrine Neoplasia Type 2 (MEN2)

MEN2 is characterized by inherited forms of medullary carcinoma of the thyroid (MTC) and has three subtypes. In type 2a, MTC is accompanied by phaeochromocytoma and parathyroid tumours, and by phaeochromocytoma and mucocutaneous neuromas in type 2b. Some families only develop familial MTC (FMTC). The biology of the MTC varies with the subtype; for example in MEN2b it develops earlier and pursues a more aggressive course than in MEN2a.

The gene involved is the *RET* proto-oncogene, localized to chromosome 10q11.2; this was cloned and sequenced in 1993. It consists of 20 exons, and encodes a receptor tyrosine kinase. The receptor consists of a large glycosylated extracellular domain containing a number of clustered cysteine residues and calcium-binding motifs, a single hydrophobic transmembrane domain and a cytoplasmic domain with tyrosine kinase activity. Receptor signalling requires dimerization. The ligand has recently been shown to be glial-cell-line-derived neurotrophic factor (GDNF), but full characterization of the interaction is awaited. In contrast to the *MEN1* gene, a finite number of mutations have been identified, and there is a fairly strong genotype–phenotype correlation, which makes familial screening easier. Almost all MEN2a patients have mutations at one of the cysteine residues on the extracellular domain, mostly at codon 634. This is thought to lead to spontaneous dimerization and activation of the receptor. A cysteine → arginine transposition appears to confer a higher risk of developing parathyroid disease. In MEN2b, the mutation is in the intracellular domain, activating tyrosine kinase even in the absence of dimerization. Genetic screening programmes based on analysis of these hotspots are now available. The identification of specific mutations can permit counselling on specific levels of risk for the individual components of the syndrome and a sensible approach to treatment. For example, thyroidectomy can be undertaken at an earlier age in individuals with the mutation linked to MEN2b.

The *RET* gene is also involved in the pathogenesis of Hirschsprung's disease, where there are losses of function mutations. This would fit with a role in neural/neuroendocrine signalling. The possible role of *RET* translocations seen in a subset of papillary carcinomas of the thyroid is, at present, less clear.

Further Reading

Agarwal SK, Lee Burns A, Sukhodolets KE, Kennedy PA, Obungu VH, Hickman AB, *et al.* Molecular pathology of the MEN1 gene. *Ann N Y Acad Sci* 2004; **1014**: 189–198.

Ichihara M, Murakumo Y, Takahashi M. RET and neuroendocrine tumors. *Cancer Lett* 2004; **204**(2): 197–211.

Santoro M, Melillo RM, Carlomagno F, Fusco A, Vecchio G. Molecular mechanisms of RET activation in human cancer. *Ann N Y Acad Sci* 2002; **963**: 116–121.

SUMMARY

- Most diseases of endocrine glands are uncommon, but they are important to recognize as many can be treated.
- Patients present in one of two ways. They may develop syndromes caused by secretion of too much, or too little, hormone or they may have an increase in size of the gland due to tumour or hyperplasia. This may be noticed by the patient or may cause pressure effects.
- It is very important to integrate the clinical, biochemical and pathological findings when reaching the final diagnosis.
- Some endocrine tumours occur in a familial setting, including multiple endocrine neoplasia types 1 and 2 in which recognized combinations are found. Over 20% of phaeochromocytomas and paragangliomas are familial.
- Autoimmune endocrine disease is most probably caused by interactions between the inherited aspects of an individual's immune system and environmental factors.
- Diabetes mellitus is not a single disease, but is the pathological and metabolic state caused by inadequate insulin action. Type 1 is insulin-dependent (IDDM), whereas type 2 is non-insulin-dependent (NIDDM).

FURTHER READING

Adeghate E, Saadi H, Adem A, Obineche E. *Diabetes Mellitus and Its Complications: Molecular Mechanisms, Epidemiology, and Clinical Medicine.* Oxford: Blackwell Publishing, 2006.

Chrousos EP, Tsigos C. *Stress, Obesity and Metabolic Syndrome.* Oxford: Blackwell Publishing, 2006.

DeLellis RA, Lloyd RV, Heitz PU, Eng C. *World Health Organization Classification of Tumours. Pathology and Genetics of Tumours of Endocrine Organs.* Lyon: IARC Press, 2004.

Rosai J. *Rosai and Ackerman's Surgical Pathology,* 9th edn, Chapters 9, 10, 15, 16, 29. London: Mosby, 2004.

18 THE SKIN

Alan T Evans and Wolter J Mooi

NORMAL SKIN STRUCTURE AND FUNCTION

The skin is the largest organ of the body, and in a 70-kg human has a total weight of 4–5 kg. The epithelial components (epidermis, sweat glands and pilosebaceous units) originate from the ectodermal layer of the embryo, while the mesenchymal tissues of the dermis are derived from mesoderm.

Normal Functions of Skin

The skin is a structurally complex organ which performs several vital functions (Table 18.1, Figure 18.1)

TABLE 18.1 **The functions of the skin**

- Strong mechanical barrier to microorganisms and antigens
- Thermoregulation (dermal vessels and sweat glands)
- Fluid and electrolyte balance (sweat glands)
- Endocrine function (UV-dependent synthesis of vitamin D)
- UV protection (melanin pigment from melanocytes)
- Immune function (epidermal Langerhans' cells)
- Sensory function (touch, temperature, pressure, pain)

Normal Epidermal Structure

The epidermis is a stratified, keratinising squamous epithelium with several distinct layers of keratinocytes (Figure 18.1B). These include:

- the basal layer of proliferative cells
- the prickle cell layer of polygonal cells with prominent desmosomal attachments
- the granular cell layer of flattened cells rich in keratohyalin granules
- the corneal layer of differentiated keratinocytes which are shed from the surface approximately 28 days after their production.

In addition to keratinocytes, the epidermis contains other important cell types:

- Melanocytes are highly dendritic cells found amongst basal layer keratinocytes (Figure 18.2). These synthesize melanin pigment responsible for UV protection, and are the precursor cells of melanocytic naevi and malignant melanoma.
- Langerhans' cells are dendritic bone marrow-derived cells located in the mid and upper epidermis. They process antigens and are important in various inflammatory dermatoses. They are not identified by routine microscopy, but can be demonstrated immunochemically (Figure 18.2) and by using electron microscopy.
- Merkel cells are neuroendocrine cells responsible for mechanoreception. They are invisible in routinely stained sections, but can be demonstrated immunochemically. They give rise to rare neuroendocrine carcinomas.

The Dermis

The dermal connective matrix is composed largely of type I collagen together with type III collagen and elastic fibres embedded in ground substance (mainly hyaluronic acid and chondroitin sulphate). The dermis has two distinct areas. The papillary dermis is a thin, superficial layer of loosely textured fibres that is rich in small nerves and capillaries orientated at right-angles to the skin surface. The underlying reticular dermis is more substantial, with thick bundles of type I collagen lying parallel to the skin surface. Within the

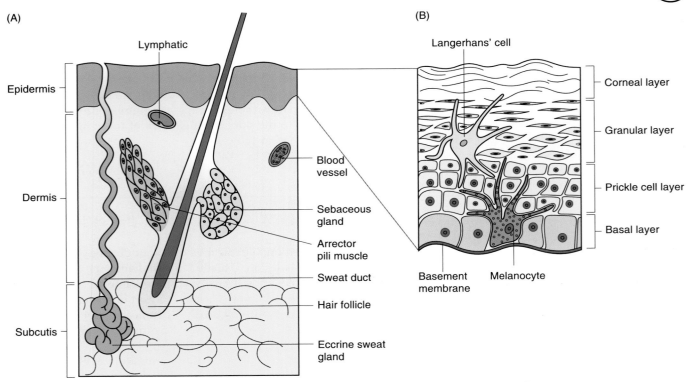

FIGURE 18.1 Diagram depicting the various components of normal skin (A) and, in greater detail, the normal epidermis (B).

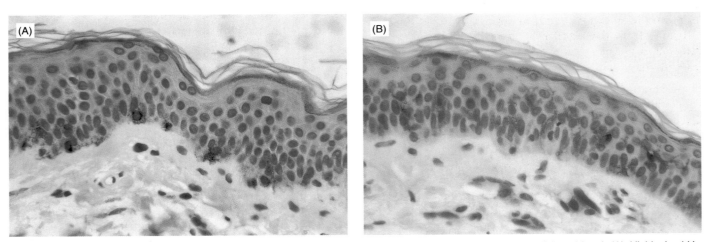

FIGURE 18.2 Immunohistochemical staining for S-100 protein demonstrates melanocytes amongst the basal keratinocytes of the epidermis (A). Highly dendritic Langerhans' cells (shown immunohistochemically by staining for the CD1a antigen) are present throughout the epidermis (B).

reticular dermis are the appendage structures (sweat glands and pilosebaceous units). Recently, many of the dermal spindle cells have been found to be highly dendritic with phagocytic function. These 'dermal dendrocytes' are morphologically similar to epidermal Langerhans' cells, and are also thought to have antigen-presenting function.

DISEASES OF THE SKIN

Skin diseases are common in both general and hospital practice. Over 1000 skin disorders have been described,

and new entities continue to be reported. Many skin diseases (especially the inflammatory dermatoses) have complex and confusing names based on macroscopic descriptions of the rash at a time when the aetiology of the condition was completely unknown. Recent progress in our understanding of the aetiology and pathogenesis of skin disease may lead to a more rational classification and nomenclature system, although many confusing terms remain entrenched in the literature. It is fortunate that some 10 skin diseases account for two-thirds of all dermatology practice!

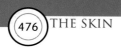

This chapter concentrates largely on primary skin disorders, and has three main sections:

1. non-infective inflammatory disorders
2. infective disorders
3. neoplasms.

Conditions that merit inclusion may be very common, for example eczema, psoriasis and the epidermal tumours.

Other rarer conditions, for example pemphigus vulgaris and bullous pemphigoid, are included because they illustrate important pathogenetic mechanisms.

Some conditions (e.g. lupus erythematosus and necrobiosis lipoidica) may act as useful pointers to underlying systemic disease. Many skin conditions are induced by drugs.

Dermatopathology employs a number of terms that are specific to the skin, and a glossary of those in common use is provided in Table 18.2.

TABLE 18.2 A glossary of the terminology used in skin pathology

Term	Description
Macroscopic term	
Macule	A circumscribed impalpable area of colour change
Papule	A small palpable lesion. Usually <5 mm diameter
Nodule	A larger palpable lesion. Usually >5 mm diameter
Plaque	A raised flat topped lesion. Usually >5 mm diameter
Vesicle	A small fluid filled blister. Usually <5 mm diameter
Bulla	A larger fluid filled blister. Usually >5 mm diameter
Pustule	A vesicle containing pus
Crust	Dried plasma proteins often with inflammatory cells and blood
Scale	Dry flaky or powdery surface due to thickened corneal layer
Excoriation	Deep (usually self-inflicted) scratch
Lichenification	Thickened skin with prominent markings resembling tree bark
Purpura	Extravasation of erythrocytes into dermis
Alopecia	Loss of hair from normally hirsute area
Microscopic term	
Acanthosis	Epidermal thickening due largely to hyperplasia of prickle cell layer
Hyperkeratosis	Thickened corneal layer
Parakeratosis	Retained nuclear staining characteristics in corneal layer
Dyskeratosis	Premature keratinization of epidermal cells
Spongiosis	Intraepidermal oedema
Acantholysis	Loss of keratinocyte cohesion
Lichenoid	Describes inflammation attacking the basal layer
Cytoid body	A homogeneous eosinophilic apoptotic keratinocyte

Non-infective Inflammatory Disorders

It is perhaps impossible to provide a comprehensive classification system that is easy to understand and use, for such a large group of diverse diseases. Most disorders selected for presentation in this section involve the epidermis, which has a limited repertoire of reaction patterns to inflammatory insult. Accordingly, a classification system utilizing the epidermal reaction pattern provides a straightforward method of categorizing these conditions. Key examples of inflammatory disorders that typify each reaction pattern are provided in Table 18.3. In effect, these key examples define the essential core content for this area of study.

Some non-infective inflammatory disorders are not centred on the epidermis, but on other skin components including dermal collagen, dermal blood vessels, appendage

TABLE 18.3 Epidermal reaction patterns

- **Spongiotic reaction pattern** (intraepidermal oedema)
  Key example is eczematous dermatitis
- **Psoriasiform reaction pattern** (epidermal hyperplasia with regular rete ridge elongation)
  Key example is psoriasis vulgaris
- **Lichenoid reaction pattern** (basal layer damage)
  Key examples are lichen planus and lupus erythematosus
- **Vesiculobullous reaction pattern** (intra- or subepidermal blistering)
  Key examples are pemphigus vulgaris and bullous pemphigoid

structures and subcutaneous fat. These diseases are less important in terms of core knowledge, although a few examples will be discussed briefly (pp. 489–490).

The Spongiotic Epidermal Reaction Pattern

Eczematous Dermatitis

> **Key Points**
>
> Eczematous dermatitis:
>
> - is a reaction pattern not a specific disease
> - may be hereditary (e.g. atopy) or due to environmental causes (e.g. contact dermatitis)
> - may have acute and chronic stages
> - may be complicated by superimposed infection.

General

The terms eczema and dermatitis are used interchangeably. Eczema is favoured by dermatologists, and dermatitis by pathologists. It is unusual that 'dermatitis' is reserved for describing the pathological changes of eczema when it could be applied to any of several hundred inflammatory skin disorders. However, such generalization is not encouraged in the study of skin disease. Together, the dermatologist and pathologist strive (often with difficulty) to give the non-eczematous inflammatory dermatoses a precise diagnosis rather than the generic label of 'dermatitis'.

Clinical Features

Eczema is not a specific disease entity, but rather is a very common cutaneous reaction pattern occurring in response to diverse insults (Figure 18.3). The acute stage is characterized by an itchy papulovesicular rash with surface oozing and crust. With chronicity, the lesions become thickened with surface scale and accentuated surface markings in the process called lichenification (this is especially likely if there has been repeated rubbing and scratching). The clinical and histological features of eczema can also be complicated by bacterial and viral infection (see Case History 18.1, p. 488).

Microscopic Features

Microscopic features of eczematous dermatitis include:

- upper dermal perivascular lymphocytic infiltrate
- spongiosis
- vesiculation
- chronicity leading to acanthosis, surface scale and dermal fibrosis
- subacute lesions show both acute and chronic features.

Clinical Subtypes

Irrespective of the underlying cause, the lesions of eczema show similar pathological features. However, the dermatologist is often able to classify eczema as being either endogenous (due mainly to hereditary factors) or exogenous (due to environmental factors). The most commonly encountered example of endogenous eczema is atopic dermatitis. Recently it has been demonstrated that mutations in the filament aggregating protein filaggrin (responsible for aggregating keratin filaments into granules of keratohyalin) is the cause of the common inherited disorder of keratinization known as ichthyosis vulgaris (a condition characterized by dry scaly skin). More importantly, it has been demonstrated that mutations in the filaggrin gene are associated strongly with atopic dermatitis and also with asthma suggesting a prominent role for the epidermal barrier in atopic disease in general. Good examples of exogenous eczema are primary irritant dermatitis and allergic contact dermatitis.

Atopic Dermatitis

Atopic dermatitis shows the following general characteristics:

- it is a common childhood condition
- it is a type I (IgE-mediated) hypersensitivity disorder
- decreased suppressor T-cell activity is also described
- it begins in early infancy
- it usually improves spontaneously in late childhood
- it may be widespread, but the flexures are often more severely affected
- patients are prone to secondary bacterial and viral infection
- some 50% of patients have other atopic disorders (hay fever and asthma).

Primary Irritant Dermatitis

In primary irritant dermatitis:

- the epidermis is damaged directly
- the condition may be induced by 'physical' stimuli, for example direct rubbing, or secondary to radiation
- the condition may be induced by exposure to chemicals, for example acids, alkalis, detergents, or urine.

Allergic Contact Dermatitis

Allergic contact dermatitis:

- is a type IV (delayed-type) hypersensitivity reaction (Figure 18.4)
- requires topical exposure to a sensitizing agent
- common sensitizers are nickel, rubber, plants and ointments
- topical antigens are processed by epidermal Langerhans' cells (Figure 18.5)
- the processed antigen is presented to the T cells
- re-exposure to antigen provokes helper T cells to release inflammatory mediators
- patch testing with common allergens is useful in diagnosis

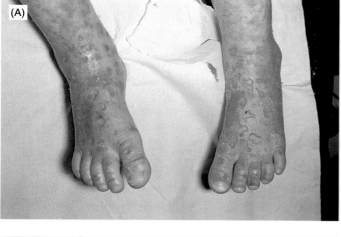

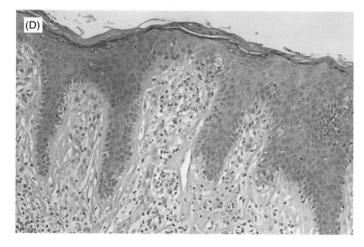

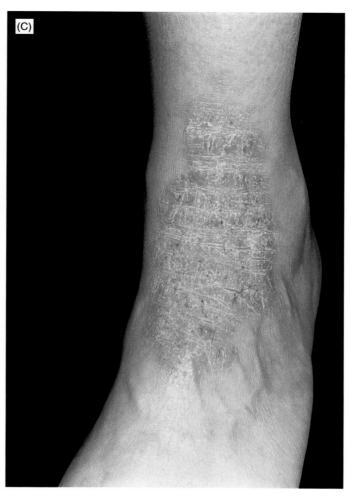

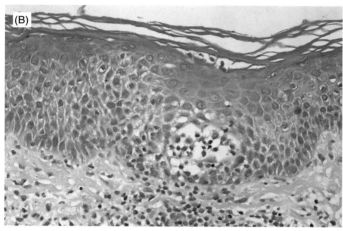

FIGURE 18.3 Acute eczema. Note the blisters oozing oedema fluid (A). The hallmarks of acute eczema are spongiotic oedema (which pushes apart individual keratinocytes) and intraepidermal collections of lymphocytes and oedema fluid known as vesicles (B). Chronic eczema. Here, the skin shows markings resembling tree bark. This appearance is termed lichenification (C). In chronic eczema the epidermis is acanthotic with surface scale. Lymphocytic inflammation is present within the rather fibrotic dermis; however, there is now little evidence of epidermal inflammation and spongiosis (D).

Many other variants of eczema are described. Worthy of note is photoallergic dermatitis, which occurs on sun-exposed sites in response to a topically applied or ingested photosensitizing agent (often a drug). In addition, a huge range of drugs act as antigens or haptens. Subsequent re-exposure to the drug provokes a dermatitis reaction which remits when the drug administration is discontinued. The presence of eosinophils amongst dermal inflammatory cells suggests a drug-based aetiology.

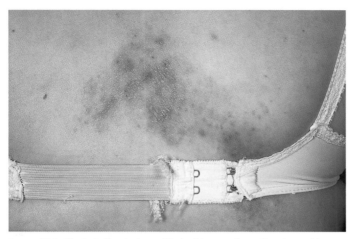

FIGURE 18.4 Contact allergic dermatitis. In this case, the patient is sensitive to nickel in clothes fasteners.

The Psoriasiform Epidermal Reaction Pattern

Psoriasis

> **Key Points**
>
> Psoriasis:
>
> - is a common dermatosis that affects 1–2% of the population
> - has a strong genetic predisposition
> - is characterized by increased epidermal turnover
> - has a relapsing and remitting course.

Clinical Features

Psoriasis is a common inflammatory dermatosis which affects 1–2% of the population. The gender-related incidence is equal, and whilst the condition tends to present in early adulthood the condition may develop at any age. The most common type of psoriasis (psoriasis vulgaris) is characterized by well-defined, pinkish red oval plaques bearing a fine, silver scale. If a few scales are scraped off, then multiple small bleeding points appear on the exposed surface

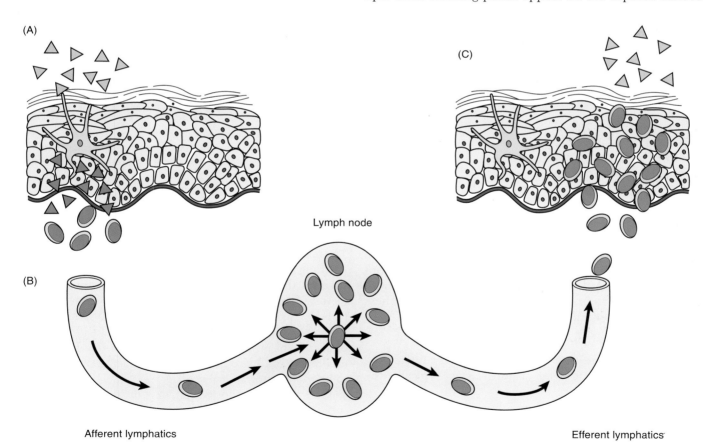

FIGURE 18.5 Contact allergic dermatitis. The immunopathogenesis of this delayed-type hypersensitivity reaction is presented diagrammatically. Langerhans' cells process antigens (pale blue triangles) applied to the epidermal surface. During processing, the antigen is modified (dark blue triangles) which enhances its immunogenicity before being presented to T lymphocytes (green discs) (A). T lymphocytes exposed to antigen then migrate to regional lymph nodes, where there is clonal expansion of specifically sensitized cells (B). Subsequent exposure to the antigen results in chemical signalling which stimulates the proliferation of specifically sensitized T lymphocytes. Cell adhesion molecules allow these lymphocytes to home into the area of re-exposed epidermis where they elaborate the cytokines responsible for eliciting spongiotic dermatitis (C).

(Auspitz's sign). Psoriasis follows a chronic relapsing and remitting course. Relapses can be precipitated by a number of factors including infections, stress and drugs. Plaque development may also be triggered by local trauma (e.g. in the skin bordering a surgical incision). This effect is known as the Koebner phenomenon, the pathogenetic mechanism for which is unclear.

Some patients with chronic psoriasis show nail involvement that varies from minor pitting to extensive destruction (onycholysis) (Figure 18.6); sometimes there is nail loss. Approximately 5% of patients develop a seronegative arthropathy (see Chapter 12) (clinically similar to rheumatoid disease) with involvement of the small joints of the fingers and toes and destruction of the distal interphalyngeal joints. In a small proportion of sufferers the arthritis is exceptionally severe, resulting in marked joint deformity and disability.

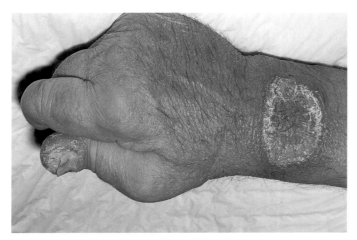

FIGURE 18.6 Psoriasis. This well-defined scaly plaque is typical of psoriasis. Note the dystrophic nail changes.

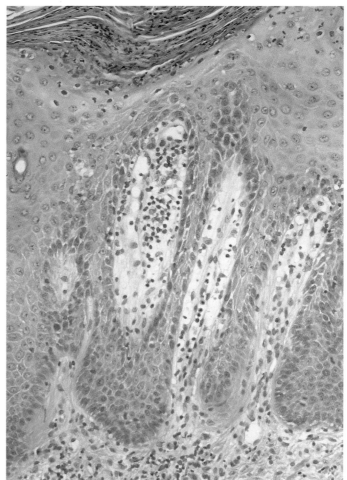

FIGURE 18.7 Psoriasis. The epidermis is acanthotic with evidence of clubbing and fusion of rete ridges. Large numbers of neutrophil polymorphs are apparent within parakeratotic surface scale forming Munro microabscesses.

Several other variants of psoriasis have been described, although all show broadly similar histological changes. In generalized pustular psoriasis, fever and systemic upset accompany the appearance of small sterile pustules on an erythematous background. Rarely, psoriasis presents with generalized erythroderma which may be difficult to distinguish clinically from cutaneous T-cell lymphoma. These unusual variants of psoriasis may be life-threatening.

Microscopic Features

The microscopic features of psoriasis largely reflect the rapid keratinocyte turnover (Figure 18.7). Typically, the following are seen:

- hyperkeratosis
- parakeratosis
- rete ridge elongation
- suprapapillary plate thinning
- frequent suprabasal mitoses
- dilated dermal capillaries
- Munro microabscesses (collections of neutrophils) in the stratum corneum.

Aetiology and Pathogenesis

The aetiology and pathogenesis of psoriasis remain unclear. A strong association with certain human leucocyte antigens suggests that the disease is determined partly by genetic factors. The risk is greatest with human leucocyte antigen (HLA) Cw6, whilst those patients with psoriatic arthropathy have a higher incidence of HLA B27. The identification of agents that trigger psoriasis supports a role for environmental factors. In essence, the aetiology of psoriasis appears to be multifactorial.

One theory proposes that, in genetically predisposed subjects, endogenous or exogenous damage to the stratum corneum leads to the unveiling of antigenic material. An autoantibody response ensues, which culminates in immune complex formation within the stratum corneum and activation of the complement cascade. Components of the complement pathway act as chemoattractant factors for neutrophils, which migrate into the stratum corneum to form characteristic Munro microabscesses.

Established plaques show prominent epidermal hyperplasia due to rapid keratinocyte turnover. In normal skin, the keratinocytes take approximately 28 days to traverse the epidermis prior to being shed. In psoriatic skin, this journey is completed in as few as 3 days. It seems that the inflammatory process is associated with the release of proliferative factors which stimulate epidermal growth. Indeed, keratinocytes from plaques show enhanced surface expression of the receptor for epidermal growth factor and the natural ligand for this receptor (transforming growth factor α) has also been demonstrated in psoriatic skin.

Other Psoriasiform Dermatoses

Psoriasis is the key example of a dermatosis displaying the psoriasiform epidermal reaction pattern (characterized by regular rete ridge elongation). A number of other skin diseases can show this morphological pattern. For example, a proportion of patients with Reiter's syndrome develop mucocutaneous lesions which are difficult to distinguish both clinically and histologically from pustular psoriasis. Psoriasiform epidermal hyperplasia may also be seen in some cases of subacute and chronic eczema (p. 477), superficial dermatophyte infections (p. 495) and in association with the cutaneous T-cell lymphoma mycosis fungoides (p. 505).

The Lichenoid Epidermal Reaction Pattern

Lichen Planus

Clinical Features

This common skin disease is the best example of an inflammatory dermatosis showing a lichenoid pattern of inflammation centred on the basal epidermis. The disease usually presents between the ages of 30 and 60 years, with spontaneous resolution after 1–2 years. The skin lesions are characterized by itchy scaly violaceous papules (Figure 18.8), often with fine white surface markings called Wickham's striae. Lesions develop most commonly on the forearms, wrists, hands and glans penis. The cutaneous lesions often exhibit a symmetrical distribution.

Many patients (up to 70%) have coexisting oral lesions which may be papular, like those on the skin, but may appear as white net-like areas. Some patients with oral lichen planus never develop cutaneous lesions. Oral lesions are often persistent, and chronically ulcerated oral lichen planus is associated with a slightly increased risk of squamous cell carcinoma. Less commonly, there is involvement of other mucous membranes including the upper respiratory tract and anus. Occasionally, lichen planus predominantly involves hair follicle epithelium (lichen planopilaris), leading to destruction of follicular units and alopecia.

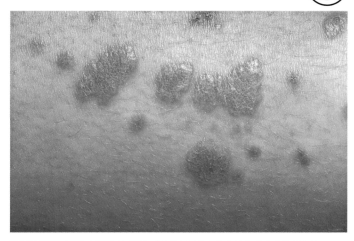

FIGURE 18.8 Lichen planus. Itchy, flat topped, polygonal and violaceous papules are typical of lichen planus.

Microscopic Features

The microscopic features of lichen planus include (Figure 18.9):

- an irregular, 'saw-toothed' acanthosis with hyperkeratosis
- a dense band of lymphocytes at the dermoepidermal junction
- liquefaction degeneration of the basal layer
- the appearance of cytoid bodies in the upper dermis
- melanin pigment incontinence, when melanin released from the damaged basal layer accumulates in the dermis and is phagocytosed by macrophages.

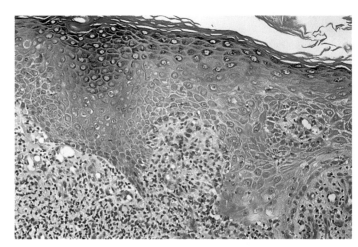

FIGURE 18.9 Lichen planus. The epidermis shows hyperkeratosis, hypergranulosis and irregular acanthosis. Within the upper dermis there is a dense band-like infiltrate of lymphocytes lying in close association with the basal epidermis.

Aetiology and Pathogenesis

The aetiology of lichen planus is unknown, although there appears to be a genetic component as affected individuals are more likely to be HLA DRI- or Dqw1-positive. The pathogenesis is almost certainly immune in nature, with several studies showing increased numbers of epidermal (antigen-presenting) Langerhans' cells, a marked excess of T-helper lymphocytes within the band-like infiltrate and immunoreactants around the dermoepidermal junction and within cytoid bodies. In summary, lichen planus probably represents a cell-mediated hypersensitivity reaction to an unknown epidermal antigen.

Other Lichenoid Dermatoses

Lichen planus is the key example of a dermatosis with a lichenoid pattern of inflammation. Many other conditions show similar features, for example some drugs provoke lichenoid eruptions very similar to lichen planus. Other important examples discussed briefly include lupus erythematosus and erythema multiforme. Graft-versus-host disease – a lichenoid dermatosis seen in a well-defined clinical setting – is presented in Special Study Topic 18.1, p. 484.

Lupus Erythematosus

> **Key Points**
>
> Lupus erythematosus:
>
> - is an autoimmune disorder that occurs mainly in young women
> - is associated with antinuclear and anti-DNA antibodies
> - has predominantly cutaneous (DLE) or multisystem variants (SLE).

Lupus erythematosus (LE) is an autoimmune disorder of early to mid adult life which occurs mainly in females (gender ratio, 2:1). The condition is characterized by the production of autoantibodies directed against 'self' antigens, most of which are nuclear. Circulating antinuclear antibodies (ANA) can be detected by immunofluorescence in 90% of patients. In 50% of cases, antibodies to double-stranded DNA are demonstrated (these are associated with renal involvement (p. 387), and their titres reflect disease activity). A small subset of patients elaborate an antibody (antiRo/SSA) against a cytoplasmic antigen within epidermal keratinocytes. AntiRo/SSA is particularly associated with subacute lupus (see below).

Once the circulating immune complexes localize in the tissues, complement activation is triggered and inflammation results. The mechanism stimulating autoantibody production in LE is unclear. It is proposed that deregulated T-suppressor lymphocytes promote B-lymphocyte over-activity and the overproduction of antibodies against 'self' antigens. Genetic factors appear important in view of an association with several HLA types, whilst environmental agents (e.g. drugs, viruses or UV light) may act as the initiating event by provoking cellular DNA damage and antigen exposure. As for many skin diseases, the aetiology is probably multifactorial.

Three major clinical patterns of LE are described, the most common variant being discoid lupus erythematosus (DLE). This condition characteristically causes scaly red patches in a 'butterfly distribution' over the nose and cheeks (Figure 18.10). Lesions heal slowly with scarring, and scalp involvement results in alopecia. Only 5% of patients with DLE progress to systemic lupus erythematosus (SLE).

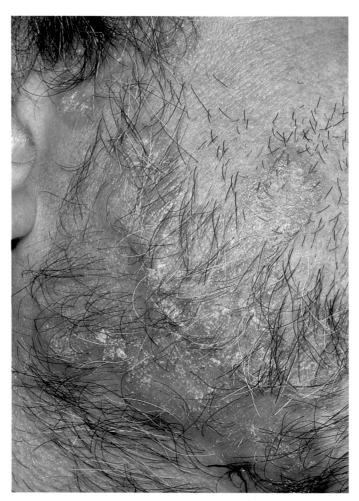

FIGURE 18.10 Chronic discoid lupus erythematosus (CDLE). This is a large plaque of chronic lupus, associated with marked scarring, on the cheek. Sometimes the lesions have a symmetrical 'butterfly' distribution involving the nasal bridge and both cheeks.

Microscopic Features

The microscopic features of LE include (Figure 18.11):

- epidermal atrophy and hyperkeratosis
- follicular plugging

- superficial and deep perivascular and periappendigeal lymphocytic infiltrate
- a lichenoid pattern of basal layer liquefaction degeneration
- basement membrane thickening (with chronicity)
- most patients show granular basement membrane deposition of IgG, M or C₃ on immunofluorescence.

of drugs, and neoplasms. In 50% of cases a trigger is not identified.

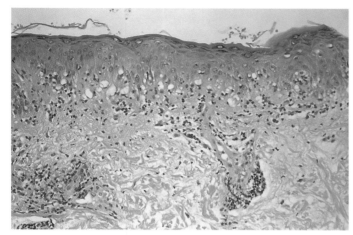

FIGURE 18.11 Chronic discoid lupus erythematosus (CDLE). In this active lesion of lupus the epidermis is atrophic and hyperkeratotic. Numerous lymphocytes are apparent close to the basal epidermis, and this is associated with striking liquefaction degeneration.

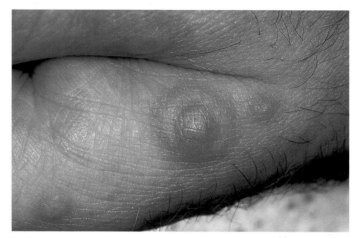

FIGURE 18.12 Erythema multiforme (EM). This is a classic 'target' lesion of EM. Note the central discrete area of blistering.

Systemic lupus erythematosus is a chronically remitting and relapsing multisystem disorder which may involve the skin, causing DLE-type changes. However, the involvement of other tissues (e.g. kidney, joints, heart, lung, CNS and serosal surfaces) dominates the clinical picture. With immunosuppressive treatment, the 10-year survival rate now exceeds 90%. Subacute LE (associated with antiRo/SSA) presents as a recurring photosensitive rash on the face, trunk and upper limbs. Visceral involvement is rare.

Erythema Multiforme

This fairly common self-limiting and sometimes recurrent dermatosis may present as macules, papules and blisters. The classic variant begins with erythematous maculopapular lesions which develop into 'target lesions' with a red margin and a dusky, blistered centre (Figure 18.12). Severe cases with oral and conjunctival involvement (Stevens–Johnson syndrome) may prove fatal.

A number of factors can precipitate erythema multiforme by provoking a cell-mediated immune response. Triggers include viral infection (e.g. herpes simplex), bacterial infection (particularly *Mycoplasma pneumoniae*), a range

Microscopy

Microscopy of erythema multiforme includes (Figure 18.13):

- a lichenoid pattern of inflammation
- lymphocytes extending into the epidermis
- vacuolar changes at the dermoepidermal junction
- subepidermal blistering
- cytoid bodies above the basal layer
- epidermal necrosis.

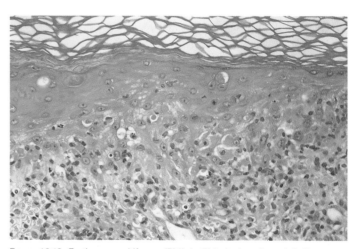

FIGURE 18.13 Erythema multiforme (EM). In EM, the lymphocytic infiltrate tends to obscure the dermoepidermal junction. Lymphocytes infiltrate the epidermis, and scattered eosinophilic cytoid bodies are evident within both the basal and suprabasal layers.

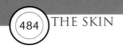

GRAFT-VERSUS-HOST DISEASE (GVHD)

This condition usually develops in an immunocompromised patient given histo-incompatible lymphocytes from an immunocompetent donor. Consequently, GVHD is usually seen in patients receiving a bone marrow transplant for treatment of marrow aplasia, leukaemia or one of the primary immunodeficiency states. Acute GVHD ensues in approximately 50% of patients who have received an HLA-matched allogeneic bone marrow transplant. The syndrome is thought to be due to competent donor cytotoxic T lymphocytes attacking recipient epithelial cells which express unmatched minor histocompatibility antigens.

GVHD affects primarily the skin and mucous membranes, gastrointestinal tract and liver. The cutaneous lesions of acute GVHD are erythematous macules and papules which may be widespread, but often affect the palms and soles most severely. Microscopy reveals features similar to erythema multiforme, with vacuolar degeneration of the basal epidermis and scattered necrotic eosinophilic keratinocytes involving all of the epidermal layers (Figure 18.14). Typically, one or more lymphocytes can be seen lying in close approximation to a degenerate keratinocyte (this phenomenon is referred to as 'lymphocyte-associated apoptosis' or 'satellite cell necrosis').

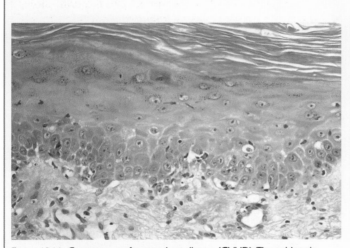

FIGURE 18.14 Cutaneous graft-versus-host disease (GVHD). The epidermis shows marked hyperkeratosis, and there is a sparse infiltrate of lymphocytes extending into the epidermis. Note the close relationship between the intrusive lymphocytes and the eosinophilic apoptotic keratinocytes ('satellite cell necrosis').

Chronic GVHD supervenes in 10% of patients who have received an allogeneic bone marrow transplant. In the chronic phase, cutaneous and oral lesions resembling lichen planus develop. Ultimately, the skin displays marked dermal fibrosis resembling the sclerodermatous skin changes of progressive systemic sclerosis.

The gastrointestinal tract and liver are commonly involved in GVHD. The oesophagus may become inflamed and, in the chronic phase, fibrosis and stricture formation ensue. Colonic involvement manifests primarily as diarrhoea which reflects lymphocyte-induced apoptosis of the crypt epithelium (Figure 18.15). The liver exhibits a periportal lymphocytic infiltrate with damage to the epithelial cells lining the bile ducts and to the hepatocytes (Figure 18.16).

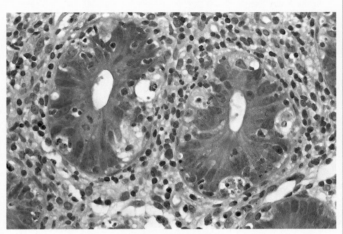

FIGURE 18.15 Gastrointestinal tract GVHD. In this section from the colon there is nuclear debris around the periphery of the glands. This debris originates from epithelial cells undergoing lymphocyte-associated apoptosis.

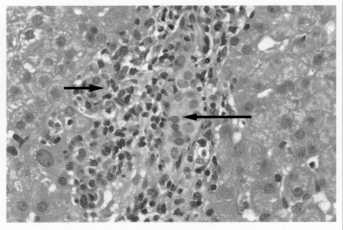

FIGURE 18.16 Hepatic GVHD. The bile ducts arrows in this portal tract are surrounded by lymphocytes. A few lymphocytes infiltrate between the ductal epithelial cells, some of which are undergoing apoptosis.

GVHD is associated with a high morbidity and mortality, and patients with this condition are especially prone to overwhelming opportunistic infection.

Further Reading

Aractingi S, Chosidow O. Cutaneous graft-versus-host disease. *Arch Dermatol* 1998; **134**:602–612.

The Vesiculobullous Epidermal Reaction Pattern

General

> **Key Points**
>
> In bullous disorders:
>
> - blisters may follow injury due to heat, infections and drug reactions
> - specific autoimmune disorders are characterized by attack on epidermal cell adhesion molecules
> - the specific location of loss of cell adhesion and immunofluorescence staining allows precise diagnoses to be made.

A range of skin conditions are associated with the formation of blisters (more correctly termed vesicles or bullae). Examples include thermal injury, insect-bite reactions, drug reactions and various cutaneous infections by viruses, bacteria and fungi. Some of the inflammatory dermatoses already discussed can cause vesicles and bullae. For example, in eczematous dermatitis the degree of intraepidermal spongiotic oedema may be sufficiently marked to produce macroscopic vesicles. Similarly, many of the lichenoid disorders (particularly lichen planus and erythema multiforme) can cause blisters reflecting damage to the basal keratinocytes which anchor the epidermis to the underlying basement membrane and dermis.

The remainder of this section concentrates on the major primary vesiculobullous disorders, namely pemphigus vulgaris, bullous pemphigoid and dermatitis herpetiformis. These three acquired conditions share an autoimmune pathogenesis, although the target antigen in each is different. The study of these conditions has furthered greatly our knowledge of the molecules that hold skin together (Figure 18.17).

Epidermal keratinocytes are held together by adhesion molecules. The intracellular domains of these molecules are linked to the actin and keratin filaments of the cytoskeleton, whilst the extracellular portions are homophilic and bind to other adhesion molecules of the same family or, at the basal layer, to extracellular matrix molecules of the basement membrane.

Of prime importance in maintaining epidermal cell adhesion are the family of calcium-dependent adhesion molecules called the *cadherins*, that are found within desmosomes. One desmosomal cadherin (desmoglein 3) located primarily within the prickle cell layer is the target antigen in pemphigus vulgaris.

The integrin family of cell adhesion molecules also plays a role in keratinocyte–keratinocyte cohesion, but these are mainly of interest because of their location in the hemidesmosomes which bind basal keratinocytes to basement membrane matrix molecules such as epiligrin, fibronectin and laminin. Integrins are heterodimers composed of an α and a β chain. Although various chains exist, the subtype $\alpha6/\beta4$, which is found within the hemidesmosomes of basal cells, is crucial in maintaining epidermal–dermal adhesion because of its affinity for the extracellular matrix ligand laminin. Lying in close association with $\alpha6/\beta4$ integrin are the major (230 kDa) and minor (180 kDa) target antigens for bullous pemphigoid. These antigens are distinct from $\alpha6/\beta4$ integrin, although it appears to be destroyed by the intensity of the immunologically mediated attack on its neighbours. Disruption of $\alpha6/\beta4$ integrin–laminin binding plays a major role in generating the subepidermal bullae seen in pemphigoid.

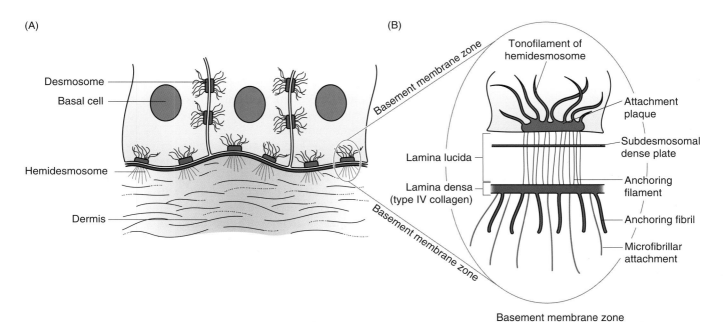

FIGURE 18.17 Diagram illustrating the mechanisms responsible for epidermal–epidermal adhesion (A) and epidermal–dermal adhesion (B).

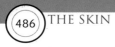
Pemphigus Vulgaris

Four variants of pemphigus are described – all are rare, although pemphigus vulgaris is the most common, accounting for 80% of cases. This disease of the middle-aged and elderly often commences with painful oral blisters and erosions. After weeks or months, fragile bullae develop on the trunk (Figure 18.18), axillae, groins, scalp and face. Lesions may also involve the conjunctiva, the membranes of the upper aerodigestive tract, the lower genitourinary tract and the anus.

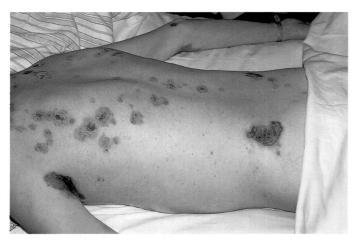

FIGURE 18.18 Pemphigus vulgaris. The fragile blisters of pemphigus vulgaris are often disrupted, leaving shallow erosions.

The blisters of pemphigus are easily traumatized, leaving shallow erosions which ooze blood and then crust over. New lesions can be induced by gentle friction over apparently normal skin (Nikolsky's sign). Treatment with immunosuppressive agents such as corticosteroids and azathioprine is generally successful. The mortality rate of 5–15% usually reflects overwhelming infection complicating steroid therapy or biochemical derangements seen in very extensive disease.

In pemphigus vulgaris the immune system elaborates an IgG autoantibody against desmoglein 3 which maintains desmosomal attachments in the prickle cell layer. Once antibody–antigen complexes form on the cell surface, the desmosomes are disrupted by components of the complement cascade, and also by proteases liberated from epidermal cells; this results in acantholysis and loss of epithelial integrity. Direct immunofluorescence on fresh biopsy material demonstrates a meshwork of intraepidermal IgG, and most patients have circulating pemphigus antibody which can be demonstrated using monkey oesophagus or human skin as an *in-vitro* substrate.

The pathogenetic mechanism resulting in the epidermal blistering of pemphigus vulgaris is now established, although the factors which initiate autoantibody production are unclear. Trauma, radiation, burns, chemicals and drugs may lead to exposure of desmoglein 3 to the immune system. However, an excess of certain HLA types (A10,

A26, Bw38 and DR4) suggest that genetic factors are also relevant.

Microscopy

In pemphigus vulgaris:

- the classic lesion is a suprabasal blister (Figure 18.19)
- basal keratinocytes remain attached to the basement membrane
- the bulla contains scattered acantholytic keratinocytes (Figure 18.19)
- inflammation is sparse
- direct immunofluorescence shows deposition of IgG between epidermal keratinocytes (Figure 18.21A).

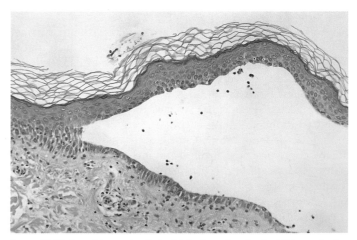

FIGURE 18.19 Pemphigus vulgaris. In this bullous disorder the blister cavity lies above the basal layer, which remains attached to the basement membrane.

Bullous Pemphigoid

Bullous pemphigoid is a chronic bullous disorder of the elderly. Although rare, the condition is more common than pemphigus vulgaris, and has a more benign course. Blisters develop over the abdomen, groins and flexor surfaces of the limbs. Oral involvement occurs in only 10% of cases, and other mucous membranes are affected rarely. The blisters of bullous pemphigoid are larger than those of pemphigus vulgaris and are more resistant to trauma (reflecting their subepidermal location), and the Nikolsky sign is negative. Lesions may develop on previously normal skin or on erythematous itchy macules which precede blistering by weeks or months.

In bullous pemphigoid, IgG autoantibodies are targeted against a major and/or a minor antigen of the hemidesmosomes which fix basal cells to basement membrane. These antigens colocalize with $\alpha6/\beta4$ integrin–laminin complexes which suffer collateral damage when immune complexes activate complement, resulting in eosinophil chemotaxis and proteinase release. The mechanisms triggering the formation of autoantibodies to hemidesmosome antigens are unknown, although the suspected factors are similar to those implicated in causing pemphigus vulgaris (i.e. trauma, burns, radiation and a range of drugs). In 80% of patients the presence of circulating IgG autoantibodies can be demonstrated, although their titre does not correlate with disease severity or activity.

Microscopy

In bullous pemphigoid:

- the subepidermal bulla contains fibrin and eosinophils
- the blister roof comprises full-thickness epidermis
- there is upper dermal oedema
- there is dermal inflammation with lymphocytes and eosinophils (Figure 18.20)
- direct immunofluorescence shows linear IgG and/or C_3 at the dermoepidermal junction (Figure 18.21B).

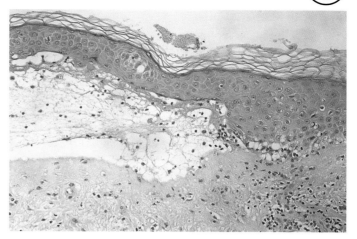

FIGURE 18.20 Bullous pemphigoid. In this condition the blister cavity lies beneath the full thickness of the epidermis. Note the large numbers of eosinophil leucocytes within the dermis and bulla.

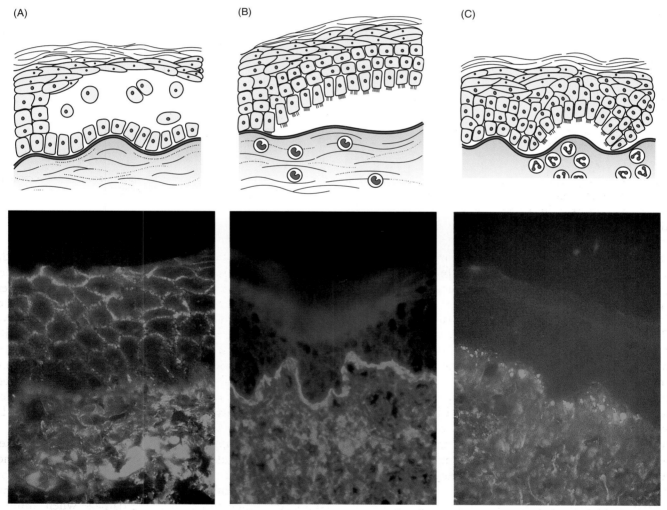

(A)   (B)   (C)

FIGURE 18.21 Pemphigus vulgaris. (A) Direct immunofluorescence demonstrates a 'chickenwire' pattern of IgG deposition within the epidermis. The line drawing emphasizes the suprabasal site of bulla formation with preservation of the basal layer. (B) Bullous pemphigoid. Direct immunofluorescence demonstrates a linear band of IgG deposition along the basement membrane zone. The line drawing illustrates that the bulla is subepidermal; however, the basement membrane does remain attached to the dermis and forms the floor of the blister – this is not obvious on routine histology. Eosinophils are often the predominant cell type in the inflammatory infiltrate. (C) Dermatitis herpetiformis. Direct immunofluorescence shows coarse granules of IgA deposited in the papillary dermis. The line drawing shows a discrete focus of subepidermal blistering associated with an infiltrate of neutrophil polymorphs.

Dermatitis Herpetiformis

This rare, chronic blistering disease usually presents in early adulthood. The eruption is characterized by crops of intensely itchy papules and vesicles which typically develop over the elbows and knees in a symmetrical distribution. Other common sites include the scalp, neck, shoulders and buttocks. Due to scratching and excoriation, intact vesicles are seen infrequently. Large bullae occur rarely.

Dermatitis herpetiformis is of particular interest because of its strong association with gluten-sensitive enteropathy (p. 245). Up to 90% of patients with skin lesions have histological evidence of gluten-sensitive enteropathy on small-bowel biopsy, although most are asymptomatic. The pathogenesis of dermatitis herpetiformis is unknown, although direct immunofluorescence studies reveal granular deposits of IgA in the dermal papillae (Figure 18.21C). It is proposed that IgA antibodies targeted against the gliadin component of gluten also react with connective tissue matrix proteins of the dermal papillae. Once the immune complexes are formed, the complement cascade is activated, generating neutrophil chemotaxins. Neutrophil microabscesses at the tips of the dermal papillae are the microscopic hallmark of dermatitis herpetiformis (see Case History 18.1).

18.1 CASE HISTORY

BLISTERING RASH

A 68-year-old man was referred to the dermatology department complaining of intensely pruritic lesions over his elbows (Figure 18.22). Examination demonstrated excoriated papulovesicles over the extensor aspects of both forearms. Dermatitis herpetiformis (DH) was thought most likely. A fresh (i.e. not formalin-fixed) skin biopsy was submitted for direct immunofluorescence and histopathology investigations. Blood for antigliadin and antiendomysial antibodies was sent to the immunopathology department. Meanwhile, the patient received a course of dapsone, with rapid relief of pruritis.

Microscopy shows subepidermal blistering with papillary dermal microabscesses typical of DH (Figures 18.23 and 18.24). Granular deposits of IgA within the

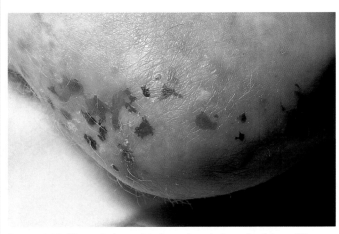

FIGURE 18.22 The typical excoriated papulovesicular rash of dermatitis herpetiformis.

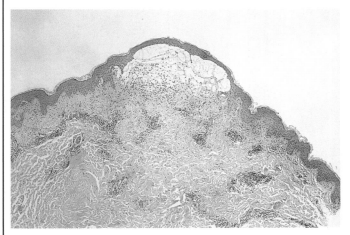

FIGURE 18.23 Scanning magnification demonstrates a discrete focus of subepidermal vesiculation.

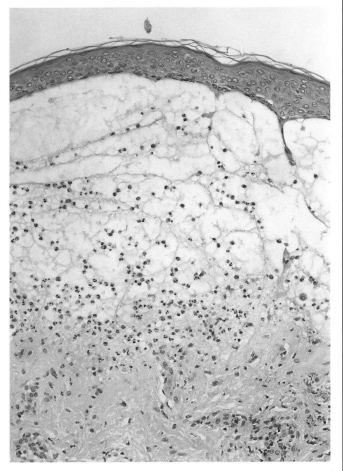

FIGURE 18.24 At higher magnification, large numbers of neutrophil polymorphs are apparent within the blister cavity and within the floor of the blister.

18.1 CASE HISTORY

papillary dermis (similar to those shown in Figure 18.21C) and positive serology supported this diagnosis.

Although the patient was free of gastrointestinal symptoms, an endoscopic biopsy of his distal duodenum revealed subtotal villous atrophy with excessive intraepithelial lymphocytes compatible with gluten-sensitive enteropathy (Figure 18.25). A gluten-free diet was introduced, and the skin lesions regressed slowly after several months, allowing the dose of dapsone to be reduced.

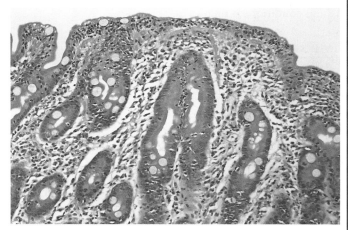

FIGURE 18.25 A biopsy of the distal duodenum demonstrates subtotal villous atrophy together with crypt hyperplasia and a marked increase in intraepithelial lymphocytes. These features are compatible with gluten-sensitive enteropathy.

INFLAMMATION OF THE DERMIS AND SUBCUTIS

General

The inflammatory disorders presented so far have centred on the epidermis. However, a range of conditions primarily involve the various components of the dermis or the subcutaneous fat. An example of a disease for each component is presented in Table 18.4.

TABLE 18.4 Examples of inflammatory conditions that primarily affect the dermis and subcutis

Skin component affected	Disorder
Dermal connective tissue	Granuloma annulare
Pilosebaceous units	Acne vulgaris
Dermal blood vessels	Leucocytoclastic (allergic) vasculitis
Subcutaneous fat	Erythema nodosum

Dermal Connective Tissue

Granuloma Annulare

This common condition of children and young adults causes raised annular lesions on the dorsal aspects of the fingers and hands. Microscopy demonstrates a central zone of collagen degeneration bounded by a rim of palisading macrophages (Figure 18.26). A subcutaneous variant (mainly seen on the lower legs of children) may mimic closely a rheumatoid nodule. Necrobiosis lipoidica, whilst similar histologically, differs by causing firm reddish yellow plaques on the lower legs of middle-aged females. Some 60% of patients with necrobiosis

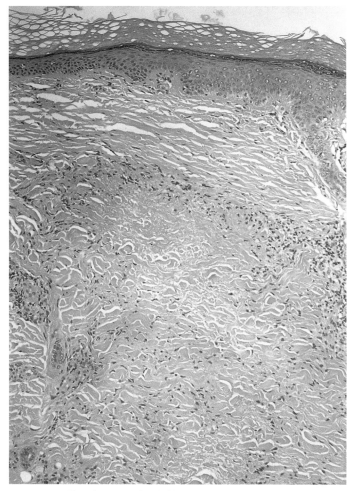

FIGURE 18.26 Granuloma annulare. Within the dermis there is a zone of amorphous and eosinophilic collagen degeneration. A rim of histiocytes surrounds the area of collagen degeneration (forming a palisading granuloma).

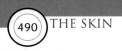
lipoidica have, or will develop, diabetes mellitus. The cause of these conditions is unknown.

Pilosebaceous Units

Acne Vulgaris

This common inflammatory disorder of the pilosebaceous units of the face and trunk is, to varying degrees, experienced by most adolescents. At puberty, the pilosebaceous units appear particularly sensitive to increased levels of circulating androgens. This stimulatory effect promotes increased keratin production within the pilosebaceous ducts (which become plugged, leading to comedones), whilst enhanced sebum production results in cystic dilatation of the remaining unit. Subsequent colonization of plugged units by *Corynebacterium acnes* may invoke an acute inflammatory response. Rupture of plugged, distended and infected units releases debris into the dermis, eliciting an intense foreign body granulomatous reaction which may heal with scarring.

Dermal Blood Vessels

Leucocytoclastic (Allergic) Vasculitis

An acute vasculitis of the small dermal blood vessels is a common cause of purpura. This condition is mediated by immune complex deposition, and common precipitating factors include infections, drugs and underlying malignancy. Some children with Henoch–Schönlein purpura (a variant of allergic vasculitis) have systemic involvement evidenced by joint pain, gastrointestinal pain and haemorrhage, and glomerulonephritis.

In allergic vasculitis, circulating immune complexes are deposited in the walls of small venules. This leads to complement activation and the production of neutrophil chemotaxins. The neutrophils release lysosomal enzymes, which damage the venules leading to endothelial cell swelling, thrombosis, fibrinoid necrosis and red cell leakage (purpura) (Figure 18.27). Many of the neutrophils undergo karyorrhexis. Direct immunofluorescence of early lesions may reveal immunoglobulin and C_3 within the walls of damaged vessels.

Subcutaneous Fat

Erythema Nodosum

This panniculitis presents as tender red nodules which appear over the lower legs and resolve slowly over a period of several weeks. The condition, which is more common in females, occurs in association with infections (*Streptococcus* and *Yersinia*), chronic inflammatory bowel disease, sarcoidosis and some drugs. Microscopy reveals chronic inflammation of the subcutaneous tissue, particularly the fibrous septae which divide the fat into lobules. Frequently,

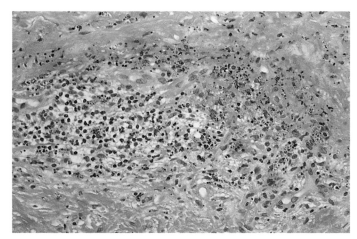

FIGURE 18.27 Leucocytoclastic (allergic) vasculitis. The dermal capillary blood vessels are surrounded by an intense infiltrate of neutrophil polymorphs. Capillary endothelial cells appear swollen and the presence of abundant nuclear debris is in keeping with leucocytoclasis.

there is evidence of venulitis with associated haemorrhage. The aetiology is unclear, with no compelling evidence that the condition is immune complex-mediated. A rarer condition is erythema induratum (or nodular vasculitis) which, in some cases, represents an immune response to underlying tuberculosis (a tuberculid reaction). The inflammation in erythema induratum involves both the fat lobules and septal connective tissue; it is often granulomatous, and vasculitis is a major feature.

INFECTIVE DISORDERS

General

A wide spectrum of organisms is capable of infecting the skin. Some cutaneous infecting organisms, such as the superficial dermatophyte which causes athlete's foot, are very common pathogens, whilst others are rare. Precisely what constitutes core knowledge for the reader will largely depend on geography. Nevertheless, a combination of inexpensive air travel and holiday packages to remote destinations ensures that even the most exotic of cutaneous infections will be encountered occasionally. Discussion of infections generally encountered in tropical regions (e.g. protozoa and helminths) is beyond the scope of this text, but some of these are discussed in Chapter 19.

Healthy skin is resilient to pathogens unless its integrity is compromised, or the immunocompetence of the host is diminished. The types of infection to be discussed include:

- viral infections
- bacterial infections
- fungal infections
- arthropod infestations.

Viral Infections

Key Points

Viral infections:

- may cause a short-lasting rash which is often vesicular
- overwhelming infection may occur in immunosuppressed patients, or in those with eczema
- some viruses are capable of latent infections, with subsequent reactivation
- some viruses cause the formation of tumours, benign or malignant.

Herpesvirus Infections

General

The herpesvirus family comprises several biologically and serologically distinct members. Understanding of this group continues to evolve, with human herpesvirus-8 recently being identified as the causative agent of Kaposi's sarcoma (p. 504). Three members of this family are associated commonly with skin disease (Table 18.5).

TABLE 18.5 The spectrum of skin conditions associated with the herpesvirus family

Herpes virus type	Main clinical association
Herpes simplex (type 1)	Recurrent herpes labialis (cold sores)
Herpes simplex (type 2)	Recurrent genital herpes
Varicella zoster virus	Primary infection is varicella (chickenpox)
	Reactivation of latent virus causes zoster (shingles)

Herpes Simplex Virus Type 1

Herpes simplex virus type 1 (HSV-1) is associated with a mild or asymptomatic primary oropharyngeal infection in childhood. At the time of primary infection, the virus passes along sensory nerves to infect and lie dormant within the neuronal cells of sensory ganglia. Latent HSV-1 infection is very common, with 80% of the population harbouring the virus within the trigeminal ganglion. Latent virus can be reactivated by several factors such as febrile illnesses, sunburn, menstruation, trauma and stress. Once reactivated, the virus passes down the sensory nerves, producing tingling and discomfort and followed soon after by crops of painful vesicles which resolve in about 1 week without scarring. Typically, the vesicles develop around the lips (herpes labialis) and are known commonly as 'cold sores'. Severe disseminated infection may occur in immunocompromised patients. Widespread primary infection of the skin (eczema herpeticum) is seen occasionally in patients with atopic eczema. This is a severe condition with fever and constitutional upset which may prove fatal. Eczema herpeticum and the histological features of HSV-1 infection are discussed in more detail in Case History 18.2.

Herpes Simplex Virus Type 2

Herpes simplex virus type 2 (HSV-2) preferentially causes genital lesions, and is transmitted primarily by sexual contact. HSV-2 also lies dormant within sensory ganglia, leaving the host prone to developing intermittent crops of painful vesicles. The factors which trigger reactivation are broadly similar to those for HSV-1. Neonatal HSV-2 infection occurs in 10% of children delivered to women with active herpetic lesions. This severe and potentially fatal infection can be avoided by caesarean section.

Varicella Zoster Virus

Varicella zoster virus (VZV; herpes virus type 3) causes the very common acute vesicular eruption known as varicella

VIRAL SKIN INFECTION

A 19-year-old woman, with a long history of flexural atopic eczema requiring topical steroids, was referred urgently to the dermatology department with an extensive eruption over the right foot and ankle (Figure 18.28), in association with fever and lethargy. Examination confirmed ulcerating papulovesicular lesions and tender groin lymphadenopathy. Eczema herpeticum was suspected, and a diagnostic biopsy was submitted for confirmation. The patient was commenced on the oral antiviral drug, acyclovir.

The biopsy demonstrated vesiculation and an intense lymphocytic infiltrate (Figure 18.29). Many keratinocytes exhibit classic changes of herpesvirus infection with multinucleation and nuclear pallor

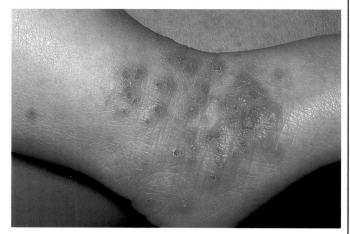

FIGURE 18.28 Numerous ulcerated vesicles are evident over the ankle.

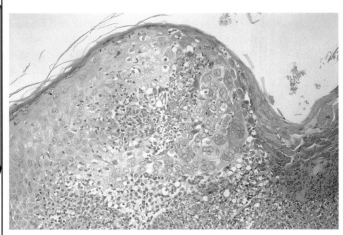

FIGURE 18.29 Scanning magnification shows intense inflammation involving the dermis and epidermis. Loss of nuclear staining and multi-nucleation can be appreciated even at this power.

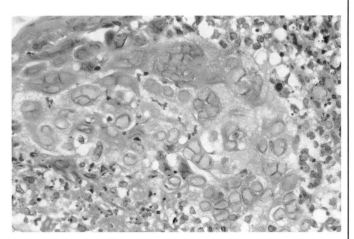

FIGURE 18.30 At higher magnification, the characteristic cytopathic effects of herpesvirus infection are clearly demonstrated. Margination of nuclear chromatin results in the nuclei appearing 'empty', and many of the keratinocytes are multinucleated.

(Figure 18.30). After a few days, a secondary bacterial infection developed, and *Staphylococcus aureus* was cultured from a swab. Treatment with oral flucloxacillin was instituted, and the lesions healed completely after 3 weeks.

(chickenpox). This highly infectious childhood condition is characterized by crops of vesicles and pustules at varying stages of crusting and healing. When acquired in adulthood the disease is often more severe, although widespread dissemination with potentially fatal encephalitis or pneumonitis is usually restricted to immunocompromised hosts.

VZV also has the ability to lie dormant within sensory ganglia. Reactivation causes herpes zoster ('shingles'), a fairly common condition seen in adults. Reactivation becomes more likely with increasing age, perhaps reflecting a reduced pool of memory T-cells specific for the virus. Patients with immunodeficiency are especially prone to developing herpes zoster, which rarely may disseminate (with potentially fatal results).

The onset of herpes zoster is heralded by pain and discomfort in the affected dermatome. After a short period the skin becomes erythematous, and crops of vesicles appear. The vesicles often become pustular, crust over and heal after approximately 14 days. These lesions are mildly infectious, and non-immune individuals (usually children) may contract varicella following exposure to an adult with herpes zoster. Herpes zoster mainly causes lesions on the trunk and abdomen, although cranial involvement is not uncommon. Involvement of the ophthalmic branch of the trigeminal nerve results in ocular complications (including blindness) in 30% of cases. Herpes zoster may be associated with severe persistent pain.

The histopathological changes seen in VZV infection are very similar to those of HSV-1 and HSV-2.

Human Papillomavirus Infections (HPV)

General

The HPV family of DNA-containing viruses incorporates more than 60 subtypes responsible for various warty lesions. Transmission of HPV occurs by direct inoculation of infected desquamated cells onto host skin. HPV replication occurs in the superficial prickle and granular cell layers where infected cells remain shielded from the blood supply (and immune system), allowing lesions to persist for months or years. Eventually, warts tend to regress spontaneously – an event which is associated with lymphocytic infiltration reflecting a cell-mediated immune response. Patients with diminished cellular immunity are especially prone to HPV infection, the resulting lesions being persistent and refractory to treatment.

Specific HPV subtypes are associated with different verrucous lesions (Table 18.6).

TABLE 18.6 The clinical distribution of skin warts typically associated with specific subtypes of the human papilloma virus (HPV) family

HPV type	Main clinical association
HPV-1	Plantar warts
HPV-2 (less often 1, 4 and 7)	Common warts
HPV-3 (less often 10)	Plane warts
HPV-6 (less often 11)	Anogenital warts
HPV-16 (less often 18)	Anogenital warts at risk of neoplastic transformation

Common Warts

The common wart (verruca vulgaris) is seen most frequently on the dorsal aspects of the hands and fingers, and on the face. Warts appear as keratotic papules that are 1–10 mm in diameter, and spontaneous involution ensues within months or a few years. Malignant transformation is very rare, except in the verrucae developing in immunosuppressed renal transplant patients.

Microscopy

Microscopy of common warts (Figure 18.31) typically shows:

- hyperkeratosis and parakeratosis
- irregular epidermal acanthosis and papillomatosis
- superficial vacuolated koilocytes (HPV-infected keratinocytes)
- clumping of keratohyalin granules
- lymphocytic infiltration (if regressing).

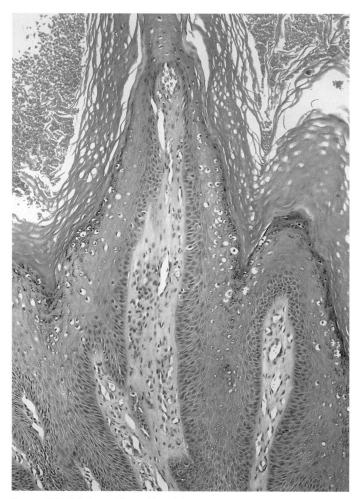

FIGURE 18.31 Viral wart. The epidermis is thrown into folds (papillomatosis), and there is marked hyperkeratosis. Within the superficial layers of the epidermis many of the keratinocytes display nuclear pyknosis and perinuclear halos. These koilocytes indicate the presence of papillomavirus infection.

Plantar Warts

This common type of wart occurs on the sole of the foot. Infection is seen in young individuals, and it is probably acquired in communal changing rooms and swimming pools. The lesions resemble common warts, except that they have an endophytic growth pattern and lie largely beneath the markedly hyperkeratotic skin surface.

Plane Warts

These fleshy, flat-topped warts develop in the same areas as common warts, but show less marked filiform acanthosis. Plane warts have a tendency to occur at sites of trauma (the Koebner phenomenon), and crops of lesions may develop in areas of scratching.

Anogenital Warts

HPV infection of the anogenital skin is seen primarily in young, sexually active adults. Lesions vary in size from small inconspicuous papules up to large fleshy condylomata. Malignant transformation is unusual with HPV types 6 and 11, whilst HPV types 16 and 18 are associated with a significant risk of progression (via dysplasia) to invasive squamous cell carcinoma. Perineal HPV infection is the principal cause of carcinoma of the anal region and vulva. Females with perineal condylomata should have regular smears as they frequently have concurrent HPV infection and dysplasia of the vulva and cervix (pp. 402–404).

Poxvirus Infections

General

The most famous member of this family is variola (smallpox), which is of historic interest only following its eradication. The poxvirus infection seen most commonly is molluscum contagiosum. Much less common is Orf, an endemic poxvirus infection of sheep, which occasionally causes large necrotic skin lesions on the hands and forearms of sheephandlers.

Molluscum Contagiosum

This common poxvirus infection is associated with dome-shaped, umbilicated papules on the face and limbs of young children. In adulthood, genital lesions occur, reflecting sexual transmission. The lesions typically regress spontaneously within a few months. Extensive crops of persistent lesions may occur in patients with impaired cellular immunity.

Microscopy

Microscopy of molluscum contagiosum (Figure 18.32) includes:

- endophytic hyperplasia of the epidermis
- a central crater
- large eosinophilic viral inclusion bodies
- inclusions (molluscum bodies) which replace the entire cell and are shed onto the surface.

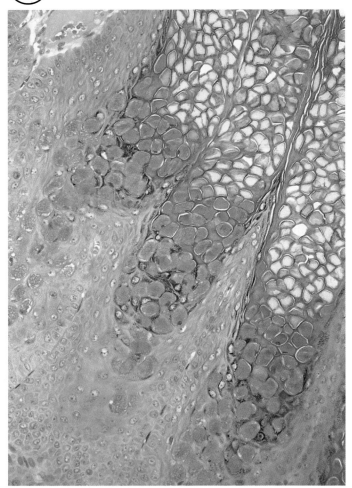

FIGURE 18.32 Molluscum contagiosum. Large eosinophilic intracytoplasmic viral inclusions are present within the superficial layers of the epidermis.

Bacterial Infections

Key Points

Bacterial infections:

- are usually due to non-resident flora
- pyogenic organisms cause localized abscesses or rapidly spreading cellulitis
- mycobacteria cause important world-wide chronic infections, for example leprosy.

General

The large number of commensal bacteria which colonize the skin surface only occasionally assume pathogenic importance. Of greater importance are bacteria that do not form part of the resident flora and which are generally acquired by person-to-person contact. A simple method of classifying the more commonly encountered bacterial infections is presented in Table 18.7.

TABLE 18.7 Examples of skin conditions associated with various types of bacterial infection

Bacterium	Main clinical associations
Coccobacilli	
Staphylococcus aureus	Impetigo
	Staphylococcal scalded skin syndrome
	Furuncles and carbuncles
β-Haemolytic streptococci	Erysipelas
	Cellulitis
	Necrotizing fasciitis
Mycobacteria	
Mycobacterium leprae	Leprosy
Mycobacterium tuberculosis	Various lesions
Mycobacterium marinum	Swimming pool granuloma
Spirochaetes	
Trichomonas pallidum	Syphilis
Borrelia burgdorferi	Erythema chronicum migrans

Staphylococcal Infections

Impetigo

This acute superficial pyogenic infection of the upper epidermal layers, seen most commonly in young children, presents as a pustular eruption on the face or extremities with crusted golden exudate. Impetigo is generally caused by *Staphylococcus aureus*, although group A β-haemolytic streptococci are sometimes isolated.

Staphylococcal Scalded Skin Syndrome

This rare condition of infants and young children is caused by a specific *Staphylococcus aureus* (group 2, phage type 71). This organism elaborates an epidermolytic toxin causing widespread erythema and desquamation. After several days, antibodies neutralize the toxin and facilitate healing. In some individuals (particularly adults), potentially fatal staphylococcal septicaemia ensues.

Furuncles and Carbuncles

These common lesions reflect staphylococcal infection of hair follicles. A furuncle (boil) involves a solitary follicular unit, whereas a carbuncle involves several adjacent follicles. Purulent exudate may discharge through the follicular ostium, although in some cases surgical drainage is required. Furuncles and carbuncles are more common in diabetics.

β-Haemolytic Streptococcal Infections

Erysipelas and Cellulitis

Erysipelas is a sharply demarcated and rapidly spreading infection of the superficial dermis. The preferential sites are the legs and, less often, the face. Cellulitis is a less well-demarcated and more deeply sited infection of the dermis and subcutaneous fat.

Necrotizing Fasciitis

This rare and exceptionally severe form of cellulitis is associated with necrosis of the skin, subcutis, fascial connective tissue and underlying skeletal muscle. The leg and perineum are the usual sites of occurrence and scrotal involvement may occur (Fournier's gangrene). The causal β-haemolytic streptococcus often acts in association with anaerobic bacteria, leading to gas formation in the deep tissues. This rapidly progressive and often fatal infection necessitates early and vigorous surgical treatment.

Mycobacterial Infections

Mycobacterial infection is associated with chronic granulomatous inflammation within the dermis. Leprosy affects 15 million people in tropical countries. Cutaneous infection with *M. tuberculosis* is now very rare in developed countries. Skin infection with atypical mycobacteria is, in many non-tropical countries, the most common type of mycobacterial infection. A good example is *M. marinum*, which is found in swimming pools and aquaria and causes persistent warty nodular lesions on the extremities. Infection remains localized to the cooler peripheral skin, reflecting the organism's inability to multiply at body temperature.

Spirochaetal Infections

Syphilis is sexually transmitted, with the primary ulcerated chancre developing at the point of inoculation (usually the anogenital region). Erythema chronicum migrans describes a sharply defined spreading lesion caused by infection with the spirochaete, *Borrelia burgdorferi*. This organism is transmitted by a tick bite and, when left untreated, the infection may spread to joints, the nervous system and heart (Lyme disease). More recently, it has been proposed that borrelial infection may be associated with some low-grade cutaneous lymphomas in a manner similar to the relationship between *Helicobacter* infection and primary gastric lymphoma (p. 243).

Fungal Infections

Key Points

Fungal infections:

- superficial infections involving epidermis, hair and nail infections are common
- deep mycoses affect the dermis and subcutaneous fat, and are uncommon in temperate climates

General

A wide range of fungi can cause skin infection. The most simple method of classification is into two groups. The first group includes fungi which infect the superficial layers of the skin together with the hair and nails (Table 18.8). While a second group comprises the deep mycoses that infect the dermis and subcutaneous fat (these are uncommon in temperate climates, and are not discussed further).

TABLE 18.8 Examples of common superficial fungal skin infections

Fungus (dermatophytes)	Main clinical associations
Epidermophyton spp.	Tinea pedis and cruris
Microsporum spp.	Tinea capitis
Trichophyton spp.	Tinea pedis, cruris, corporis, capitis; nail infection

The diagnosis of superficial fungal infection may be possible on clinical grounds, although skin scrapings and, in some cases, a biopsy are required. Deeply sited fungal infection is usually diagnosed on biopsy material. Fungi stain magenta pink with periodic acid–Schiff (PAS) (Figure 18.33), and this facilitates their detection in tissue sections.

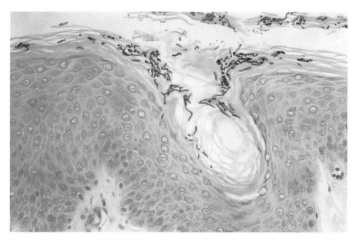

FIGURE 18.33 Superficial dermatophyte infection. Large numbers of fungal hyphae are present within the stratum corneum. (PAS.)

Tinea

The various types of dermatophyte infection are classified according to the site involved:

- Tinea capitis is the term given to dermatophyte infection (usually *Trichophyton tonsurans* or *Microsporum canis*) of the scalp which causes slight scaliness and mild hair loss. A minority of cases develop marked suppurative folliculitis (kerion).
- Tinea corporis reflects the infection of non-hirsute skin, tinea cruris affects the groin region, and tinea pedis (or athlete's foot) – the most common dermatophytosis – causes itchy, macerated fissures in the interdigital spaces. These three variants are usually caused by infection with *Trichophyton rubrum*, *Trichophyton mentagrophytes* or *Epidermophyton floccosum*.
- Fungal infection of the nail (onychomycosis) results in a thickened brittle nail showing yellow-brown discoloration. Onychomycosis is generally due to infection with *T. rubrum* or *T. mentagrophytes*, although *Candida albicans* may infect the fingernails (often following an episode of candidal paronychia).

Candidosis

Candida albicans – a normal commensal of the oropharynx, gut and vagina – does not usually colonize normal skin. The most common cutaneous infection with *C. albicans* occurs in the intertriginous folds, and is especially likely in obese individuals or in hot humid climates. Chronic mucocutaneous candidosis which affects the mucous membranes, skin and nails is generally seen in children with defective cell-mediated immunity. In adults, the syndrome is rarer and may point to the presence of an underlying tumour (especially thymoma). Disseminated candidosis involves multiple organs, with skin lesions being seen in a minority of cases. It is a disease that is associated particularly with immunosuppression, intravenous drug abuse and broad-spectrum antibiotic treatment.

Pityriasis Versicolor

This describes a common superficial infection with the unicellular commensal yeast *Malassezia furfur*. Pathogenicity is only acquired when budding occurs in warm humid conditions. Lesions appear as small scaly hypo- or hyperpigmented macules over the torso and upper arms.

Arthropod Infestations

General

An enormous array of arthropods are capable of causing human disease. Many members are venomous (e.g. spiders, scorpions, wasps and bees), others act as vectors for microbes (e.g. tick-borne borellial infection), and some (e.g. the scabies mite and various types of lice) infest the skin.

Scabies

This contagious condition is due to infestation with the mite *Sarcoptes scabiei*, with transmission being facilitated by close physical contact. After mating, gravid female mites tunnel into the corneal layer leaving burrows containing faeces and eggs (Figure 18.34). Infestation results in an itchy papulovesicular rash involving the interdigital skin, palms, wrists, inframammary folds and genitals. The itch associated with infestation reflects an allergic reaction to the mite. The complex relationship that exists between the mite and host immune system is emphasized by cases of extensive infestation with crusting and secondary bacterial infection (Norwegian scabies) seen in immunosuppressed and debilitated patients.

Pediculosis

Lice are blood-sucking insects, the saliva of which elicits an intensely itchy allergic reaction. Three species of louse cause different patterns of infestation:

- *Pediculus humanus capitis* infests the scalp, with outbreaks occurring commonly in schools. The lice and hair shafts bearing attached eggs (nits) are readily identifiable.

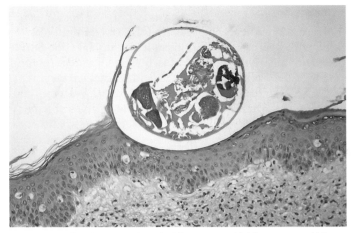

FIGURE 18.34 Scabies. A scabies mite (*Sarcoptes scabiei*) is apparent within the stratum corneum.

- *Phthirus pubis* infests any areas of coarse hair including pubic, axillary and trunk hair. Transmission is generally by intimate contact.
- *Pediculus humanis corporis* (the body louse) is rarer, except in circumstances of gross overcrowding and poor hygiene (e.g. in times of war). The faeces from this species are an important vector of diseases such as the rickettsial infection causing typhus. This louse is larger than the other species, and it differs by laying its eggs in the seams of clothing rather than cementing them to hair shafts.

NEOPLASTIC DISEASES

Key Points

Skin tumours:

- most skin tumours are benign
- tumours can arise from surface epithelium, adnexae, melanocytes, neuroendocrine cells and dermal constituents
- ultraviolet light is the main aetiological factor in most skin cancers
- awareness and early detection of skin tumours lead to better cure rates.

Of all the tissues of the body, the skin is most directly exposed to the outside world and its plethora of tissue-damaging and mutagenic influences. Not surprisingly, neoplasms of the skin are common and, as a reflection of the complex histology of the skin, constitute an extremely varied group. Patients with DNA repair deficiencies, such as the rare inherited disorder called xeroderma pigmentosum (see p. 506), are especially prone to developing multiple skin tumours.

Fortunately, the large majority of skin tumours are benign, and the most common malignant ones (basal cell carcinoma and squamous cell carcinoma) are usually cured by simple surgical excision. A number of malignant skin cancers, however, are potentially life-threatening: the most important of these is melanoma. The much rarer angiosarcoma, Merkel cell carcinoma and some malignant lymphomas are also high-risk malignancies.

Since the skin is more easily inspected than practically any other tissue of the body, most cutaneous tumours can be identified when they are small. Indeed, in recent decades, awareness of the benefits of early cancer detection has led to the increasingly early treatment of skin cancers, which is reflected in steadily improving cure rates.

Benign Epidermal Tumours

Benign epidermal tumours are a highly heterogeneous group of lesions. Some are entirely inconsequential, but others have a certain premalignant potential; some are easy to recognize for what they are, but others may mimic malignancy. Indeed, as a group, these tumours constitute a major challenge to the student (who needs to become acquainted with the main types), the clinician (who must diagnose them or decide on the need for histological diagnosis and treatment), and the pathologist (who needs to provide the definitive diagnosis). Here, we shall limit the discussion to the two most important types.

Seborrhoeic Keratosis

The typical characteristics of seborrhoeic keratosis are that:

- it is a common, benign epidermal tumour
- it protrudes above skin surface
- it is usually pigmented
- it occurs most commonly in middle-aged and elderly subjects
- the sudden emergence of large numbers of lesions may indicate visceral cancer (the Leser–Trélat sign).

This benign tumour of the epidermis occurs most commonly on the trunk of middle-aged or elderly individuals, and usually presents as a pigmented, sharply circumscribed growth with a coarsely granular surface (Figure 18.35). It often protrudes above the skin surface in its entirety, so that it appears to have been 'stuck on' the skin. The sudden emergence of large numbers of seborrhoeic keratoses may be caused by internal malignant neoplasms: this so-called Leser–Trélat sign should incite a search for a possible visceral malignancy.

Histologically, a seborrhoeic keratosis consists of a proliferation of epidermal-type squamous epithelium with some degree of maturation impairment, so that the number of basal-type epidermal keratinocytes is disproportionately increased. Accordingly, the term 'basal cell papilloma' is commonly used as a synonym. In its most common form, the epithelial proliferation assumes an exophytic growth pattern with many keratin-filled 'horn cysts' (Figure 18.36). Clinically, these lesions are usually inconsequential, since malignant transformation is exceptionally rare. If the lesion troubles the patient, it can be removed by simple excision, which is curative.

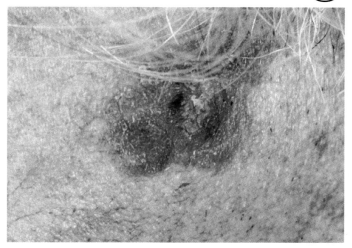

FIGURE 18.35 Seborrhoeic keratosis. This slightly raised and brownish benign skin tumour is common in late adult life. This particular example is only slightly raised and brownish; others are dark, broad-based papillomas.

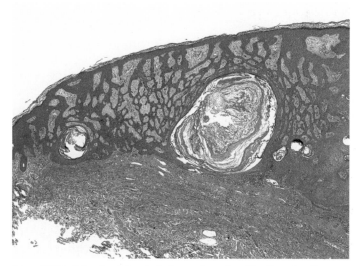

FIGURE 18.36 Seborrhoeic keratosis. An exuberant proliferation of well-circumscribed sheets and strands of epithelium resulting in thickening of the involved skin is characteristic.

Keratoacanthoma

The typical characteristics of keratoacanthoma are that:

- it is a benign epidermal tumour
- it has a central, keratin-filled crater that is bordered by proliferating squamous epithelium
- there is a characteristic rapid initial growth, followed by stabilization and eventual regression
- the lesion has a close histological resemblance to well-differentiated squamous cell carcinoma.

This hyperkeratotic skin nodule most commonly arises in sun-exposed skin and grows rapidly, reaching a size of over 1 cm diameter within a few months. The lesions closely resemble squamous cell carcinoma, both clinically and histologically. However, unlike carcinoma, which continues to grow relentlessly when left untreated, the initial quick growth of keratoacanthoma is followed by a period of stability and, subsequently, regression. The histopathologist, whose task it is to distinguish between keratoacanthoma and squamous cell carcinoma, mainly relies on a few subtle characteristics of tissue architecture. The presence of an exuberant but regular proliferating squamous epithelium surrounding a keratin horn mass on all sides characterizes keratoacanthoma.

Premalignant Epithelial Lesions of the Epidermis

As at many other body sites, the emergence of carcinoma of the skin is preceded by more or less well-defined and recognizable 'precursor' lesions. The recognition of these premalignant neoplastic lesions is of obvious importance in order to prevent the damaging and potentially life-threatening effects of cancer. The two main examples – actinic keratosis and Bowen's disease – will be considered briefly here.

Actinic Keratosis

The typical characteristics of actinic keratosis include:

- an area of epidermal dysplasia with overlying parakeratosis
- the lesions occur either singly or multiply on sun-damaged skin
- if left untreated, some may progress to carcinoma.

This skin lesion arises in chronically sun-exposed skin (hence its synonym: solar keratosis) in white adults. It presents as a somewhat scaly brownish or erythematous macule, generally under 1 cm in size. Multiple lesions are common. Histologically, the key features are those of epidermal dysplasia, evidenced by nuclear atypia associated with impaired epidermal maturation (Figure 18.37). Although not an integral part of the lesion, the dermis characteristically exhibits marked degenerative changes resulting from chronic solar ('actinic') damage. Invasive growth of the atypical epithelium is absent by definition: indeed, its development hallmarks the emergence of squamous carcinoma.

When left untreated, some actinic keratoses ultimately evolve into invasive squamous cell carcinomas. To prevent this, excision, cauterization, freezing or another type of superficial treatment is generally instituted. Such simple treatment is generally curative; however, the keratosis may recur and new ones may emerge, so that regular review is advocated.

Bowen's Disease

Typically, Bowen's disease of the skin:

- equates with squamous cell carcinoma *in situ*
- occurs in middle-aged and elderly subjects
- the typical site is the lower leg, but lesions also occur on the head, trunk and genitalia
- microscopy shows high-grade cellular atypia and architectural disorder
- if left untreated, some lesions progress to invasive squamous carcinoma.

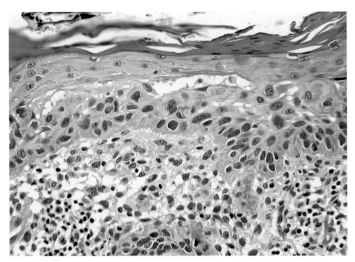

FIGURE 18.37 Actinic keratosis. The epidermis exhibits irregular orientation and increased variation in size and shape of keratinocytes. This is associated with parakeratosis (the presence of blue-staining nuclei in the stratum corneum) and an inflammatory infiltrate within the underlying dermis.

Like actinic keratosis, Bowen's disease of the skin is an epidermal neoplastic lesion which has not yet acquired the potential to invade the underlying tissues. Presenting clinically as a local reddish discoloration, the lesion is characterized histologically by a pronounced degree of nuclear atypia and disordered maturation, including the presence of abnormal mitotic figures and dyskeratotic cells. The degree of nuclear and architectural atypia markedly exceeds that typically seen in actinic keratosis. Bowen's disease of the epidermis may affect sun-damaged skin, when it is sometimes referred to as Bowenoid actinic keratosis, or covered skin lacking clinical and histological evidence of solar damage. The causative factors responsible for the latter examples remain obscure.

Carcinoma of the Skin

The majority of skin carcinomas arise in the epidermis, the component which is most directly exposed to the mutagenic influences of the outside world. Carcinomas of skin adnexae are far less common: they are briefly considered on pages 505 and 506. However, in the common basal cell carcinoma (see below), the origin from epidermal versus adnexal epithelium is in fact often unclear.

Basal Cell Carcinoma

Typically, basal cell carcinoma:

- is a slow-growing malignant tumour of keratinocytes
- is common, especially in the sun-exposed skin of white people
- shows a typical 'basaloid' appearance of tumour cells
- shows palisading of nuclei around the periphery of tumour nests
- causes local tissue destruction by invasive growth.

This non-metastasizing but locally aggressive epithelial neoplasm commonly arises in sun-exposed skin of middle-aged or elderly white individuals. In its most typical form, it appears as a slightly shiny and pearly nodule, at times with central ulceration (so-called 'rodent ulcer') (Figure 18.38). Other examples form slowly spreading, ill-defined patches of cutaneous thickening or reddish discoloration. Histologically, the tumour cells most commonly form irregular strands and nodules, often with characteristic peripheral tumour cell palisading (Figure 18.39). Basal cell carcinoma derives its name from the histological resemblance of the tumour cells to the basal cells of the epidermis. Variants include a superficial spreading variant, and a poorly circumscribed spindle-cell variant (morphoeic type), which has a bad reputation for extending beyond the clinically apparent borders of the lesion, and an associated tendency to recur locally.

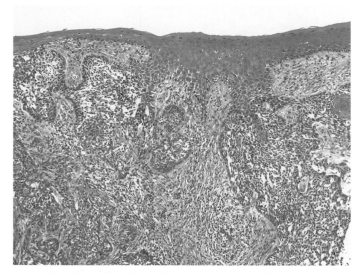

FIGURE 18.38 Basal cell carcinoma. This example manifests itself as a shiny, pigmented skin papule.

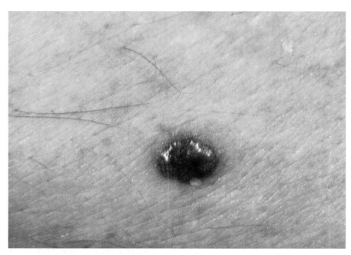

FIGURE 18.39 Basal cell carcinoma. Irregular strands of small darkly stained epithelial cells extend into the dermis. Although there may be a superficial resemblance to seborrhoeic keratosis (Figure 18.36), the strands are more irregular and the cellular details (not visible at this magnification) also differ.

Basal cell carcinoma is generally cured by simple total excision. It is very important to obtain tumour-free surgical margins, since basal cell carcinoma almost never metastasizes but may produce extensive local destruction of tissues if the treatment is inadequate. Especially on the face, local recurrence and outgrowth of basal cell carcinoma may ultimately necessitate extensive and mutilating surgery.

Squamous Cell Carcinoma

Squamous cell carcinoma:

- is a common type of epidermal carcinoma
- arises commonly in the sun-damaged skin of white subjects
- some tumours arise in burn scars, in chronic ulcers, or after exposure to chemical carcinogens
- the histological features are of squamous epithelium, with frequent keratinization, and irregular growth
- the tumour is locally aggressive
- may metastasize to regional lymph nodes, and also to distant sites.

Squamous carcinoma arises from the epidermal squamous epithelium, presumably from its basal cell layer. However, it differs from basal cell carcinoma morphologically as well as clinically; the most important difference is the metastatic potential of squamous cell carcinoma.

Again, solar irradiation appears to be a major causative factor, since these tumours arise most commonly in the sun-damaged skin of middle-aged or elderly white subjects (Figure 18.40). In addition, chronic ulcers, burn scars and direct exposure of the skin surface to certain industrial carcinogens are important causative factors in some populations.

Clinically, squamous cell carcinoma most commonly presents as a hyperkeratotic nodule or area of induration. In

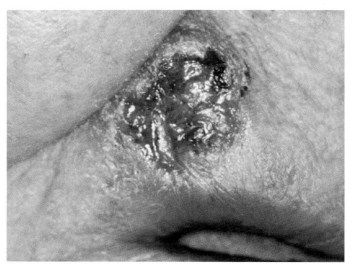

FIGURE 18.40 Squamous cell carcinoma, manifesting itself as an irregular ulcer near the upper lip of an elderly patient.

more advanced stages, ulceration and destruction of underlying tissues may be evident. Histologically, the tumour consists of irregular strands and nodules of atypical squamous epithelium (Figure 18.41), which penetrate the underlying tissues and induce a desmoplastic stromal response. If there is a predisposing factor such as a chronic ulcer, the diagnosis of carcinoma may be very difficult, since reactive epidermal proliferation and hyperkeratosis at the ulcer margin may closely mimic carcinoma, both clinically and histologically.

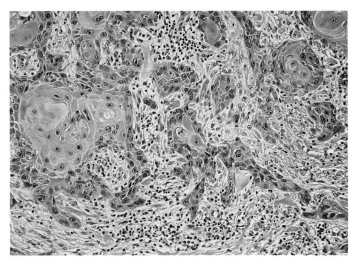

FIGURE 18.41 Squamous cell carcinoma, forming highly irregular strands of atypical epithelial cells, invading the skin and inducing an inflammatory response.

Usually, squamous cell carcinoma of the skin is easily cured by local excision. Metastases are rare, except in cases associated with a chronic ulcer, where metastasis may occur in up to one-third of cases.

Some squamous cell carcinomas – designated verrucous carcinomas – consist of very well-differentiated squamous epithelium, and do not form the characteristically irregular cellular strands and nests. Large cell masses, with a 'pushing' rather than an 'infiltrating' pattern of growth give the erroneous impression that true invasive growth is absent. However, such tumours do grow progressively and destructively, without halting at natural tissue borders, so that there is no doubt that these tumours are capable of true invasive growth.

Merkel Cell Carcinoma

Merkel cell carcinoma is a highly aggressive carcinoma of the skin, thought to arise from the rare epidermal neuroendocrine Merkel cells, which are considered to play a role in the reception of mechanical stimuli, and also exert trophic effects on epidermal and neural cells of the skin. Merkel cell carcinoma readily metastasizes to regional nodes and distant sites. It should be distinguished from a variety of tumours, most importantly from skin metastasis of an extracutaneous neuroendocrine carcinoma. This distinction is important, since radical surgery of the skin tumour has the potential of cure if the tumour is primary, but not if it is a metastasis from an occult visceral primary.

Melanocytic Naevus

The melanocytic naevus – otherwise known as a 'naevus' or 'mole' – is a benign, melanocytic neoplasm which usually arises in the epidermis and often subsequently extends into the dermis. Many variants of this lesion, which is extremely common in white races, have been recognized, but only the most common and clinically important ones will be considered here.

Common Acquired Naevus

Common acquired naevus is typically:

● very common in white subjects
● a small, symmetrical, well-circumscribed hyperpigmented macule or papule
● a melanocytic proliferation which arises in the epidermis and then spreads to the dermis (Figure 18.42)
● with time, the epidermal component and subsequently the entire naevus, disappears.

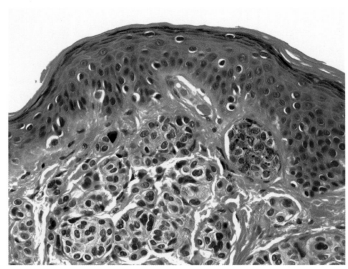

FIGURE 18.42 Common acquired naevus. Round to oval nests of melanocytes are present at the dermoepidermal junction, and extend into the upper dermis. The epidermis shows a reactive lengthening of the rete ridges and slight hyperkeratosis.

Melanocytic naevi of the usual type are very common in Caucasians, but are rare in coloured races. At birth, naevi are usually absent (except for the so-called congenital naevi; see below). Most naevi emerge in childhood and adolescence, but some arise in adulthood. After a period of growth, the naevus stabilizes in size and appearance, and after many years gradually loses its pigmentation, diminishes in size and ultimately disappears so that in old age, naevi are again absent or scarce. Their main significance derives from their cosmetic effect and from the fact that at least half of all cutaneous melanomas (see below) arise in naevi.

The causative factors responsible for the emergence and disappearance of these very common but enigmatic lesions remain largely obscure. Sunlight certainly plays a role: marked sun exposure – and especially a history of sunburn in childhood – is associated with increased numbers of naevi, and naevi are uncommon on areas of doubly covered skin, such as the buttock area. Most currently available evidence suggests that they are benign neoplasms; the mechanisms by which they at some stage lose their proliferative potential is currently a subject of great interest.

The common acquired naevus arises from epidermal melanocytes, which are situated at the junction between the epidermis and the underlying dermis. In the first phase of its development, a proliferation of these melanocytes emerges, first in an arrangement of solitary cells arranged side-to-side, later in the form of cell nests (junctional naevus). The melanocytes of this and subsequent stages of naevus development are often designated 'naevus cells'. Macroscopically, an early naevus presents as a brown, flat, usually symmetrical and well-circumscribed macule, reaching a size of up to several millimetres. After some time, the naevus cells extend into the superficial dermis, where they continue to form nests and sheets. It is important to note that this migration into the dermis should not be equated with invasive growth of malignant tumours, since in naevi it is a clinically innocent phenomenon. The lesion is now designated a compound naevus, as it involves both the junction and the dermis proper.

After a number of years – and for reasons unknown – the junctional component disappears, so that all naevus cells are now intradermal (intradermal naevus). At the base of the naevus, the melanocytes usually become smaller and/or elongated and lose their pigmentation (so-called 'maturation'). After further passage of time, the intradermal naevus cells also gradually diminish in number and disappear altogether, so that ultimately, the skin returns to normal.

Spitz Naevus

This naevus type, which is most common in childhood and adolescence but which may also occur later in life, most often presents as a symmetrical reddish or skin-coloured nodule, with a predilection for the face and extremities. Its importance lies in its close histological resemblance to melanoma, which may easily lead to overdiagnosis and overtreatment of this essentially innocent lesion. Several variants of Spitz naevus have been recognized: these include the pigmented spindle cell naevus (also known as Reed naevus) which, in its most characteristic form, presents as a small, symmetrical, pitch-black nodule, raising clinical suspicion of nodular melanoma (see below) – a suspicion which may be compounded by the somewhat alarming histology of this exuberant and densely cellular naevus. However, like the classical Spitz naevus, the Reed naevus is harmless.

Congenital Naevus

At birth, about 1% of new-born Caucasians have a clinically detectable melanocytic naevus. In contrast to acquired naevi – which are usually smaller than 1 cm across – these congenital naevi are much more variable in size and shape, and occasionally cover large parts of the body (so-called giant congenital naevi) (Figure 18.43).

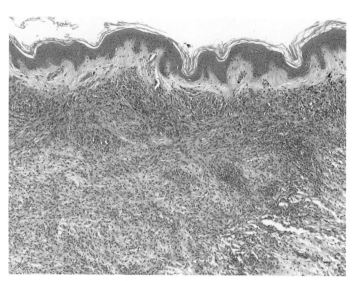

FIGURE 18.43 Congenital naevus. Large numbers of naevus cells occupy almost the entire thickness of the dermis. Such deep penetration of tissues is common in congenital naevi, but rare in acquired naevi.

Clearly, extensive congenital naevi cause significant cosmetic problems and in addition, there is a small risk of malignant transformation. Various surgical procedures are currently used in order to eradicate as much as possible of the giant congenital naevus, preferably within the first few weeks or months of life.

Blue Naevus

In contrast to the naevus types discussed so far, this enigmatic melanocytic tumour appears to arise within the dermis rather than the epidermis. The naevus is often slightly bluish when viewed from the skin surface, since the pigmentation is deeply located in the skin and is covered by the opaque normal overlying skin tissue (the resultant colour shift toward blue is known as the Tyndall effect). In contrast to most intradermal naevus cells, some melanocytes of blue naevi possess slender dendrites and actively produce melanin.

Melanoma

Characteristically:

- melanoma is a malignant tumour of melanocytes
- at least half of these tumours arise in a melanocytic naevus
- the treatment is primarily surgical
- the chance of cure is closely related to tumour thickness

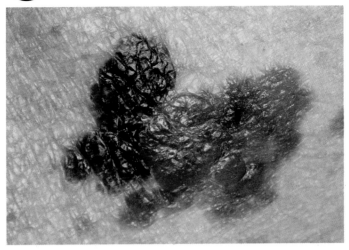

FIGURE 18.44 Superficial spreading melanoma. This lesion shows several of the key features of melanoma: irregular shape, marked variation in colour, and irregular surface with loss of skin lines in some places.

- metastases occur in nearby skin and subcutis (satellites/in-transit metastases), regional lymph nodes and distant sites
- there are four main subtypes: superficial spreading melanoma; nodular melanoma; lentigo maligna melanoma; and acral lentiginous melanoma.

Malignant melanoma, or simply melanoma – the adjective 'malignant' being omitted as there is no such thing as a benign melanoma – is a malignant tumour of melanocytes. Clinically, melanomas are flat or raised lesions, and are often irregular in shape and colour. They occasionally bleed, and may produce an itching or burning sensation. These signs, or a history of recent change in a previously stable mole, call for excision and histological evaluation.

Melanomas vary widely in macroscopical and histological appearance. Four main subtypes are recognized (Table 18.9). Superficial spreading melanoma in its most characteristic form presents as an irregularly shaped and coloured, slowly growing lesion with a flat periphery (Figure 18.44). Part of the lesion may become raised, and in the course of time may show accelerated growth and ulceration. Typical histology is shown in Figure 18.45. Nodular melanoma usually grows rapidly from the start, forming a nodule which is commonly – but not always – pigmented. If the tumour is totally devoid of pigment (amelanotic

melanoma), it is often not recognized as such clinically, so that initially it is often considered to be a trivial, benign lesion. Lentigo maligna melanoma arises in the sun-exposed skin of middle-aged or elderly Caucasians, and is most common on the face and the dorsa of hands. The melanoma derives its name from the precursor lesion, lentigo maligna (also known as 'Hutchinson's freckle'), a proliferation of atypical melanocytes within the atrophic epidermis of sun-damaged skin, which produces a slowly enlarging, irregularly shaped pigmentation. Acral lentiginous melanoma arises in the skin of the palms of hands, soles of feet, or subungually. It is the main type of melanoma occurring in coloured races.

The treatment of melanoma is primarily surgical, and the prognosis primarily depends on tumour stage (the presence or absence of regional or distant metastases). In the absence of any signs of metastatic disease, ulceration of the tumour and its thickness (measured in millimetres – Breslow's thickness) predict prognosis. Ulcerated or thicker tumours do worse.

Melanoma has a propensity to produce small tumour deposits in the direct vicinity of the primary tumour. In order to avoid the outgrowth of these so-called 'satellites' – which

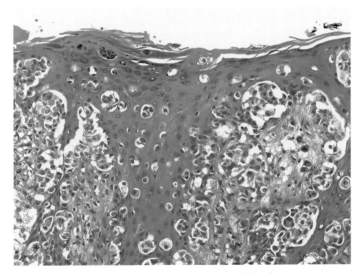

FIGURE 18.45 Superficial spreading melanoma. Atypical melanocytes are seen throughout the thickness of the epidermis, which contrasts with the more regular nests of melanocytes at the dermoepidermal junction, seen in most naevi (compare with Figure 18.42).

TABLE 18.9 The clinical and aetiological characteristics of melanoma

Melanoma type	Site	Remarks
Superficial spreading melanoma	Anywhere	Most common type of melanoma in whites
Nodular melanoma	Anywhere	Usually rapidly growing
Lentigo maligna melanoma	Sun-damaged skin of elderly whites	Precursor lesion: lentigo maligna (Hutchinson's freckle)
Acral lentiginous melanoma	Volar skin or nail bed	Most common type of melanoma in coloured races

may be undetectable at the time of resection of the primary tumour – melanoma is excised with a wide margin of surrounding skin and subcutis. Usually, a skin margin of 1 cm is used for all invasive melanomas with a thickness up to 2 mm; for thicker melanomas, even wider margins are used.

Metastases occur primarily in regional lymph nodes and pass via the bloodstream to a wide variety of organs. Superficial metastases which occur between the primary tumour and the regional nodes, and which are presumably caused by outgrowth of tumour emboli within lymph vessels, are known as 'in-transit metastases'.

Familial Dysplastic Naevus Syndrome

In some families, a high incidence of melanoma is found; the melanoma patients – or those who later develop melanoma – often show an abnormally large number of naevi, which vary markedly in size, shape and colour, and which occur at sites where naevi are normally rare. Histologically, these so-called dysplastic naevi show a number of distinctive features, the most important of which are cytological and architectural atypia and some associated inflammation and fibrosis. Family members with such large numbers of clinically and histologically abnormal naevi have a markedly increased life-time risk of melanoma, so that close follow-up is essential. Any change in a previously stable naevus is suspicious of malignant change, necessitating removal. In this way, many 'early melanomas' can be removed, which results in a markedly improved life expectancy of these patients.

It is important to note that very similar dysplastic naevi also occur as solitary lesions in individuals with a negative family history for melanoma and that in this context, melanoma risk hardly exceeds that of the general population.

SUSPICIOUS MOLE

A 35-year-old woman visited her general practitioner because she had recently noticed a dark mole on her upper thigh; the mole was enlarging and gave a slightly burning sensation (Figure 18.46). The patient's father had a history of melanoma on the back, which had been removed 2 years previously.

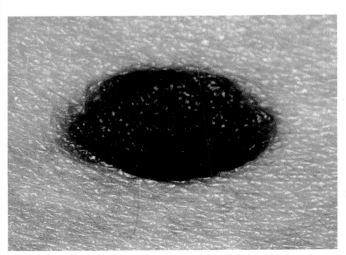

FIGURE 18.46 The skin lesion of this patient manifested itself as a raised, darkly pigmented, symmetrical nodule. Because of the pitch-black colour, there was some concern that the lesion could be a heavily pigmented nodular melanoma.

On inspection, a pitch-black, symmetrical, oval, non-ulcerating papule of 0.8 cm diameter was seen. The number and features of the patient's other naevi were considered to be within normal limits. The lesion was considered to be suspicious of nodular melanoma and was excised with a margin of 2 mm, in order to obtain a histological diagnosis.

A histological examination revealed the characteristic features of a pigmented spindle cell naevus (PSCN) (Figure 18.47). This naevus subtype can present as a pitch-black papule that is clinically indistinguishable from a small nodular pigmented melanoma. The burning sensation was probably derived from the mild inflammatory response caused by the shedding of melanin pigment from the lesion. The general practitioner reassured the patient that the lesion was entirely benign, and that there was no relation to her father's history of melanoma.

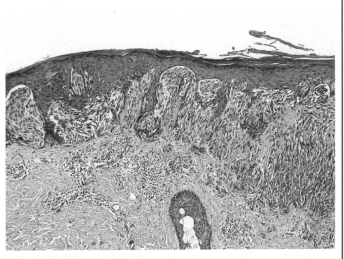

FIGURE 18.47 Histology of the lesion shows many confluent nests and sheets of melanocytes at the dermoepidermal junction, associated with epidermal hyperplasia and hyperkeratosis. The histology is characteristic of pigmented spindle cell naevus (PSCN), a benign lesion.

An on-going hunt for the genes responsible for the hereditary dysplastic naevus syndrome has resulted in the identification of a number of loci and candidate genes. It has become apparent that the dysplastic naevus syndrome phenotype may result from different genotypes. Particularly intriguing is the finding of involvement of the *P16INK4A* gene in some families, since the P16 protein is a potent proliferation inhibitor (acting by blocking CDK4's proliferation-promoting kinase activity) that is abundantly present in the large majority of common naevi, but is absent from many melanomas. Further evidence incriminating P16 in melanomagenesis derives from recent studies of P16 knockout mice which, under certain conditions, exhibit an increased incidence of melanoma.

Various other Skin Tumours

Dermatofibroma

This common and innocent intradermal proliferation of mesenchymal cells with characteristics of histiocytes as well as fibroblasts (hence its alternative designation, cutaneous fibrous histiocytoma) presents as a firm, skin-coloured or slightly hyperpigmented nodule, usually under 1 cm in size, and most commonly located on the extremities. There has been dispute as to whether the lesion represents a true neoplasm or is an exuberant response to tissue damage, but the recent identification of karyotypic aberrations in a substantial number of these lesions argues strongly in favour of neoplasia. It is important not to confuse dermatofibroma with the rare dermatofibrosarcoma protuberans, which shares some of its histological features, but which diffusely invades surrounding tissues and has a notorious propensity for local recurrence and relentless local invasive growth.

Vascular Tumours

Haemangioma

Haemangiomas of the skin are benign tumours of endothelium, which are especially common in childhood. Capillary haemangiomas produce large numbers of small vessels (Figure 18.48); cavernous haemangiomas consist of large, gaping vascular spaces. Large and flat congenital haemangiomas are commonly referred to as port wine stains. In contrast, the so-called 'strawberry haemangioma' of the neonate is a raised lesion, which sometimes grows rapidly to produce a disfiguring exophytic lesion, but it generally regresses spontaneously after a number of years so that a conservative approach is warranted. Pyogenic granuloma, which is a haemangioma rather than a granuloma, produces a reddish nodule with wet surface, caused by erosion of the overlying epidermis. Some of these lesions arise after trauma, and it is still a matter of debate, whether these represent true neoplasms or exuberant reactive local endothelial proliferations.

Kaposi's Sarcoma

Kaposi's sarcoma is a locally aggressive endothelial tumour (Figure 18.49) which occurs in several clinical settings, the

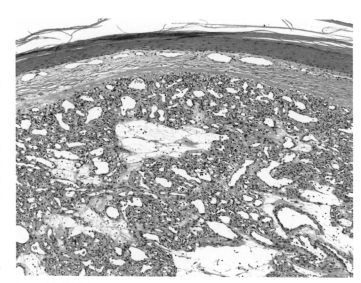

FIGURE 18.48 Skin tumour composed of endothelial cells. This haemangioma is a benign tumour characterized by an accumulation of regular vessels which may be small or large, and lined by (usually) flat endothelial cells.

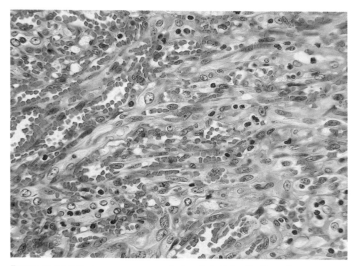

FIGURE 18.49 Skin tumour composed of endothelial cells. Kaposi's sarcoma, especially when it has progressed to the nodular phase, shows an irregular mass of elongated atypical endothelial cells alternating with slit-like spaces filled with blood.

best known of these being the association with AIDS. However, the tumour may also affect HIV-negative individuals, especially elderly males, transplant patients, and children in certain regions of Africa. The tumour is closely associated with the presence of the human herpesvirus type 8, which plays an important causal role in its pathogenesis.

Clinically, the lesion often presents initially as one or several small macules, but may later progress to mass lesions (nodular phase) which may lead to ulceration of the overlying epidermis. Involvement of internal organs, such as the respiratory and digestive tracts, is common.

Angiosarcoma

Angiosarcoma of the skin is a rare, malignant tumour of vascular endothelium, which most commonly arises on chronically sun-exposed skin in the elderly. The tumour usually presents as an ill-defined area of cutaneous thickening, induration and discoloration, but later develops protuberant and locally aggressive masses. The tumour often extends far beyond the clinically apparent borders, responds poorly to therapy and, because of these properties, carries a dismal prognosis. Other cutaneous angiosarcomas arise on the basis of chronic lymphoedema, such as may develop in the arm after axillary lymph node dissection and radiotherapy for breast carcinoma (Stewart–Treves syndrome). Again, the prognosis is poor.

Cutaneous Lymphoma

Cutaneous lymphoma may be of either T cell or B cell origin. The main type of primary cutaneous T-cell lymphoma is mycosis fungoides (MF) (p. 203). The initial stage of MF – which may last for many years – is characterized by the formation of patches, which are vexingly difficult to distinguish clinically and histologically from a number of inflammatory skin diseases. Permeation of the epidermis by monoclonal atypical T cells constitutes the essential diagnostic feature. The early, patch stage of MF is followed by the emergence of indurated plaques and, later, nodular lesions and tumours. A variant of cutaneous T-cell lymphoma, characterized by generalized skin reddening (erythroderma) and involvement of lymph nodes and blood, is known as the Sezáry syndrome. A variety of other lymphoma types including B-cell lymphomas may arise, or may become manifest clinically, in the skin: these rare tumours fall outside the scope of this chapter.

Metastasis to the Skin

It should be borne in mind that carcinomas of internal organs may grow into, or metastasize to, the skin. Breast cancer may involve the skin by local extension or lymphatic spread. Skin metastasis of renal carcinoma is of special significance: for unknown reasons, renal carcinoma more commonly metastasizes to the skin than carcinomas of many other organs. Since the primary tumour of renal carcinoma may not produce symptoms for a long period of time, metastases rather than the primary tumour may cause the first manifestation of the tumour.

Tumours of Skin Appendages

Characteristically, the tumours of skin appendages:

- comprise a highly heterogeneous group
- the large majority are benign
- some are associated with specific syndromes.

The hair follicles and sweat glands give rise to an extraordinary variety of neoplasms. The large majority are benign, and precise subtyping of these generally is of little consequence – which explains why general designations such as 'benign eccrine sweat gland tumour' are commonly used. The significance of some variants derives mainly from the possible confusion with malignant tumours, or from the association with some specific syndromes. Some adnexal tumours (the carcinomas in the list below) are malignant.

The basis of the histological classification of these neoplasms is by way of their phenotypic resemblance to adnexal structures, from which they have presumably arisen. Thus, there are eccrine and apocrine sweat gland tumours, and tumours of the pilosebaceous unit.

Adnexal structure	Tumour presumably arising from it
Eccrine sweat gland	Syringoma Nodular hidradenoma Microcystic adnexal carcinoma
Apocrine sweat gland	Cylindroma Apocrine carcinoma
Pilosebaceous unit	Infundibular cyst ('epidermal cyst') Trichofollicular cyst Pilomatrixoma ('Malherbe's tumour') Pilar tumour ('proliferating tricholemmal cyst')

Eccrine Sweat Gland Tumours

Syringomas usually present as multiple small papules on the upper cheek. Histologically, they are found to consist of a proliferation of small epithelial cells arranged in small islands and strands, resulting in a superficial resemblance to basal cell carcinoma. Nodular hidradenoma – which probably arises from the distal portion of the sweat duct – produces a solitary nodule consisting of large masses of epithelium. Malignant eccrine sweat gland tumours are rare and comprise a varied group of lesions, including microcystic adnexal carcinoma, most of which occur on the face and have a bad reputation for local recurrence and destructive growth, so that early complete surgical removal is essential.

Apocrine Sweat Gland Tumours

Situated mainly in areas where apocrine glands are numerous (axillae, groins, midline of back), these rare neoplasms exhibit a baffling variability of appearances. Cylindromas occur multiply on the skin of the face (usually forehead) and scalp, but in contrast to syringomas of the face, which remain small, these tumours can grow to form disfiguring masses ('turban tumour'). Histologically, closely adjacent islands of small epithelial cells, with little interjacent stroma, result in a jigsaw-like appearance. Apocrine carcinomas are exceedingly rare.

Tumours of the Pilosebaceous Unit

Simple epithelial cysts within the dermis or subcutis, lined by an attenuated layer of stratified squamous epithelium, are often designated 'epidermal cysts': however, these lesions do not originate from the epidermis but from the

SPECIAL STUDY TOPIC

XERODERMA PIGMENTOSUM AND DNA REPAIR

The basic defect in the rare inherited disorder xeroderma pigmentosum (XP) is a failure to repair DNA damage by nucleotide excision. This defect uncovers the devastating effects of the genetic damage which the skin incurs naturally, but which in healthy individuals is repaired quickly and effectively, so that it does not lead to significant cell and tissue damage. The fact that most of this damage is sun-induced is evident from the extreme photosensitivity of the skin in XP patients and the approximately 2000-fold increase in the incidence of skin cancers, including squamous cell carcinomas, basal cell carcinomas and melanomas. Some of these malignant tumours appear at an early age, even in childhood. The distribution of lesions reflects the aetiological role of sunlight exposure – the face, dorsa of hands but also arms and legs being most severely affected. In these patients, the extensive skin damage and multiple tumours often necessitate major surgical procedures. Avoidance of sun exposure is obviously an essential part of the clinical management.

The basic molecular mechanisms underlying this rare disease have been the subject of intense research interest. It has become clear that, at the genetic level, a variety of defects may cause very similar phenotypic effects: at least seven genetically distinct subgroups of XP have thus far been identified. This is a reflection of the fact that nucleotide excision repair is not a single enzyme activity, but is brought about by a multiprotein complex, each component of which needs to function adequately in order to achieve effective nucleotide excision repair.

Although at first sight, the link between genotype (defective nucleotide excision repair resulting in accumulation of UV-induced mutations) and phenotype (emergence of large numbers of sunlight-induced cancers) appears straightforward, some intriguing riddles remain to be solved. For example, another very rare form of defective nucleotide excision repair, Cockayne's syndrome, is not associated with an elevated skin cancer risk. This apparent paradox illustrates that the very complex mechanisms of DNA repair and their phenotypic effects are still incompletely understood. They are currently a main focus of interest in molecular cancer research.

hair follicle infundibulum, and are therefore properly termed infundibular *cysts*. The cyst wall may rupture, inducing an inflammatory response. The resultant swelling and pain may draw attention to the lesion. A histologically similar cyst, which most commonly involves the scalp but which is characterized by tricholemmal rather than epidermal-type keratinization, is known as a tricholemmal *cyst*.

Pilomatrixoma or Malherbe's tumour is a benign hair follicle tumour that may be recognized clinically because, as a result of extensive calcification, it is as hard as stone. Finally, the rare so-called pilar tumour, or 'proliferating tricholemmal cyst' is of interest, since it may produce an alarming large tumour of the scalp, usually in elderly females, and histologically may be misdiagnosed as carcinoma if a small biopsy is taken from the centre. However, the tumour is entirely benign, as becomes evident when the expansile growth pattern of the edge of the tumour is appreciated.

Hypertrophy and hyperplasia of sebaceous glands of the skin of the nose, of a poorly understood but probably non-neoplastic nature, results in a disfiguring nasal swelling known as rhinophyma. The benign sebaceous adenoma and malignant sebaceous carcinoma are both very rare.

SUMMARY

Dermatopathology can appear to be a daunting subject with a myriad of seemingly obscure diagnoses compounded by complex terminology and pathogenetic mechanisms that often remain poorly understood. At a basic level it is reassuring to know that a relatively small group of well defined disorders account for the bulk of dermatology practice.

As is the case in all areas of pathology, the subject becomes infinitely more manageable when diseases with similar morphological characteristics are grouped together in a classification. For example, there are many hundreds of non-infective inflammatory disorders but the majority can be placed into one of only a few broad groups according to the morphological reaction pattern displayed by the epidermis (Table 18.3). The logical classification for cutaneous neoplastic disease, like other organ systems, reflects the cell of origin and examples of tumours derived from the epidermal cells (principally the keratinocytes and melanocytes), dermal constituents, adnexal structures and lymphoid elements have been presented.

Currently, the classification of most cutaneous disease relies largely on histological and clinical characteristics but this is likely to change in the future as the detailed molecular genetic abnormalities underpinning disorders are unraveled, linking conditions formerly believed to be unrelated. For example, mutations in the filaggrin gene recently found to be responsible for a common inherited type of dry scaly skin (ichthyosis vulgaris) are now implicated strongly in the pathogenesis of the clinically distinct conditions atopic dermatitis and asthma.

It is crucial to remember that accurate diagnosis of cutaneous disease demands close correlation of the pathological findings with the clinical picture and also with the results of other investigations such as microbiology, immunofluorescence studies and molecular genetics. Diseases with diverse but distinctive clinical patterns can share very similar histological features and it is therefore fortunate that there is no other area of medicine where the organ of interest is so accessible to inspection. At the very least the pathologist needs to be made aware of several pieces of information including the site of the biopsy, any relevant history (such as a recent infection or exposure to drugs) together with the duration, distribution and description of the abnormality. Specialist multidisciplinary meetings with clinical colleagues where diagnoses can be reviewed (and if necessary revised) in the light of more detailed information is now central to effective patient management.

FURTHER READING

McKee PH, Calonje JE, Granter SR. *Pathology of the Skin, with Clinical Correlations*, 3rd edn. Edinburgh: Elsevier, 2005.

Weedon D. *Skin Pathology*. Edinburgh: Churchill Livingstone, 2002.

TABLE 19.6 Protozoal infections and their habitat

Habitat	Infection
Lymph node and systemic	*Toxoplasma gondii*
	Leishmania species
Skin and systemic	*Leishmania* species
Intraerythrocytic, CNS	*Plasmodium falciparum*
Intestine	*Entamoeba histolytica*
	Cryptosporidium parvum
	Giardia lamblia
Liver	*Entamoeba histolytica*

TABLE 19.7 Helminth infections and their habitat

Habitat	Infection
Bladder, liver and gut	*Schistosoma* species
Intestine	*Necator* and *Ankylostoma* species (hookworms)
	Ascaris lumbricoides (gut roundworms)
	Trichuris trichiura (whipworm)
	Strongyloides stercoralis
	Enterobius vermicularis (pinworm)
Any organ	*Echinococcus granulosus* (hydatid cyst)

TABLE 19.8 Causes of immunosuppression that predispose to infections

Primary inherited conditions	Acquired conditions
Agammaglobulinaemia	HIV/AIDS
Common variable immunodeficiency	Malnutrition
Isolated IgA deficiency	Extremes of age
Di George syndrome (thymic deficiency)	Cirrhosis
Severe combined (SCID) immunodeficiency disease	Cancer (solid, lymphoma and leukaemia)
Wiskott–Aldrich syndrome	Steroid therapy, anticancer chemotherapy and transplant immunosuppressive therapy
	Autoimmune diseases
Inherited complement deficiencies	
Inherited leucocyte function defects	Diabetes mellitus

mucosal surfaces (such as conjunctiva, airways and gut). Behind these physical barriers are complex systems of interacting cells and their secretions such as antibodies and cytokines, and the complement system. It is not an exaggeration to state that most of these internal defence systems have evolved in response to infectious challenges from the environment. Thus, when these defences malfunction, as a result of either inherited or acquired defects, infection is the consequence and the major focus of clinical management.

Immunosuppression may be classified as primary (inherited) and acquired, the latter category being by far the more important. The primary conditions also include genetically determined malfunctions of the complement system and leucocytes (Tables 19.8 and 19.9).

Overview of Viral Infections

Viruses are intracellular pathogens that use the host cell metabolism for their replication. There are hundreds of species of viruses which contain either RNA or DNA in their core. The viruses vary in size from 20 to 30 nm, and they tend to infect certain cells, that is they exhibit tissue tropism. Once inside host cell, the infection may be either abortive (viral replication is incomplete), latent (the infection persists but without continuous replication) or persistent (replication produces new virions). Viruses cause disease in many ways, and these are summarized in Table 19.10.

TABLE 19.9 Immunodeficiency conditions and consequent infections – some representative examples

Defect	Infections more common and severe
Reduced number of polymorphonuclear neutrophils	Pyogenic bacteria (*Staphylococcus, Pseudomonas*); fungi (*Candida, Aspergillus*)
Defective oxidative burst in leucocytes (chronic granulomatous disease)	Pyogenic bacteria; mycobacteria: many species
Interferon-γ receptor deficiency	Mycobacteria: many species
Complement defect	*Neisseria* infections (gonococcus, meningitis)
B-cell defect (defective IgG production)	Pyogenic bacteria (*Haemophilus, Staphylococcus, Streptococcus*)
Isolated IgA deficiency	Intestinal giardiasis
CD4 +ve T-helper cell	Virus: CMV, herpes Bacteria: pyogenic bacteria Mycobacteria: many species Fungi: *Candida, Cryptococcus, Pneumocystis jirovecii* Protozoa: *Leishmania donovani*
Iatrogenic immunosuppression (e.g. transplantation, steroids)	Mycobacteria – many species Pyogenic bacteria Fungi: *Aspergillus* species Protozoa: *Entamoeba histolytica* Worms: *Strongyloides stercoralis*

TABLE 19.10 Pathogenesis of viral diseases

- Entry into a cell via a receptor
- Replication using host cell enzymes or by incorporation into the cell nuclear DNA
- Interference with host cell metabolism (e.g. polio)
- Damage to the host cell membrane (e.g. measles, HIV, HSV)
- Direct cytolytic effect of the virus, killing the cell (e.g. CMV, HIV, HSV)
- Damaging mucosal cells, permitting secondary infection (e.g. influenza, measles)
- Damaging host immune cells, permitting opportunistic infections (e.g. HIV)
- Presentation of viral antigen on host cell surface, inducing attack by host lymphocytes (e.g. hepatitis B)
- Induction of cell proliferation and transformation, producing cancer (e.g. EBV)

HIV/AIDS

Key Points

Typically, HIV/AIDS:

- is caused by a retrovirus, the human immunodeficiency virus (HIV)
- is a global pandemic
- HIV destroys the cell-mediated immune system
- permits opportunistic infections, in addition to Kaposi's sarcoma and lymphomas
- AIDS is ultimately fatal, although HIV can temporarily be controlled using chemotherapy.

History and Epidemiology of the HIV/AIDS Pandemic

AIDS is a disease that is characterized by profound immuno-suppression which leads to opportunistic infections, secondary neoplasms and neurological disorders. In 1981,

TABLE 19.11 Modes of transmission of HIV infection

- Heterosexual intercourse (bidirectional)
- Anal sexual intercourse
- Mother-to-child transplacental and perinatal transmission
- Intravenous drug users who share contaminated needles
- Blood transfusion and infected blood products (e.g. Factor VIII concentrates)
- Accidental percutaneous injury with infected blood (e.g. to healthcare workers)
- To infant via breast feeding

clinicians in the USA noted unusual frequencies of hitherto rare conditions – *Pneumocystis jirovecii* pneumonia and Kaposi's sarcoma – in previously well men. These subjects were homosexual, and were suffering these fatal diseases as a consequence of depleted T-helper cells (CD4+ phenotype): the disease complex was termed the 'acquired immunodeficiency syndrome', or AIDS. By 1984, the aetiology of this immunosuppression had been determined as a retrovirus, the modes of viral transmission described (Table 19.11), and the geographical spread of the infection was being investigated.

The viruses causing AIDS are the human immunodeficiency viruses (HIV), of which type 1 (HIV-1) is globally distributed, and the second much less frequent type (HIV-2) is mainly restricted to West African countries or people therefrom.

This fatal disease is pandemic. In the year 2006, about 40 million people are living infected with HIV, and over 90% of them live in sub-Saharan Africa, south and east Asia, and South America. Approximately 4.3 million people were infected with HIV in 2006. In many parts of Africa, one-quarter of the adult population is infected with HIV, and parts of Asia are similarly affected. In such hyperendemic areas, life expectancy is decreasing, as a consequence of increasing numbers of young adults and infected babies dying of AIDS. In the UK over 6000 new infections are registered annually, and up to 64 000 of the population are infected.

 19.1 SPECIAL STUDY TOPIC

PATHOGENESIS OF HIV/AIDS

Most adult infections are from the transmucosal passage of HIV virions in body fluids, across the cervical, penile and rectal mucosae. HIV has a surface glycoprotein molecule, gp120, which binds to the CD4 receptor on

host cells. More recently, two coreceptors for gp120 have been described, the binding of one of which is also necessary for HIV infection to occur: CCR5 which is present on macrophages, Langerhans' cells and CD4+ T cells; and CXCR4 which is restricted to T cells. There are polymorphisms in the CCR5 receptor which may account for the very small number of persons who have been significantly exposed to HIV infection yet do not appear to be

SPECIAL STUDY TOPIC CONTINUED...

susceptible. M-tropic HIV strains use CCR5, while T-tropic strains use the CXCR4 receptor.

An M-tropic virus enters a susceptible mucosal Langerhans' dendritic (antigen-presenting) cell via the surface CD4 and CCR5 receptors; a CD4+ T cell fuses with the dendritic cells and becomes infected; the infected

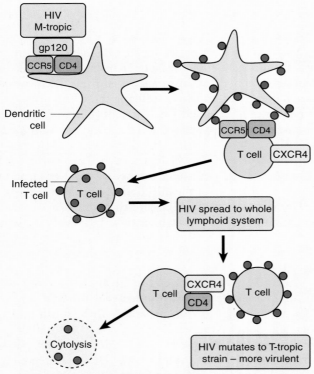

FIGURE 19.1 Human immunodeficiency virus (HIV) infection. HIV enters the Langerhans dendritic cell, via gp120 binding to the receptors CD4 and CCR5; HIV then spreads to the T cells via the same receptors, and throughout the lymphoid system. Over time, the virus mutates and enters T cells via CD4 and CXCR4 receptors.

T cell passes to the local lymph nodes where it activates and infects more CD4+ T lymphocytes, and within days the infection is widely disseminated to lymphoid tissue throughout the body. The other main cell infected by HIV is the macrophage, also via its CD4 surface receptor. This is how infection can spread to the brain, through the microglia (brain macrophage) cells (Figure 19.1).

Vertical transmission occurs in up to 25% of pregnancies in HIV-infected mothers in the absence of anti-HIV treatment; this may be via the placenta or the fetal mucosae. In infections by blood, HIV virions directly infect CD4+ T cells.

Once inside a susceptible cell, the HIV RNA genome is transcribed into a matching DNA via a reverse transcriptase enzyme. This can remain in the cytoplasm, but when the cell divides the HIV DNA enters the nucleus and becomes integrated into the host cell DNA as a provirus. Transcription, productive infection and then host cell death occur when the cell is activated by cytokines or antigen. Infected T cells die by cytolysis, although the precise mechanisms are unclear.

Immune resistance to HIV infection involves B-cell activation (with lymph node hyperplasia) and NK cells killing infected T cells by apoptosis, but these do not eliminate the infection, which progressively destroys the cell-mediated immune system by destruction of T-helper cells faster than they can be replaced. The huge turnover of HIV and T cells is indicated in Table 19.12. It promises that anti-HIV chemotherapy can reduce productive infection and retard the disease, but cannot eliminate the infection completely.

TABLE 19.12 Kinetics of HIV in the latent phase of infection

- 10^{10} HIV viral particles produced per day in the body
- 10^9 CD4+ T cells produced and destroyed per day
- A large pool of infected CD4+ T cells with half life of 1 day (viral DNA integrated)
- A small pool of CD4+ cells latently infected with half life of >7 days (DNA not integrated)
- A small pool of very long-lived latently infected CD4+ T cells (half life >4 months) with integrated DNA
- Long lived HIV-infection in brain microglia (DNA integrated)

Whilst the HIV destroys the T-cell system, patients are asymptomatic but can infect others. The peripheral blood CD4+ T-cell count is used as a surrogate marker of bodily cell-mediated immunocompetence. The normal values are 500–2000 per mm^3; the count drops transiently during acute infection, and then progressively during the latent phase. Conversely, blood viral loads peak during acute infection then drop, and rise again after the latent phase (Figure 19.2).

Over time, the HIV in a person mutates from a M-tropic to a T-tropic strain. This is significant because T-tropic strains are more virulent and T-cell-cytolytic.

SPECIAL STUDY TOPIC CONTINUED . . .

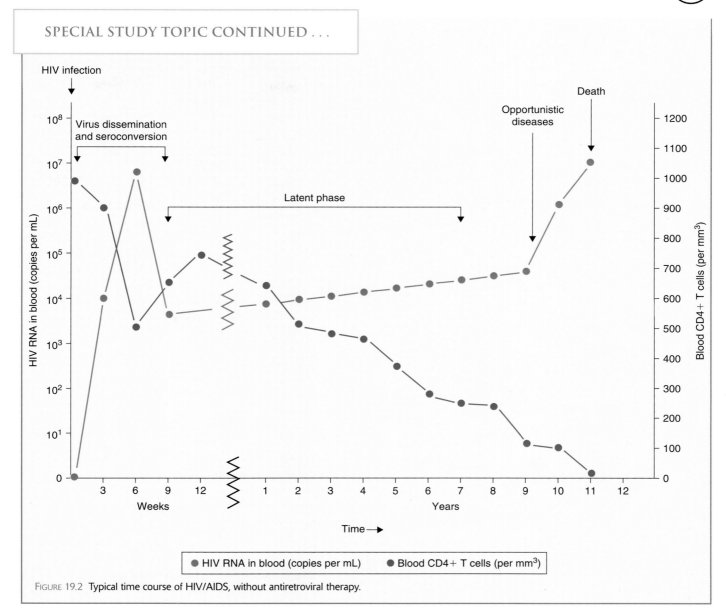

FIGURE 19.2 Typical time course of HIV/AIDS, without antiretroviral therapy.

Natural History and Clinical Features of HIV/AIDS

The natural history of HIV/AIDS is summarized in Figure 19.3. About half of those subjects infected have a seroconversion illness which mimics acute infectious mononucleosis. During the latent phase, a proportion develop persistent generalized lymphadenopathy (PGL), which is a reactive hyperplasia affecting all lymph nodes. Histologically, there is follicular germinal cell hyperplasia of the B-cell follicles, reacting to virus in the follicle dendritic cells. The lymph nodes later atrophy.

General constitutional symptoms develop years after infection, with weight loss, lassitude, fever and diarrhoea. These may result from the HIV viral damage to various organs (e.g. gut mucosal HIV infection), but are also attributable to one or more secondary infections: once there is an identified opportunistic disease, the patient is said to have AIDS, indicating a state of severe cellular immunosuppression. Without treatment, survival is no more than months. Opportunistic diseases are of varying virulence, and Figure 19.4 outlines how the more virulent (e.g. tuberculosis) present earlier, when patients have a less-damaged immune system.

Patients may present at several time-points during the HIV/AIDS sequence (see Table 19.13).

The list of opportunistic infections and tumours that are important in HIV-infected adults and children is long, and every organ may be involved. Multiple pathologies are common in the terminal phase of the disease (Table 19.14).

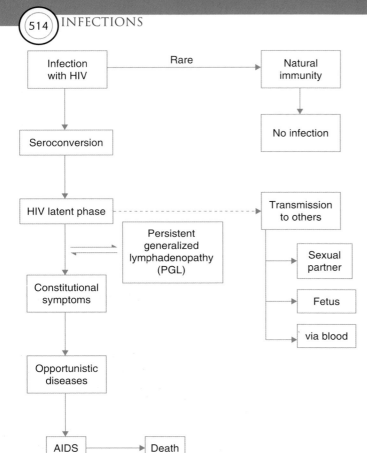

FIGURE 19.3 Overview of HIV infection and clinical outcome.

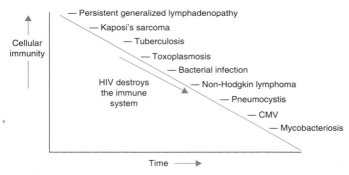

FIGURE 19.4 The progression of HIV disease. As the immune system is destroyed, the more virulent opportunist infections (e.g. tuberculosis) develop earlier, and the less virulent (e.g. *M. avium-intracellulare*) later.

TABLE 19.13 How people present with HIV disease

- Primary infection, seroconversion illness
- Asymptomatic through incidental HIV screening
- With persistent generalized lymphadenopathy (PGL)
- With non-specific constitutional illness
- With a specific opportunistic infection, neoplasm or HIV-dementia
- As they are dying of opportunistic disease and wasting
- If infants: failure to thrive, and opportunistic infections

TABLE 19.14 Important opportunistic diseases in HIV/AIDS

Viral infections
- Cytomegalovirus
- Herpes simplex
- JC virus
- Molluscum contagiosum

Bacterial infections
- *Mycobacterium tuberculosis*
- *Mycobacterium avium-intracellulare*
- *Streptococcus pneumoniae*
- Non-typhoid *Salmonella* infections
- *Treponema pallidum* (syphilis)

Fungal infections
- *Pneumocystis jirovecii*
- *Candida albicans*
- *Cryptococcus neoformans*

Protozoal infections
- *Cryptosporidium parvum*
- *Leishmania* species
- *Toxoplasma gondii*
- Microsporidia

HIV-associated tumours
- Kaposi's sarcoma
- B-cell non-Hodgkin lymphoma: cerebral and extracerebral
- Mucosal squamous carcinomas: cervix, anus, conjunctiva

Other HIV-associated diseases
- Central nervous system: HIV encephalitis and dementia
- Gut: mucosal HIV infection and malfunction
- Kidney: HIV-associated nephropathy (HIVAN)

The Pathological Features of HIV/AIDS

Viral Infections

Cytomegalovirus

Key Points

Cytomegalovirus:

- is a latent infection, which is reactivated in HIV/AIDS
- infects endothelial and epithelial cells
- causes damage to the gut, lung, retina and brain.

Cytomegalovirus (CMV) is a DNA herpes virus, and latently infects most people. It is acquired transplacentally, during infancy, by respiratory droplet infection, and via sexual intercourse. It reactivates in states of immunosuppression – particularly HIV/AIDS – and also in transplant recipient patients. By infecting the endothelial and epithelial cells it causes cytolytic cell damage and focal necrosis. Common presentations in HIV/AIDS are a pneumonitis, intestinal lesions with diarrhoea, confusional states from encephalitis and, importantly, visual defects. Retinal CMV infection is a significant cause of blindness in HIV disease, and is the reason why many patients are given prophylactic anti-herpes virus therapy. Morphologically, the nucleated layers of the retinal epithelium show the characteristic CMV nuclear and cytoplasmic inclusions, with necrosis.

CMV infection is diagnosed by finding the viral inclusions in biopsies (Figure 19.5) and virological identification in samples of blood and cerebrospinal fluid (CSF).

Herpes Simplex

This is representative of the large group of human herpes DNA viruses which includes herpes simplex virus (HSV) types 1 and 2, herpes zoster, CMV, Epstein–Barr virus (EBV) and HHV8 (the cause of Kaposi's sarcoma).

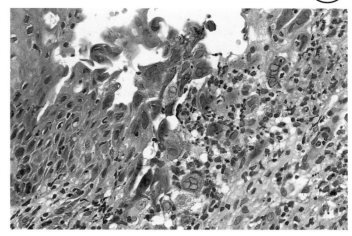

FIGURE 19.6 Herpes simplex virus (HSV) of the penis: eroded squamous mucosa with multinucleated cells, the nuclei containing blocks of HSV virions.

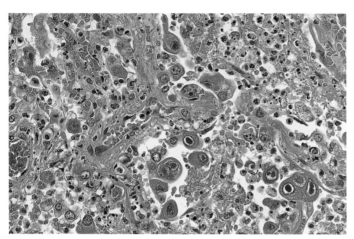

FIGURE 19.5 Cytomegalovirus (CMV) pneumonitis: large intranuclear viral inclusions in alveolar epithelial cells.

HSV is transmitted by direct contact with infected lesions, mainly from sexual intercourse. It primarily affects the genital skin and mucosae, but it is also neurotropic, and can disseminate to internal organs. Whether or not there is clinical primary infection, latent infection is thereafter life-long, and HSV reactivates in immunosuppression.

The skin and mucosal lesions are painful and erosive. Typically, they are on the penis, vulva and around the mouth ('cold sore'). Pathologically, the epithelial cells contain characteristic nuclear inclusions of virus (Figure 19.6), associated with cytolytic necrosis and inflammation. Similar pathology is seen in the skin lesions of chicken pox, caused by herpes zoster.

In HIV/AIDS, severe HSV skin and mucosal ulceration can occur, involving the genitalia, mouth and oesophagus. It can also cause necrotizing encephalitis and ulcerating conjunctival keratitis; both these lesions also occur in people without evident immunosuppression.

JC Virus

This is a papovavirus that everyone acquires as a latent infection in childhood. In late HIV disease it can reactivate, and cause a characteristic cytolytic infection of brain oligo-dendrocytes. This results in white matter necrosis.

Molluscum Contagiosum

This is a poxvirus infection that produces multiple small white nodules on the skin. It is normally common in childhood, and is more florid in people with HIV.

Bacterial Infections

The mycobacterial infections (*M. tuberculosis* and *M. avium-intracellulare*) are described in later sections of this chapter. Streptococcal infection causes both pneumonia and septicaemia; non-typhoid *Salmonella* infections cause enteritis and septic shock.

Fungal Infections

Pneumocystis jirovecii (carinii)

This is a ubiquitous fungus in the environment (although it was once classified as a protozoan parasite) to which everyone is exposed. Like many infections of very low virulent potential, it causes disease only in those significantly immunosuppressed (Table 19.15; see also Figure 19.4). Whilst it is now seen mainly in those with HIV infection (adults and children) and transplant patients (especially renal transplant), there have been epidemics in infancy that relate to malnutrition.

TABLE 19.15 Predisposing conditions to *Pneumocystis jirovecii (carinii)* pneumonia

- HIV infection
- Malnutrition in infancy
- Steroid and anticancer chemotherapy
- Immunosuppression for preventing organ transplant rejection

The infection can present rapidly with shortness of breath and prostration. Chest X-radiography shows fluffy fine shadows in the perihilar zones or throughout the lung fields.

On pathological examination, the lung in *Pneumocystis* pneumonia is solid, pale brown and dry (Figure 19.7). Microscopically, the alveoli are filled with masses of cysts, thus preventing gas exchange. The cysts are 3–4 μm in diameter, and contain small nuclei (Figure 19.8). There is often a mild interstitial lymphoplasmacytic infiltrate (interstitial pneumonitis). Aided by chemotherapy, macrophages phagocytose the fungi to clear the alveoli. However, if the infection persists or returns, there is progressive intra-alveolar organization and interstitial fibrosis. The diagnosis of *Pneumocystis* pneumonia is made by identifying the organisms in sputum or bronchial lavage specimens, or by lung biopsy. Standard treatment is with co-trimoxazole, which enables the lung to return to normal. However, in those with continuing immunosuppression, prophylactic therapy needs to be maintained. If and when pneumocystosis returns, it tends to cause progressive lung damage, with fibrosis and even cavitation.

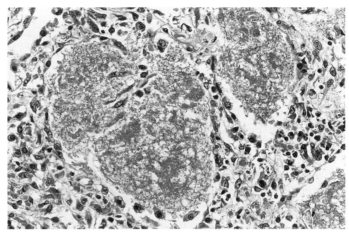

FIGURE 19.8 *Pneumocystis jirovecii* pneumonia: the alveoli are filled with numerous tiny cysts with nuclear dots. Interstitial inflammation is present.

Cryptococcus neoformans

Key Points

Cryptococcus:

- is a ubiquitous fungus in the environment
- infects humans via the respiratory tract
- disseminates in people with cell-mediated immune defects
- spreads from the lungs to the brain, lymphoreticular system and skin
- is a common cause of cerebral confusional states in HIV/AIDS
- is usually fatal if not treated.

This fungus is present globally in bird droppings and the soil. Infection is acquired by inhalation, but clinical disease is uncommon in people who are not immunocompromised. The primary lesion is a pneumonia: it may be localized (a 'cryptococcoma' that can present as a mass on chest X-radiography) or, more commonly, as a diffuse process causing breathlessness. HIV-infected patients are prone to developing cryptococcal meningo-encephalitis, presenting with confusion or focal neurological signs.

Pathologically, in HIV disease, the fungus elicits a minimal cellular reaction, so within the consolidated lung one sees alveoli filled with yeast. The brain shows milky, thick meninges and mucoid holes in the grey and white matter (resembling Swiss cheese; Figure 19.9). Histologically, the fungal yeasts have a mucoid capsule; they lie in unactivated macrophages or free in parenchyma and spaces around vessels.

Diagnosis is based on seeing the yeasts in tissue samples (e.g. CSF or biopsies), supported by antibody detection of antigen in blood or CSF (the CrAg test). Modern antifungal therapy can clear the disease, but it always recurs if prophylactic therapy is not continued.

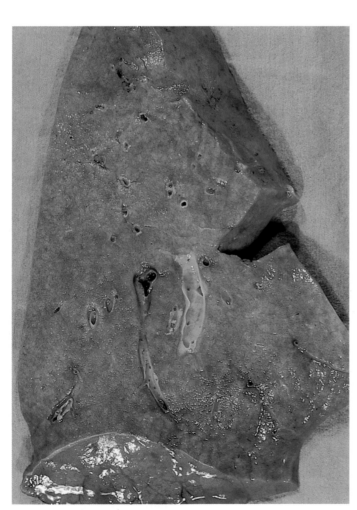

FIGURE 19.7 *Pneumocystis jirovecii* pneumonia: complete consolidation of the lung.

Protozoal Infections

Leishmania- and *Toxoplasma*-mediated infections are described elsewhere in this chapter (see pp. 532–534 and 537–538).

Cryptosporidium

Cryptosporidium parvum is a gut parasite of cattle that can be transmitted to man via contaminated water. In non-immuno-compromised people it causes self-limiting diarrhoea. However, in immunocompromised patients, chronic cholera-like diarrhoea results, with malabsorption. *C. parvum* infects the small and large bowel mucosae, the parasites residing in large numbers just within the enterocyte surface membrane; small intestinal villi are blunted, and there is an enteritis.

Several species of microsporidia (e.g. *Enterocytozoon bieneusi*) have been newly described in people with severe HIV-associated immunosuppression, and globally are a common cause of diarrhoea. The parasites reside within the enterocyte cytoplasm. As with *Cryptosporidium*, the exact pathogenesis of the diarrhoeal disease is unclear.

Diagnosis of both infections is by finding the parasites in faeces, or by gut biopsy (see Figure 19.12). No specific therapy is available, but anti-HIV chemotherapy often eradicates the infections.

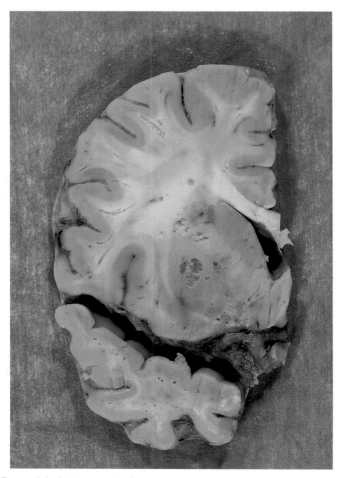

FIGURE 19.9 Cryptococcal CNS disease: within the white and grey matter are 'holes' – these are large accumulations of *Cryptococcus neoformans*.

HIV-associated Tumours

Kaposi's Sarcoma

Kaposi's sarcoma (KS) – which was first described in 1872 – is a peculiar proliferation of endothelial cells affecting the skin, mucosal surfaces, lymph nodes and many internal organs. Although HIV infection greatly increases the frequency of KS, it is not a necessary factor in the lesion's development. In 1994 a virus, human herpesvirus type 8 (HHV8), was found to be the significant factor; this is globally distributed and is transmitted by sexual intercourse, and vertically to children.

In all organs, KS (see Chapter 18, p. 504) develops as a red flat lesion (macule on the skin), and then thickens to plaques and infiltrative red nodules (Figure 19.10). It behaves as a space-occupying lesion and causes significant local oedema (e.g. in the subcutis and lung). Histologically, the mature lesion is a spindle-cell tumour with red blood cells between the endothelial tumour cells.

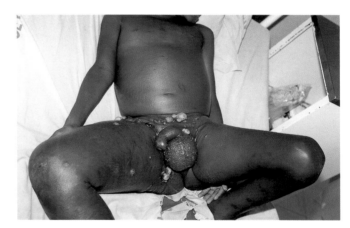

FIGURE 19.10 Kaposi's sarcoma: widespread nodular lesions around the pelvis, with leg oedema, in an HIV-infected young man.

Lymphoma

HIV-associated lymphomas comprise B-cell, high-grade tumours (see Chapter 8, p. 202), located in extranodal sites. They are 100-fold more common in HIV-infected people than in the normal population, and many are associated with EBV infection. Cerebral lymphoma (p. 318) presents with focal neurological signs and confusion; pathologically, there are one or more tumour masses within the brain, the malignant cells spreading out from the blood vessel walls. Elsewhere, tumours present as oral and intestinal ulcerating lesions, and with pulmonary and retroperitoneal masses. A common histological pattern is high-grade B-cell lymphoma similar to that of Burkitt lymphoma.

Mucosal Squamous Cell Neoplasms

Intraepithelial and invasive squamous cell neoplasms of the cervix and anus are aetiologically associated with human papilloma virus (HPV) infections (p. 418). People who are coinfected with HIV have a significant risk of developing dysplasia and *in-situ* carcinoma at these sites, which are often detected by screening. However, invasive malignant lesions are less frequent than expected. In central Africa, conjunctival carcinoma (associated with UV light exposure) is also more common in those with HIV infection.

Neurological Disease in HIV/AIDS

In addition to common central nervous system (CNS) diseases such as toxoplasmosis, cryptococcosis, progressive multifocal leucoencephalopathy (PML) and lymphoma, HIV-associated dementia is a late phenomenon (p. 299). It appears to be caused by cortical neuronal loss and abnormalities of the dendritic connections. Morphologically, there is cerebral atrophy, and the characteristic HIV encephalitis comprises multiple nodules of infected microglia and microglial giant cells in the white matter (Figure 19.11). By secreting toxic cytokines, these lesions also affect neural function.

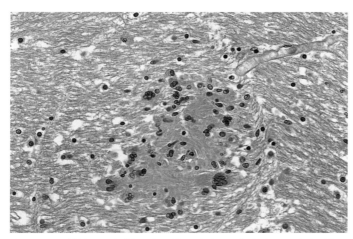

FIGURE 19.11 HIV encephalitis: microglia and giant cells in the cerebral white matter.

Skin Disease in HIV/AIDS

The skin lesions in HIV/AIDS include herpetic ulceration, molluscum contagiosum nodules, cryptococcal nodules, mycobacterial infections, lymphoma, Kaposi's sarcoma, and a pruritic maculopapular rash (particularly in Africans).

Renal Disease in HIV/AIDS

Many opportunistic diseases can affect the kidney (e.g. cryptococcosis, CMV infection of the tubules, pyaemic bacterial infection, tuberculosis, lymphoma), but one specific entity is important – HIV-associated nephropathy (HIVAN). Clinically, this condition presents with renal failure and nephrotic syndrome. Pathologically, it is characterized by focal segmental glomerulosclerosis (FSGS) and interstitial inflammation with tubular atrophy and dilatation. It appears to be caused directly by HIV, and is significant

because it is an ethnically-restricted opportunistic disease in HIV/AIDS: it occurs only in ople of African descent.

Paediatric HIV Disease

This is common in many poor parts of the world since, without antiretroviral chemotherapy during pregnancy and delivery, about 25% of fetuses are infected if the mother is HIV-infected. The clinical and pathological features are listed in Table 19.16. Without specific treatment, the mortality in children is 50% by the age of 3 years, and few survive 5 years. Malaria is not aggravated by HIV infection.

TABLE 19.16 Features of paediatric HIV disease

- Failure to thrive
- Lymphadenopathy (PGL)
- Diarrhoea and wasting, with opportunistic parasitic infections
- *Pneumocystis jirovecii* pneumonia
- Bacterial infections, particularly pneumonia
- Lymphoid interstitial pneumonia (LIP) and measles pneumonitis
- Thymic atrophy
- HIV encephalitis and neurodevelopmental delay

Treatment of HIV/AIDS

This hugely complex area comprises specific antiretroviral therapy (ART), for example by inhibiting the reverse transcriptase enzyme, in addition to specific therapy for opportunistic infections and tumours, and prophylaxis against opportunistic infections. The major clinicopathological points of HIV therapy are listed in Table 19.17.

TABLE 19.17 HIV therapy

- Antiretroviral therapy (ART) slows down HIV virion production and prolongs life
- ART permits partial restoration of CD4+ T cell counts and immune status
- ART prevents or enables the patient to eliminate many opportunistic diseases
- Specific prophylaxis (e.g. co-trimoxazole against *Pneumocystis jirovecii*) prolongs life
- All of these therapies have potentially severe toxic side effects (e.g. marrow suppression, liver damage, atherogenesis, redistribution of body fat stores)

BACTERIAL INFECTIONS

Mycobacterial Infections

Mycobacteria are aerobic Gram-positive bacilli with a thick waxy cell wall. They are often referred to as acid-fast bacilli

HIV/AIDS IN AFRICA

A 35-year-old African male presented to his local hospital in West Africa with a 6-month history of weight loss and intermittent diarrhoea with watery stools (not bloody). Direct examination of the faeces showed oocysts of *Cryptosporidium* (Figure 19.12), and serology confirmed the clinical suspicion of infection with HIV-1. His blood CD4+ T-cell count was 55 per mm^3. He thus had AIDS.

Being relatively wealthy, the patient could afford to be treated with antiretroviral drugs; his diarrhoea ceased and he put on weight. His CD4 count rose to 200 per mm^3, but he became intolerant of the anti-HIV drugs and stopped them. He also stopped taking regular co-trimoxazole prophylaxis therapy. After 2 months his weight had fallen again, and he was readmitted with fever and a cough. Chest X-radiography showed a pneumonia, and blood culture indicated a *Streptococcus pneumoniae* bacteraemia. Antibiotics suppressed this infection.

Six months later, he was admitted for the last time, fitting and in coma. Despite empirical antitoxoplasmosis therapy, the patient died. At autopsy, the swollen brain showed a large haemorrhagic mass in the basal ganglia; histology confirmed *Toxoplasma gondii* as the cause (Figure 19.13).

Clinicopathological Points

1. Treating HIV infection and reducing the viral infection load permits partial recovery of the cell-mediated immune system, and thereby indirectly treats several of the opportunistic infections, including cryptosporidiosis for which there is no specific therapy.
2. Simple prophylactic antibiotics – if taken consistently – can prevent several bacterial infections, *Pneumocystis* pneumonia, and reactivation of toxoplasmosis.
3. During the course of HIV disease, patients suffer from multiple pathologies.

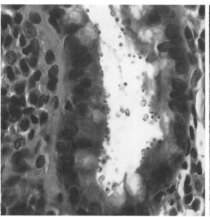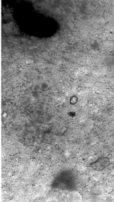

FIGURE 19.12 Cryptosporidiosis. Right: oocysts of *Cryptosporidium* in the faeces (Ziehl–Neelsen staining). Left: rectal crypt lined by numerous parasites.

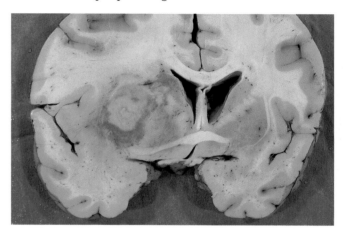

FIGURE 19.13 Cerebral toxoplasmosis: haemorrhagic necrotic lesion compressing the brain.

(AFB) because once a stain colour has bound to the wall, it is resistant to decolorization by acid. The standard stain is red carbol fuchsin, the basis of the classical Ziehl–Neelsen (ZN) stain for mycobacteria (see Figure 19.21, p. 524). Most mycobacteria are environmental saprophytes (including *M. avium-intracellulare*) and reside in water and soil. However, two species are essentially human-adapted, are transmitted directly from man to man, and are the cause of much human disease: these are *M. tuberculosis* and *M. leprae*, the aetiological agents of tuberculosis and leprosy respectively.

Tuberculosis

Epidemiology

Tuberculosis is a typical epidemic infection which affects large numbers in a susceptible population with high mortality, and then becomes less virulent over decades and centuries as man adapts to it. Thus, it accounted for one-quarter of adult deaths in the mid-nineteenth century in British cities. Although the incidence was greatly reduced (Table 19.18), since the early 1990s the frequency of UK cases has risen again, due to overseas immigrants being infected with tuberculosis, in addition to HIV co-infection and poverty. In tropical countries, tuberculosis has, for more than a century, been a major cause of mortality, but this has now been made even worse by the HIV/AIDS pandemic.

Sequence and Pathogenesis of Tuberculosis Infection

Acquisition of tuberculosis is usually by inhalation of bacilli from a patient with pulmonary cavitating tuberculosis, and this gives rise to primary tuberculosis (see Figure 19.14).

TABLE 19.18 Epidemiology of tuberculosis

- 2 billion people infected (one-third of the global population)
- 8 million new cases each year globally
- 3 million deaths each year
- in England and Wales, 8000 new cases per year (and rising)

The lung lesion is in any lobe, and is usually subpleural. The initial polymorphonuclear leucocyte inflammatory response cannot contain the bacilli, at which point monocyte-derived macrophages phagocytose them. Within hours, bacilli are carried in cells to the draining hilar lymph nodes, and in both lung and nodes, the characteristic inflammatory reaction develops (the primary complex; Figure 19.14). There is necrosis of the lesions which macroscopically are yellowish

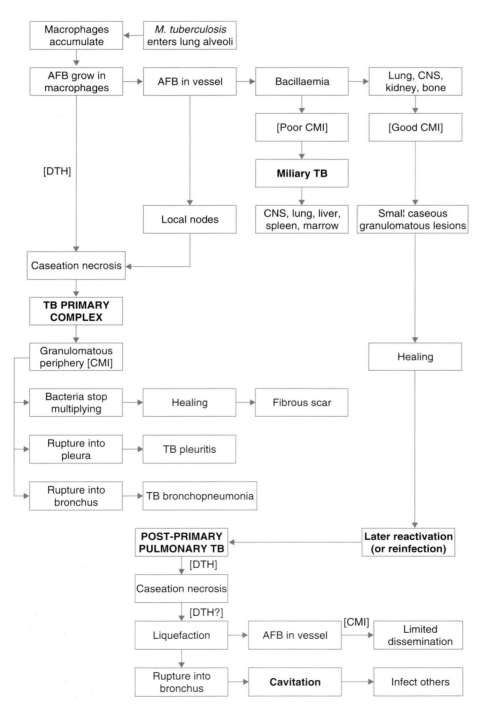

FIGURE 19.14 The typical development of tuberculosis (TB); primary complex, miliary TB and subsequent post-primary pulmonary TB. The immunopathological inputs are indicated: CMI (cell-mediated immunity) and DTH (delayed-type hypersensitivity). AFB = acid-fast bacilli.

and are thus termed 'caseous (cheesy) necrosis' (Figure 19.15). The factors responsible for this necrosis are unclear, but they involve delayed-type hypersensitivity phenomena (Table 19.19) and coincide with skin test positivity for tuberculous infection. Around the necrosis are formed granulomas, a product of cell-mediated immunity (CMI) where, following antigenic stimulation and copresentation with MHC class II molecules, T-helper cells secrete cytokines to active macrophages. Activated macrophages – which morphologically are known as epithelioid cells – have more potent products that are able to kill or neutralize virulent agents such as *M. tuberculosis* (oxide radicals and proteases; Figures 19.16 and 19.17).

Primary Tuberculosis

Tuberculous disease that occurs within 5 years of infection is classified as 'primary tuberculosis'. The primary lung/node complex is usually subclinical, and heals spontaneously with fibrous scarring and even dystrophic calcification.

As part of the primary infection there is a bacillaemia with dissemination of infection to many organs (see Figure 19.14).

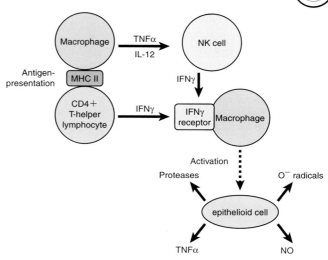

FIGURE 19.16 Schematic outline of cell-mediated immunity. Macrophages present antigens to a CD4+ T cell via MHC class II molecules, while cytokines activate macrophages to epithelioid cells. The alternative activation route via NK cells is indicated. IFN = interferon; IL = interleukin; TNF = tumor necrosis factor.

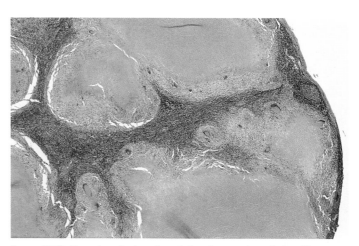

FIGURE 19.17 Caseation of a lymph node in primary tuberculosis, with surrounding giant cell granulomas.

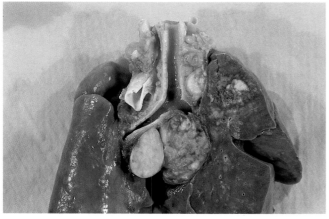

FIGURE 19.15 Primary tuberculosis in a child: the small lung lesion near the left apex, and the large hilar node caseating masses are seen.

TABLE 19.19 Immunopathological responses to *M. tuberculosis* infection

A. Cell-mediated immunity (CMI)
- activation of macrophages to epithelioid cells, forming granulomas
- requires T cells
- effective in controlling mycobacteria, or killing them
- prevents dissemination of bacilli

B. Delayed-type hypersensitivity (DTH)
- appears at the time of caseation in primary infection
- also manifests as positive skin test to tuberculoprotein
- causes mass necrosis of *M. tuberculosis* infected tissue
- rapidly controls spread of infection, but at cost of mass tissue necrosis
- is responsible for liquefaction necrosis of lung lesions
- pathogenesis not well understood, but involves different T-cell subsets than those operating CMI

These also usually heal, but they may progress or reactivate later to cause 'end-organ tuberculosis'. Bone, adrenal gland, kidney and brain are typical sites, with caseous granulomatous destructive lesions: if they form a tumour-like mass of necrosis, they are called 'tuberculoma'.

The lung apex zone is frequently a site of such dissemination, and bacilli here may remain latent in macrophages for years and even decades. Subsequently, they may reactivate to cause post-primary pulmonary tuberculosis. Pleuritis and progressive bronchopneumonic disease can occur in a small proportion of those with primary tuberculosis, but this occurs more frequently if they are coinfected with HIV.

If there is a heavy bacillaemia in primary infection and CMI is poor, miliary tuberculosis may result (it is called 'miliary' because the lesions resemble seeds; see Figure 19.19). This represents multiorgan haematogenous dissemination of infection, forming 1–3-mm necrotic foci with a poor granulomatous CMI response. The lungs are typically involved. If there is meningeal spread, then death always occurs in the absence of treatment.

Post-primary Pulmonary Tuberculosis

This is the characteristic form of adult pulmonary tuberculosis, and such patients are the source of *M. tuberculosis* infection – they have 'open TB'. The pathogenesis is either reactivation of a previous lesion, or reinfection with a new bacillus, or *M. tuberculosis* infection for the first time. These proportions depend on environmental circumstances. Some 5–10% of those with healed pulmonary primary lesions reactivate later in life, often precipitated by a change in immunological status (Table 19.20). Patients present with cough, often haemoptysis, and feeling generally ill. The chest X-radiograph usually has upper zone shadows, and sometimes also cavitation.

The pathological features are as follows. Typically, the lesions are in the apex of the lung, the site of a previous seeding of infection. There is an aggressive necrotizing granulomatous pneumonia, and crucially the necrotic material becomes liquefied. If the material communicates with an airway, the necrotic debris is coughed up, along with large numbers of AFB. This leaves a cavity in the lung, lined by granulomatous inflammation (Figure 19.18). Peripheral to this is a fibrotic lining, and the whole lesion is termed 'fibrocaseous tuberculosis'. There is some passage of bacilli from the lung to local nodes and other internal organs, but this is much less prominent than occurs in primary infection.

The Koch Phenomenon

Robert Koch – who discovered the tubercle bacillus – described a feature of tuberculosis infection in guinea pigs that helps to explain the difference between primary and post-primary lung lesions. When *M. tuberculosis* is injected into the hind limb of a guinea pig, a local nodule develops and the draining lymph nodes enlarge with caseation. If a second subcutaneous infection is injected into the other hind limb 4–6 weeks later, a nodule develops rapidly, ulcerates and sloughs off; the local node is unaffected. Thus, the tissue reaction is more aggressive the second time round, indicating greater delayed-type hypersensitivity (DTH). A similar phenomenon occurs if the second injection is not live bacilli but is sterile tuberculoprotein.

Adults acquiring tuberculosis for the first time also tend to develop a post-primary rather than a primary type response, unless they are HIV-infected.

TABLE 19.20 Conditions predisposing to reactivation of tuberculosis lesions

- HIV infection
- Alcoholism and liver cirrhosis
- Malnutrition
- Diabetes
- Steroid and immunosuppressive therapy
- Old age

With proper antituberculous treatment, the mortality of adult pulmonary tuberculosis is less than 10%. Although the granulomatous inflammation subsides, the cavities and scarring remain. Full antituberculosis therapy takes several months to complete. Failure to complete the course may permit renewal of infection and, worse, the development of drug-resistant strains of *M. tuberculosis*.

It is important to identify and treat the disease rapidly, since the lung cavity lining is a rich source of bacilli that can infect others. One complication is massive haemoptysis as the inflammation may erode into a bronchial artery. Chronically, colonization of the cavity by an aspergilloma (see later) may occur.

Diagnosis of Tuberculosis

The main diagnostic methods are direct examination of sputum, tissue, CSF, etc. for AFB and culture of suspected material (culture has the higher sensitivity and provides species identification of the *Mycobacterium*). Tissue is obtained by knife biopsy, fine needle aspiration of peripheral nodes, and computed tomography (CT)-guided biopsy of (for example) deep lymph nodes. It is essential that such material be submitted for culture as well histology. Increasingly, polymerase chain reaction (PCR) technology is used for rapid sensitive diagnosis on fresh tissue material and, further, for the rapid identification of sensitivity to rifampicin, the main antituberculosis drug.

Tuberculosis in HIV/AIDS

HIV is now the major risk factor for reactivation of previous tuberculosis infection: indeed, instead of a lifetime risk

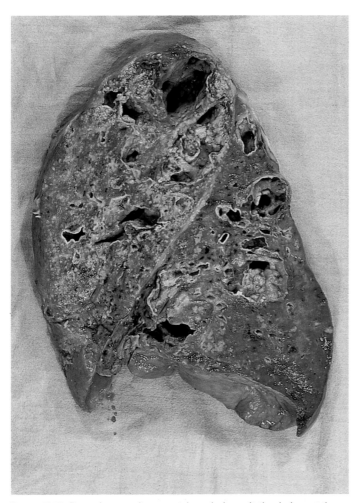

FIGURE 19.18 Post-primary pulmonary tuberculosis: cavitating lesions at the apex and elsewhere.

of 5–10% reactivation, it is a 10% per annum risk of disease. Similarly, primary infections in HIV-infected people are much more aggressive than in non-infected people.

Patients present with fever, severe malaise, weight loss and diarrhoea, and the tuberculous disease is usually disseminated. Any organ can be affected, including the lung with miliary nodular disease, lymph nodes, intestine and meninges. If presentation is relatively early during the course of HIV disease, the pathology is granulomatous and AFB are relatively sparse. However, in the state of terminal immunosuppression, the lesions are non-reactive ('anergic TB'): there are no epithelioid cells, giant cells or granulomas, just necrotic macrophages and huge numbers of bacilli (Figures 19.20 and 19.21). Patients die in a state of toxic shock, probably related to release of the cytokine tumor necrosis factor alpha (TNFα).

This pathology is not unique to those with HIV infection. It also occurs in people severely immunosuppressed by other means (see Tables 19.8 and 19.9).

Mycobacterium avium-intracellulare (MAI)

The patterns of MAI clinical pathology are listed in Table 19.21.

Man is constantly infected with MAI through food and water supplies, but until the HIV pandemic, clinical disease was uncommon. Pre-AIDS, the major disease was a granulomatous necrotizing lymphadenitis affecting the cervical nodes, mainly in children, which exactly resembled tuberculosis pathologically. Infection is acquired by mouth. Treatment – following culture identification of the pathogen – is surgical drainage, but chemotherapy is not required.

Chronic bronchopulmonary infection occurs in already damaged lungs (e.g. by tuberculosis or bronchiectasis). The MAI colonize poorly drained or aerated lung zones, causing granulomatous necrotizing inflammation similar to tuberculosis itself, with progressive lung destruction. The preferred treatment is surgery plus chemotherapy.

The most frequent MAI disease is now part of HIV/AIDS. Towards the terminal phase of disease (see Figure 19.4), such patients present with fever, diarrhoea and lymphadenopathy. The standard work-up includes bone marrow biopsy and blood culture to look for MAI infection, for there is bacillaemia and AFB are present within macrophages throughout the lymphoreticular system: bone marrow, lymph nodes, gut

TUBERCULOSIS IN A HOMELESS INTRAVENOUS DRUG USER

A 35-year-old unemployed white male lived in a central London doorway and was known to be injecting heroin regularly. He had not been seen for several days until he was found by the police, slumped on a park bench. He was incoherent, and was taken to the police station where initially he was thought to be on a heroin 'high'. However, when next morning his conscious level was worse and his breathing was obviously fast and shallow, he was brought to the hospital casualty department.

He was very thin. Chest X-radiography showed widespread fine nodularity: the differential diagnosis was bacterial or tuberculous lung disease. His blood pressure was 80/55 mmHg. A sample of sputum had numerous AFB on Ziehl–Neelsen staining. The blood toxicology showed traces of heroin metabolites, but this was insufficient to account for the man's mental status. Because of his lifestyle and presumed tuberculosis infection, the blood was also tested for HIV and hepatitis B and C virus infections: he was HIV-negative, but HCV- and HBV-positive.

He was commenced on intravenous antituberculosis therapy and oxygen by mask. He appeared to improve, with rising blood pO$_2$ and blood pressure, but on the fifth day of treatment he went into cardiorespiratory failure, and then asystole. Despite resuscitation measures – which were undertaken despite his being a tuberculosis risk to healthcare workers – the man died.

At autopsy, he had miliary tuberculosis of the lung (Figure 19.19) and hilar nodes. Histology showed poor

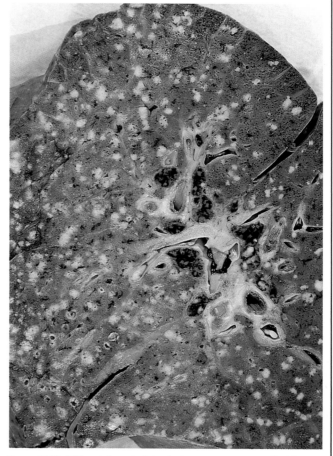

FIGURE 19.19 **Miliary tuberculosis in the lung: numerous small white necrotic lesions in parenchyma and the hilar node.**

granuloma formation and abundant AFB in the lesions (Figures 19.20 and 19.21); the lung was very oedematous. There were no old calcified lung lesions. The liver appeared macroscopically normal, but on histology there was stage 3 fibrosis and chronic portal inflammation, consistent with HCV infection at the precirrhotic phase. The results of the sputum culture were returned 2 weeks later and showed the presence of *M. tuberculosis*, with normal drug sensitivity.

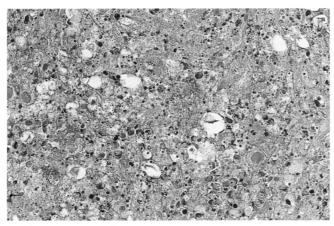

FIGURE 19.20 Pulmonary lesions: necrotic macrophages, and no granulomas.

Clinicopathological Points

1. Malnourished intravenous drug users are at high risk of acquiring tuberculosis.
2. This patient's infection had the morphology of severe primary tuberculosis, rather than a reactivation lesion.
3. Despite appropriate chemotherapy, patients with advanced tuberculosis may die in shock – perhaps due to an excessive immunological reaction initiated by the anti-tuberculosis drugs rapidly killing the large bacillary load.
4. Incoherence in drug users may be due to medical illness, and not to toxic substances.

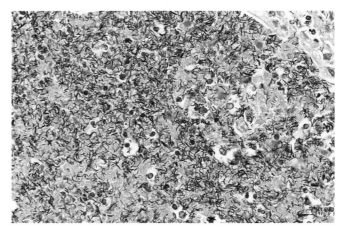

FIGURE 19.21 Acid-fast staining to show vast numbers of tubercle bacilli. (Ziehl–Neelsen.)

TABLE 19.21 Patterns of MAI clinical pathology

- Immunocompetent patients: neck lymph node infection
- Immunocompetent patients with damaged lungs: necrotizing bronchopneumonia
- Immunosuppressed patients (e.g. HIV): widespread infection of macrophages

mucosa, spleen and liver. Nodules and sheets of highly parasitized cells without granuloma formation are seen. As MAI is of low virulence, there is usually no necrosis (Figure 19.22). Antibiotic treatment is both difficult and expensive.

Leprosy

Key Points

Leprosy:

- is caused by *Mycobacterium leprae*
- is the most common global cause of peripheral neuropathy
- is characterized by infection of the peripheral nerves and skin
- has an immunopathological spectrum of disease
- is treatable and curable if diagnosed early.

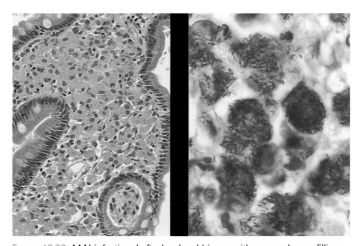

FIGURE 19.22 MAI infection. Left: duodenal biopsy with macrophages filling the lamina propria. (Haematoxylin and eosin staining.) Right: the cells contain many acid-fast bacilli (AFB). (Ziehl–Neelsen.)

Today, leprosy is uncommon in the UK (up to 30 new patients present each year), but globally there are still up to one million sufferers in the tropics and subtropics, with 600 000 new cases a year, particularly in India. This is markedly fewer than two decades ago, due to determined global case-finding and treatment, and mass Bacille

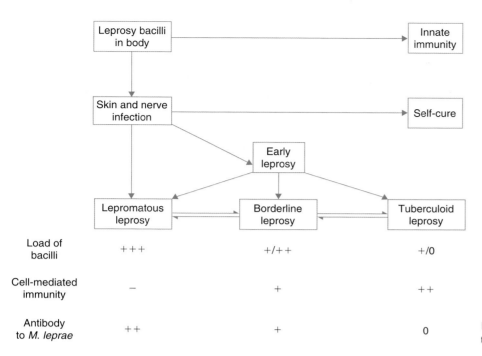

	Lepromatous leprosy	Borderline leprosy	Tuberculoid leprosy
Load of bacilli	+++	+/++	+/0
Cell-mediated immunity	–	+	++
Antibody to *M. leprae*	++	+	0

FIGURE 19.23 Leprosy: outcome of infection and the basic immunopathology.

Calmette-Guérin (BCG) vaccination (BCG may not prevent tuberculosis in the tropics, but it is effective in preventing leprosy). Leprosy is important because it is the most common cause of peripheral nerve disease and, if diagnosed early, is curable and the feared deformities are preventable.

Leprosy is the result of infection by *Mycobacterium leprae* which, apart from a few monkeys and armadillos in the wild, only affects man. This bacillus has never been cultivated in the laboratory, although the mouse footpad supports growth and may be used for drug resistance testing. The habitat and mode of infection of the bacterium are still unclear, but it is probable that bacilli are inhaled from secretions from the respiratory tract of patients with the lepromatous form of the disease (see below).

The leprosy bacillus targets Schwann cells of the peripheral nerves, and is also phagocytosed by macrophages. Control of bacillary replication is via classical CMI, and many of those infected never develop clinical disease (Figure 19.23). Those who develop the clinical disease (with an incubation period of several years) generally have either:

● lepromatous leprosy: this disease has large numbers of organisms and little CMI, indicating a specific immune defect to leprosy
● tuberculoid leprosy: this disease has granuloma formation (i.e. good CMI) and few or no evident infectious organisms.

Clinical Features

In lepromatous leprosy there are multiple symmetrical reddish patches and nodules on the skin, which may be tender, but not itchy. The peripheral nerves are progressively thickened and damaged, producing glove-and-stocking anaesthesia of the hands and feet (Figure 19.24A).

In contrast, in tuberculoid leprosy the skin lesions are few and asymmetrical, with a raised margin and hypopigmented centre; they are often anaesthetic (see Figure 19.24B). The peripheral nerves are thickened; damage may be acute with relatively sudden anaesthesia or motor damage.

In advanced leprosy, the surface lesions may be destructive (e.g. of the nose) and disfiguring, but the effects of nerve damage are more important. Sensory anaesthesia permits trauma to feet and hands, secondary ulceration and osteomyelitis; motor nerve damage causes paralyses such as ulnar nerve palsy and claw hand.

Pathology

Lepromatous leprosy has abundant mycobacteria in masses of macrophages in the skin, and also often in dermal and peripheral nerve Schwann cells (Figures 19.25 and 19.26). The bacilli are non-toxic, and can be detected by incising a skin lesion, smearing some of the dermal 'juice' onto a slide, and staining for AFB (this is called 'taking a slit skin smear').

Nerves in this form of the disease may undergo progressive fibrosis, resulting in 'glove and stocking anaesthesia'. Other organs may also be infected by leprosy bacilli, such as the testes (with chronic atrophy causing gynaecomastia), the iris (causing iritis) and the larynx.

Tuberculoid leprosy – so called because it shares some histopathological features with tuberculosis – is characterized by granulomas in and around nerves in the skin (Figure 19.27), and bacilli are detected only with difficulty. Destructive granulomas affect the endoneurium of peripheral nerves, causing anaesthesia and motor damage, while in some patients a major peripheral nerve may undergo caseous-type necrosis causing irreparable damage.

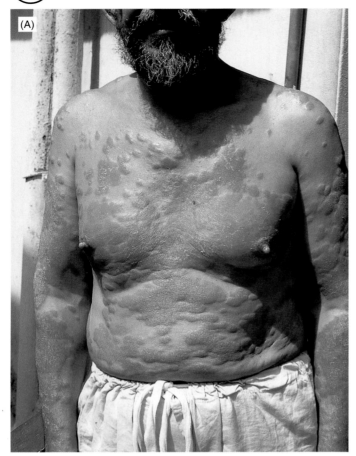

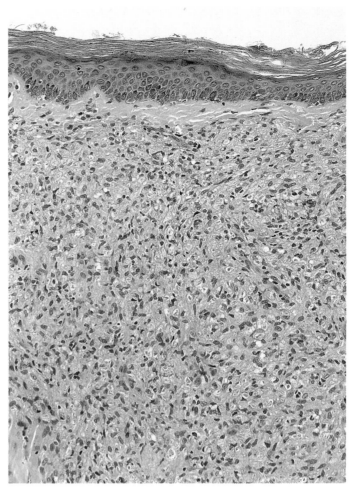

FIGURE 19.25 Lepromatous leprosy of the skin: packed macrophages under the epidermis.

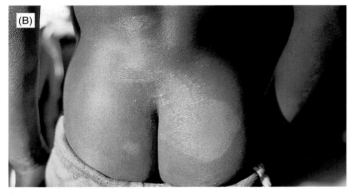

FIGURE 19.24 Clinical leprosy. (A) Lepromatous widespread nodular lesions. (B) Tuberculoid leprosy with few, hypopigmented flat lesions.

Management

The disease may be diagnosed from the typical skin and neurological features, supported by slit skin smears. For patients in industrialized countries, a skin or nerve biopsy is always performed for proper confirmation and accurate subtyping of the disease.

Proper treatment of leprosy involves multidrug therapy with rifampicin and other mycobactericidal or static drugs. Most of the bacteria are rapidly killed, but it may take years for all the leprosy bacillus antigen in lepromatous patients to be cleared. In those patients with chronic disabilities due

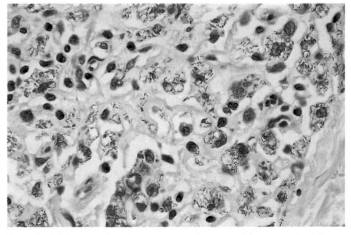

FIGURE 19.26 Lepromatous leprosy: macrophages contain many acid-fast leprosy bacilli. (Wade–Fite.)

to neuropathy, plastic surgery may be beneficial (e.g. tendon transfer), and good care of anaesthetic feet can prevent ulceration.

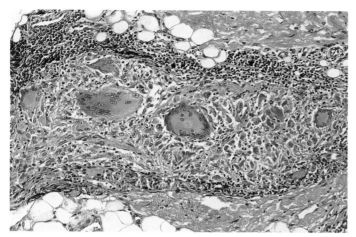

FIGURE 19.27 Tuberculoid leprosy: skin biopsy showing a deep nerve disrupted by a giant cell granulomatous infiltrate.

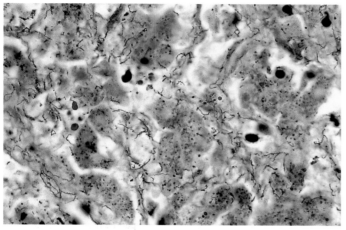

FIGURE 19.28 Spirochaetes of *Treponema pallidum* in congenital syphilis. (Warthin–Starry.)

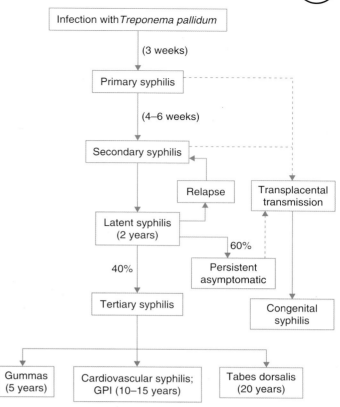

FIGURE 19.29 Sequelae of events in untreated syphilis, with time scales and approximate proportions. GPI = general paralysis of the insane.

Syphilis

Syphilis is a systemic infection caused by the *Treponema pallidum*. It is transmitted mainly by sexual intercourse (venereal syphilis), and less commonly via the placenta (congenital syphilis).

The organism is a spirochaete, of length 4–14 μm and diameter 0.2 μm, which cannot be grown in culture (Figure 19.28). It invades the penile and vulvovaginal mucosae directly, and at that site the primary lesion – a chancre – develops. Within hours of infection, spirochaetes disseminate via lymphatics and bloodstream, and reactive lymphadenopathy develops. Thereafter, the disease sequence is unpredictable, but a proportion of patients go on to develop secondary and tertiary syphilis, which have distinct clinical pathologies (Figure 19.29).

Clinical and Pathological Features

The primary lesion or chancre is a punched-out ulcer which heals within weeks, with minimal scarring. Histologically, there is associated epithelial hyperplasia, plasmacytic perivascular inflammatory infiltrate, oedema, and abundant spirochaetes. A characteristic feature of primary and secondary syphilis lesions is a reactive swelling of vascular endothelial cells: this is termed 'endarteritis obliterans' (and is also found in other infections such as tuberculosis).

In secondary syphilis, the mucosal surfaces develop erythematous rashes (condylomata lata), with generalized lymphadenopathy, representing a reaction to the initial haematogenous infection spread. Histologically, they resemble primary lesions.

There are three basic forms of tertiary lesions: the gumma; cardiovascular lesions; and neurosyphilis. Gummas are necrotic lesions of varying size (up to centimetres) that appear in the skin, testis, liver and bones (e.g. the nose, with collapse). Histological examination shows the presence of necrotic granulomas, similar to those of tuberculosis, and spirochaetes are rarely identified.

The *cardiovascular lesions* are arteritis affecting the media of large vessels; there is chronic inflammation and destruction of the elastic elements critical for maintenance of the artery diameter. Thus, the classical lesion is proximal thoracic aortitis which can manifest as an aneurysm (the rupture of which is usually fatal), dilatation of the aortic valve ring with aortic regurgitation, or coronary artery stenosis with myocardial ischaemia.

Neurosyphilis (p. 297) comprises meningitis, tabes dorsalis, and general paralysis of the insane (GPI). The meningovascular inflammation is an example of endarteritis obliterans, and can cause ischaemic cerebral lesions. There may also be small meningeal gummas. Tabes is a degeneration of the posterior spinal columns and dorsal nerve roots; it results from chronic inflammation of the nerve roots. GPI is a cerebral atrophy characterized by loss of neurones, a microglial cell reaction, and visible spirochaetes in the tissues.

Congenital syphilis is rare, but is a standard cause of abortion, fetal hydrops, or newborns with hepatosplenomegaly and pneumonia. Abundant spirochaetes are present in the lesions. Later CNS, bone and mucocutaneous lesions may develop.

Diagnosis

Whilst the primary and secondary lesions have distinct histopathology and usually evident spirochaetes, the mainstay of diagnosis is serological. The screening tests are the rapid plasma reagin (RPR) and Venereal Disease Research Laboratory (VDRL) tests – these detect autoantibodies, and are not specific. Specific tests are the treponemal haemagglutination assay (TPHA) and treponemal immobilization test (TPI).

FUNGAL INFECTIONS

Most fungi are saprophytes living in the soil, and man is constantly exposed to infection, particularly through the respiratory tract. A few potential pathogens, such as *Candida*, are also part of the normal human flora. In nature they usually grow in a mycelium composed of elongated branching cells 5–10 μm across, called hyphae; in man, they may change their growth morphology and form rounded cell yeasts.

Candida

Candida albicans is part of the normal flora of the mouth and gut, and some 10% of women have the infection in the vagina. Clinical disease is common and is precipitated by a wide range of immunological defects (Table 19.22). The more common superficial infections involve the mouth, vagina and oesophagus. The fungus proliferates in and invades into the squamous epithelium, causing local irritation and even ulceration. Grossly, the mucosal surfaces are thickened and pale (Figure 19.30). Histologically, *Candida* is characterized by having both hyphae and yeast forms in tissue (Figure 19.31).

TABLE 19.22 Conditions associated with candidiasis

- Diabetes
- Oral contraceptive pill
- Pregnancy
- Insufficient neutrophil polymorphs
- Phagocyte defects
- Anticancer and transplantation therapy
- Leukaemia
- HIV disease

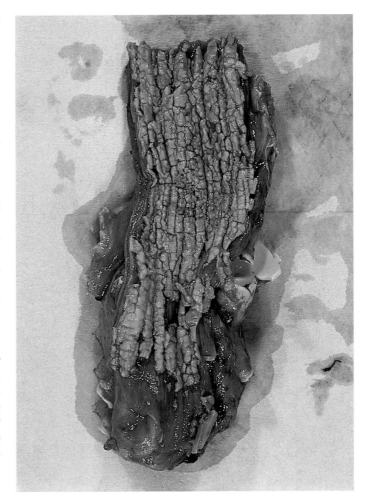

FIGURE 19.30 Oesophageal candidiasis: note the thick coat of fungus on the mucosa.

In severe infections, there is haematogenous dissemination of *Candida*; this is particularly common in leukaemic patients, and is a cause of septic shock. The main organs involved are the kidney, liver, lung, brain and meninges. There are multiple small abscesses within which are clumps of yeasts.

Aspergillus

There are many *Aspergillus* species in the environment, of which *A. flavus* is the most common pathogen. Infection is by inhalation. Clinical disease only occurs if the patient has abnormal defences against infection, or has a structurally abnormal lung. The three main clinicopathological patterns of aspergillosis are indicated in Table 19.23.

Aspergilloma is a mass of fungal hyphae growing in a lung cavity that communicates with the airways; it does not invade the lung. The aetiology of the cavity is most commonly previous tuberculosis. The condition presents with cough and haemoptysis, and the only curative treatment is to resect the cavity.

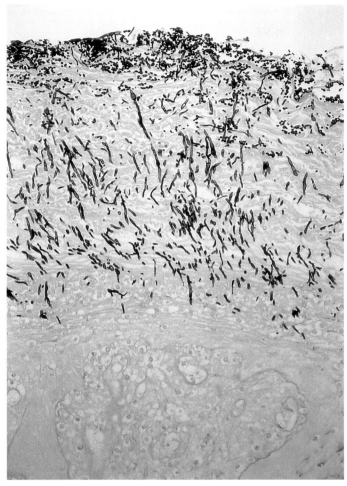

FIGURE 19.31 Oesophageal candidiasis: fungal hyphae invading the mucosa. (Grocott silver.)

TABLE 19.23 Clinicopathological patterns of aspergillosis

- Aspergilloma in a lung cavity
- Bronchopulmonary aspergillosis
- Invasive aspergillosis

Bronchopulmonary aspergillosis is a type 3 immune reaction (antigen–antibody) taking place across the bronchial epithelium, reacting to fungal antigens in the airways. Clinically, patients suffer from asthma and eventually bronchiectasis. The airways are plugged with mucus and eosinophils, and the mucosa is oedematous and inflamed.

Invasive aspergillosis occurs in patients with depleted neutrophil leucocytes, for example leukaemics and those receiving cancer chemotherapy. The condition presents with poor lung function, infiltrates on chest X-radiography, and septic shock. The infection is highly necrotizing, with large clusters of *Aspergillus* hyphae invading the bronchial mucosa (Figure 19.32) and pulmonary arteries, which thrombose, leading to lung infarction. Haematogenous spread may affect other organs, producing areas of necrosis.

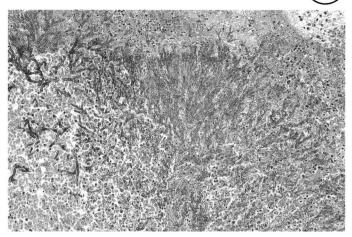

FIGURE 19.32 Invasive aspergillosis: fungal hyphae infiltrating the bronchial wall.

Mycetoma

Mycetoma is a subcutaneous fungal disease that is caused by certain environmental fungi, and contracted by injury through the skin, mainly in tropical countries. It is a chronic soft tissue infection that gradually spreads with swelling and dysfunction of the affected limb. There are deep abscesses and fibrosis, sinuses that discharge through the skin, and osteomyelitis if the underlying bone is involved (Figure 19.33). Visible grains of fungi discharge through

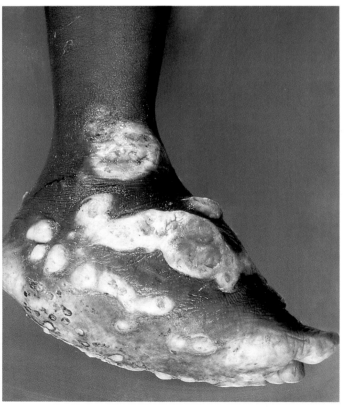

FIGURE 19.33 Mycetoma of the foot: swelling and discharging sinuses.

the skin sinuses, which may be taken and viewed directly under the microscope to make the diagnosis.

PARASITIC INFECTIONS

Parasitic diseases result from infection by protozoa (single cell organisms), helminths (worms) and some arthropods. They range from the rapidly fatal through the chronically morbid, to the incidental and asymptomatic. About 20 genera of protozoa afflict man, and about 100 species of worms. Some infections are restricted to man, and others are zoonoses (infections of animals), where man is infected incidentally but not at a critical stage in the parasite's lifecycle. One protozoal infection alone, *Plasmodium falciparum*, is a major public health problem for one-third of the world's population, and in Africa it kills an estimated million children each year.

Parasitic diseases are not synonymous with tropical diseases, which incorporate the natural results of poverty, overcrowding, malnutrition, lack of clean water and adequate disposal of excreta. In industrialized countries many parasites are endemic at low levels (e.g. amoebae and hydatid cyst), and several at high level (e.g. *Toxoplasma gondii* and threadworms). Each year, one-fifth of the global population flies to distant countries: visitors to endemic zones can bring back their newly acquired parasites before the incubation period is over, and present clinically at home.

Parasite Pathophysiology

The intensity of infection often determines whether an infection is symptomatic, or not. In the absence of effective host resistance, protozoa can replicate within the host and can build up fatal intensities, for example in cerebral malaria. Conversely, most worms do not multiply in the human host, but increase in numbers by repeated infections (the lifecycles are not detailed here, but details may be found in standard texts on parasitology).

Resistance to parasitic infection is a vast and complex subject. Many intracellular protozoal infections are subject to control by host cell-mediated immunity; extracellular infections tend to elicit antibody responses that modulate the degree of infection. In worm infections, both cell-mediated and antibody-mediated immune mechanisms are important – examples are strongyloidiasis and schistosomiasis.

The pathogenetic mechanisms by which parasites cause disease vary greatly. For example, in schistosomiasis the damage is immunopathological, with secondary scarring. The lesions of amoebiasis are entirely due to direct cytotoxic tissue damage.

A few parasites are associated with the development of malignant tumours: examples are *Schistosoma haematobium* with squamous cell carcinoma of the bladder, and *Plasmodium falciparum* malaria with Burkitt lymphoma (high-grade B-cell lymphoma). The parasites do not directly produce any carcinogenic agent; rather they appear to act as tumour promoters, or cause immunosuppression.

Protozoal Infections

Malaria

> **Key Points**
>
> Malaria:
>
> - is a mosquito-transmitted infection
> - is endemic in tropical regions, but travellers can present anywhere
> - *Plasmodium falciparum* infects only the red blood cells
> - causes anaemia by red cell rupture
> - causes cerebral malaria (coma) with significant mortality.

The main and most pathogenic of human malarias is that caused by *Plasmodium falciparum*. This disease was once endemic in Europe, but the UK now has about 2000 imported cases of falciparum malaria each year, with a fatality rate of about 1%. In the tropics – and particularly in Africa and southeast Asia – more than two billion people live in zones at risk for malaria. About 90% of deaths from malaria occur in Sub-Saharan Africa.

In malarial zones, at birth there is maternal antibody-mediated immunity from infection. Thereafter, in areas of regular transmission, children are the main sufferers (malaria is a major cause of childhood mortality in the tropics), and survivors acquire immunity, the nature of which is not well understood. By adulthood, clinical episodes of infection are uncommon, unless the person loses his or her immunity by moving away from an endemic zone. In contrast, visitors (e.g. European tourists) to malarial areas have no immunity, and unless they take antimalarial prophylaxis they are liable to become infected. The clinical features of malaria are detailed in Table 19.24 (see also Figure 19.34).

TABLE 19.24 Clinical features of malaria (see also Figure 19.34)

- Fever: classically, a peak occurs every 2 days
- Normocytic anaemia
- Hepatosplenomegaly
- Prostration
- Renal failure and shock
- Pulmonary oedema
- Hypoglycaemia and acidosis
- Cerebral malaria, coma leading to death
- In pregnancy: increased abortion, stillbirth, maternal death, and small fetuses
- Effects of chronic infection: Burkitt lymphoma, massive splenomegaly

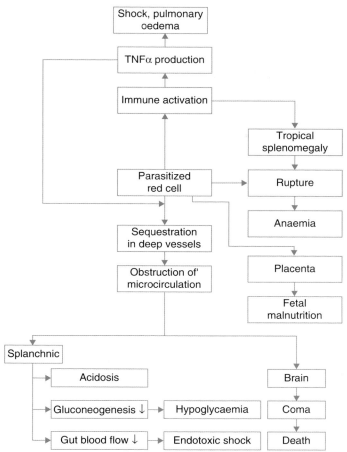

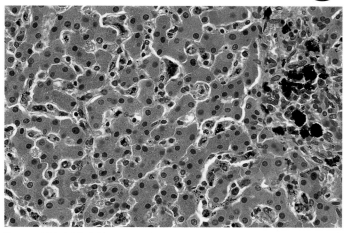

FIGURE 19.35 Malarial liver: note the extensive brown haemozoin pigment in Kupffer cells and portal macrophages.

FIGURE 19.34 Sequelae of infection with *Plasmodium falciparum* causing malaria. TNF = tumour necrosis factor.

The Lifecycle of *Plasmodium falciparum*

The anopheline mosquito is the vector for malaria. The multiplication of parasites occurs in the liver (without clinical effects), and then by repeated intraerythrocytic cycles of division (schizogony) and red cell rupture. The incubation period is about 2 weeks, but this may be prolonged.

Pathology and Pathogenesis of Malaria

Malaria is an intraerythrocytic infection. As a result of red cell rupture at schizogony, there is haemolytic anaemia, the haemoglobin level often falling below 5 g/dL. Parasitaemia rates may be up to 50% of circulating red cells, the trophozoites being visible as small rings, accompanied by some dark brown haemozoin pigment (Figure 19.35; see also Figure 19.39). This pigment is the product of the parasite's metabolism of haemoglobin.

The liver and spleen are moderately enlarged, and dark in colour. The colour derives from the accumulation of haemozoin pigment in the macrophages, phagocytosed from ruptured red cells (see Figure 19.35). Macrophage hyperplasia accounts for some of the organomegaly, along with congestion of the small vessels and sinusoids. The hypoglycaemia that is particularly prominent in children with malaria is associated with reduced glycogen stores in the liver.

The kidney and lung may fail in severe falciparum malaria. The kidneys may show the effects of shock (acute tubular necrosis; see 'Septic shock', p. 543), and some very sick patients also develop 'blackwater fever', with haemoglobinuria that colours the urine dark red, and casts of haemoglobin visible in the tubules.

The pulmonary alveoli may become oedematous, and in some sick patients there is shock lung (hyaline membrane disease). There is no specific alveolitis or pneumonia in malaria, and the manifestations are part of the systemic cytokine-mediated effects of shock.

The parasite has a particular affinity for the maternal sinuses of the placenta, and high parasite counts are noted there. This adversely affects fetal nutrition, with resulting high fetal mortality and low birth weight.

Cerebral malaria is the key pathogenetic puzzle in falciparum malaria, and is a major cause of death in infected children and adults. Clinically, there is a rapidly deteriorating conscious level and coma, sometimes with focalizing signs. With effective treatment and support, recovery may be equally rapid, with no evidence of residual neurological damage in most patients.

In those who die from cerebral malaria, the brain is mildly swollen, very congested, and on slicing it often shows multiple petechial haemorrhages in the white matter (Figure 19.36). Histologically, the small vessels are packed with parasitized red blood cells, and some vessels have ruptured to cause the haemorrhages. This vascular packing phenomenon is termed 'sequestration'. The probable pathogenesis is indicated in Figure 19.37. The parasitized cells develop 'knobs' on the surface membrane, comprising cell and parasite proteins (Figure 19.38). These bind to adhesion molecules on the endothelial cells; the most studied of these is intercellular adhesion molecule-1 (ICAM-1). This is up-regulated in malaria, perhaps as a

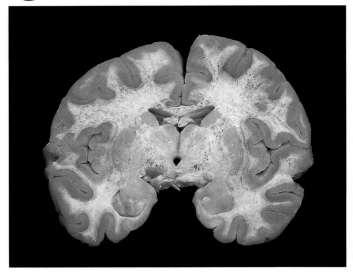

FIGURE 19.36 Cerebral malaria in a child: mild swelling, grey cortex (from the haemozoin pigment) and petechial haemorrhages in the white matter.

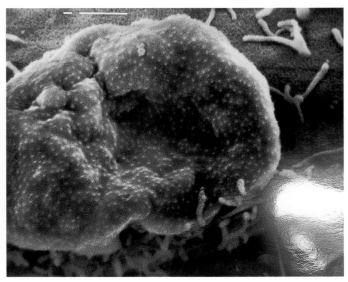

FIGURE 19.38 Red cell with falciparum malaria: this scanning electron micrograph shows the tiny knobs on the red cell surface.

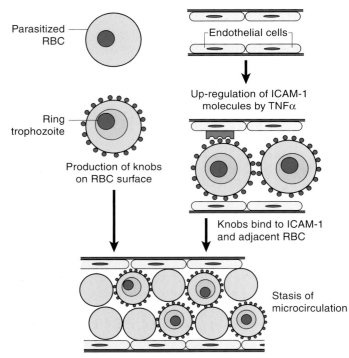

FIGURE 19.37 Pathogenesis of sequestration in falciparum malaria. ICAM = intercellular cell adhesion molecule; RBC = red blood cell; TNF = tumour necrosis factor.

result of increased systemic TNFα production. The result is stagnation of blood flow and secondary ischaemia of the brain, producing coma. If the stagnation is severe enough, the capillary ruptures and a petechial haemorrhage results.

Chronic Effects of Falciparum Malaria

Children in Africa who are chronically infected by falciparum malaria are liable to develop a high-grade B-cell lymphoma (Burkitt lymphoma) if they are also infected early in life with EBV. The latter virus causes B-cell proliferation and transformation if it is not controlled, and malaria contributes to reduced cell-mediated control of EBV.

Some adults in endemic zones may develop massive splenomegaly with secondary hypersplenism (anaemia and cytopenias). This is essentially a lymphoreticular reactive hyperplasia to chronic infection that is idiosyncratic (there is an inherited tendency). There are high immunoglobulin levels in the blood, but parasite numbers are very scant. This condition is also referred to as 'tropical splenomegaly syndrome'.

Diagnosis and Treatment

Diagnosis of acute malaria is by microscopic examination of the blood film. Treatment requires one or more antimalarial drugs to which the parasite is not resistant (resistance to the cheaper drugs such as chloroquine is spreading). In the UK, patients with high blood parasite counts are often also given an exchange transfusion of blood.

Leishmaniasis

Leishmaniasis is group of diseases caused by protozoa of the genus *Leishmania*. With few exceptions, these are zoonoses (the main hosts being canines and small mammals), and transmission is from the bite of sandflies, the vector of infection. The distribution is tropical and subtropical, but includes the Mediterranean littoral; this is why many cases are imported by travellers to the UK.

IMPORTED MALARIA

A 60-year-old English woman visited the East African coast for a 2-week holiday, and took chloroquine as antimalarial prophylaxis only for the duration of the trip. Two weeks after returning to UK, she felt unwell and feverish. Whilst her general practitioner considered influenza, not knowing about her Africa visit, she was admitted to hospital in coma that developed over one morning. A blood sample taken in casualty showed *Plasmodium falciparum* trophozoites in her red blood cells (a 30% parasitaemia) (Figure 19.39).

Immediate intravenous quinine was started, followed by an exchange blood transfusion; this reduced the malaria parasitaemia to 1% within 2 days. However, the woman died from cardiorespiratory failure on the third day, without having regained consciousness. At autopsy, the liver and spleen were found to be enlarged and dark brown in colour, the heart flabby (but not infarcted), and the lungs oedematous. The brain was swollen, with flattening of gyri, and was plum-coloured. On coronal slicing, the brain showed ventricular compression and numerous petechial haemorrhages in the white matter. Microscopy confirmed cerebral malaria, with parasitized red cells packed in the capillaries and venules (Figure 19.40).

Clinicopathological Points

1. Falciparum malaria in East Africa (and elsewhere) is often chloroquine-resistant; thus the prophylaxis was inadequate.
2. Effective antimalarial chemotherapy and exchange transfusion reduces the parasite load in the circulation, but does not immediately flush out the sequestered parasitized red cells in the brain vessels.
3. Fatality can be rapid as here, through microvascular ischaemia and impaired nutrition of the brain.

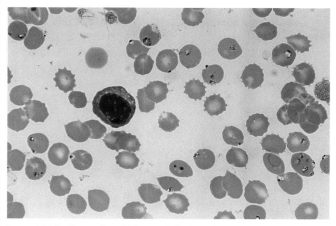

FIGURE 19.39 *Plasmodium falciparum* infection of red cells: the blood smear shows many ring forms in red cells. (Giemsa.)

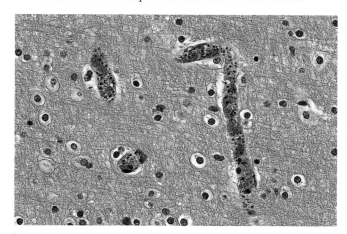

FIGURE 19.40 Cerebral malaria: capillaries with sequestration of parasitized red cells.

Three broad groups of diseases are apparent (see Table 19.25). Morphologically, the parasites are identical, but the species does determine in part the pattern of disease. All are intracellular parasites, and the control of infection is by cell-mediated immunity, similar to what happens with *M. tuberculosis* infection (see Figure 19.16). Hence, HIV/AIDS will alter the clinical pathology of leishmaniasis.

The parasites – which are known as amastigotes in the human part of the lifecycle – are 2–3 μm in size, and divide by binary fission in macrophages.

Cutaneous leishmaniasis is a localized, self-healing condition. At the site of the infected bite, an ulcer develops. The parasites multiply and the inflammatory response is necrotizing. Cell-mediated immunity then develops with a granulomatous response, the parasites are controlled and eliminated, and the ulcer heals with scarring some weeks or months after infection. The diagnosis is confirmed by finding parasites in smears and biopsies from the lesion, with in-vitro cultivation and PCR available to confirm the species. Chemotherapy is still with antimonials, and is effective in reducing the scarring of skin by accelerating healing.

TABLE 19.25 Leishmaniasis: the diseases, parasite species and geographical distribution

Disease	Parasite	Distribution
Cutaneous leishmaniasis	*L. infantum*	Mediterranean
	L. major	Middle East, Asia
	L. mexicana	South and Central America
Mucocutaneous leishmaniasis	*L. brasiliensis*	South and Central America
Visceral leishmaniasis (kala azar)	*L. donovani*	Africa, Asia, Mediterranean

Mucocutaneous leishmaniasis is a variant of cutaneous leishmaniasis, caused specifically by *L. brasiliensis*. In some patients, there is spread of the skin infection to a squamo-mucosal junction, characteristically on the lips and nose. The resulting inflammation can be very destructive and cause gross disfigurement by bone, soft tissue and skin necrosis.

Visceral leishmaniasis (VL) – also known as kala azar – affects only a small proportion of the many people infected with *L. donovani*: these are persons who have not generated sufficient specific cell-mediated immune response to suppress the infection initially. Thus, VL represents a relatively anergic state and the parasites disseminate throughout the macrophages of the lymphoreticular system. In this it has a parallel with disseminated *Mycobacterium avium-intracellulare* infection in immunosuppressed patients. Clinically, there is hepatosplenomegaly, lymphadenopathy, fever and cachexia, with anaemia and pancytopenia (Table 19.26). In infected patients the spleen can weigh up to 3 kg; indeed, VL is one of the few causes of massive splenomegaly (see Table 19.27). As a consequence of both splenomegaly and marrow involvement, there is anaemia and cytopenia (hypersplenism).

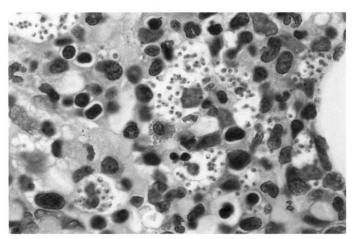

FIGURE 19.41 Visceral leishmaniasis: bone marrow biopsy with many parasites in the macrophages.

TABLE 19.26 Pathology of visceral leishmaniasis

- Macrophages filled with parasites
- Organs involved: liver (Kupffer cells), spleen, lymph nodes, bone marrow and gut mucosa
- Anaemia and pancytopenia
- Hypergammaglobulinaemia (B-cell stimulation) of IgG and IgM
- Secondary bacterial infections: pneumonia and septic shock

TABLE 19.27 Differential diagnosis of massive splenomegaly

- Visceral leishmaniasis
- Chronic myeloid leukaemia and myelofibrosis
- Lymphoma
- Storage diseases, e.g. Gaucher's disease
- Chronic falciparum malaria
- Hydatid cyst

The incubation period for leishmaniasis is several months and, if untreated, the patient usually dies from secondary bacterial infection. Because of the high parasite loads, the macrophage defence system is effectively paralysed, permitting sepsis.

The diagnosis of VL is made by identifying parasites in spleen (e.g. splenic aspirate), liver or bone marrow biopsy (Figure 19.41). Serological identification of specific antibody is usually positive. Chemotherapy is effective.

Not surprisingly, persons coinfected with HIV and *Leishmania* suffer severe acute visceral leishmaniasis, which is virtually impossible to cure in the face of absent CMI. However, immunosuppression from HIV and other causes (e.g. chronic lymphocytic leukaemia, steroid therapy) can also result in latent *Leishmania* infections becoming clinically overt. This can occur years or decades after infection, the parasites having presumably remained within macrophages in small, subclinical numbers. Both cutaneous and visceral disease can result from this re-emergence of infection.

Giardiasis

Key Points

Giardiasis:

- is caused by *Giardia lamblia*
- appears as a lumenal infection of the upper small bowel
- does not invade tissues
- causes diarrhoea and malabsorption
- may mimic coeliac disease
- is readily diagnosable and treatable.

Infection with *Giardia lamblia* is common, and cosmopolitan. It is important as a treatable cause of acute and chronic diarrhoea and weight loss. The transmission route is faecal–oral, that is people ingest oocysts from the faeces of infected persons via contaminated food and water (including water supplies), and homosexual practices. The lifecycle is vegetative, with binary fission of the parasites in the upper small bowel lumen. The organism does not invade tissues. The trophozoites measure $20 \times 15\,\mu$m, and the cysts in faeces are smaller.

Only a minority of those patients with *Giardia* are symptomatic. They have abdominal pain and diarrhoea of varying severity; a proportion may also suffer from malabsorption. Children and those with IgA deficiency are particularly susceptible.

The parasites attach to the small bowel enterocyte brush border, and can be present in large numbers (Figure 19.42).

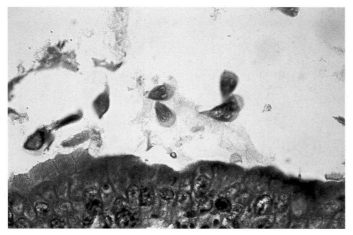

FIGURE 19.42 Giardiasis: six pear-shaped parasites near the enterocyte surface.

The gut villi may be normal or blunted, but only rarely are as flat and as inflamed as in coeliac disease. The pathogenesis of giardiasis is unclear; the damage to the mucosa may be mechanical, there may be toxic damage, or an immune injury may play a role.

In diagnosis, the cysts may be found in the faeces, but this is unreliable. A duodenal biopsy, performed in the work-up of patients with upper gastrointestinal tract and malabsorption symptoms, is a common means of obtaining the diagnosis.

Amoebiasis (Entamoeba histolytica)

Key Points

Amoebiasis:

- is caused by distinct invasive and non-invasive (benign) species of *Entamoeba*
- causes proctocolitis with bloody diarrhoea
- can spread to the liver to cause liver abscess
- the gut and liver symptoms can mimic those of many other diseases
- is treatable and curable.

Amoebiasis is a potentially severe disease caused by *Entamoeba histolytica*, an infection of the large bowel that is transmitted via the faecal–oral route. About 10% of the global population is infected, with higher prevalences in the tropics and subtropics, but the disease is endemic at all latitudes. However, only a small proportion of those infected have significant disease. The explanation has recently become evident. Although the parasites are morphologically identical, there are two genetically distinct species of *Entamoeba*; one species never invades tissues, is now termed *E. dispar*, and is the more common infection; the other species can invade the gut epithelium and is called *E. histolytica*. The lifecycles are vegetative, with binary fission and release of infective cysts into the faeces. The trophozoites in the gut lumen and liver are 20–30 μm in size, and the cysts are smaller.

Clinical Features

Entamoeba dispar may be asymptomatic, or a cause of mild lower gut diarrhoea. It is commonly identified in homosexual men. Conversely, *E. histolytica* is potentially fatal, causing painful diarrhoea with blood in the stool; this mimics idiopathic inflammatory bowel diseases such as ulcerative colitis and Crohn's disease, and bacterial colitis. This may resolve spontaneously, or persist and progress to more severe mucosal ulceration. If untreated, up to 5% of patients – and especially those who are pregnant or receiving steroids – suffer colon perforation and peritonitis, which has a high mortality.

If the parasites spread to the liver via the portal veins (Figure 19.43), one or more liver abscesses will develop. There is tender hepatomegaly, fever, leucocytosis and cholestatic jaundice. Clinically, the symptoms and signs are very similar to those of a bacterial liver abscess or hepatocarcinoma. If untreated, a liver abscess is fatal, as it perforates through the liver capsule into the peritoneum, or less commonly across the diaphragm into the pleural cavity. It is important to note that the absence of current colonic disease does not exclude liver amoebiasis; some gut infections are subclinical.

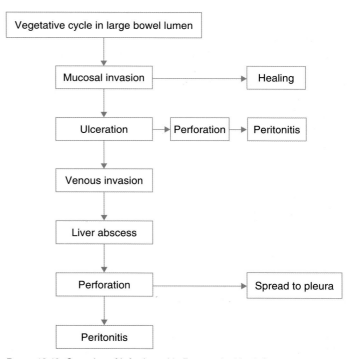

FIGURE 19.43 Sequelae of infection with *Entamoeba histolytica*.

Pathological Features

The colorectal lesions are focal erosions or deeper ulcers that undermine the mucosa (Figure 19.44). Ulcers may become very large with only residual islands of oedematous mucosa, and they may perforate through the muscularis into the serosa and into the peritoneal cavity. The amoebae are seen on the surface epithelium, damaging enterocytes, and at the advancing edge (Figure 19.45). They do not

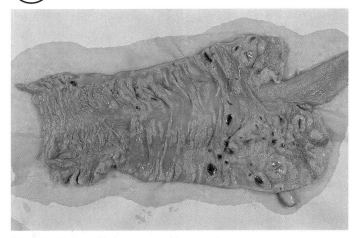

FIGURE 19.44 Amoebiasis: caecum with many ulcers.

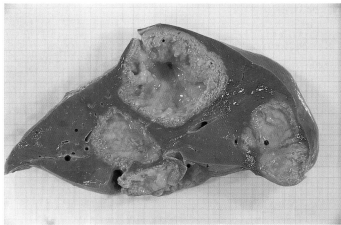

FIGURE 19.46 Amoebiasis: four liver abscesses are indicated.

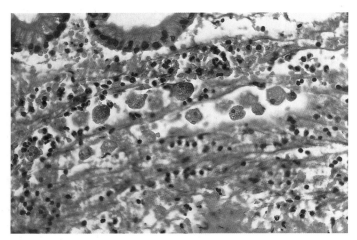

FIGURE 19.45 Amoebiasis: trophozoites (many with phagocytosed red cells) invading under the colon mucosa.

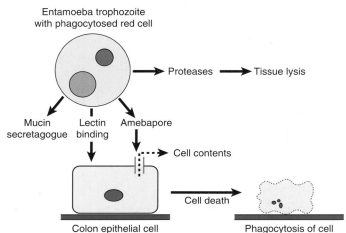

FIGURE 19.47 The pathogenesis of intestinal amoebiasis: the parasites secrete a potent ionophore ('amebapore') which results in lysis of the cell.

induce an acute inflammatory response. Characteristically they phagocytose erythrocytes. An important difference at colonoscopy between amoebic ulcers and those of ulcerative colitis and bacterial dysentery is that they are focal, rather than being a diffuse mucosal disease; conversely, they can mimic Crohn's disease.

In the liver, the abscess does not contain true pus (i.e. no polymorphonuclear leucocyte accumulation), but rather comprises dead liver tissue, fluid and fibrin exudate and blood; hence it resembles anchovy sauce in texture. Abscesses are 4–12 cm in diameter, with a necrotic, irregular periphery (Figure 19.46). The amoebic trophozoites destroy and phagocytose hepatocytes.

Pathogenesis of Amoebiasis

Pathogenic amoebae cause direct tissue damage by secreting an ionophore called 'amebapore' (a 28-kDa protein). This is released following direct contact with host cells' receptors, and causes a 2-nm membrane lesion through which cell contents and ions are able to leak (Figure 19.47). The cell dies and may be phagocytosed by the parasite. In addition, the parasites secrete tissue proteases which also enable invasion and the entry into small veins. There appears to be no immunopathological component to amoebic disease. However, there are some unresolved puzzles; whilst those patients receiving steroids suffer severe disease, amoebiasis is neither more common nor more severe in persons with HIV/AIDS.

Diagnosis and Treatment

Although antibodies to *E. histolytica* are present in serum of most patients with invasive gut and liver disease, the main diagnostic tools are examination of faeces for parasite trophozoites or cysts, a colorectal biopsy, or a surface scrape of a rectal ulcer and direct microscopical examination. For suspected liver abscess, a fine aspirate or biopsy identifies the parasites (or provides an alternative diagnosis). Metronidazole is used effectively to treat the invasive condition. A liver abscess may also need to be aspirated if it is considered to be near to the point of rupture.

Toxoplasmosis

Key Points

Toxoplasmosis:

- toxoplasmosis due to *Toxoplasma gondii* is acquired from undercooked meat, or from cat faeces
- it is a common infection globally
- the primary infection is usually asymptomatic or is a cervical lymphadenitis
- a latent infection may reactivate because of immunosuppression (e.g. HIV)
- reactivated toxoplasmosis causes cerebral lesions and myocarditis.

Infection with *Toxoplasma gondii* is one of the frequent opportunistic infections in patients with HIV/AIDS. It is a common latent infection around the world, with evidence of infection in between 10 and 90% of the adult population (about 40% prevalence in UK).

The lifecycle is complex. The sexual phase of the cycle takes place in the mucosal lining of the intestine of felines, with the excretion of oocysts in faeces. A wide range of intermediate hosts ingest the oocysts, which form latent cysts in many tissues including muscle (cells contain hundreds of 2-μm parasites). Man is infected by eating cysts in undercooked infected meat, or by oocysts direct from cats and possibly from contaminated water supplies.

Clinical Pathology

The pathological forms of toxoplasmosis are outlined in Figure 19.48.

The most common consequence is a subclinical latent infection, where tissue cysts reside in brain and muscle where they cause no significant pathology, but they may reactivate if the person becomes immunosuppressed. Acute acquired toxoplasmosis presents as fever, malaise, lymphadenopathy and splenomegaly. As suspicion of lymphoma is common, lymph node biopsy is frequently performed in tandem with serology. Characteristically, the node shows reactive follicular hyperplasia and numerous small non-necrotic granulomas, but rarely – if ever – any detectable parasites. Congenital toxoplasmosis follows transplacental transmission in about 30% of women who acquire *Toxoplasma* infection in pregnancy. During the first trimester this results in abortion, and as pregnancy progresses the risk of severe fetal disability declines. The classic tetrad is hydrocephalus or microcephaly, chorioretinitis and cerebral calcification. Histologically, there is an encephalitis reaction against the parasites. Milder sequelae include mental retardation and epilepsy.

Ocular toxoplasmosis occurs following congenital toxoplasmosis, or as a reactivation in immunocompromised hosts. The retina and choroid are mainly involved, causing blurred vision and pain. There is acute retinal necrosis.

Toxoplasmosis in the immunocompromised host reflects the reactivation of latent infection in tissue cysts when CMI declines. Currently, the most common cause is HIV/AIDS, and CNS disease is the major focus. The prevalence of cerebral toxoplasmosis depends on the infection level in the population coinfected with HIV. Patients present with focal cerebral lesions or confusion. Imaging can suggest the diagnosis supported by serology, but often treatment is given empirically. The main differential diagnosis is cerebral lymphoma. Grossly, the acute lesions are haemorrhagic, necrotic, space-occupying lesions that, with oedema, cause cerebral compression (see Figure 19.13). Histologically, there are cysts, free parasites, necrosis and vasculitis (Figure 19.49). With treatment, the lesions

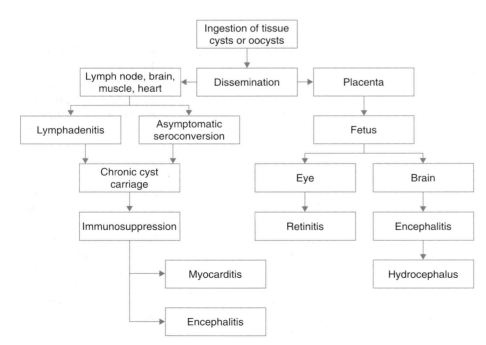

FIGURE 19.48 **Sequelae of infection with** *Toxoplasma gondii.*

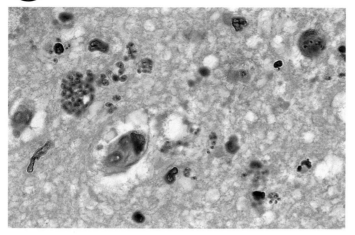

FIGURE 19.49 Cerebral toxoplasmosis: a cyst breaking up (left), with many tiny parasites, spreading through the brain.

regress. Toxoplasmosis can also present in HIV/AIDS as a myocarditis with heart failure.

The diagnosis of toxoplasmosis is made by a combination of clinical, imaging, morphological and serological investigations. Parasites may be visible in tissues – and confirmed by immunocytochemical labelling. Serology detects both IgM (evidence of active infection) and IgG (chronic/past infection) antibodies, but has yet to provide high sensitivity and specificity.

HELMINTH INFECTIONS

There are more than 100 parasitic worm infections of man; these may be subclassified into roundworms (nematodes), trematodes (flatworms, flukes) and cestodes (tapeworms). Globally, the most common are the parasites of the intestinal lumen: hookworms, ascarids and whipworms in the tropics; pinworms in temperate zones (see Table 19.7). The clinicopathological effects of intestinal nematode worms are summarized in Table 19.28. The infections that will be discussed in more detail are those with more systemic clinical pathology; namely, schistosomiasis, hydatid disease and strongyloidiasis.

TABLE 19.28 Pathology of the major intestinal nematode worm infections

Parasite	Location	Effect
Hookworms	Small bowel	Mucosal erosion and bleeding, normocytic anaemia
Ascaris	Small and large bowel	Intestinal obstruction
Whipworms	Colo-rectum	Dystentery, anaemia
Pinworms	Appendix, colorectum	Perianal pruritis
Strongyloides	Small bowel	Diarrhoea

Schistosomiasis

> **Key Points**
>
> Schistosomiasis:
>
> - is caused by the blood flukes *S. haematobium, S. mansoni* and *S. japonicum*
> - the disease is caused by the effects of eggs deposited in the tissues
> - results in cystitis, enteritis and chronic liver disease
> - is the common cause of portal hypertension in the tropics
> - is the common cause of bladder cancer in endemic zones.

The three major schistosome worms affect 10% of the world population in the tropics and Middle East, and are significant causes of chronic gut, bladder and liver disease. The lifecycle is complex as snails are required as an intermediate host. Man is infected through the skin from small cercariae (larvae) in fresh water, which pass to the lungs and mature; worms then migrate via the bloodstream to their main location in deep veins. The lifecycle is completed when eggs are excreted in faeces or urine into water, taking about 40 days from infection. The adult worms are 10–15 mm long, and feed on red cell haemoglobin. Males fertilize female worms, and hundreds of eggs are excreted by each female per day. The eggs are 90–160 µm long, depending on the species.

Clinical and Pathological Features

After infection, there may be a local dermatitis where the cercariae penetrated the skin. Once the worms start egg-laying, some people infected for the first time develop an acute systemic disease (Katayama syndrome) (Table 19.29). This is a serum-sickness-type illness that is associated with a humoral antibody response to new egg antigens.

Schistosomiasis is mainly a chronic disease, and the clinical pathology depends on the species involved (Figure 19.50).

Schistosoma haematobium Infection

This species is found in the Middle East and Africa. It classically causes painful cystitis with haematuria. New lesions are the foci of inflammation around eggs as they traverse the urothelial mucosa. Histologically, there are many eosinophils around the eggs (Figure 19.51). As the lesions become more chronic, cystoscopy reveals nodules and 'sandy patches'; these

TABLE 19.29 Acute schistosomiasis (Katayama syndrome)

- Fever and blood eosinophilia
- Abdominal pain
- Diarrhoea
- Cough and infiltrates on chest X-radiography
- Urticaria
- Lymph node, liver and spleen enlargement

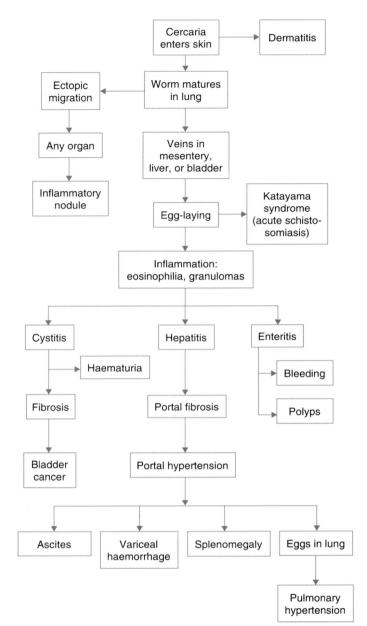

FIGURE 19.50 Sequence of clinicopathological events in schistosomiasis.

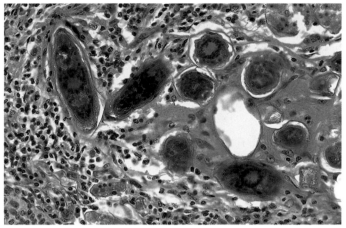

FIGURE 19.51 *Schistosoma haematobium*: live eggs in a mucosa.

TABLE 19.30 Clinical pathology of *Schistosoma haematobium*

- Cystitis with haematuria
- Proctitis and distal colitis
- Progressive bladder fibrosis
- Ureteric obstruction by granulomatous inflammation
- Bladder squamous cell carcinoma in chronically infected people

wall. Its pathogenesis is probably through bacterial cystitis, squamous metaplasia of urothelium, and catabolism of dietary nitrates/nitrites into carcinogenic nitrosamines.

Schistosoma mansoni and *S. japonicum*

Patients present with gut and or liver disease (Table 19.31). These infections cause bloody diarrhoea: the eggs cross the mucosa, and erosions results. Focally, infection intensities can build up with formation of inflammatory polyps containing large numbers of eggs.

TABLE 19.31 Clinical pathology of *Schistosoma mansoni* and *S. japonicum*

- Small and large bowel inflammatory erosions
- Portal hepatitis
- Chronic liver fibrosis (but not cirrhosis)
- Portal hypertension
- Splenomegaly
- Variceal haemorrhage.

The most important condition is the liver disease, hepatosplenic schistosomiasis. Eggs that are carried to the liver induce granulomas in the small portal veins, with hepatomegaly. There is haemozoin pigment (similar to that formed in malaria) in the macrophages and Kupffer cells. The granulomas cause fibrosis of the portal tracts in a characteristic pattern still known as Symmers' clay pipestem fibrosis (Figures 19.52 and 19.53). However, this is not true cirrhosis as the architecture of the liver lobules is intact.

represent granuloma formation, secondary fibrosis, and calcification of eggs that have not been excreted. In chronic severe infections, the bladder wall becomes so fibrosed that it does not empty properly, and bacterial bladder infections persist.

Ureteric obstruction may arise from inflammation around eggs laid in the lower ureter, and may cause hydronephrosis. Intestinal disease is similar to that caused by *S. mansoni*.

The most important complication of chronic infection is squamous cell carcinoma of the bladder, not the standard transitional cell carcinoma of industrialized countries (Table 19.30). A major disease in those parts of the world endemic for *Schistosoma haematobium* (Egypt, Middle East, tropical Africa), this condition usually presents late, filling the bladder space and with invasion through the muscle

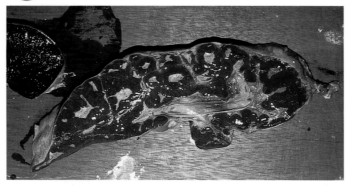

FIGURE 19.52 *Schistosoma mansoni*: chronic liver infection has caused marked fibrosis around the main portal tracts.

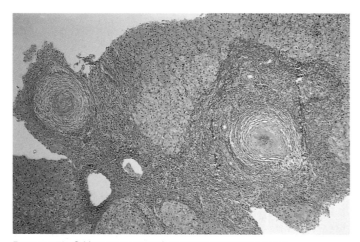

FIGURE 19.53 *Schistosoma mansoni*: chronic liver infection with two granulomas surrounded by concentric fibrous rings, and increased portal fibrosis tissue linking them. (van Gieson.)

The clinical effects in chronic infection are those of portal hypertension, and variceal haemorrhage is common. However, unlike in cirrhosis where the vascular architecture is damaged, in this disease liver metabolism is better preserved, so hepatic coma does not result from the breakdown of blood in the gut.

Schistosomiasis is not associated with the development of liver or intestinal cancer.

As a product of portal hypertension and portosystemic venous anastomoses, eggs laid in mesenteric veins can pass to the lungs. There, they lodge in the pulmonary arterioles, induce granuloma formation and fibrosis, and thereby can cause pulmonary hypertension.

More importantly, adult worms do not always migrate to veins in the 'classical' body locations around the bladder, intestine and upstream from liver. Rather, they can locate in 'ectopic' sites such as the brain and spinal cord, skin, retroperitoneum, lymph nodes and genitalia. As a consequence, schistosomal granulomatous nodules may be found in various places, often mimicking a neoplasm. The most serious of these ectopic schistosomiases are space-occupying lesions in the brain, and inflammatory lesions in and around

the spinal cord. The latter are not uncommon and are a cause of spinal paralysis.

Pathogenesis

The pathology in schistosomiasis comes essentially from the host reaction to parasite eggs. The adult worms elicit no reaction because they coat themselves in host red cell antigens. The eggs live for only 3 weeks, and around half are excreted and half are retained in the body. In the process of excretion or retention they cause the disease spectrum. The main determinants of disease severity are the intensity and chronicity of infection. Travellers who acquire schistosomiasis do not develop chronic severe disease, in contrast to those who build up infection levels from years of exposure (Table 19.32).

TABLE 19.32 Pathogenesis of schistosomiasis

- Host reaction to eggs in tissues
- Acute inflammatory response with eosinophils
- Erosion of mucosal surfaces as eggs are excreted
- T-cell-mediated response with granuloma formation around eggs
- Subsequent fibrosis related to healing of granulomas
- Organ dysfunction secondary to fibrosis

Diagnosis and Treatment

The diagnosis is made by identifying the eggs in samples of faeces, urine or tissue biopsies. Schistosome serology is specific and useful, but remains positive after effective therapy. Treatment with praziquantel is standard for all species; this kills the adult worms but does not affect the host reaction to eggs in tissues.

Hydatid Disease

Key Points

Hydatid disease:

- is caused by larvae of the tapeworm *Echinococcus granulosus*
- results in cysts in the liver, peritoneum and lung
- the cysts act as space-occupying lesions
- the diagnosis is confirmed by radiology and fine-needle aspiration
- is treated by surgery and chemotherapy.

Echinococcus granulosus is a tapeworm that is widely prevalent, irrespective of latitude. It is endemic at low levels in the UK and at high levels in Africa and the Middle East.

This is a zoonosis where man is accidentally infected and develops the intermediate cystic stage of the lifecycle of the tapeworm. The definitive hosts are canines, with worms in the intestine and eggs excreted in the faeces. The usual intermediate hosts are bovines, sheep and camels;

when their offal, containing cysts, is eaten by dogs, the life-cycle continues.

Ingested tapeworm eggs hatch in the duodenum and pass to the liver via the portal veins. Growing at a rate of up to 2 cm a year, a hydatid cyst develops which may reach over 20 cm in final size (Figure 19.54). The eggs can also reach other organs and result in cysts (Table 19.33).

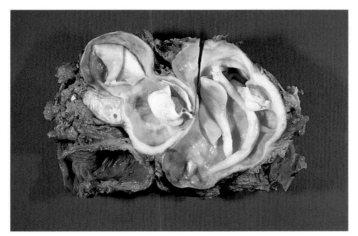

FIGURE 19.54 Hydatid cysts in the mesentery, causing intestinal obstruction.

TABLE 19.33 Organs affected by hydatid disease, and the effects

- Liver (>70% of patients): enlargement, discomfort, bile duct obstruction
- Peritoneal cavity: abdominal swelling, adhesions and intestinal obstruction
- Lung: shortness of breath, abnormal chest X-radiography
- Brain: cerebral compression, epilepsy
- Kidney: compression, hydronephrosis
- Spleen: moderate to massive splenomegaly
- Bone: fracture, collapse
- Any organ (in endemic zones, this is in the differential diagnosis of all tumours)

Pathology

The form of hydatid cyst is similar in all organs. The parasite generates a soft white laminated acellular membrane which is 1–2 mm thick. Outside this, the host reacts with a fibrous wall that helps contain the cyst and stop it from rupturing. Within the membrane is a thin germinal membrane from which bud myriads of scolices (singular = scolex), which are the heads of future adult tapeworms (Figure 19.55). The scolices have characteristic suckers and a ring of curved hooklets. Often, a cyst membrane generates internal daughter cysts, and the whole structure contains much colourless watery fluid.

The cyst acts like a benign expanding tumour. Over many years or decades, if untreated, cysts die and collapse. Spontaneous, traumatic or iatrogenic rupture may occur, with secondary spread of infection to adjacent organs or body cavities. There is a risk of a type 1 anaphylactic shock

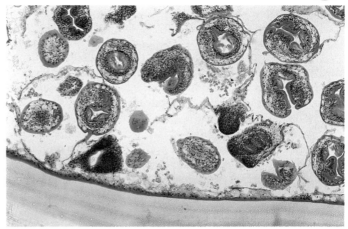

FIGURE 19.55 Hydatid cyst: the pale-staining laminated membrane (bottom), germinal membrane (red line) and numerous scolices within the cyst.

reaction, which is potentially fatal, if hydatid cyst antigen enters the bloodstream to react with specific antibodies. This risk modifies the approach to treatment, but it is not a bar to performing fine needle aspiration (FNA) of suspected cysts for diagnosis: large studies have demonstrated the safety of the procedure.

Diagnosis and Treatment

Clinical suspicion and radiology are the main indicators of hydatid cyst. Serology is reasonably sensitive and specific. Fine needle aspiration is often used to confirm the diagnosis, and often makes it when unsuspected. The scolices and hooklets are readily identified on cytological preparations.

The ideal management is to remove the cyst if possible; single liver cysts form a major presentation. Care is taken when opening the cyst not to spill its contents, prior to sucking the parasitic material out. If cysts are multiple, or in the peritoneal cavity, bone or lung, then chemotherapy (albendazole) is available but is slow in effect, and it is uncertain whether it ultimately sterilizes a hydatid cyst.

Strongyloidiasis

Key Points

Strongyloidiasis:

- is caused by *Strongyloides stercoralis*
- infects intestinal mucosa
- is almost unique among worms by proliferating in man, with life-long infection
- causes diarrhoea
- during immunosuppression, it can disseminate in the body and precipitate septic shock.

Strongyloidiasis is caused by the nematode *Strongyloides stercoralis*. This worm is endemic in the tropics and subtropics and, because of its lifecycle, it can be a life-long infection and is potentially fatal. Importantly, people infected previously (e.g. soldiers in the Far East during the Second World War) can present decades later with acute illness for the first time. Man is infected by larvae in the soil, deposited from human faeces. The larvae penetrate the skin and migrate to the small intestine and lodge in mucosal crypts. The female lays eggs which immediately hatch into larvae in the bowel lumen. These are able to re-invade the bowel or perianal skin, so keeping an auto-infection cycle going. Should the patient become immunosuppressed (Table 19.34), this auto-infection cycle can rapidly generate massive infection with millions of parasites throughout the whole intestine, and haematogenous dissemination of larvae to all organs including liver, lungs and meninges.

TABLE 19.34 Conditions that predispose to hyperinfection with *Strongyloides stercoralis*

- Steroid therapy
- Organ transplantation and therapeutic immunosuppression
- Old age (a common cause for decline in immunity)
- HTLV-1 coinfection
- Cancer, particularly HTLV-1-associated T-cell lymphoma
- Malnutrition

Clinical Features

The infection may be asymptomatic, or the cause of periodic skin itch. If the gut infection intensity builds up, it causes diarrhoea and weight loss. If there is massive infection ('hyperinfection'), it precipitates multiple organ failure with fulminant diarrhoea, septic shock, pneumonia, and meningitis, accompanied by a high blood eosinophil count.

The sequelae of infection with *Strongyloides* infection are indicated in Figure 19.56.

Pathology

With mild infection there are focal erosions of small bowel mucosa, with adult worms in the mucosal crypts accompanied by chronic inflammation and local eosinophilia. Adult worms are typically 2.5 mm long. The disease may be segmental in the bowel, reminiscent of Crohn's disease.

In hyperinfection, the intestine is extensively ulcerated and there are abundant worms (Figure 19.57). Acute pneumonia and shock lung, inflammation and enlargement of the liver and meningitis follow. Some of this is in reaction to the larvae (250 µm long) which are disseminated in blood vessels; the intestinal lesions also permit the entry of Gram-negative bacteria, producing bacteraemia and septic shock.

One notable and intriguing coinfection is that of HTLV-1 (human T-lymphotropic virus type 1) and *Strongyloides*. This is important in West Africa and the Caribbean, and in people who have originated from those areas. HTLV-1 is the cause of a high-grade T-cell lymphoma in a proportion of those infected; it appears that *Strongyloides* coinfection can accelerate the malignant transformation. Conversely, the immunological damage of HLTV-1 infection can precipitate hyperinfection in those with subclinical *Strongyloides* infection.

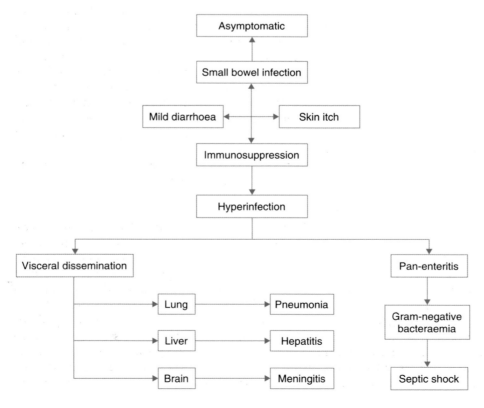

FIGURE 19.56 Sequelae of infection with *Strongyloides stercoralis*.

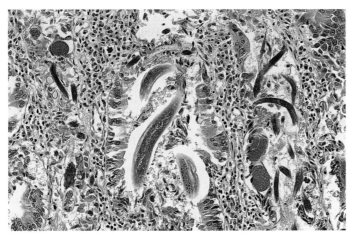

FIGURE 19.57 *Strongyloides* hyperinfection: small bowel with heavy infection of adult and larval worms in the mucosa.

SEPTIC SHOCK

Shock is the end-result of many clinical processes, and is defined as the hypoperfusion of critical organs such that their function and integrity is compromised. This may be either reversible or irreversible (and then generally fatal). Because modern hospital medicine sustains sick patients who might previously have died without interventions, older and frailer patients undergo major operations, more patients undergo organ transplantation with subsequent immunosuppression, and intensive care facilities are expanding in size and complexity, an increasing number of patients are encountered in various states of shock. This section deals with the pathogenesis of one such type – septic shock (Table 19.35). Further details on shock in general may be found in Chapter 6, pp. 128–131.

TABLE 19.35 Classification of shock: the five major types

- Cardiogenic: from ventricular failure (e.g. infarction, tamponade)
- Hypovolaemic: from haemorrhage or plasma loss (e.g. burns)
- Septic: from infection, usually bacterial
- Anaphylactic: from type-1 immunological hypersensitivity reactions
- Neurogenic: from spinal cord injury

Aetiology

The aetiology of septic shock is most commonly infection by Gram-negative bacilli that produce endotoxins (hence the term 'endotoxic shock'). These include *Escherichia coli*, *Pseudomonas*, *Klebsiella* and *Enterobacter* species. Initially, the infection is localized to an organ or cavity, such as appendicitis, pneumonia, or peritonitis following bowel surgery. If the host defences and medical interventions such as antimicrobial drugs and surgical resection are unable to contain the infection, the systemic inflammatory and cytokine effects then involve other organs, and there is often dissemination of infection with bacteraemia and then septicaemia ('bacteraemia' indicates bacterial infection in the blood without major clinical disease, whilst 'septicaemia' involves shock as well). Gram-positive bacteria, some systemic fungal infections, and severe falciparum malaria infection also initiate similar pathophysiological processes to Gram-negative septic shock.

Pathogenesis

Shock caused by endotoxin-producing Gram-negative bacteria has been the most comprehensively studied. Endotoxin is a lipopolysaccharide (LPS) structural component of the outer cell wall of these bacilli. In contrast to bacterial exotoxins (e.g. that produced by *Clostridium perfringens*, a cause of tissue gangrene) which are secreted by intact bacteria, LPS is released as the bacilli disintegrate. LPS comprises a long-chain toxic fatty acid (lipid A) which is common to all Gram-negative bacteria, and a variable polysaccharide carbohydrate chain that includes the O antigens, unique to each species. Similar LPS-like complex molecules are present in the walls of other bacteria and fungi.

LPS binds to circulating monocytes, tissue macrophages, and to endothelial cells, and activates them. This is obviously a useful evolutionary adaptation in the cellular defence against infection. The key event that turns a local infection into septic shock is the progressive production of TNFα by LPS-activated macrophages. TNFα causes macrophages and many other cells in the body (e.g. liver) to secrete interleukin 1 (IL-1) which, depending on the concentration, is directly tissue damaging. Thereafter a series of cytokine cascades generates further interleukins (IL-6 and IL-8), with production of the acute phase responses and nitric oxide (NO), and can activate the clotting system to initiate disseminated intravascular coagulation (DIC). The cardiac output falls due to pump failure, the peripheral vascular resistance falls, the tissues are underperfused, the capillaries leak resulting in tissue oedema, and the critical capillary/epithelium interface in the lung alveoli is damaged (Figure 19.58).

The features of septic shock can be reproduced by the injection of endotoxin LPS alone.

Clinical Features

As can be predicted from the pathophysiology, the clinical aspects of septic shock comprise fever, systemic hypotension, increasing oxygen requirement to maintain blood pO_2, infiltrates on chest X-radiography, generalized oedema, oliguric renal failure, and jaundice. Chronologically there is a division into three stages. In the initial phase, the body's normal compensatory mechanisms maintain critical organ perfusion. This is succeeded by a progressive phase where tissue hypoperfusion results in organ failure, particularly cardiorespiratory, exacerbated by toxic endothelial damage and fluid leakage; metabolic acidosis and renal shutdown occur. Patients can recover from

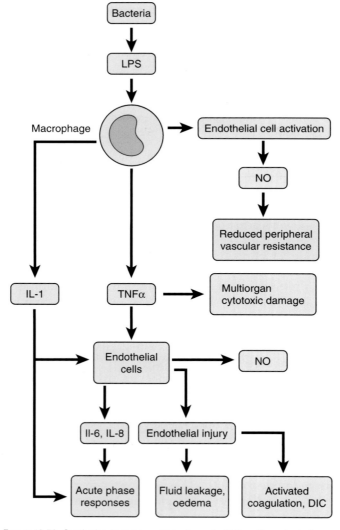

FIGURE 19.58 Septic shock: the sequelae of events. DIC = disseminated intravascular coagulation; IL = interleukin; LPS = lipopolysaccharide; NO = nitric oxide; TNF = tumour necrosis factor.

unique to septic shock, and may be seen in shock from the other aetiologies. In the case of the lung, shock lung has a broadly similar morphology whether it follows from sepsis, drug toxicity or external trauma such as high-pressure ventilation and oxygen toxicity. Regarding the heart, the clinical syndrome of 'electromechanical dissociation (EMD)' is a common pre-death observation. The ECG records electrical impulses, but the cardiac output measured both clinically and by echocardiography is slight. This results from overt ischaemic damage to myocytes and probably from direct toxic functional damage by TNF and other cytokines. Finally, as the result of the overactivation of the cytokine and cellular defence systems in the progressive and final stages of septic shock, there is an increased susceptibility to more bacterial infections (e.g. bronchopneumonia).

Whether the patient can recover from septic shock will depend on control of the initiating and subsequent infection events, the degree of damage suffered by the critical organs, and their capacity to recover with cellular regeneration. Kidney tubular damage (acute tubular necrosis), pulmonary alveolar damage and liver necrosis are, in principle, recoverable lesions provided that appropriate intensive care support is available. If the integrity of the intestinal mucosa is damaged, the consequent invasion by Gram-negative bacteria from the lumenal faeces perpetuates and worsens the septic shock. The loss of heart myocytes from ischaemic and toxic damage, and loss of cerebral cortex neurones are, of course, irreversible.

Outcome of Septic Shock

The mortality of septic shock ranges from 25 to 75% according to age (the older the patient, the poorer the outcome), the underlying cause, and patient management. In clinical practice, the outcome is often determined by the degree of acute cardiac muscle damage (on top of any pre-existing heart disease) and the capacity of the lung alveolar lining cells to regenerate whilst the fibrosing response is inhibited. It must be remembered that modern intensive care itself, with positive-pressure ventilation, high inhaled oxygen concentrations and powerful toxic drugs including inotropes, can incur and may reinforce the pathology of shock: the balance between undertreatment and overtreatment is often difficult to negotiate.

this phase. The final, irreversible, phase follows when critical organ cellular injury is too severe for regeneration or compensation, even if the organs were to be reperfused adequately.

Pathological Features

The critical organs damaged in shock are the lungs, heart, kidneys, intestine, liver and brain. The morphologies are not

SEPTIC SHOCK

A 67-year-old female had mitral stenosis with reduction of cardiac output. About 20 years ago, she had a mitral valvotomy to relieve the stenosis, but a definitive artificial valve replacement was now required. The operation was technically successful, but she was slow in waking up from anaesthesia.

In intensive care, 2 days after surgery, her respiratory function deteriorated, requiring increasing concentrations of oxygen and ventilation pressures to maintain the pO_2 in blood. Chest X-radiography showed diffuse infiltration. Her blood pressure fell, and increasing doses of inotropic drugs were needed to keep the systolic blood pressure at 100 mmHg. Daily blood cultures were made, and on the fourth postoperative day a Gram-negative *Pseudomonas* bacillus was isolated. The patient developed oliguric renal failure and despite antibiotic therapy she died from cardiorespiratory failure seven days after surgery.

At autopsy, the mechanical mitral valve was properly *in situ*, without any superimposed endocarditis. The kidneys had pale and oedematous cortices, characteristic of acute tubular necrosis. The lungs were heavy, consolidated and mucoid in appearance, with multiple 1–2-mm grey foci. The liver had micronodular cirrhosis. Histologically, the lungs were bronchopneumonic; numerous small pulmonary arteries were thickened due to dense intramural infiltration of Gram-negative bacilli; there was secondary lumenal thrombosis and surrounding infarction of the lung (Figure 19.59). The kidneys showed DIC (Figure 19.60). The undiagnosed cirrhosis (a recognized infection risk factor) predisposed her to septic shock.

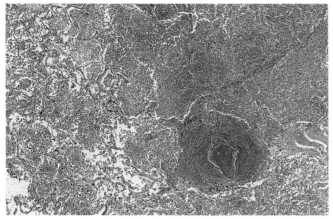

FIGURE 19.59 Lung: the pulmonary arteriole (lower half) is thickened from infiltrating *Pseudomonas* bacilli, and thrombosed; the surrounding lung is infarcted.

Clinicopathological Points

1. The undiagnosed liver cirrhosis (probably alcoholic in aetiology) was the reason the patient did not clear the anaesthetic drugs rapidly, so delaying recovery.
2. The *Pseudomonas* bacteraemia was probably acquired from nosocomial infection of the intravascular lines necessary for intensive care support.
3. *Pseudomonas* characteristically causes a vasculitis, resulting in occlusive thrombosis and infarction.
4. The septic shock precipitated DIC, which contributed to renal failure.

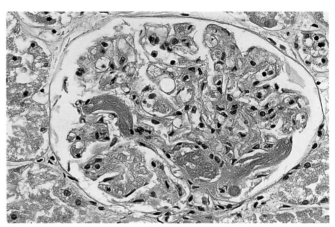

FIGURE 19.60 Kidney: thrombi in the glomerular capillaries, indicating disseminated intravascular coagulation.

SUMMARY

This chapter outlines the basic clinicopathological features and epidemiological aspects of a range of infectious diseases that doctors encounter in Europe. Virus infections (particularly HIV and its complications), bacteria, fungi and parasitic protozoa and worms are included. Because of increasing travel and migration, it is important that certain diseases that are only acquired outside Europe are understood, as well as the global infections. The emphasis throughout is on pathogenesis, i.e. understanding why the infections affect some people but not others, and how they cause disease and sometimes death.

FURTHER READING

Cohen J, Powderly WG. *Infectious Diseases*, 2nd edn. Edinburgh: Mosby, 2004.

Herrington CS, Douek DC. Infection and disease: cause and cure. *J Pathol* 2006; **208**: 131–138.

Mandell GL, Bennett JE, Dolin R. *Mandell, Douglas and Bennett's Principles and Practice of Infectious Diseases*, 6th edn. Edinburgh: Elsevier, 2005.

Timbury MC, McCartney AC, Thakker B, Ward KN. *Notes on Medical Microbiology*. Edinburgh: 2002.

INDEX

Numbers in **bold** indicate the location of a figure/table

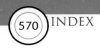